AF412997

RHINITIS

Compliments of

AstraZeneca

A research-based pharmaceutical
company committed to bringing you
innovative respiratory medications.

160073   8/99

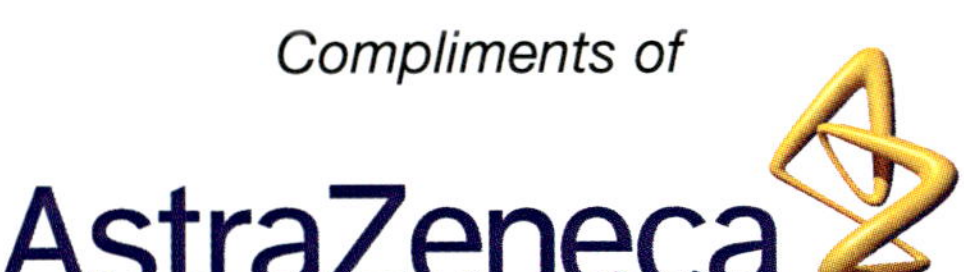

LUNG BIOLOGY IN HEALTH AND DISEASE

Executive Editor

Claude Lenfant
Director, National Heart, Lung and Blood Institute
National Institutes of Health
Bethesda, Maryland

ADDITIONAL VOLUMES IN PREPARATION

Lung Tumors, *edited by Christian Brambilla and Elisabeth Brambilla*

The Lung at Depth, *edited by Claes Lundgren and John N. Miller*

Diagnostic Pulmonary Pathology, *edited by Philip T. Cagle*

Immunotherapy of Asthma, *edited by Jean Bousquet and Hans Yssel*

Air Pollutants and the Respiratory Tract, *edited by David L. Swift and Michael Foster*

Viral Infections of the Lung, *edited by Raphael Dolin and Peter F. Wright*

Pediatric Asthma, *edited by Shirley J. Murphy, H. William Kelly, and Bennie C. McWilliams*

LAM and Other Diseases Characterized by Smooth Muscle Proliferation, *edited by Joel Moss*

GERD and Airway Disease, *edited by Mark R. Stein*

Neurobiology of Sleep and Circadian Rhythms, *edited by Fred Turek and Phyllis Zee*

Multimodality Treatment of Lung Cancer, *edited by Arthur T. Skarin*

Cytokines in Pulmonary Infectious Disease, *edited by Steven Nelson and Thomas Martin*

Asthma's Impact on Society: The Social and Economic Burden, *edited by Kevin B. Weiss, A. Sonia Buist, and Sean D. Sullivan*

Interleukin 5: From Molecule to Drug Target for Asthma, *edited by Colin J. Sanderson*

Control of Breathing in Health and Disease, *edited by Murray D. Altose and Yoshikazu Kawakami*

Exercise-Induced Asthma, *edited by E. Regis McFadden, Jr.*

The opinions expressed in these volumes do not necessarily represent the views of the National Institutes of Health.

RHINITIS
MECHANISMS AND MANAGEMENT

Edited by

Robert M. Naclerio

*University of Chicago
Chicago, Illinois*

Stephen R. Durham

*National Heart and Lung Institute
London, England*

Niels Mygind

*University Hospital of Aarhus
Aarhus, Denmark*

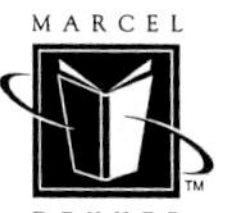

MARCEL DEKKER, INC.   NEW YORK · BASEL · HONG KONG

ISBN 0-8247-0189-5

This book is printed on acid-free paper.

MARCEL DEKKER, INC.
270 Madison Avenue, New York, New York 10016
http://www.dekker.com

Current printing (last digit):
10 9 8 7 6 5 4 3 2 1

PRINTED IN THE UNITED STATES OF AMERICA

INTRODUCTION

Where do the airways begin: in the nose, or lower in the respiratory tract? There have been many discussions and debates about this question but, to be candid, I wonder whether it really matters. In their Preface, the editors of this volume make a very powerful point: ''Rhinitis can have a significant impact on the quality of life of the patients.'' Should one have any doubt about the veracity of this statement, one needs only to observe city pedestrians sneezing and sniffling in early spring!

The nose, inside and out, has always been an organ of considerable interest. Its configuration, especially its length, was somewhat glorified by the French dramatist and poet Edmond Rostand in his play *Cyrano de Bergerac* presented in 1918.

Fortunately for patients affected by rhinitis, others have concentrated their efforts on the inside of the nose. History tells us that endoscopy appears to have been conceived during the later years of the eighteenth century. Initially laryngoscopy was the main interest, but eventually rhinoscopy became the standard by which to diagnose disorders of the nasal passage. M. Mackenzie in 1865 and C. Wagner in 1881 became the champions and advocates of this procedure as reported in their publication *The Use of the Laryngoscope in Diseases of the Throat with an Appendix on Rhinoscopy* (Mackenzie) and *Diseases of the Nose* (Wagner).

As described in the first chapter of this volume, the nasal cavities have an important physiological function, that is, to condition the inspired air. To this, we can add filtering, that is, to retain some of the particles that are in the inspired air. This, of course, is what results in some of the disorders that have such an impact on our quality of life.

The Preface of this volume also makes the statement that ''asthma is a more serious disease than rhinitis.'' The accuracy and relevance of this statement will be explored in this volume. Drs. Naclerio, Durham, and Mygind are giving patients and clinicians a major contribution that will help them all. In addition, the authors of the chapters raise questions and thus challenge the research community to do further work on rhinitis, a major public health problem.

When the editors of this monograph approached me to include it in the *Lung Biology in Health and Disease* series I knew that this would be a remarkable and important addition. The end product exceeds my expectations. The participants at the workshop that led to this volume are experts in their respective fields. All together, they present the views from many countries, thus making this volume a landmark in this area.

To the editors and the contributors, I express my gratitude for this contribution.

Claude Lenfant, M.D.
Bethesda, Maryland

PREFACE

The mucous membrane of the nose is a part of the airway mucous membrane, and rhinitis and asthma are parallel manifestations of allergic and infectious airway diseases. There are many more monographs on asthma than on rhinitis, which is understandable because asthma is the more serious disease. However, rhinitis can have a significant impact on the quality of life of patients, and with regard to this parameter, rhinitis ranks between moderately severe and severe asthma. In addition, the number of rhinitis patients outnumbers that of asthma patients. The nose is the entrance to the airways and it acts as a filter for the lower airways, resulting in antigen deposition and antigen presentation in the nose both in rhinitis and in asthma patients. This may partially explain why nasal inflammation can inversely affect the asthma disease and intranasal anti-inflammatory treatment can have a beneficial effect on asthma.

For the above reasons, we have found it relevant to publish a monograph on rhinitis in this prestigious series, *Lung Biology in Health and Disease*. This book was conceived by a group of experts from America and Europe who met at the University of Chicago to discuss issues related to this common but under-studied disease. The participants' expertise spanned the disciplines of otorhinolaryngology, allergy, pediatrics, and pulmonary medicine and related basic sciences. Their hard work and depth of understanding are reflected in the quality of the chapters. We are proud of having gathered a number of scientists who in our opinion are the leading experts in this field of research, and we hope that this volume will be of interest for readers dealing with both rhinitis and asthma patients.

This project would not have been possible without a generous grant-in-aid from Astra Draco, Lund, Sweden. We want to acknowledge the essential support of Erik Lanner, who realized that support of a publication about good basic and clinical science is of mutual interest to university researchers and pharmaceutical companies, and ultimately for the patients. Carol Colabelli did a superb job in organizing the meeting.

We hope this book will provide a state-of-the-art review of allergic and nonallergic rhinitis and point the way for future research.

Robert M. Naclerio
Stephen R. Durham
Niels Mygind

CONTRIBUTORS

Fuad M. Baroody, M.D.   Assistant Professor, Department of Otolaryngology, Head and Neck Surgery, and Pediatrics, Pritzker School of Medicine, University of Chicago, Chicago, Illinois

Rebecca Bascom, M.D.   Department of Pulmonary, Allergy, and Critical Care Medicine, The Pennsylvania State College of Medicine and Penn State Geisinger Health System, Hershey, Pennsylvania

Peter Borum, M.D., Ph.D.   Chairman of the Board, ENT Department, Roskilde Hospital, Roskilde, Denmark

Jean Bousquet, M.D., Ph.D.   Professor, Department of Respiratory Medicine, Montpellier University, Montpellier, France

William W. Busse, M.D.   Professor, Department of Medicine, University of Wisconsin Medical School, Madison, Wisconsin

Ronald Dahl, M.D.   Professor, Department of Respiratory Medicine, University of Aarhus, Aarhus, Denmark

Pascal Demoly, M.D., Ph.D.   Assistant Professor, Department of Respiratory Diseases, Hôpital Arnaud de Villeneuve, Montpellier, France

Anne Des Roches   Clinique de Maladies Respiratoires, Hôpital Arnaud de Villeneuve, Montpellier, France

Stephen R. Durham, M.D., F.R.C.P.   Reader, Department of Upper Respiratory Medicine, Imperial College School of Medicine at the National Heart and Lung Institute, London, England

Ronald Eccles, Ph.D., D.Sc.   Professor, Common Cold Centre, School of Molecular and Medical Biosciences, Cardiff University, Cardiff, Wales, England

Philippe A. Eigenmann   School of Medicine, University of Geneva School of Medicine, Geneva, Switzerland

Philip Fireman, M.D.   Professor, Section of Allergy and Immunology, Children's Hospital of Pittsburgh and University of Pittsburgh School of Medicine, Pittsburgh, Pennsylvania

Peter H. Howarth, B.Sc., D.M., F.R.C.P.   Senior Lecturer, Department of University Medicine, University of Southampton, Southampton, England

Alfredo A. Jalowayski, Ph.D.   Specialist and Respiratory Physiologist, University of California, San Diego, California

Elizabeth F. Juniper, M.C.S.P., M.Sc.   Associate Professor, Department of Clinical Epidemiology and Biostatistics, McMaster University Medical Centre, Hamilton, Ontario, Canada

David W. Kennedy, M.D., F.R.C.S.I.   Professor and Chair, Department of Otorhinolaryngology, Head and Neck Surgery, University of Pennsylvania Medical Center, Philadelphia, Pennsylvania

Ian S. Mackay, F.R.C.S.   Department of Otorhinolaryngology, Charing Cross Hospital and Royal Brompton Hospital, London, England

Eli O. Meltzer, M.D.   Clinical Professor, Allergy and Asthma Medical Group and Research, University of California, San Diego, California

François-Bernard Michel, M.D.   Professor, Department of Respiratory Diseases, Hôpital Arnaud de Villeneuve, Montpellier, France

Niels Mygind, M.D.   Associate Professor, Department of Respiratory Diseases, University of Aarhus, Aarhus, Denmark

Robert M. Naclerio, M.D.   Professor and Chief, Otolaryngology Head and Neck Surgery, University of Chicago, Chicago, Illinois

H. Alice Orgel, M.D., Ph.D.   Clinical Associate Professor, University of California, San Diego, California

Thomas A. E. Platts-Mills, M.D., Ph.D. Professor, Department of Internal Medicine, University of Virginia, Charlottesville, Virginia

Hugh A. Sampson, M.D. Professor, Department of Pediatrics, Chief, Allergy and Immunology, The Mount Sinai School of Medicine, New York, New York

Robert P. Schleimer, Ph.D. Professor, Department of Medicine, Asthma and Allergy Center, The Johns Hopkins University School of Medicine, Baltimore, Maryland

Brent A. Senior, M.D. Senior Staff Otolaryngologist, Henry Ford Health System, Detroit, Michigan

Dennis Shusterman Division of Occupational Medicine, University of California, San Francisco, California

F. Estelle R. Simons, M.D., F.R.C.P.C. Professor and Head, Section of Allergy and Clinical Immunology, Department of Pediatrics and Child Health, University of Manitoba, Winnipeg, Manitoba, Canada

Jeanne Montgomery Smith, M.D. Associate Professor, Department of Internal Medicine, University of Iowa Hospitals and Clinics, Iowa City, Iowa

Heinz R. Stammberger, M.D. Professor and Head, Department of General ENT, Head and Neck Surgery, ENT—Hospital University Medical School, Graz, Austria

Alkis Togias, M.D. Associate Professor, Divisions of Clinical Immunology and Respiratory and Critical Care Medicine, The Johns Hopkins University, Baltimore, Maryland

Paul van Cauwenberge, M.D., Ph.D. Professor and Chairman, Department of Otorhinolaryngology, University Hospital Ghent, Ghent, Belgium

De-Yun Wang, M.D., Ph.D. Director of Rhinology Research, Department of Otorhinolaryngology, University Hospital Ghent, Ghent, Belgium

Lisa M. Wheatley, M.D. Assistant Professor, Department of Internal Medicine, University of Virginia, Charlottesville, Virginia

S. James Zinreich, M.D. Associate Professor, Department of Radiology and Otolaryngology and Head and Neck Surgery, The Johns Hopkins University, Baltimore, Maryland

CONTENTS

1

Anatomy and Physiology

FUAD M. BAROODY

University of Chicago
Chicago, Illinois

I. Introduction

When discussing allergic and nonallergic rhinitis and the different influences that
our environment has on the nose and its function, it is essential to have a clear
understanding of the anatomy and physiology of the nasal cavity. This chapter
is designed to provide such an understanding of both nasal structure and function
and therefore facilitate the appreciation of impacts of different diseases and treatments discussed in subsequent chapters of this book.

II. External Framework

The external bony framework of the nose consists of two oblong, paired nasal
bones located on either side of the midline that merge to form a pyramid (Fig.
1). Lateral to each nasal bone is the frontal process of the maxilla, which contributes to the base of the nasal pyramid. The piriform aperture is the bony opening
that leads to the external nose.

  The cartilaginous framework of the nose consists of the paired upper lateral,
the lower lateral, and the sesamoid cartilages (Fig. 1). The upper lateral cartilages

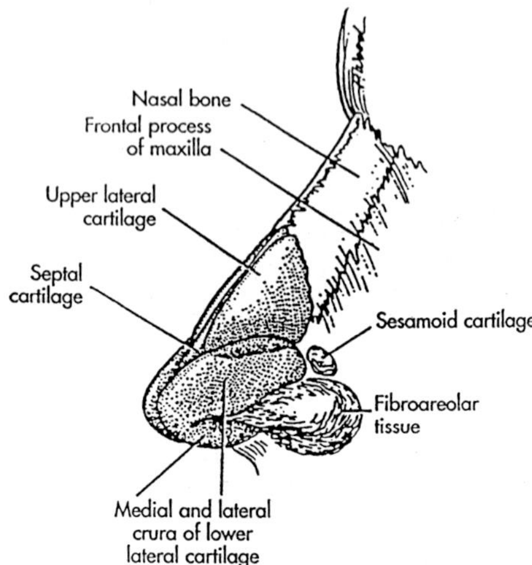

Figure 1 External nasal framework. (From Drumheller GW. Topology of the lateral nasal cartilages: the anatomical relationship of the lateral nasal to the greater alar cartilage, lateral crus. Anat Rec 1973; 176:321, with permission of Wiley-Liss.)

are attached to the undersurface of the nasal bones and frontal processes superiorly and their inferior ends lie under the upper margin of the lower lateral cartilages. Medially, they blend with the cartilaginous septum. Each lower lateral cartilage consists of a medial crus, which extends along the free caudal edge of the cartilaginous septum, and a lateral crus, which provides the framework of the nasal ala, the entrance to the nose (Fig. 1). Laterally, between the upper and lower lateral cartilages, are one or more sesamoid cartilages and fibroadipose tissue.

III. Nasal Septum

The nasal septum divides the nasal cavity into two sides and is composed of cartilage and bone. The bone receives contributions from the vomer, perpendicular plate of the ethmoid, maxillary crest, palatine bone, and anterior spine of the maxillary bone. The main supporting framework of the septum is the septal cartilage, which forms the most anterior part of the septum and articulates posteriorly with the vomer and the perpendicular plate of the ethmoid bone. Inferiorly, the cartilage rests in the crest of the maxilla, whereas anteriorly, it has a free border when it approaches the membranous septum. The latter separates the medial crura of the lower lateral cartilages from the septal cartilage.

The perpendicular plate of the ethmoid bone forms the posterosuperior portion of the septum and the vomer contributes to its posteroinferior portion. In a recent study of cadaveric specimens, Van Loosen and colleagues showed that the cartilaginous septum increases rapidly in size during the first years of life with the total area remaining constant after the age of 2 years (1). In contrast, endochondral ossification of the cartilaginous septum resulting in the formation of the perpendicular plate of the ethmoid bone starts after the first 6 months of life and continues until the age of 36 years.

The continuous, albeit slow, growth of the nasal septum until the third decade might explain frequently encountered septal deviations in adults. Other causes for septal deviations may be spontaneous or as a result of previous trauma. Deviations can involve any of the individual components of the nasal septum and can lead to nasal obstruction because of impairment to airflow within the nasal cavities. In addition to reduction of nasal airflow, some septal deviations obstruct the middle meatal areas and can lead to impairment of drainage from the sinuses with resultant sinusitis.

Severe anterior deviations can also prevent the introduction of intranasal medications to the rest of the nasal cavity and therefore interfere with the medical treatment of rhinitis (2). It is important to examine the nose in a patient with complaints of nasal congestion to rule out such deviations. It is also important to realize that not all deviations lead to symptoms and that surgery should be reserved for those deviations that are thought to contribute to the patient's symptomatology.

IV. Nasal Vestibule

The nasal vestibule, located immediately posterior to the external nasal opening, is lined with stratified squamous epithelium and numerous hairs (or vibrissae) that filter out large particulate matter.

The vestibule funnels air toward the nasal valve, which is a slit-shaped passage formed by the junction of the upper lateral cartilages, the nasal septum, and the inferior turbinate. The nasal valve accounts for approximately 50% of the total resistance to respiratory airflow from the anterior nostril to the alveoli. The surface area of this valve, and consequently resistance to airflow, is modified by the action of the alar muscles. An increase in the tone of the dilator naris muscle, innervated by the facial nerve, dilates the nares, increases the cross-sectional area of the nasal valve, and thus decreases resistance to airflow. This occurs in labored breathing, such as during exercise, and is a physiological mechanism to increase nasal airflow. On the other hand, the nasal valve and the vestibule collapse depending on the pressure gradient between ambient and respired air. As negative pressure in the nose increases to increase airflow, the cartilages collapse in spite of the opposing action of the dilator muscles. An example of

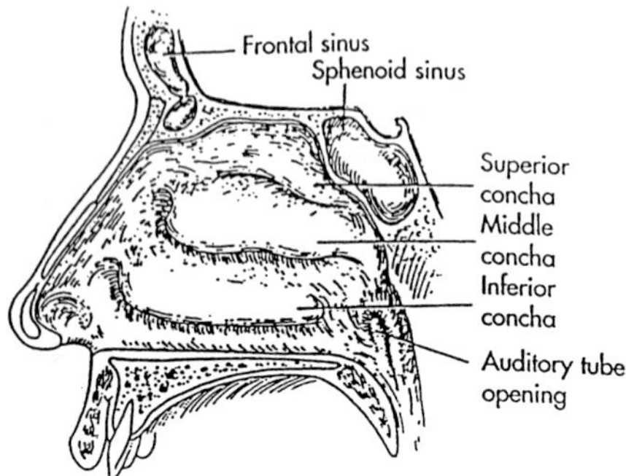

Figure 2 Sagittal section of the lateral nasal wall, showing the three turbinates or conchae, the frontal and sphenoid sinuses, and the opening of the eustachian tube in the nasopharynx. (From Cummings CW, Fredrickson JM, Harker LA, et al. Otolaryngology-Head and Neck Surgery, 2nd ed. St. Louis: Mosby-Year Book, 1993.)

these paradoxical actions occurs during sniffing where resistance to airflow increases across the vestibule/nasal valve complex.

Aging results in loss of strength of the nasal cartilages with secondary weakening of nasal tip support and the nasal valve with resultant airflow compromise (2).

V. Lateral Nasal Wall

The lateral nasal wall commonly has three turbinates, or conchae, the inferior, middle, and superior (Fig. 2). The turbinates are elongated laminae of bone attached along their superior borders to the lateral nasal wall. Their unattached inferior portions curve inward toward the lateral nasal wall resulting in a convex surface that faces the nasal septum medially. They not only increase the mucosal surface of the nasal cavity to about 100–200 cm^2 but regulate airflow by alternating their vascular content and, hence, thickness through the state of their capacitance vessels (3).

The large surface area of the turbinates and the nasal septum allows intimate contact between respired air and the mucosal surfaces thus facilitating humidification, filtration, and temperature regulation of inspired air.

Under and lateral to each of the turbinates are horizontal passages or meati. The inferior meatus receives the opening of the nasolacrimal duct whereas the middle meatus receives drainage originating from the frontal, anterior ethmoid,

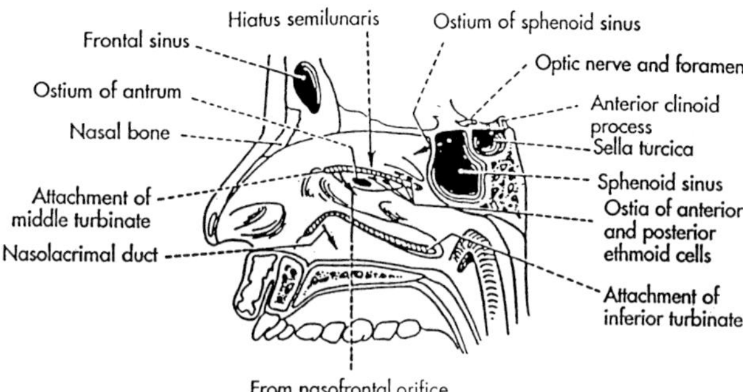

Figure 3 Detailed view of the lateral nasal wall. Parts of the inferior and middle turbinates have been removed to allow visualization of the various openings into the inferior, middle, and superior meati. (From Montgomery WW. Surgery of the Upper Respiratory System. Philadelphia: Lea & Febiger, 1979.)

and maxillary sinuses (Fig. 3). The sphenoid and posterior ethmoid sinuses drain into the sphenoethmoid recess, located below and posterior to the superior turbinate.

The middle meatus is an important anatomical area in the pathophysiology of sinus disease. It has a complex anatomy of bones and mucosal folds, often referred to as the osteomeatal complex, in which drain the frontal, anterior ethmoid, and maxillary sinuses. Anatomical abnormalities or inflammatory mucosal changes in the area of the osteomeatal complex can lead to impaired drainage from these sinuses, which can, at least in part, be responsible for acute and chronic sinus disease. Endoscopic sinus surgery is targeted at restoring the functionality of this drainage system in patients with chronic sinus disease that is refractory to medical management.

VI. Nasal Mucosa

A thin, moderately keratinized, stratified squamous epithelium lines the vestibular region. The anterior tips of the turbinates provide a transition from squamous to transitional and finally to pseudostratified columnar ciliated epithelium, which lines the remainder of the nasal cavity except for the roof, which is lined with olfactory epithelium (Fig. 4) (3). All cells of the pseudostratified columnar ciliated epithelium contact the basement membrane, but not all reach the epithelial surface. The basement membrane separates the epithelium from the lamina propria, or submucosa.

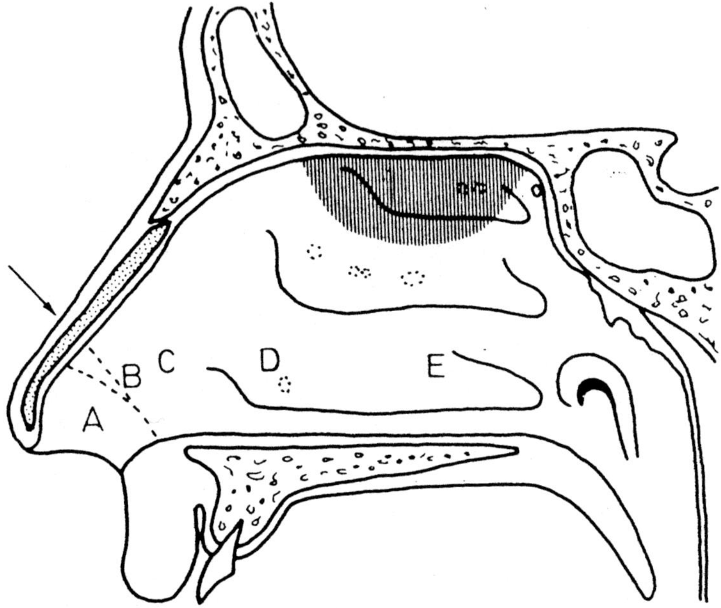

Figure 4　Distribution of types of epithelium along the lateral nasal wall. The hatched region represents the olfactory epithelium. The arrow represents the area of the nasal valve. (A) Skin; (B) squamous epithelium without microvilli; (C) transitional epithelium; (D) pseudostratified columnar epithelium with few ciliated cells; (E) pseudostratified columnar epithelium with many ciliated cells. (From Proctor DF, Andersen I, eds. The Nose. Upper Airway Physiology and the Atmospheric Environment. Amsterdam: Elsevier Biomedical Press, 1982.)

A.　Nasal Epithelium

Within the epithelium, three types of cells are identified: basal, goblet, and columnar, which are either ciliated or nonciliated.

Basal Cells

Basal cells lie on the basement membrane and do not reach the airway lumen. They have an electron-dense cytoplasm and bundles of tonofilaments. Among their morphological specializations are desmosomes, which mediate adhesion between adjacent cells, and hemidesmosomes, which help anchor the cells to the basement membrane (4). These cells have long been thought to be progenitors of the columnar and goblet cells of the airway epithelium, but recent experiments in rat bronchial epithelium suggest that the primary progenitor cell of airway epithelium might be the nonciliated columnar cell population (5). Currently, basal cells are believed to help in the adhesion of columnar cells to the basement membrane. This is supported by the fact that columnar cells do not have hemidesmosomes and attach to the basement membrane only by cell-adhesion molecules, i.e., laminin.

Goblet Cells

The goblet cells arrange themselves perpendicular to the epithelial surface (6). The mucous granules give the mature cell its characteristic goblet shape, in which only a narrow part of the tapering basal cytoplasm touches the basement membrane. The nucleus is situated basally, with the organelles and secretory granules that contain mucin toward the lumen. The luminal surface, covered by microvilli, has a small opening, or stoma, through which the granules secrete their content. The genesis of goblet cells is controversial with some experimental studies supporting a cell of origin unrelated to epithelial cells and others supporting either the cylindrical nonciliated columnar cell population or undifferentiated basal cells as the cells of origin (6). There are no goblet cells in the squamous, transitional, or olfactory epithelia of adults, and they are irregularly distributed, but present, in all areas of pseudostratified columnar epithelium (6).

Columnar Cells

These cells are related to neighboring cells by tight junctions apically and, in the uppermost part, by interdigitations of the cell membrane. The cytoplasm contains numerous mitochondria in the apical part. All columnar cells, ciliated and nonciliated, are covered by 300–400 microvilli, uniformly distributed over the entire apical surface. These are not precursors of cilia but are short and slender finger-like cytoplasmic expansions that increase the surface area of the epithelial cells, thus promoting exchange processes across the epithelium. The microvilli also prevent drying of the surface by retaining moisture essential for ciliary function (3). In humans, ciliated epithelium lines the majority of the airway from the nose to the respiratory bronchioles, as well as the paranasal sinuses, the eustachian tube, and parts of the middle ear.

Inflammatory Cells

Different types of inflammatory cells have been described in the nasal epithelium obtained from normal, nonallergic subjects. Using immunohistochemical staining, Winther and colleagues identified consistent anti-HLA-DR staining in the upper portion of nasal epithelium as well as occasional lymphocytes interspersed between the epithelial cells (7). There appeared to be more T than B lymphocytes and more T-helper than T-suppressor cells. The detection of HLA-DR antigens on the epithelium suggested that the airway epithelium may be potentially participating in antigen recognition and processing. Bradding and colleagues observed rare mast cells within the epithelial layer and no activated eosinophils (8).

B. Nasal Submucosa

The nasal submucosa lies beneath the basement membrane and contains a host of cellular components in addition to nasal glands, nerves, and blood vessels.

In a light microscopy study of nasal biopsies of normal individuals, the predominant cell in the submucosa was the mononuclear cell, which includes lymphocytes and monocytes (9). Much less numerous were neutrophils and eosinophils (9). Mast cells were also found in appreciable numbers in the nasal submucosa as identified by immunohistochemical staining with a monoclonal antibody against mast cell tryptase (8).

Winther and colleagues evaluated lymhocyte subsets in the nasal mucosa of normal subjects using immunohistochemistry (7). They found T lymphocytes to be the predominant cell type with fewer scattered B cells. The ratio of T-helper cells to T-suppressor cells in the lamina propria averaged 3:1 in the subepithelial area and 2:1 in the deeper vascular stroma with the overall ratio being 2.5:1, similar to the average ratio in peripheral blood. Natural killer cells were very rare constituting less than 2% of the lymphocytes.

Recent interest in inflammatory cytokines prompted Bradding and colleagues to investigate cells containing IL-4, IL-5, IL-6, and IL-8 in the nasal mucosa of patients with perennial rhinitis and normal subjects (8). The normal nasal mucosa was found to contain cells with positive IL-4 immunoreactivity with 90% of these cells also staining positive for tryptase, suggesting that they were mast cells. Immunoreactivity for IL-5 and IL-6 was present in 75% of the normal nasal biopsies and IL-8-positive cells were found in all the normal nasal tissue samples. A median 50% of IL-5$^+$ cells and 100% of the IL-6$^+$ cells were mast cells. In contrast to the other cytokines, IL-8 was largely confined to the cytoplasm of epithelial cells.

From the above studies, it is clear that the normal nasal mucosa contains a host of inflammatory cells the role of which is unclear. In allergic rhinitis, most of these inflammatory cells increase in number (10), and eosinophils, a large portion of which are activated (as identified by positive staining with antibodies against EG2), are also recruited into the nasal mucosa (8). Furthermore, cells positive for IL-4 increase significantly in patients with allergic rhinitis compared to normal subjects (8).

C. Nasal Glands

There are three types of nasal glands: anterior serous, seromucous, and intraepithelial. They are located in the submucosa and epithelium.

Anterior Serous Glands

These serous glands have ducts (2–20 mm in length) that open into small crypts located in the nasal vestibule. The ducts are lined by one layer of cuboidal epithelium. Bojsen-Müller found 50–80 crypts anteriorly on the septum and another 50–80 anteriorly on the lateral nasal wall (11). He suggested that these glands play an important role in keeping the nose moist by spreading their serous secretions backward, thus moistening the entire mucosa. Tos, however, was able to find only 20–30 anterior nasal glands on the septum and an equal number on the lateral wall (6). He deduced that the contribution of these glands to the total production of secretions is minimal and that they represent a phylogenetic rudiment.

Seromucous Glands

The main duct of these glands is lined with simple cuboidal epithelium. It divides into two side ducts that collect secretions from several tubules lined with either serous or mucous cells. At the ends of the tubules are acini, which may similarly be serous or mucous. Serous acini predominate over mucous acini by a ratio of about 8:1.

The glands first laid down during development grow deep into the lamina propria before dividing and thus develop their mass in the deepest layers of the mucosa with relatively long ducts. The glands that develop later divide before growing down into the mucosa and thus form a more superficial mass with short ducts. Vessels, nerves, and fibers develop in between, giving rise to two glandular layers: superficial and deep. The mass of the deep glands is larger than that of the superficial ones and the total number of these glands is approximately 90,000.

Intraepithelial Glands

These glands are located in the epithelium and consist of 20–50 mucous cells arranged radially around a small lumen. Some intraepithelial glands exist in nasal polyps. Compared to seromucous glands, intraepithelial glands produce only a small amount of mucus and thus play a minor role in the physiology of nasal secretions.

VII. Vascular and Lymphatic Supplies

The nose receives its blood supply from both the internal and external carotid circulations via the ophthalmic and internal maxillary arteries, respectively (Fig.

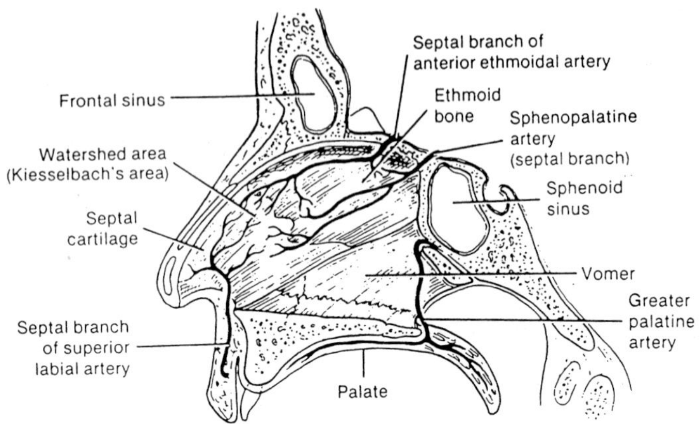

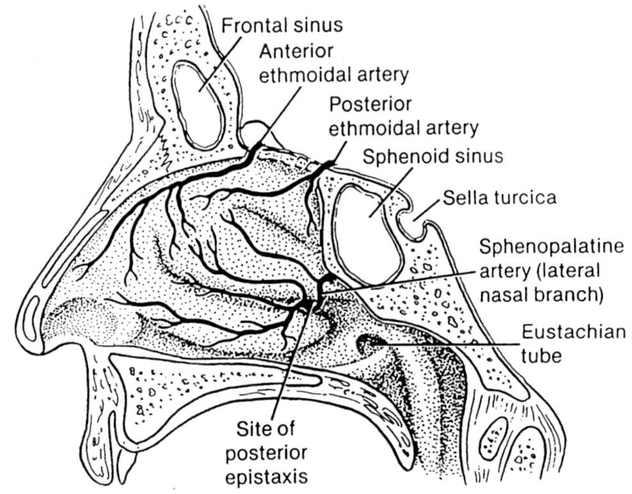

Figure 5 Nasal blood supply. (Top) the supply to the nasal septum; (bottom) the supply to the lateral nasal wall. (From Cummings CW, Fredrickson JM, Harker LA, et al. Otolaryngology-Head and Neck Surgery. St. Louis: CV Mosby, 1986.)

5). The ophthalmic artery gives rise to the anterior and posterior ethmoid arteries, which supply the anterosuperior portion of the septum, the lateral nasal walls, the olfactory region, and a small part of the posterosuperior region. The external carotid artery gives rise to the internal maxillary artery, which ends as the sphenopalatine artery, which enters the nasal cavity through the sphenopalatine foramen behind the posterior end of the middle turbinate. The sphenopalatine artery gives origin to a number of posterior lateral and septal nasal branches. The posterolateral branches proceed to the region of the middle and inferior turbinates and to the floor of the nasal cavity. The posterior septal branches supply the corresponding area of the septum, including the nasal floor. Because it supplies the majority of blood to the nose and is often involved in severe epistaxis, the sphenopalatine artery has been called "the rhinologist's artery." The region of the vestibule is supplied by the facial artery through lateral and septal nasal branches. The septal branches of the sphenopalatine artery form multiple anastomoses with the terminal branches of the anterior ethmoidal and facial arteries giving rise to Kisselbach's area, located at the caudal aspect of the septum and also known as Little's area. Most cases of epistaxis occur in this region (12).

The veins accompanying the branches of the sphenopalatine artery drain into the pterygoid plexus. The ethmoidal veins join the ophthalmic plexus in the orbit. Part of the drainage to the ophthalmic plexus proceeds to the cavernous sinus via the superior ophthalmic veins and the other part to the pterygoid plexus via the inferior ophthalmic veins. Furthermore, the nasal veins form numerous anastomoses with the veins of the face, palate, and pharynx. The nasal venous system is valveless, predisposing to the spread of infections and constituting a dynamic system reflecting body position.

The subepithelial and glandular zones of the nasal mucosa are supplied by arteries derived from the periosteal or perichondrial vessels. Branches from these vessels ascend perpendicularly toward the surface, anastomosing with the cavernous plexi (venous system) before forming fenestrated capillary networks next to the respiratory epithelium and around the glandular tissue (13). The fenestrae always face the respiratory epithelium and are believed to be one of the sources of fluid for humidification (14).

The capillaries of the subepithelial and periglandular network join to form venules that drain into larger superficial veins. They, in turn, join the sinuses of the cavernous plexus. The cavernous plexi, or sinusoids, consist of networks of large, tortuous, valveless, anastomosing veins mostly found over the inferior and middle turbinates but also in the midlevel of the septum. They consist of a superficial layer formed by the union of veins that drain the subepithelial and glandular capillaries and a deeper layer where the sinuses acquire thicker walls and assume a course parallel to the periosteum or perichondrium. They receive venous blood from the subepithelial and glandular capillaries and arterial blood from arteriovenous anastomoses.

The arterial segments of the anastomoses are surrounded by a longitudinal smooth muscle layer that controls their blood flow. When the muscular layer contracts, the artery occludes; when it relaxes, the anastomosis opens, allowing the sinuses to fill rapidly with blood. Because of this function, the sinusoids are physiologically referred to as capacitance vessels. Only endothelium interposes

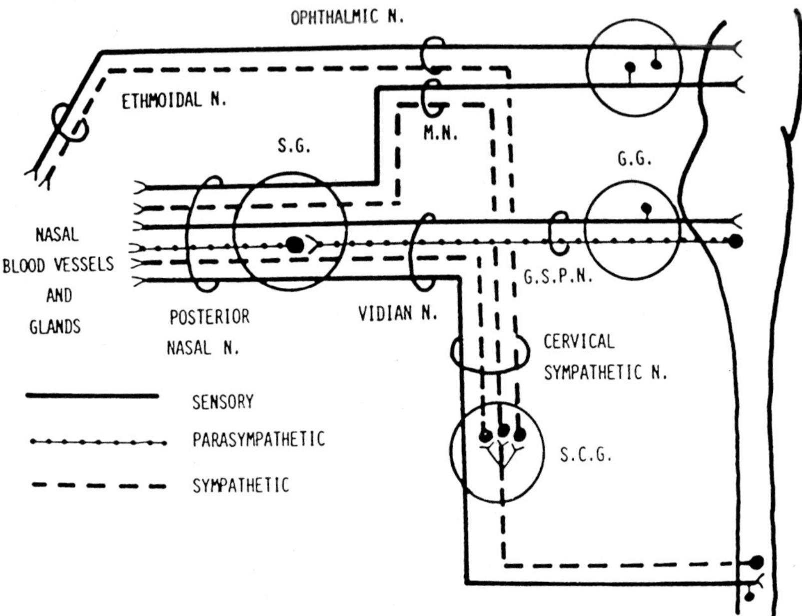

Figure 6   Nasal neural supply: sensory, sympathetic, and parasympathetic. SG, sphenopalatine ganglion; MN, maxillary nerve; GG, geniculate ganglion; GSPN, greater superficial petrosal nerve; SCG, superior cervical ganglion. (From Proctor DF, Andersen I, eds. The Nose. Upper Airway Physiology and the Atmospheric Environment. Amsterdam: Elsevier Biomedical Press, 1982.)

between the longitudinal muscles and the blood stream, making them sensitive to circulating agents. The cavernous plexi change their blood volume in response to neural, mechanical, thermal, psychological, or chemical stimulation. They expand and shrink, altering the caliber of the air passages and, consequently, the speed and volume of airflow.

Lymphatic vessels from the nasal vestibule drain toward the external nose, whereas the nasal fossa drains posteriorly. The first-order lymph nodes for posterior drainage are the lateral retropharyngeal nodes, whereas the subdigastric nodes serve that function for anterior drainage.

VIII. Neural Supply

The nasal neural supply is overwhelmingly sensory and autonomic (sympathetic, parasympathetic, and nonadrenergic noncholinergic) (Fig. 6). The sensory nasal innervation comes via both the ophthalmic and maxillary divisions of the trigeminal nerve and supplies the septum, the lateral walls, the anterior part of the nasal floor, and the inferior meatus.

The parasympathetic nasal fibers travel from their origin in the superior salivary nucleus of the midbrain via the nervus intermedius of the facial nerve to the geniculate ganglion where they join the greater superficial petrosal nerve, which, in turn, joins the deep petrosal nerve to form the vidian nerve. This nerve travels to the sphenopalatine ganglion where the preganglionic parasympathetic fibers synapse and postganglionic fibers supply the nasal mucosa.

The sympathetic input originates as preganglionic fibers in the thoracolumbar region of the spinal cord, which pass into the vagosympathetic trunk and relay in the superior cervical ganglion. The postganglionic fibers end as the deep petrosal nerve, which joins the greater superficial nerve to form the vidian nerve. They traverse the sphenopalatine ganglion without synapsing and are distributed to the nasal mucosa.

Nasal glands receive direct parasympathetic nerve supply, and electrical stimulation of parasympathetic nerves in animals induces glandular secretions that are blocked by atropine. Furthermore, stimulation of the human nasal mucosa with methacholine, a cholinomimetic, produces an atropine-sensitive increase in nasal secretions (15). Parasympathetic nerves also provide innervation to the nasal vasculature and stimulation of these fibers causes vasodilatation.

Sympathetic fibers supply the nasal vasculature but do not establish a close relationship with nasal glands, and their exact role in the control of nasal secretions is not clear. Stimulation of these fibers causes vasoconstriction and a decrease in nasal airway resistance. Adrenergic agonists are commonly used, both topically and orally, to decrease nasal congestion.

The presence of sympathetic and parasympathetic nerves and their transmitters in the nasal mucosa has been known for decades but recent immunohistochemical studies have established the presence of additional neuropeptides. These are secreted by unmyelinated nociceptive C-fibers (tachykinins; calcitonin gene-related peptide, CGRP; neurokinin A, NKA; gastrin-releasing peptide), parasympathetic nerve endings (vasoactive intestinal peptide, VIP; peptide histidine methionine), and sympathetic nerve endings (neuropeptide Y).

Substance P (SP), a member of the tachykinin family, is often found as a cotransmitter with NKA and CGRP and has been found in high density in arterial vessels, and to some extent in veins, gland acini, and surface epithelium (16). SP receptors (NK1 receptors) are located in epithelium, glands, and vessels (16). CGRP receptors are found in high concentration on small muscular arteries and arterioles in the nasal mucosa (17). The distribution of VIP fibers in human airways corresponds closely to that of cholinergic nerves (18). In the human nasal mucosa, VIP is abundant and its receptors are located on arterial vessels, submucosal glands, and epithelial cells (19).

IX. Nasal Mucus and Mucociliary Transport

A thin layer of mucus covers the nasal surface epithelium (20). It is slightly acidic, with a pH between 5.5 and 6.5. The mucous blanket consists of two layers: a low viscosity, periciliary layer (sol phase) that envelops the shafts of the cilia, and a more viscous layer (gel phase) riding on the periciliary layer. The gel phase can also be envisioned as discontinuous plaques of mucus.

The distal tips of the ciliary shafts contact these plaques when they are fully extended. Insoluble particles caught on the mucous plaques move with them as a consequence of ciliary beating. Soluble materials like droplets, formaldehyde, and CO_2 dissolve in the periciliary layer (21–23).

The sources of nasal secretions are multiple and include anterior nasal glands, seromucous submucosal glands, epithelial secretory cells (goblet cells), tears, and exudation from blood vessels.

Exudation increases in pathological conditions as a result of the effects of inflammatory mediators that increase vascular permeability. A good example is the increased vascular permeability seen in response to allergen challenge of subjects with allergic rhinitis as measured by increasing levels of albumin in nasal lavages after provocation (24). Albumin and immunoglobulins make up the bulk of the protein in mucus; other substances in nasal secretions include lactoferrin, lysozyme, antitrypsin, transferrin, lipids, histamine and other mediators, cytokines, antioxidants, ions (Cl^-, Na^+, Ca^{2+}, K^+), cells, and bacteria.

Mucus functions in mucociliary transport, and substances will not be cleared from the nose without it, despite adequate ciliary function. Furthermore, mucus provides immune and mechanical mucosal protection and its high water content plays a significant role in humidifying inspired air.

Mucociliary transport is unidirectional based on the unique characteristics of cilia. Cilia in mammals beat in a biphasic, or to-and-fro, manner. The beat consists of a rapid effective stroke during which the cilium straightens, bringing it in contact with the gel phase of the mucus, and a slow recovery phase during which the bent cilium returns in the periciliary or sol layer of the mucus, thus propelling it in one direction (Fig. 7).

Metachrony is the coordination of the beat of individual cilia that prevents collision between cilia in different phases of motion and results in the unidirectional flow of mucus. Ciliary beating produces a current in the superficial layer of the periciliary fluid in the direction of the effective stroke. The mucous plaques move as a result of motion of the periciliary fluid layer and the movement of the extended tips of the cilia into the plaques. Thus, the depth of the periciliary fluid is the key factor in mucociliary transport. If excessive, the extended ciliary tips fail to contact mucous plaques, and the current of the periciliary fluid provides the only means of movement.

Mucociliary transport moves mucus and its contents toward the nasophar-

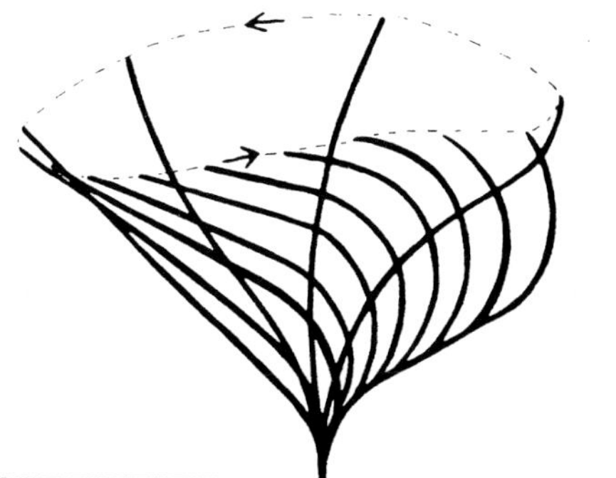

Figure 7 Schematic diagram of motion of a single cilium during the rapid forward beat and the slower recovery phase. (From Proctor DF, Andersen I. The Nose. Upper Airway Physiology and the Atmospheric Environment. Amsterdam: Elsevier Biomedical Press, 1982.)

ynx, with the exception of the anterior portion of the inferior turbinates, where transport is anterior. This anterior current prevents many of the particles deposited in this area from progressing further into the nasal cavity. The particles transported posteriorly toward the nasopharynx are periodically swallowed. Mucociliary transport, however, is not the only mechanism by which particles and secretions are cleared from the nose. Sniffing and nose blowing help in moving airway secretions backward and forward, respectively. Sneezing results in a burst of air, accompanied by an increase in watery nasal secretions that are then cleared by nose blowing and sniffing.

Respiratory cilia beat about 1000 times per minute, which translates to surface materials being moved at a rate of 3–25 mm/min. Both the beat rate and propelling speed vary. Several substances have been used to measure nasal mucociliary clearance; the most frequently utilized are saccharin, dyes, or tagged particles.

The dye and saccharin methods are similar, consisting of placing a strong dye or saccharin sodium on the nasal mucosa on the inferior turbinate or septal wall and recording the time it takes to reach the pharyngeal cavity; this interval is termed "nasal mucociliary transport time." With saccharin, the time is recorded when the subject reports a sweet taste, whereas with a dye, when it appears in the pharyngeal cavity. Combining the two methods reduces the disadvantages of both—namely, variable taste thresholds in different subjects when using saccharin and repeated pharyngeal inspection when using the dye—and makes them more reliable.

The use of tagged particles involves placement of an anion exchange resin particle about 0.5 mm in diameter tagged with a ^{99}Tc ion on the anterior nasal mucosa, behind the area of anterior mucociliary movement, and following its subsequent clearance with a gamma camera or multicollimated detectors. This last method permits continuous monitoring of movement.

Studies of several hundred healthy adult subjects by the tagged particle or saccharin methods have consistently shown that 80% exhibit clearance rates of 3–25 mm/min (average 6 mm/min), with slower rates in the remaining 20% (25). The latter subjects have been termed ''slow clearers.'' The finding of a greater proportion of slow clearers in one group of subjects living in an extremely cold climate raises the possibility that the differences in clearance may be related to an effect of inspired air (25). In diseased subjects, slow clearance may be due to a variety of factors, including the immotility of cilia, transient or permanent injury to the mucociliary system by physical trauma, viral infection, dehydration, or excessively viscid secretions secondary to decreased ions and water in the mucus paired with increased amounts of DNA from dying cells, as in cystic fibrosis.

X. Nasal Airflow

The nose provides the main pathway for inhaled air to the lower airways and offers two areas of resistance to airflow (provided there are no gross deviations of the nasal septum): the nasal valve and the state of mucosal swelling of the nasal airway.

The cross-sectional area of the nasal airway decreases dramatically at the nasal valve to reach 30–40 mm^2. This narrowed area separates the vestibule from the main airway and accounts for approximately half of the total resistance to respiratory airflow from ambient air to the alveoli.

After bypassing this narrow area, inspired air flows in the main nasal airway, which is a broader tube bounded by the septal surface medially and the irregular inferior and middle turbinates laterally. The variable caliber of the lumen of this portion of the airway is governed by changes in the blood content of the capillaries, capacitance vessels, and arteriovenous shunts of the lining mucosa and constitutes the second resistive segment that inspired air encounters on its way to the lungs.

Changes in the blood content of these structures occur spontaneously and rhythmically resulting in alternating volume reductions in the lumen of the two nasal cavities, a phenomenon referred to as the ''nasal cycle.'' This occurs in approximately 80% of normal individuals and the reciprocity of changes between the two sides of the nasal cavity maintains total nasal airway resistance unchanged (26). The duration of one cycle varies between 50 min and 4 hr and is interrupted by vasoconstrictive medications or exercise, which leads to a marked reduction of

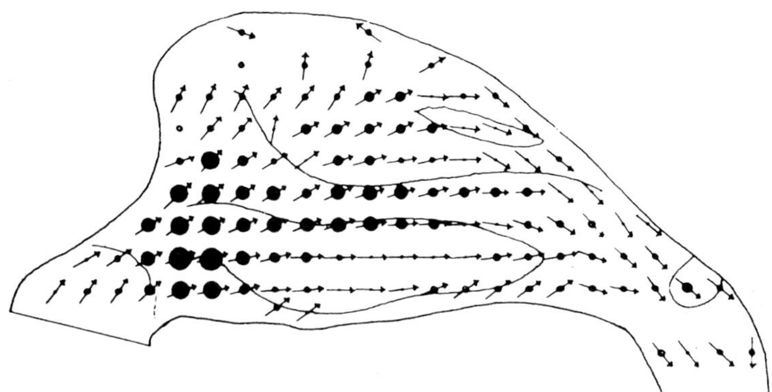

Figure 8 Schematic diagram of the direction and velocity of inspired air. The size of the dots is directly proportional to velocity and the arrows depict direction of airflow. (From Proctor DF, Andersen I, eds. The Nose. Upper Airway Physiology and the Atmospheric Environment. Amsterdam: Elsevier Biomedical Press, 1982.)

total nasal airway resistance. Kennedy and colleagues observed the nasal passages using T2-weighted magnetic resonance imaging and demonstrated an alternating increase and decrease in signal intensity and turbinate size over time in a fashion consistent with the nasal cycle (27). The nasal cycle can be exacerbated by the increase in nasal airway resistance caused by exposure to allergic stimuli and explains why some allergic individuals complain of alternating exacerbations of their nasal obstructive symptoms.

Swift and Proctor presented a detailed description of nasal airflow and its characteristics (Fig. 8) (28). Upon inspiration, air first passes upward into the vestibules in a vertical direction at a velocity of 2–3 m/sec, then converges and changes its direction from vertical to horizontal just prior to the nasal valve, where, due to the narrowing of the airway, velocities reach their highest levels (up to 12–18 m/sec). After passing the nasal valve, the cross-sectional area increases, and velocity decreases concomitantly to about 2–3 m/sec.

The nature of flow changes from laminar, before and at the nasal valve, to more turbulent posteriorly. As inspiratory flow increases beyond resting levels, turbulent characteristics commence at an increasingly anterior position and, with mild exercise, are found as early as the anterior ends of the turbinates. The airstream increases in velocity to 3–4 m/sec in the nasopharynx, where the direction again changes from horizontal to vertical as air moves down through the pharynx and larynx to reach the trachea. Turbulence of nasal airflow minimizes the presence of a boundary layer of air that would exist with laminar flow and maximizes interaction between the airstream and the nasal mucosa. This, in turn, allows the nose to perform its functions of heat and moisture exchange and of cleaning inspired air of suspended or soluble particles.

XI. Nasal Conditioning of the Temperature and Humidity of Inspired Air

Inspiratory air is rapidly warmed and moistened mainly in the nasal cavities and, to a lesser extent, in the remainder of the upper airway down to the lungs (29). Inspired air is warmed from a temperature of around 20°C at the portal of entry to 31°C in the pharynx and 35°C in the trachea. This is facilitated by the turbulent characteristics of nasal airflow, which maximize the contact between inspired and expired air and the nasal mucosal surface (30).

After inspiration ceases, warming of the nasal mucosa by the blood is such a relatively slow process that, at expiration, the temperature of the nasal mucosa remains lower than that of expired air. As expiratory air passes through the nose, it gives up heat to the cooler nasal mucosa. This cooling causes condensation of water vapor and, thus, a 33% return of both heat and moisture to the mucosal surface. Since recovery of heat from expiratory air occurs mainly in the region of the respiratory portal, blood flow changes that take place in the nasal mucosa affect respiratory air conditioning more markedly in this region (31).

Ingelstedt and Ivstam showed that the humidifying capacity of the nose is greatly impaired in healthy volunteers after a subcutaneous injection of atropine (29,32). They thus concluded that atropine-inhibitable glandular secretion is a major source of water for humidification of inspired air. In contrast, Kumlien and Drettner failed to show any effect of intranasal ipratropium bromide, another anticholinergic agent, on the degree of warming and humidification of air during passage in the nasal cavity in a small clinical trial using normal subjects and a group of patients with vasomotor rhinitis (33).

In addition to glandular secretions, other sources provide water for humidification of inspired air and these include water content of ambient air, lacrimation via the nasolacrimal duct, secretion from the paranasal sinuses, salivation (during oronasal breathing), and secretions from goblet cells and seromucinous glands of the respiratory mucosa, and passive transport against an ionic gradient in the paracellular spaces (32,34). Not inhibited by atropine, but also probably important as a source of water for humidification of inspired air, is exudation of fluid from the blood vessels of the nose. Impairment of the humidifying capacity of the nose is further accentuated when the nasal mucosa is chilled, leading, along with condensation, to the nasal drip so often seen in cold weather.

XII. Olfaction

One of the important sensory functions of the nose is olfaction. The olfactory airway is 1–2 mm wide and lies above the middle turbinate just inferior to the cribriform plate between the septum and the lateral wall of the nose. The olfactory mucosa has a surface area of 200–400 mm^2 and contains numerous odor-receptor cells with thin cilia that project into the covering mucus layer and increase the surface area of the epithelium (35). The olfactory mucosa also contains small, tubular, serous Bowman's glands situated immediately below the epithelium. Each receptor cell is connected to the olfactory bulb by a thin, nonmyelinated nerve fiber that is slow conducting but short, making the conduction time as low as 50 m/sec. The impulses from the olfactory bulb are conveyed to the olfactory cortex, which in humans is part of the thalamus, which also receives taste signals.

The area where the olfactory epithelium is located is poorly ventilated as most of the inhaled air passes through the lower aspect of the nasal cavity. Therefore, nasal obstruction, as documented by elevations in nasal airway resistance, leads to an elevation in olfactory thresholds (36). This may be secondary to several factors such as septal deviations, nasal polyposis, nasal deformities, or increased nasal congestion, one of the characteristic symptoms of allergic rhinitis. Sniffing helps the process of smell by increasing the flow rate of inhaled air and, consequently, raising the proportion of air reaching the olfactory epithelium by 5–20%. This results in increasing the number of odorant molecules available to the olfactory receptors and proportionally enhancing odor sensation.

In addition to crossing the anatomical barriers of the nose, the odorant molecules must have a dual solubility in lipids and water to be able to reach the olfactory receptors. To penetrate the mucus covering the olfactory mucosa, they solubilize to a certain extent in water. Lipid solubility, on the other hand, enhances their interaction with the receptor membrane of the olfactory epithelial cilia. Finally, olfactory sensitivity normally decreases with age as evidenced by a recent longitudinal study of men and women between the ages of 19 and 95 followed over a 3-year period (37).

XIII. Vomeronasal Organ

Many vertebrate species including many mammals have a small chemosensory structure in the nose called the vomeronasal organ, which is dedicated to detecting chemical signals that mediate sexual and territorial behaviors. A similar structure appears to exist in the human nose and is described as two small sacs about 2 mm deep that open into shallow pits on either side of the nasal septum. In vertebrates, the pair of small sacs is lined by sensory neurons, tucked inside the vomer bone where the hard palate and nasal septum meet. In mice and rats, the vomeronasal organ is connected to the brain through a neural pathway that is independent from the olfactory pathway, but it is not clear whether the human vomeronasal organ is connected to the brain. There is recent renewed interest in researching the anatomy and function of this organ in humans and this effort is primarily funded by the perfume industry (38).

XIV. Conclusions

As detailed in this chapter, the nose is an intricate organ with important functions that include filtration, humidification, and temperature control of inspired air in preparation for transit to the lower airways. It is also important in providing the sense of olfaction. It has an intricate network of nerves, vessels, glands, and inflammatory cells, which all help to modulate its function. Chronic inflammation affects multiple end-organs within the nasal cavity and will lead to diseases such as rhinitis (allergic and nonallergic) as well as sinusitis. The overview of the anatomy and function of the nose provided in this chapter will serve as a useful prelude to the following chapters where different diseases of the nose are discussed along with the effects of the different available therapeutic agents that are used to treat these nasal disorders.

References

1. Van Loosen J, Van Zanten GA, Howard CV, et al. Growth characteristics of the human nasal septum. Rhinology 1996; 34:78.
2. Gray L. Deviated nasal septum. III. Its influence on the physiology and disease of the nose and ears. J Laryngol 1967; 81:953.
3. Mygind N, Pedersen M, Nielsen M. Morphology of the upper airway epithelium. In: Proctor DF, Andersen I, eds. The Nose. Amsterdam: Elsevier Biomedical Press, 1982.
4. Evans MJ, Plopper GG. The role of basal cells in adhesion of columnar epithelium to airway basement membrane. Am Rev Respir Dis 1988; 138:481.
5. Evans MJ, Shami S, Cabral-Anderson LJ, et al. Role of nonciliated cells in renewal of the bronchial epithelium of rats exposed to NO_2. Am J Pathol 1986; 123:126.
6. Tos M. Goblet cells and glands in the nose and paranasal sinuses. In: Proctor DF, Andersen I, eds. The Nose. Amsterdam: Elsevier Biomedical Press, 1982.
7. Winther B, Innes DJ, Mills SE, et al. Lymphocyte subsets in normal airway mucosa of the human nose. Arch Otolaryngol Head Neck Surg 1987; 113:59.
8. Bradding P, Feather IH, Wilson S, et al. Immunolocalization of cytokines in the nasal mucosa of normal and perennial rhinitic subjects. J Immunol 1993; 151:3853.
9. Lim MC, Taylor RM, Naclerio RM. The histology of allergic rhinitis and its com-

parison to cellular changes in nasal lavage. Am J Respir Crit Care Med 1995; 151:136.

10. Varney VA, Jacobson MR, Sudderick RM, et al. Immunohistology of the nasal mucosa following allergen-induced rhinitis. Am Rev Respir Dis 1992; 146:170.

11. Bojsen-Müller F. Glandulae nasales anteriores in the human nose. Ann Otol Rhinol Laryngol 1965; 74:363.

12. Cauna N. Blood and nerve supply of the nasal lining. In: Proctor DF, Andersen I, eds. The Nose. Amsterdam: Elsevier Biomedical Press, 1982.

13. Dawes JDK, Prichard M. Studies of the vascular arrangement of the nose. J Anat 1953; 87:311.

14. Cauna N, Hinderer KH. Fine structure of blood vessels of the human respiratory mucosa. Ann Otol Rhinol Laryngol 1969; 78:865.

15. Baroody FM, Wagenmann M, Naclerio RM. A comparison of the secretory response of the nasal mucosa to histamine and methacholine. J Appl Physiol 1993; 74:2661.

16. Baraniuk JN, Lundgren JD, Mullol J, et al. Substance P and neurokinin A in human nasal mucosa. Am J Respir Cell Mol Biol 1991; 4:228.

17. Baraniuk JN, Castellino S, Merida M, et al. Calcitonin gene related peptide in human nasal mucosa. Am J Physiol 1990; 258:L81.

18. Laitinen A, Partanen M, Hervonen A, et al. VIP-like immunoreactive nerves in human respiratory tract. Light and electron microscopic study. Histochemistry 1985; 82:313.

19. Baraniuk JN, Okayama M, Lundgren JD, et al. Vasoactive intestinal peptide (VIP) in human nasal mucosa. J Clin Invest 1990; 86:825.

20. Wilson WR, Allansmith MR. Rapid, atraumatic method for obtaining nasal mucus samples. Ann Otol Rhinol Laryngol 1976; 85:391.

21. Andersen I, Lundqvist G, Proctor DF. Human nasal mucosal function under four controlled humidities. Am Rev Respir Dis 1979; 119:619.

22. Fry FA, Black A. Regional deposition and clearance of particles in the human nose. Aerosol Sci 1973; 4:113.

23. Lippmann M. Deposition and clearance of inhaled particles in the human nose. Ann Otol Rhinol Laryngol 1970; 79:519.

24. Baumgarten C, Togias AG, Naclerio RM, et al. Influx of kininogens into nasal secretions after antigen challenge of allergic individuals. J Clin Invest 1985; 76:191.

25. Proctor DF. The mucociliary system. In: Proctor DF, Andersen I, eds. The Nose: Upper Airway Physiology and the Atmospheric Environment. Amsterdam: Elsevier Biomedical Press, 1982.

26. Hasegawa M, Kern EB. The human cycle. Mayo Clin Proc 1977; 52:28.

27. Kennedy DW, Zinreich SJ, Kumar AJ, et al. Physiologic mucosal changes within the nose and the ethmoid sinus: Imaging of the nasal cycle by MRI. Laryngoscope 1988; 98:928.

28. Swift DL, Proctor DF. Access of air to the respiratory tract. In: Brain JD, Proctor DF, Reid LM, eds. Respiratory Defense Mechanisms. New York: Marcel Dekker, 1977.

29. Ingelstedt S, Ivstam B. Study in the humidifying capacity of the nose. Acta Otolaryngol (Stockh) 1951; 39:286.

30. Aharonson EF, Menkes H, Gurtner G, et al. The effect of respiratory airflow rate on the removal of soluble vapors by the nose. J Appl Physiol 1974; 37:654.

31. Scherer PW, Hahn II, Mozell MM. The biophysics of nasal airflow. Otolaryngol Clin North Am 1989; 22:265.

32. Ingelstedt S, Ivstam B. The source of nasal secretion in normal condition. Acta Otolaryngol (Stockh) 1949; 37:446.

33. Kumlien J, Drettner B. The effect of ipratropium bromide (Atrovent) on the air conditioning capacity of the nose. Clin Otolaryngol 1985; 10:165.

34. Togias AG, Proud D, Lichtenstein LM, et al. The osmolality of nasal secretions increases when inflammatory mediators are released in response to inhalation of cold, dry air. Am Rev Respir Dis 1988; 137:625.

35. Berglund B, Lindvall T. Olfaction. In: Proctor DF, Andersen I, eds. The Nose. Amsterdam: Elsevier Biomedical Press, 1982.

36. Rous J, Kober F. Influence of one-sided nasal respiratory occlusion of the olfactory threshold values. Arch Klin Ohren Nasen Kehlkopfheilk 1970; 196:374.

37. Ship JA, Pearson JD, Cruise LJ, et al. Longitudinal changes in smell identification. J Gerontol 1996; 51:M86.

38. Taylor R. Brave new nose: sniffing out human sexual chemistry. J NIH Res 1994; 6:47.

2

Definition and Classification

ROBERT M. NACLERIO

University of Chicago
Chicago, Illinois

NIELS MYGIND

University of Aarhus
Aarhus, Denmark

I. Rhinitis

Symptoms referable to the nose cause tremendous morbidity throughout the world (Chapter 3). These symptoms include those primarily referable to the nose, such as sneezing, irritation, anterior discharge, hyposmia/anosmia, and stuffiness, and those possibly secondary to nasal disease, such as headache, facial pain, ear popping, dry throat, postnasal drip, cough, and eye symptoms. Another important characteristic of the symptomatology are the systemic effects that interfere with the quality of our lives, e.g., sleep disturbances (see Chapter 4). The persistence of these symptoms is often referred to as rhinitis. The common cold, also a major cause of morbidity, is a self-limited form of rhinitis and is not discussed in this book.

The suffix ''itis'' in the term ''rhinitis'' implies inflammation. Unfortunately, the pathophysiology of many forms of rhinitis is not understood. The pathophysiology of allergic rhinitis, the focus of the majority of basic and clinical investigations, continues to evolve (Chapter 7). Similarly elucidating the nature and molecular structure of the allergens that provoke allergic rhinitis (Chapter 6) continues to improve. Whereas little is known about the pathophysiology of most forms of nonallergic rhinitis, the presence of inflammation has not even been documented in most instances.

Classifying rhinitis into rigid categories risks being simplistic and might overlook many important considerations, especially that some nasal problems are not even associated with inflammation to deserve the suffix "itis." An example is an anatomical problem such as septal deviation that causes symptoms such as nasal stuffiness.

When do normal physiological responses become rhinitis? When do the increased demands to warm and humidify outdoor air in the winter become rhinitis: when the patient complains, when glandular secretions become triggered by neural reflexes? What are the normal changes associated with aging and what is disease? Weakened cartilage supporting the nasal valve associated with aging causes morbidity and can be treated with mechanical support. Is this a disease? Furthermore, rhinitis, a familiar term, does not accurately reflect all issues associated with nasal dysfunction. Rhinitis limits the problem to the nose. Does that exclude involvement of the sinuses or the eustachian tube? Studies by Gwaltney and colleagues (1) showed that a common cold causes radiographic changes within the sinuses that resolve with resolution of the cold. Should the term "rhinosinusitis" be introduced?

Since the list of issues with the term "rhinitis" is long, is it time to define a new term? Currently there is no acceptable alternative. Furthermore, the familiarity with the term "rhinitis," like familiarity with the term "hay fever," causes it to persist and thus we chose to keep it in the title of this book. While the term "hay fever" is inaccurate for two reasons (it is not caused by hay and there is no fever associated with it), "rhinitis" is only partially incorrect in a small number of nasal disorders.

As research into our understanding of nasal function in health and disease expands, more specific causes of nasal symptoms will be defined. For example, the pathophysiology of anterior nasal discharge associated with eating, a form of nonallergic rhinitis referred to as gustatory rhinitis, has become understood and is treatable with anticholinergic agents (Chapter 15). As we better understand disorders of the nose, like gustatory rhinitis, then the large group referred to as nonallergic rhinitis will be further subdivided.

In addition, our ability to define symptoms or signs objectively with respect to physiological alteration will also increase. Greater understanding will enable us to define nasal disorders better and subsequently provide better treatments for our patients. Better understanding will undoubtedly lead to new ways of classifying rhinitis.

II. Classification

Although problems exist with limiting disorders of the nose and their sequelae to an oversimplified classification, the fact remains that such a tool provides a means of communication between colleagues and a guideline for patient management. We must also define criteria to classify patients. Consider reading a manuscript that discusses a clinical trial for the treatment of nonallergic rhinitis. Are the criteria for classifying the patients sufficient so clinicians in different parts of the world are able to apply the results of the study to their clinical practice? For the clinician, does using criteria to classify a patient impact on management? Does knowing whether a patient has a late-phase reaction to nasal provocation affect the management of his or her allergic rhinitis? While classification, like definitions, becomes easier with increased understanding, it is a continually evolving process. The major limitation of the current classification system is the absence of multiple causes for nasal symptoms. How is the patient with allergic rhinitis and a septal deviation classified? How does pollution impact on nasal function or interact with allergic rhinitis (Chapter 8)? Sorting out the potential contributions of several factors to the patient's symptoms is difficult and remains the domain of the skilled clinician.

The enormity of the problem with rhinitis has become the focus of international interest. Consensus conferences on allergic rhinitis and sinusitis have been convened and the results of some published. While many of the authors of this book participated in a number of these meetings, this volume provides reviews of topics rather than summary statements. In some instances the writings of an author differ from consensus statements. The differences are both understandable and good. In a field in its infancy, where terminology is not always precise, differences are expected. Where pathophysiological mechanisms of disease do not always exist, how can there be absolute agreement? If opinion is uniform, then there will be no advancement of knowledge. In rhinology, we need to extend our insights.

Because allergic rhinitis (seasonal, perennial, or episodic) is easily defined, diagnosed, treated, and affects a large percentage of the population, it receives the most attention in this book. The nonallergic forms of rhinitis, the most difficult to diagnosis and manage, can be classified into those with a known etiology and those without. If we eliminate the known causes (Table 1), then a large number of patients remain to be classified. Some divide them on the presence or absence of eosinophils. Some divide them on their response to treatment. Some divide them on the basis of major symptom. There is no correct answer, but the clinician should choose a scheme that helps with the current management of his patients. Investigators should attempt to define their patients on criteria that communicate the issues to others. These issues vary with a particular study and will change with time. The chapters to follow share the state of our current knowledge as a means to manage patients now and to define issues for future investigations.

III. Evaluation of Rhinitis

An approach to patients with rhinitis and their subsequent classification are briefly outlined here with the details highlighted in the chapters that follow. The clinician

Table 1 Nonallergic Causes of Nasal Symptoms

Mechanical factors
  Foreign bodies
  Septal deviation
  Nasal polyps
  Tumors
  Choanal atresia
  Adenoidal hypertrophy
  Meningocele/encephalocele
Infectious causes
  Nasal tuberculosis
  Herpes zoster
  Klebsiella rhinoscleromatis
  Fungus
Other
  Pollution
  Occupational
  Gustatory rhinitis
  Cold, dry air–induced rhinitis (skier's nose)
  Nasal carriers of *Staphylococcus aureus*
  Rhinitis medicamentosa
  Drug-induced symptoms—aspirin/NSAIDS/antihypertensives/cocaine
  Pregnancy
  Hypothyroidism
  Wegener's granulomatosis
  Cystic fibrosis
  Nonallergic rhinitis with eosinophilia syndrome (NARES)
  Primary ciliary dyskinesia
  Sarcoidosis

begins with the patient's complaints. The constellation of symptoms usually leads to a presumptive diagnosis. The teenager with sneezing and watery nasal discharge each spring makes one think of allergic rhinitis, whereas nasal obstruction following trauma suggests a deviated septum. Next a physical examination is done. Swollen eyes, limitations of extraocular movements, forehead swelling, carious teeth, middle ear effusions, wheezing, facial numbness, and neck adenopathy all suggest serious problems. The nasal examination follows (Chapter 10). This examination based on understanding of the anatomy and physiology (Chapter 5) looks for evidence of anatomical problems, infections, polyps, and unusual findings suggestive of tumors or systemic disease. Then diagnostic procedures such as allergy testing (Chapter 12), cytology (Chapter 11), and imaging studies (Chapter 10) are performed. Once a diagnosis is suggested, treatment is instituted

(Chapters 13–20). Special considerations regarding nonallergic rhinitis, nasal polyps, sinusitis, rhinitis in children, rhinitis and asthma, and rhinitis and otitis are highlighted in Chapters 21–25. Since currently available management options do not always lead to a full resolution of symptoms, a look to the future is presented in Chapter 26.

References

1. Gwaltney J, Phillips C, Miller R, Riker D. Computed tomographic study of common cold. NEJM 1994; 330(1):25–30.

3

Epidemiology

JEANNE MONTGOMERY SMITH

University of Iowa Hospitals and Clinics
Iowa City, Iowa

I. Prevalence of Rhinitis

For most diseases epidemiological studies are the first basis on which we form our ideas about likely causes. For conditions of unknown etiology, such as those involving atopy, this should remain a primary function. This chapter will focus on observations about the occurrence and natural history of allergic rhinitis and its related conditions, in the hope that the reader will recognize that many of our basic assumptions can be questioned and that many basic questions about atopy and other possibly related conditions await answers.

The large numbers of people affected by atopic diseases worldwide and large differences from one community to another present a picture of a very important group of conditions where potentially alterable environmental factors certainly must play a major role. Since a few decades ago when some countries began to report an increase in the prevalence of asthma, other countries all over the world have been counting their cases. These studies often include skin testing and sometimes ask questions regarding hay fever. About 30 countries have reported, some having several studies. The great majority of these surveys are cross-sectional in school populations or recruits for military training. Almost all the studies where there are previous data for comparison found an increase in asthma.

Table 1 Prevalence of Asthma and Rhinitis in 55,000 Swedish
Conscripts

	1971	1981
Asthma	1.9	2.8
Rhinitis	4.4	8.4

When studied, a parallel increase in hay fever or atopy as judged by positive
skin tests was also found (1–6). Some studies, such as those in the Scandinavian
countries, show quite marked differences between regions not very far apart (1,3).
There are no reliable figures about the occurrence of rhinitis other than seasonal
allergic rhinitis. One study of subjects aged 16–65 years registered with a London
general practice estimated the prevalence of allergic rhinitis was 16% and of
nonallergic rhinitis, 11% (7).

Studies in Finland, Sweden, Australia, and Scotland have tried to match
earlier studies and have found an increase in the occurrence of asthma, hay fever,
and positive skin tests. A study in Australia comparing the number of people
complaining of hay fever in 1981 and 1990 found an increase from 21.9% to
46.7% but no change in the number of people with positive skin tests (4). The
figures shown for Swedish recruits are a good example (see Table 1). European
prevalence figures for allergic rhinitis and asthma range from a low of 4.3% for
asthma and 6% allergic rhinitis in Finnish children and teenagers to 4.5% for
asthma and 31% allergic rhinitis in the south of France (1,8).

American figures for allergic rhinitis range from 16% (excluding asthma)
to 55%. The higher figure is from Arizona, a desert area to which many families
have migrated to avoid the problems of damper climates (9).

A study from Hong Kong, Kota Kimabu in Malaysia, and Sam Bu in China
gives the following figures for secondary school children: 15.7% rhinitis and
11.6% asthma in Hong Kong, 11.2% rhinitis and 8.2% asthma in Kota Kimabu,
and only 2.1% rhinitis and 1.9% asthma in San Bu (10). Nevertheless, immigrant
populations of Chinese in America and Australia increase their rates to those of
the host country (11,12).

The prevalence of allergic rhinitis is said to peak in the late teens or young
adulthood and drop quite sharply after the age of 40. On the other hand, according
to the American National Health Surveys, complaints of ''chronic sinus disease''
climb in midlife to levels well above complaints of hay fever at their peak (13).
It is difficult to know how many of these people with chronic nasal symptoms
may have chronic allergic disease or nasal disease with similar eosinophilic inflammation. This problem with nasal disease can be compared to the situation

in asthma where, with age, it becomes more difficult to separate asthma from other forms of chronic obstructive lung disease.

One group of studies of asthma in a Third World country needs to be mentioned even though language difficulties were blamed for an inability to study allergic rhinitis (14–16). These studies are the work of several Australian authors who have been following the development of asthma in the South Fore group of New Guinea islanders (14–16). About 20 years ago the first seven cases of asthma were recognized. Six of these were in adults who had returned to the villages after working in the European-influenced community. The villages were surveyed in 1972 and two cases in adults were found in a 1500-strong population. In 1976, another survey found 20 asthmatic adults and two children among 900 adults and 14,000 children. The affected children were found in households with affected adults. Since then, there have been increasing numbers of cases. At last report, 7.3% of the adult population had asthma but as yet only 0.6% of the children. House dust mites seem to be the major allergens related to this epidemic of asthma, but it is difficult to understand why the children should be spared. Some other New Guinea groups still have little asthma. This phenomenon presents an unparalleled opportunity to study environmental factors in the development of atopy in a newly affected population, and if at all possible, an effort should be made to study nasal symptoms and seasonal allergens as well as dust mites. A 1985 study of urban Goroka, another New Guinea area, found 10 asthmatic adults and one asthmatic child of an affected family. All of the adults had either moved from or worked in the area where asthma has become endemic. In this paper the authors also remark that in the South Fore study two pairs of spouses and the child of one of these couples developed asthma within a year of one another. The authors point out that this is difficult to explain on the basis of current theories (17).

Interrelationships make it necessary to decide which conditions should really be considered in studying the epidemiology of allergic rhinitis. Allergic rhinitis and extrinsic asthma are clearly members of a group of conditions associated with atopy. "Atopy" was the name coined by allergists early in this century who recognized "a hereditary group of spontaneously appearing allergies." Robert Cooke, a pioneer in American allergy studies, felt that the term should be used to denote "spontaneously occurring long-lasting wheal reacting allergy" regardless of family history (18). That is how most allergists use the term today. It is important to recognize that IgE is produced normally and that some antigens, for example many parasites, call forth an IgE response more readily than others. Thus not all raised IgE levels or all positive skin tests are signs of atopy. For clinical and for epidemiological purposes it is important to know that positive tests can reflect IgE responses to currently met antigens and not the abnormal, long-lasting, sometimes (but not always) very high levels of atopic disease.

In the 1950s Michael Schwartz of Denmark undertook a classic study that identified the conditions that were and were not epidemiologically interconnected in the families of patients with asthma (19). These were allergic rhinitis, infantile eczema, asthma both with and without atopy, and rhinitis with nasal polyps. Schwartz's findings seemed to settle the question of interrelatedness for these conditions, but it is important to realize that his findings will be affected by the fact that his study started with an asthmatic patient population.

Most people dealing with these diseases still feel that we may be dealing with several overlapping tendencies or diseases and make efforts to define and separate them. This is particularly true when infantile eczema, rhinitis, and asthma occur without demonstrable atopy. Good modern examples of these efforts in asthma are studies by Sibbald and Turner-Warwick, in Britain (20). Of 1166 possible subjects with asthma they decided to compare the 89 with negative skin tests, late onset, and no exacerbations related to allergens with 327 allergic asthma patients who had developed symptoms at an early age. This choice of patients from the two extremes of what seems to be a spectrum left another 750 patients somewhere in between and illustrates the difficulty we have in defining groups because of clinical and epidemiological overlap. If we arranged the equivalent group of skin-test-negative, older-onset nasal disease at one end of a spectrum and the larger group of young-onset atopic disease at the other, we would probably also find that there is a large middle group with mixed characteristics.

Nasal disease with polyp formation is clearly associated with a particularly chronic form of asthma. Both nasal polyps and asthma have a family-related epidemiology, which sometimes overlaps with family atopy (21). Settipane and Chafee, in an allergy practice population, found that 2.2% of patients with allergic rhinitis or extrinsic asthma had nasal polyps, compared with 12.5% of asthmatics without demonstrable allergy (22). The 2.2% is probably greater than the general population occurrence of nasal polyps, but for comparison we have only the 0.3% of the population who reported nasal polyps in the American General Health Survey of 1980 (13).

One must be careful as to where the figures from clinical practices, or even one's own experience, come from. For example Settipane and Chafee, in an allergy practice, found that 71% of their patients with polyps had asthma, while two separate groups of otolaryngologists, Malony (23) and Drake-Lee et al. (24), found only 21% and 29% asthmatic, respectively. In the otolaryngologist experience, 2–3 times as many men had nasal polyps as women, but women with polyps were twice as likely to have asthma. In the 445 nasal polyp patients studied by Drake-Lee et al. (24), positive skin tests to pollens were found in 10.5% and another 15% reacted to dust mites. At a time when the head of our otolaryngology clinic sent all patients with polyps to us, we found that 17% of 140 had positive skin tests to seasonal allergens or animal danders or marked reactions to house dust. Less strongly positive skin tests to dusts or dust mites are common in asymptomatic populations and therefore hard to interpret.

We think of nasal polyps and intrinsic asthma as relatively late-onset conditions, but of our 140 patients with nasal polyps, 46% had their first nasal symptoms, though not necessarily polyps, before the age of 20. The inflammatory cells in nasal polyps are usually like those of allergic inflammation, and since polyps are often associated with asthma, it is tempting to suppose that they are part of the atopic disease spectrum. Currently available epidemiological information does not clearly separate the two kinds of asthma or their nasal equivalents.

It is difficult to study nasal allergy in young children because of their many viral colds. When nasal polyps are found in childhood, the child should be tested for cystic fibrosis in which about 20% of children have nasal polyps. This is another similarity between the epidemiology of nasal polyps and atopy since atopy is also more common in patients with cystic fibrosis than in the general population (25,26).

There are some families who have more eczema with their atopy than others, some families who have more hay fever than asthma, and some families where almost everyone with allergic rhinitis has asthma. Still other families have nasal polyps with or without asthma and with or without atopy. Table 1 from a study of patients joining a prepaid medical plan is a good example of this family tendency to develop similar manifestations (27).

Where the aim of epidemiology is to look for interconnections that may give clues about the cause of these diseases, it is important to study the whole group, defining each subset carefully. For epidemiological purposes, it is also important to recognize that the form taken by atopic disease can be modified by intercurrent viral infections, age at onset, excessive allergen exposure, and the nature of the allergen.

II. Risk Factors for the Development of Atopic Conditions, Nasal Polyps, and Asthma

A. The Family

There can be no doubt that the family is the single most important risk factor for the development of all these conditions in childhood. However, the influence of family diminishes sharply in adulthood, over the age of 25 in our experience.

In a study of an Iowa rural population looking at those under the age of 20 at the time of interview, 16% of the girls and 27% of the boys born into households with allergic members had developed allergic rhinitis or asthma whereas 0.8% of the girls and 1.5% of the boys born into households without allergy were affected (28).

Table 2 Allergic Rhinitis and Asthma in Relatives of Patients with Allergic Rhinitis With and Without Asthma

	Relatives' disease	
Subjects' disease	Iowa rural area, general population under age 20	Population of all ages, initial examination for a health insurance plan
Rhinitis	42% rhinitis only	41% rhinitis only
	28% rhinitis and asthma	9% rhinitis and asthma
	30% negative family	50% negative family
Rhinitis and asthma	24% rhinitis only	25% rhinitis only
	52% rhinitis and asthma	44% rhinitis and asthma
	24% negative family	31% negative family

There is a strong tendency for the form of the disease to be characteristic of a particular family (27) (Table 2). On the other hand, this can be overcome by environmental factors such as excessive allergen exposure or lower respiratory tract infection. Family allergic disease also is a determining factor for an early onset, and in turn, an early age at onset is a risk factor for the development of asthma and multiple allergies in the atopic child. Seasonal sensitivities developing in adults are more often manifested as allergic rhinitis except where exposure is heavy, as in occupational asthma (29,30). Figures from an Iowa rural survey, given in Table 3, show the most common ages at onset for rhinitis and asthma. These are fairly typical of the experience of other workers. The Iowa farming population, but not the city subjects, studied by us had somewhat more asthmatic relatives for the allergic rhinitis group, possibly because of an excess of occupational asthma in adult men (Tables 2 and 4) (27).

Table 3 Age at Onset of Seasonal Allergy

Age (years)	Male ($n = 135$)	Female ($n = 123$)
0–9	60%	39%
10–19	17%	32%
20–29	21%	24%
30–39	23%	12%
40–49	10%	8%
50–59	2%	6%
60+	2%	2%

Table 4 Age at Onset of Asthma in Subjects Drawn from General Populations

Age (years)	Urban ($n = 193$)		Rural ($n = 277$)	
	Male	Female	Male	Female
0–9	80 (75%)	51 (59%)	117 (65%)	68 (70%)
10–19	13 (12%)	18 (21%)	16 (9%)	9 (9%)
20+	14 (13%)	17 (20%)	20 (26%)	20 (21%)

B. The Role of Genetic Factors in Atopic Disease

As it is clear that the family is a very important risk factor, it has been assumed that this was entirely on genetic basis. One theory is that the genetic tendency relates to specific purified allergens. There is good evidence for this but it is also true that in the same families there are often other affected individuals allergic to other things (31,32).

Most studies find that monozygotic twins are more concordant for atopic diseases than dizotic twins, but not all studies agree (33). Of frequently quoted studies, four of 10 did not find a significant difference. Hanson et al. studied a group of twins reared apart with results suggesting support for more concordance for monozygotic pairs, but the number of pairs was small and the monozygotic twins were separated on average at 133+ to 153 days and dizigotic twins at 370+ to 498 days, periods long enough for important early environmental influences to be different (34). Thus it seems likely that genetic factors are involved in atopy, but none of these studies really settles the magnitude of the genetic factor's role completely. In view of the frequency of atopy, genetic permissiveness must be common.

Genetic studies have found a locus in the 11q13 region that seems to be involved in both atopy and asthma. This supports the involvement of genetic factors but does not define the nature of the genetic role (35). For example, an author points out that this is a region needed to supply genetic material to complete a T-cell leukemia virus (36). It has been assumed that whatever is involved in the abnormal IgE response in atopy involves genes, but the nature of the role of genes certainly remains to be clarified.

C. Allergen and Migration

Allergen exposure probably influences the nature of symptoms in atopic disease and its recognition. It is difficult to know to what extent it influences the total number of cases. Recent studies in France, Italy, and Australia each comparing populations with different allergen prevalence demonstrate the effect of allergen exposure in causing specific sensitizations, but show relatively small differences in the total occurrence of atopic disease (8,37,38). A good example of the effect of allergen exposure in the development of a specific allergy is seen in the French study comparing a mountainous area having little mite allergen with Marseilles (8). Ten percent of the mountain dwellers had positive mite skin tests compared with 27% in Marseilles. In spite of differences in allergen exposure, the prevalence of atopic diseases is also very similar in most parts of the United States except where families with allergic disease have sought refuge in desert areas like Arizona. In the most recent report from the Arizona authors, 55% of the general population being followed by Barbee et al. complain of allergic rhinitis (39). A recent repeated survey of atopy as judged by skin tests shows an increase in the number of people with positive tests, most of which is accounted for by recent migrants who develop new sensitivity soon after coming to Arizona. This can be compared with the other immigrant studies (40).

An old study of immigrants at the University of Michigan found a high rate of ragweed hay fever developing in Chinese students (12). Most of the students had not had allergic symptoms in China (11). The Australians have recently done a study of hay fever and asthma developing in Asian students comparing them with non-Asian natives and Asians born in Australia. Table 4 shows some of their results. Again there was a high rate of hay fever in the immigrants, this time to grass pollen. Here also most cases were in previously unaffected people. In these situations and others where people move to new environments, sensitivity to a single allergen is common. It seems as though new-onset allergic disease in adults is commonly related to one or very few allergens and symptoms are more often rhinitis than asthma except in occupational situations with heavy exposure.

An early age at onset is associated with strong and multiple allergies, but not all patients with an early onset of symptoms and similar inflammation have positive skin tests or probable allergy. Several studies show an increased risk for the development of pollen allergy for those born a month or so before the season (41,42). On the other hand, hay fever with positive skin tests can develop for the first time in old age, even to allergens to which there has been lifelong exposure.

Certain allergens, such as the enzymes used in laundry detergents, seem to be particularly prone to cause occupational asthma rather than just nasal symptoms. With this particular type of allergen most cases represent new symptoms in already atopic individuals and the development of altogether new cases occurs at about the same rate as new cases in a general population of adults (43). There has been little study of occupational allergic rhinitis though it is sometimes mentioned in studies such as those of laboratory animal workers or bakers in whom rhinitis usually precedes asthma (44).

In the New Guinea studies more mites were found in the blankets of households with asthmatic members and it is likely that the nature of the allergen and heaviness of exposure affect the presentation of atopic disease. This may explain the prevalence of asthma in the New Guinea population but does not explain the sparing of children (15,16).

D. Pollution

There has been a good deal of effort to study the role of pollution in the development of respiratory allergy. Smoking by parents, especially mothers, has been found to promote the development of asthma in the young child, but all studies do not agree and the effect may instead be on the respiratory infections that promote asthma (45). Animal experiments have shown an effect or irritants on the development of sensitization but there are no similar data in humans (46). Two studies, one in 1964 and another in 1989 in Aberdeen Scotland, showed an increase in hay fever from 3.2% to 11.9% and asthma from 4.1% to 10.2% and attributed the change to pollution (47). They also found the use of asthma medicines much higher in towns near power stations. Yet it is difficult to separate the effect pollution may have on asthma symptoms from effects on numbers of people who develop asthma or allergic rhinitis. A study in Japan found that Japanese cedar sensitivity had developed more often in people who lived in an urban area near a highway than in inhabitants of the cedar forest. These authors attributed this effect to pollution, but city rural differences may have other causes (48). In other experiences people living in more polluted areas have not had as much respiratory allergy as in some less polluted places. A case in point is a comparison between East and West Germany soon after reunion (49). The Eastern city of Leipzig had less respiratory allergy and less atopy in spite of much heavier pollution with sulfur dioxide and particulate matter. The Western city of Munich had more asthma and rhinitis and was less polluted except for some pollution from more automobiles. A more recent study finds East Germany beginning to catch up with the West but many other things have changed (50). These studies are good examples of the difficulty one has with confounding factors when interpreting the role of pollution in determining the number of cases of allergic disease.

E. Infection

Respiratory infection clearly affects the occurrence of asthma in the very young child, both the initial development and recurrences are often related to virus infections (51). There is also evidence that viral infections can promote IgE responses to other allergens (52). Falliers et al. made a study of two paris of monozygous twins, one of each set having severe asthma and the other only hay fever (53). Both were apparently equally atopic and the only difference was a history of lower respiratory tract infection at the onset in the asthmatic twin. A relationship between allergic rhinitis and respiratory infection may not be discernible because of the ubiquity of upper respiratory infections.

In the New Guinea studies one cannot postulate a primary role in asthma

Table 5 Hay Fever in Immigrants

Age (years)	<20 (%)	20–39 (%)	>40 (%)
Asian immigrant	28	49	40
Asian Australian	35	—	—
Non-Asian Australian	20	28	25

for the usual epidemic respiratory viruses because there is no reason why children and adults would not be equally affected by such viruses (14,17). In underdeveloped countries there has been an increase in the use of day care for young children with its increased exposure to respiratory infections. A retrospective study of 7-year-old children did not find an increase in atopic disease or more positive skin tests in children who had been in day care for at least 3 months under the age of 2, compared with children who had been cared for at home. More studies should be done to confirm this study since many more children have been in day care in recent years (54).

F. Race

Race as a factor in atopy has been difficult to separate from environmental factors. For example a study in Singapore has found more asthma in Malaysians and Indians than in Chinese. However, hay fever did not differ, and the chief differences between Chinese households and the others were fewer pets and carpets (55). Australian studies of Maoris and other Australians found no difference in the occurrence of asthma or rhinitis although mortality and severity were greater for Maoris (56). Australian authors also studied Asian immigrants and found that something in the immigration situation had increased the risk of grass pollen sensitivities for the Asians (Table 5) (11).

There are many examples of very different prevalences of atopic disease comparing racial groups, but also enough examples of different rates in the same ethnic group in different environments to make it impossible to know whether there is any real racial difference in susceptibility.

III. The Natural Course of Atopic Disease

Population studies that follow atopic patients over many years are scarce. It has long been known that people can develop atopic sensitivity in the sense of markedly positive skin tests several years before respiratory symptoms begin. It is also true that, occasionally, symptoms develop before skin tests become positive.

An example is found in a study of German baker's apprentices who were followed from the beginning of their employment in order to study the development of baker's asthma (44). Most developed skin reactivity first, but the reverse order also occurred.

Hagy and Settipane followed students with positive skin; tests but no symptoms from the beginning of their college years until their 4th year and then to 7 years. They found that the most strongly positive skin tests were predictive of symptoms (71%) but lesser reactions were less certain to predict symptoms (57). Sixty-four percent of the 1836 students originally tested 23 years ago have recently been followed up once more. Seventeen new cases of asthma have developed in the 162 subjects who previously only had hay fever (10.5%). Nineteen new cases of asthma have developed in the 528 without previous symptoms (3.2%). Subjects without symptoms but with previous positive skin tests were also somewhat more likely to have developed asthma than people with negative tests, 10.6% compared with 3.2% (58).

The prevalence of allergic rhinitis is said to peak in the late teens or young adulthood and drop quite sharply over the age of 40. On the other hand, according to the American National Health Surveys, complaints of ''chronic sinus disease'' climb in midlife to levels well above complaints of hay fever at their peak. It is difficult to know how many of these people with chronic nasal symptoms may have chronic allergic disease or nasal disease with similar eosinophilic inflammation. This problem with nasal disease can be compared to the situation in asthma where, with age, it becomes more difficult to separate asthma from other forms of chronic obstructive lung disease.

In clinical practice we require correlation of skin tests with symptoms for diagnosis, and the same requirement should apply in epidemiological studies because some of the positive skin tests may represent normal IgE from recent exposure to some allergens (59). For example, in 1952 Schwartz found 50% of subjects in a study of Danish bakers to be skin-test-positive, but only about 20% were symptomatic (19). It is probable that some of the skin test positivity represented normal IgE in response to recent allergen exposure and not the abnormal, atopic IgE response that persists long after the stimulus is gone.

An important characteristic of atopy is this long-lasting, self-perpetuating, abnormally high level of specific sensitivity without the need for further allergen exposure. Most other IgE responses are relatively short lived except when the stimulus remains.

The natural course of atopic sensitization has not received much attention. Several workers have demonstrated that abnormal IgE levels can develop in utero. Although its usefulness has been disputed, measurement of cord blood was proposed as a predictor of atopic disease (60,61). We know from clinical experience that very strong and multiple positive skin tests are mainly developed in youth (62). On the other hand, both asthma and hay fever with strongly positive skin tests (usually to only one or a very few allergens) can develop at any age, even in people who have been exposed to the same allergen all their lives.

Forty years ago it was a fairly common practice to skin-test every year to see if new allergies had developed. This was given up long ago because usually the pattern of allergies remains the same over many years. This is an important observation in need of much more study. The long-term localization of the abnormal immune response that, unlike normal IgE responses, has become self-perpetuating suggests resistance to further involvement.

We wrote to the people with respiratory allergy who had been skin-tested or treated with allergens during their years at university (63). A total of 245 (88%) of these subjects responded. Only 10 thought that they had developed a new allergy. The 10 had developed new springtime symptoms, but five of these had positive skin tests to spring pollens in our tests years before. Twenty-nine subjects thought that their problems had increased over the years and 14 of these reported nasal polyps. If these observations are correct, sensitization usually occurs over a limited period under unknown circumstances that are only rarely repeated. There is a great need for more data on the occurrence of new allergies. When we go to meetings, we ask fellow allergists how our patients do when they move to another part of the country. We forget that they will not have seen those whose condition had resolved. They will also usually not have knowledge of previous skin tests.

IV. Discussion

Probably most allergists think of the atopy-eczema-allergic rhinitis and asthma group of conditions as a collection of overlapping, genetically determined susceptibilities. For example, it has been postulated that atopy is a genetically determined tendency to mount excessive IgE responses and that excessively reactive bronchial membranes are a second inherited trait that is prone to cause asthma, to which the atopic population is particularly susceptible. There is a great deal of evidence to suggest that environmental factors must play a part in both atopic sensitization and the development of asthma.

It is also possible to explain the epidemiological interconnections if we think of atopy-eczema-allergic rhinitis and extrinsic asthma as manifestations of a single disease in which several self-perpetuating abnormalities develop over a period of time, influenced by both host factors and environmental factors. First, there is the localized long-term, specific, IgE-mediated allergy that may be evident on skin test for several weeks or several years before the development of symptoms. Then there is possible involvement of the skin, nose, and lower respiratory tract with a chronic inflammatory response in which the eosinophil plays an important role. Development of lesions in these various areas may occur simultaneously, or there may be intervals of years between the development of disease in one area and its spread to involve another. At least for asthma, the beginning of chest symptoms is often related to intercurrent viral infection, trauma to the respiratory membranes, or excessive allergen exposure. The similar inflammation of infantile eczema, rhinitis with nasal polyps, and asthma without atopy could also be manifestations of similar disease that may not be related to the atopic group.

It is important to develop and test a variety of working hypotheses clearly recognizing that the cause of atopy and related diseases is unknown. Nasal conditions, and not asthma alone, should be carefully scrutinized in epidemiological studies.

V. Conclusions

Over the past 20 years, and especially the last 10 years, there has almost certainly been a substantial increase in the occurrence of allergic nasal disease and asthma in the industrialized countries. Asthma with allergy has also been developing in some previously unaffected Third World populations. Unfortunately, nasal conditions have not been studied in these groups because of language problems. In the Nordic countries the cumulative prevalence for allergic rhinitis in the general population is about 7%. It is probably somewhat higher in North America, with prevalence figures ranging from 16 to 55%. Australia reports a very high figure of 27.6–46.7% for hay fever in children and also very high rates for asthma. It is clear that, although the family occurrence of these diseases points to a possible role for genetic susceptibility, the short-term increase within a generation must involve environmental factors. Since environmental factors are often alterable, it is of the utmost importance to determine the nature of such factors. Neither indoor nor outdoor pollution, or new allergens, explain the increasing numbers of cases, and it will be important to ask new questions if we are to get new answers.

References

1. Rimpela AH, Savonius B, Rimpela MK, Haahtela T. Asthma and allergic rhinitis among Finnish adolescents in 1977–1991. J Scand Univ Press 1995; 23:60.
2. Varonier HS, De Haller J, Schopfer C. Prevalence de L'allergie chez les enfants et les adolescents. Helv Paediatr Acta 1984; 39:129.
3. Norrman E, Rosenhall L, Nyström L, Jönsson E, Stjernberg N. Prevalence of positive skin prick tests, allergic asthma, and rhinoconjunctivitis in teenagers in northern Sweden. Allergy 1994; 49:808.
4. Peat JK, Haby M, Spijker J, Berry G, Woolcock AJ. Prevalence of asthma in adults in Busselton, Western Australia. Br Med J 1992; 305:1326.

5. Fleming DM, Crombie DL. Prevalence of asthma and hay fever in England and Wales. Br Med J 1987; 294:279.

6. Aberg N. Asthma and allergic rhinitis in Swedish conscripts. Clin Exp Allergy 1989; 19:59.

7. Sibbald B, Rink E. Epidemiology of seasonal and perennial rhinitis: clinical presentation and medical history. Thorax 1991; 46:895.

8. Charpin D, Hughes B, Mallea M, Sutra J-P, Balansard G, Vervloet D. Seasonal allergic symptoms and their relation to pollen exposure in south-east France. Clin Exp Allergy 1993; 23:435.

9. Burrows B, Lebowitz MD, Barbee RA. Respiratory disorders and allergy skin test reactions. Ann Intern Med 1976; 84:134.

10. Leung R, Ho P. Asthma, allergy, and atopy in three south-east Asian populations. Thorax 1994; 49:1205.

11. Leung RC, Carlin JB, Burdon JGW, Czarny D. Asthma, allergy and atopy in Asian immigrants in Melbourne. Med J Aust 1994; 161:418.

12. Maternouski CJ, Mathews KP. The prevalence of ragweed pollinosis in foreign and native students at a midwestern university and its implications concerning methods of inheritance of atopy. J Allergy 1962; 33:130.

13. Vital and Health Statistics. Prevalence of Selected Chronic Conditions, USA. Series 10, 1980, No. 155, p. 25.

14. Woolcock AJ, Green W, Alpers MP. Asthma in a rural highland area of Papua New Guinea. Am Rev Respir Dis 1981; 123:565.

15. Dowse GK, Turner KJ, Woolcock AJ, Alpers MP. Emerging asthma in the Okapa District of the Eastern Highlands Province of Papua New Guinea: the problem and its implications. Papua New Guinea Med J 1983; 26:33.

16. Turner KJ, Dowse GK, Stewart GA, Alpers MP, Woolcock AJ. Prevalence of asthma in the South Fore people of the Okapa district of Papua New Guinea. Int Arch Allergy Appl Immunol 1985; 77:158.

17. Dowse GK, Smith D, Turner KJ, Alpers MP. Prevalence and features of asthma in a sample survey of urban Goroka, Papua New Guinea. Clin Allergy 1985; 15:429.

18. Cooke RA. Allergy in Theory and Practice. London: WB Saunders, 1947.

19. Schwartz M. Heredity in Bronchial Asthma. Copenhagen: Munksgaard, 1952.

20. Sibbald B, Turner-Warwick M. Factors influencing the prevalence of asthma among first degree relatives of extrinsic and intrinsic asthmatics. Thorax 1979; 34:332.

21. Lockey RF, Rucknagel DL, Vanselow NA. Familial occurrence of asthma, nasal polyps and aspirin intolerance. Ann Intern Med 1973; 78:57.

22. Settipane GA, Chafee FH. Nasal polyps in asthma and rhinitis: a review of 6,037 patients. J Allergy Clin Immunol 1977; 59:17.

23. Maloney JR. Nasal polyps, nasal polypectomy, asthma and aspirin sensitivity. J Laryngol Otol 1977; 91:837.

24. Drake-Lee AB, Lowe D, Swanston A, Grace A. Clinical profile and recurrence of nasal polyps. J Laryngol Otol 1984; 98:783.

25. Rachelefsky GS, Osher A, Dooley RE, et al. Coexistent respiratory allergy and cystic fibrosis. Am J Dis Child 1974; 128:335.

26. Wönne R, Hofmann D, Posselt H-G, et al. Brochial allergy in cystic fibrosis. Clin Allergy 1985; 15:455.

27. McKee WD. The incidence and familial occurrence of allergy. J Allergy 1966; 38: 226.

28. Smith JM, Knowler LA. Epidemiology of asthma and allergic rhinitis. I. In a rural area. II. In a university-centered community. Am Rev Respir Dis 1965; 92:16.

29. Ramirez DA. The natural history of mountain cedar pollinosis. J Allergy Clin Immunol 1984; 73:88.

30. Bousquet J, Knani J, Hejjaoui A, et al. Heterogeneity of atopy. I. Clinical and immunologic characteristics of patients allergic to cypress pollen. Allergy 1993; 48: 183.

31. Marsh D, Hsu SH, Roebber M, et al. HLA-Dw2: a genetic marker for human immune response to short ragweed allergen RAS. I. Response resulting primarily from natural antigenic exposure. J Exp Med 1982; 155:1439.

32. Freidhoff LR, Ehrlich-Kautzky E, Meyers DA, Ansari AA, Bias WB, Marsh DG. Association of HLA-DR3 with human immune response to Lol p I and Lol p II antigens in allergic subjects. Tissue Antigens 1988; 31:211.

33. Bonini S, Magrini L, Rotiroti G, Ronchetti MP, Onorati P. Genetic and environmental factors in the changing incidence of allergy. Allergy 1994; 49:6.

34. Hanson B, McGue M, Roitman-Johnson B, Segal NL, Bouchard TJ, Jr, Blumenthal MN. Atopic disease and immunoglobulin E in twins reared apart and together. Am J Hum Genet 1991; 48:873.

35. Postma DS, Bleecker ER, Amelung PJ, et al. Genetic susceptibility to asthma— bronchial hyperresponsiveness coinherited with a major gene for atopy. N Engl J Med 1995; 333:894.

36. Kelleher K, Bean K, Clark SC, et al. Human interleukin-9:genomic sequence, chromosomal location, and sequences essential for its expression in human T cell leukemia virus (HTLV)-I-transformed human T cells. Blood 1991; 77:1436.

37. Britton WJ, Woolcock AJ, Peat JK, Sedgwick CJ, Lloyd DM, Leeder SR. Prevalence of bronchial hyperresponsiveness in children: the relationship between asthma and skin reactivity to allergens in two communities. Int J Epidemiol 1986; 15:202.

38. Charpin D, Kleisbauer J-P, Lanteaume A, et al. Asthma and allergy to house-dust mites in populations living in high altitudes. Chest 1988; 93:758.

39. Barbee RA, Halonen M, Kaltenborn WT, Burrows B. A longitudinal study of respiratory symptoms in a community population sample: correlations with smoking, allergen skin-test reactivity, and serum IgE. Chest 1991; 99:20.

40. Barbee RA, Kaltenborn W, Lebowitz MD, Burrows B. Longitudinal changes in allergen skin test reactivity in a community population sample. J Allergy Clin Immunol 1987; 79:16.

41. Korsgaard J, Dahl R. Sensitivity to house dust mite and grass pollen in adults. Influence of month of birth. Clin Allergy 1983; 13:529.

42. Björksten F, Suoniemi I, Koski V. Neonatal birch pollen contact and subsequent allergy to birch pollen. Clin Allergy 1980; 10:585.

43. Slavin RG, Lewis CR. Sensitivity to enzyme additives in laundry detergent workers. J Allergy Clin Immunol 1971; 48:262.

44. Thiel H, Ulmer WT. Baker's asthma: development and possibility for treatment. Chest 78:2, August, 1980 Supplement:400.

45. Halken S, Høst A, Nilsson L, Taudorf E. Passive smoking as a risk factor for devel-

opment of obstructive respiratory disease and allergic sensitization. Allergy 1995; 50:97.

46. Osebold JW, Owens SL, Zee YC, Dotson WM, Labarre DD. Immunological alterations in the lungs of mice following ozone exposure: changes in immunoglobulin levels and antibody containing cells. Arch Environ Health 1979; 34:258.

47. Ninan TK, Russell G. Respiratory symptoms and atopy in Aberdeen schoolchildren: evidence from two surveys 25 years apart. Br Med J 1992; 304:873.

48. Ishizaki T, Kazuhiro K, Ryosuke I, Ishiyama Y, Kushibiki E. Studies of prevalence of Japanese cedar pollinosis among the residents in a densely cultivated area. Ann Allergy 1987; 58:265.

49. von Mutius E, Fritzsch C, Weiland SK, Röll G, Magnussen H. Prevalence of asthma and allergic disorders among children in united Germany: a descriptive comparison. Br Med J 1992; 305:1395.

50. Schäfer T, Krämer U, Behrendt H, Vieluf D, Ring J. Skin prick test (SPT) reactivity in East and West Germany is changing. J Allergy Clin Immunol 1996; 97:217 (abstract).

51. Busse WW. The relationship between viral infections and onset of allergic diseases and asthma. Clin Exp Allergy 1989; 19:1.

52. Frick OL, German DF, Mills J. Development of allergy in children. I. Association with virus infections. J Allergy Clin Immunol 1979; 63:228.

53. Falliers CJ, Cardoso A, Bane MS, et al. Discordant allergic manifestations in monozygotic twins. J Allergy 1971; 47:207.

54. Backman, A, Björksten F, Ilmonen S, Juntunen K, Suoniemi I. Do infections in infancy affect sensitization to airborne allergens and development of atopic disease? Allergy 1984; 39:309.

55. Ng TP, Hui KP, Tan WC. Prevalence of asthma and risk factors among Chinese, Malay, and Indian adults in Singapore. Thorax 1994; 49:347.

56. Shaw R, Woodman K, Crane J, Moyes C, Kennedy J, Pearce N. Risk factors for asthma symptoms in Kawerau children. NZ Med J 1994; 107:387.

57. Hagy GW, Settipane GA. Risk factors for developing asthma and allergic rhinitis. J Allergy Clin Immunol 1976; 58:330.

58. Settipane RJ, Hagy GW, Settipane GA. Development of new asthma and allergic rhinitis in a 23-year follow-up of college students. J Allergy Clin Immunol 1991; 87:232.

59. Cserhati E, Kiss AG, Mezei G, et al. Positive skin prick tests of immediate type of non-allergic children. Acta Paediatr Hung 1983; 24:189.

60. Michel FB, Bousquet J, Greillier P, et al. Comparison of cord blood immunoglobulin E concentrations and maternal allergy for prediction of atopic diseases in infancy. J Allergy Clin Immunol 1980; 65:422.

61. Kjellman N-IM. Development and prediction of atopic allergy in childhood. Theoretical and clinical aspects of allergic diseases. In: Skandia International Symposia 1982. Stockholm: Almqvist and Wiksell, 1983:52–73.

62. Hide DW, Arshad SH, Twiselton R, Stevens M. Cord serum IgE; an insensitive method for the prediction of atopy. Clin Exp Allergy 1991; 21:739.

63. Smith JM. The long-term effect of moving on patients with asthma and hay fever. J Allergy 1971; 48:191.

4

Allergens

LISA M. WHEATLEY and THOMAS A. E. PLATTS-MILLS

University of Virginia
Charlottesville, Virginia

I. Introduction

In 1873 Charles Blackley published his findings on catarrhus aestivus, otherwise known as hay fever or seasonal rhinitis. He proved that pollen grains were the cause, invented the pollen count, proved that pollen could be airborne up to a thousand feet above the ground, and also reported nasal provocation tests (1). At the same time Wyman reported evidence that ragweed pollen was the cause of ''autumnal catarrh'' in the United States (2). By the turn of the century skin tests for immediate hypersensitivity were well established, and in 1911 Noon reported successful desensitization treatment for hay fever using allergen extracts (3). Allergic rhinitis became widely recognized, and by the 1930s a wide range of allergen sources had been demonstrated as causes of sensitization and associated with seasonal or perennial disease (4). These sources were broadly divided into pollens (always seasonal), fungal spores (often seasonal but with poorly defined seasons), and the allergens that contribute to house dust, including animal dander, insects, and some molds. These indoor allergens are generally perennial but may have seasonal increases (5,6). The techniques for extracting allergens from crude sources to make reagents for diagnostic and therapeutic applications were well established; multiple studies had defined the dates on which different plants pollinated; and excellent atlases were (and are) available on the physical properties of pollen grains (7,8).

Purification of the substances that cause atopic disease also started in 1930. It rapidly became clear that most of the substances were proteins, that these proteins were freely soluble, and that the allergens from some sources (e.g., grasses) were much more stable than others. Two other major research efforts started in the 1930s and were not successful until the 1960s. The first was the attempt to purify the active substance in serum that could passively transfer skin test reactivity; the second was to identify the source of allergens in house dust. Both of these problems were resolved over a short period between 1965 and 1970. Ishizaka and Ishizaka demonstrated that reaginic activity was dependent on a specific class of immunoglobulin, IgE, which had the unique property of binding to a high-affinity receptor on mast cells and basophils (9). Voorhorst and his colleagues established that dust mites of the genus *Dermatophagoides* were the single most important source of allergen in house dust (5). These two discoveries established the basis for modern studies on allergens.

The discovery of IgE meant that allergens were defined as those substances that induce human IgE antibodies. Many different sources contribute antigens to house dust but dust mite allergens have become the primary model for studying perennial allergic disease. In thinking about the ways in which allergens give rise to rhinitis, it is necessary to consider the sources and the particles that become airborne, as well as the proteins that produce an immune response. Such information will also facilitate development of techniques for controlling exposure and the use of allergens for immunotherapy.

Central to much of the present understanding of exposure and avoidance is the ability to measure allergen. For the outdoor allergens measurement is still dependent on pollen counts and microscopic identification of fungal spores. For indoor allergens the particles cannot be identified microscopically and can only be measured with immunoassays. The current chapter will address these issues but will also consider the ways in which allergens could be modified to make them more effective and safer for treatment of allergic disease.

II. Sources, Particles, and Proteins

In normal usage the word ''allergen'' is used both for the source, i.e., cats and cat dander or ragweed and its pollen, and also for the specific proteins, i.e., Fel d 1 from cat dander or Amb a 1 from ragweed pollen (Table 1). The terminology of the specific proteins is derived from the first three letters of the genus name and the first letter of the species, the number refers to the order in which allergens were defined. Thus, Asp f 1 is the first allergen defined from *Aspergillus fumigatus*. The primary characteristic of the allergen sources is that they give rise to

Table 1 Indoor Sources of Environmental Allergens Related to Rhinitis

Domestic mites	Mammals
Dermatophagoides pteronyssinus[a]	Cats: *Felis domesticus*
Dermatophagoides farinae[a]	Dogs: *Canis familiaris*
Euroglyphys maynei[a]	Rabbits, ferrets
Storage mites	Rodents
Blomia tropicalis	Pets: Mice, gerbils, guinea pigs,
Lepidoglyphus destructor	chinchilla, etc.
Tarsonimidae	Pests: Mice, *Mus musculus*[b]
Insects	Rats, *Rattus norvegicus*
Cockroaches	Pollens
Blattella germanica (German)	Derived from outside
Periplanetta americana	Other sources
(American)	Horsehair in furniture, kapok
Blatta orientalis (Oriental)	Food dropped by inhabitants
Other: Crickets, flies, beetles, fleas,	Spiders, silverfish, etc.
moths, midges	
Fungi[c]	
Indoors	
Multiple species including	
Penicillium, Aspergillus,	
Cladosporium (growing on	
surfaces of rotting wood)	
Outside	
Multiple species, *Alternaria*	

[a]Pyroglyphid mites.
[b]Many small rodents, including many different species of ''mice,'' become indoor pests.
[c]Many fungi which grow predominantly outdoors may have high indoor levels due to entry c̄ incoming air.

large numbers of allergen-containing particles, which are at least transiently airborne. The windborne pollen grains and the wind-dispersed fungal spores are the best-recognized outdoor allergens. The ways in which indoor allergens become airborne are more complex but it is still clear that allergens are carried on particles. No significant quantity of allergen can become airborne as molecules or on particles <0.1 μm in diameter. To make this point we have made some estimates of the concentrations of different antigens on particles, their release characteristics, and the quantities airborne (Table 2).

III. Particles

The major allergenic pollens come from plants that depend on the wind to distribute their gametes for reproduction. Although these pollens are smaller than insect

Table 2 Properties of Particles Carrying Allergens

Source	No. of particles airborne[a]	Size	Relative volume	Release of protein	Allergen per particle
Ragweed pollen (trees, grass, etc)	10–200/m³	20–30 µm	1	1–2 min	~0.2 ng
Penicillium, Aspergillus, Basidiomycetes	100–5000/m³	2–3 µm	~0.002	Slow	<0.001 ng
Dust mite fecal particles	5–100/m³	10–30 µm	1	1–2 min	~0.2 ng
Alternaria	5–200/m³	6 × 20 µm	0.2	Minutes?	~0.05
Airborne cat allergen	?	2–20 µm	0.001–1	Rapid	0.001–0.2 ng

[a]Maximum number of particles, i.e., peak season for pollen or mold spores and during domestic disturbance (e.g., vacuum cleaning) for mite and cat dander.

disseminated pollen, airborne pollen grains are "large," i.e., ≥ 10 µm in diameter. They release proteins rapidly as part of their modus operandi and, to an expert, each species is distinct. Thus, the pollen count is a remarkably accurate method of defining airborne exposure to specific pollens outdoors (1,10). For some fungi the spores are also distinctive and can be identified down to the species (11,12). However, for many other groups the spores are too similar to define even the genus. For example, the small spores (i.e., 2–3 µm diameter) of *Aspergillus* or *Penicillium* species are difficult to distinguish and are generally counted together. While the spores of the genus *Alternaria* are distinctive, the different species may be difficult to identify. Equally important fungal spores do not need to release proteins rapidly to germinate and grow.

For indoor allergens the particles carrying airborne allergens are generally not well defined and do not rely on airborne dispersal as part of their life cycle. In addition, none of the particles are sufficiently distinct under simple microscopy to allow any indoor equivalent of the pollen count. The fecal particles produced by dust mites are consistent in size but are distinctive only when seen under electron microscopy (13–15). The particles carrying airborne cat and dog allergens are even less well defined. Although the range of aerodynamic particle sizes can be defined (i.e., 2–20 µm) without visualizing the particles carrying Fel d 1, it is not possible to define the actual size of the particle or the mean quantity of allergen on each particle (17,18).

Similarly, for cockroach allergens, there is no definition of the airborne particle. The allergens may be derived from saliva and digestive enzymes as well as broken-down bodies. The debris that accumulates at the bottom of a cockroach culture (frass) contains large quantities of allergen. Aerodynamically cockroach allergens behave much like dust mite allergens; that is, they are not detectable in undisturbed conditions and become transiently airborne during disturbance such as vacuum cleaning (19–21).

IV. Solubility/Release from Particles

Although all the known inhalant allergens are readily soluble in aqueous solutions, they are not released equally rapidly from the particles that are airborne. On contact with the stigma, pollen grains release recognition proteins that trigger the formation of a pollen tube (22). Indeed, pollen grains of all species have easily visible pores that allow rapid egress of proteins, either on the stigma or in the nose (8). For ragweed or grass allergens it has generally been assumed that the pollen grain is the primary form in which the allergens become airborne. However, using immunochemical assays Reed and his colleagues in Minnesota have provided evidence that other particles derived from the ragweed plant can carry airborne Amb a 1 (23,24). This information has several potentially important consequences: (1) The pollen count may not be a complete guide to exposure, especially late in the season. (2) Ragweed allergen may at least in part be carried on particles smaller than a pollen grain that would be expected to deposit on different parts of the respiratory tract. (3) The elution of proteins from fragments of leaves or flowers may not be as rapid as that from pollen grains.

It has been known for many years that the feces of mites have a peritrophic membrane made of chitin but the function of this "membrane" is not clear. It is possible that it protects the hindgut of the mite from physical damage, that it functions as an antioxidant, or that it is important for recognition by those mites that are coprophagous. However, a more interesting role for these membranes has recently been appreciated in mosquitoes. Here the peritrophic membrane helps to prevent the malarial parasite from entering the insect (16). In mites it is possible that the membrane helps to protect the acarid from invasion by fungi or bacteria in the gut. Inherent in this role the membrane would have to allow free diffusion of proteins both into and out of the fecal ball.

In saline solution, 90% of the allergen Der p 1 is eluted from feces of the mite, *Dermatophagoides pteronyssinus*, within 2 min (13). Measurement of airborne mite allergen in houses has provided strong evidence that the allergen becomes airborne during disturbance and falls rapidly afterward (15). This suggests that little or no allergen is associated with small particles, which would tend to remain airborne. Thus, the fecal particle may be the predominant form in which mite allergen is inhaled.

Fungal spores are designed both to disperse the species and to provide a resistant form that can survive prolonged periods when conditions for growth are poor. Thus, rapid release of protein from a fungal spore is not biologically necessary. Studies on the release of the *Aspergillus* allergen, Asp f 1, from spores revealed a complex relationship (25). The protein is not present in the spores and is not released when they are wetted. Within 4 hr of contact with water the gene for Asp f 1 is expressed and production of the protein starts (25,26). For some of the basidiospores the allergens are similarly not released on contact with water and the spores need to be physically disrupted (27). In the case of *Alternaria* it is thought that the large spores (average size 14–20 μm in length) contain allergen and that release may occur as soon as the spore starts to swell, i.e., within minutes (28,29).

The study of fungal antigens has been severely limited because sensitive assays have not been available. Thus, there are very few studies on airborne fungal antigens (as distinct from counts of airborne fungal spores). For this reason it is not clear whether spores are the form in which fungal antigens become airborne. If the antigens are produced by mycelia and are secreted (for activities such as extracellular digestion), they may well become airborne on mycelial fragments or on dried material from the area where the fungus was growing. Overall, it is clear that understanding of exposure to fungal antigens either outdoors or within houses is very limited. We do not have a good index of exposure to fungal antigens inside houses, and consequently it is difficult to evaluate either the importance of fungal allergy to nasal symptoms or the effects of avoidance measures.

V. Proteins

For many years immediate hypersensitivity was an enigma because although skin test reactivity and Prausnitz-Küstner activity could be demonstrated, it was not possible to measure serum antibodies. The techniques in use at that time included precipitation and complement fixation tests. Indeed, immediate hypersensitivity was referred to as ''supersensitivity without immunity.'' This led to the view that the proteins or antigens that gave rise to this form of immunity must have special properties, and they were referred to as ''atopens.'' During the 1930s it was recognized that the pollen allergens were proteins even though some of the grass allergens were remarkably resistant to heat denaturation.

Today it is clear that all the inhaled allergens are proteins or glycoproteins. There does not appear to be anything distinctive about their composition or the amino acid sequences (Tables 3 and 4). Many of the allergens that have been sequenced have homology with known families of enzymes (30–32). However, it is not uncommon for proteins to be enzymes, and the prevalence of enzyme homology among allergens may not be greater than expected. For many years it was known that crude allergen extracts had enzymatic activity. Some fully purified allergens have enzymatic activity and it has been argued that this activity is relevant to their immunogenicity (30). However, the quantities inhaled, i.e., ng/

Table 3 Purified Indoor Allergens

		Molecular weight (kDa)	Sequence	Status[a]	Function	Monoclonal antibodies[b]	Assay
Dust mites:							
Group 1[c]	Der p 1	25	cDNA	M ⎱	Cysteine	+ +	ELISA
	Der f 1	25	cDNA	M ⎰	proteases	+ +	ELISA
	Eur m 1	25	Nucleotide	—		+	—
Group 2	Der p 2	14	cDNA	M	Unknown	+ +	ELISA
	Der f 2	14	N-terminal	M	Unknown	+ +	ELISA
Group 3	Der p 3	29	N-terminal	— ⎱	Serine	−	RIA
	Der f 3	29	N-terminal	— ⎰	proteases	+ +	RIA
Blomia tropicalis Blo t 5		14	cDNA	M	Unknown	−	RIA
Cat: *Felis domesticus*							
Fel d 1		35	cDNA	M	Unknown	+ +	ELISA
Albumin		68	—	—	Carrier protein	±	RIA
Dog: *Canis familiaris*							
Can f 1		27	cDNA	M	Unknown	+ +	ELISA
Cockroach:							
Blattella germanica							
Bla g 1		20–25	—	—	Unknown	+	ELISA
Bla g 2		36	cDNA	M	Aspartic protease	+ +	ELISA
Bla g 4		21	cDNA	M	Calycin	+ +	ELISA
Bla g 5		23	cDNA	M	Glutathione transferase		
Periplanetta americana							
Per a 1		20–25	—	?	Unknown	−	—
Rodents							
Mus musculus		19	Protein	? ⎱	Alpha-2U- globulin	+	ELISA
Rattus norvegicus		19	cDNA	M ⎰		+	RIA
Fungi							
Aspergillus, Asp f 1			cDNA	M	Cytotoxin	+ +	RIA
Alternaria, Alt a 1			cDNA	M	Unknown	+	RIA

[a]M = major allergens; i.e., ≥50% of allergic subjects react with the allergen.
[b]+ + indicates that more than one epitope has been defined.
[c]Groups 1, 2, and 3 include both Der p 1 and Der f 1, etc.

day, are such that it is unlikely that they are present in sufficient concentration in the nasal mucosa to act as enzymes. On the other hand, it is clear that many allergens can act as enzymes in the extracts.

Recently, considerable attention has been given to the ability of fungal extracts to denature mite allergens, indicating that these two extracts should not be mixed for immunotherapy. However, some mite allergens are also enzymes,

Table 4 Purified Pollen and Fungal Allergens

Source	Allergen	MW (kDa)	Sequence	Status[a]	Function
Grasses					
Lolium perenne	Lol p 1	27	cDNA	M	Unknown
	Lol p 2	11	cDNA	M	Unknown
	Lol p 3	11	cDNA	M	Unknown
	Lol p 10	12	cDNA	—	Cytochrome C
Phleum pratense	Phl p 5	15	cDNA	M	Ribonuclease?
Poa pratense	Poa p 10	12	—	—	Cytochrome
Trees					
Betula verrucosa	Bet v 1	17	cDNA	M	Unknown
Alnus incana	Aln i 1	17	—	M	Unknown
Weeds					
Ambrosia atemisi-	Amb a 1	37	cDNA/P	M	Unknown
folia (ragweed)	Amb a 2	38	—	—	Unknown
	Amb a 5	5	cDNA/P	M	Recognition protein
Salsola pestifer	Sol p 1	39	—	M	Unknown
(Russian thistle)					
Parietaria	Par j 1	—	—	—	—
Fungi					
Alternaria alternata	Alt a 1	30	Protein	M	—

[a]M = major allergens, i.e. ≥50% of allergic subjects react with the allergen.

and it is probable that proteins in a mite extract will digest other mite proteins (33), just as fungal enzymes can digest other proteins in the fungal extract. There are also some important allergens that do not have homology with known enzyme families or enzymic activity, e.g., Der p 2 and Fel d 1 (34–37). The tertiary structure is only known for a few allergens: e.g., Bet v 1 and Der p 2 (38,39). These structures derived from crystallography or nuclear magnetic resonance imaging may well provide much better understanding of the epitopes that bind to IgE antibodies but are unlikely to define a distinctive chemical or structural property of allergens.

Some of the physical properties of inhalant allergens are distinctive; in most cases the molecules are between 10 kDa and 50 kDa; they are freely soluble in aqueous solution; and most of the *major* allergens are present as a high percentage of the protein available from that source (40). Given these rather simple properties, one could conclude that the distinctive feature of allergens is that patients are exposed to small doses (i.e., 1–50 ng/day) for many weeks or months of the year. When patients are breathing through their noses, >90% of these particles will impact in the nose and the immune response will therefore occur in the lymph nodes draining the nose or in the tonsils. In mice repeated low-dose immunization in alum (not in complete Freund's adjuvant) is the best way to induce IgE antibody responses (41). Thus, natural exposure to inhalant allergens may be "ideally designed" to induce IgE antibody responses in humans.

Over the last few years many allergens have been cloned (26,31,32,35,37, 42,43). This provides a simple approach to obtaining the full amino acid and nucleotide sequences and also the ability to produce recombinant proteins. Knowledge of the sequences has led to two new approaches to immunotherapy, both of which are based on the assumption that immunotherapy is, or should be, directed at T cells. The first approach is to identify the linear epitopes in the proteins that T cells bind, and to treat patients with small peptides including these epitopes (44). The clinical studies have produced significant effects in cat-allergic patients but have been less effective than some people had hoped (45). The alternative approach is to use site-directed mutagenesis to modify small portions of otherwise intact allergens so that they do not react with IgE antibodies but retain reactivity with T cells (46). Molecules of this kind have been produced but have not yet been tested clinically. However, it seems likely that modified antigens will provide a more effective and safer form of immunotherapy.

VI. Environmental Control

Once the specific sensitivity of a patient with rhinitis has been determined, some environmental control measures are obvious: removing a cat, replacing fitted carpets to reduce mites, closing windows during the pollen season, and leaving the Midwest during August to avoid ragweed pollen. However, some avoidance regimes are neither obvious nor simple. Others become necessary because patients will not or cannot carry out the obvious changes. Considerable effort has been applied to developing techniques to control cat allergen with a cat in the house (47,48). Similarly, techniques for treating carpets to kill dust mites or denature allergen have been developed, but they are only necessary because patients keep carpets in warm, damp conditions (49–52). All avoidance measures should be antigen-specific. For the outdoor allergens only a few things can be done. The most effective measure is closing the house, using air conditioning, and staying indoors. At a simpler level it is important to advise patients not to use fans in the window, blowing into the house, as that can introduce large quantities of pollen or fungal spores into the bedroom. Reducing the concentration of pollinating plants or trees around the house may be useful but cannot prevent exposure because pollen grains travel large distances in the air (1). Fungal spores can also be dispersed widely by wind; however, local dispersal is also thought to be important. Reducing mold growth around the house, as well as within the house, should be recommended for mold-allergic patients. Avoidance measures for those indoor allergens for which immunoassays have been developed are species-specific. Indeed the first and perhaps the most important reason for testing for sensitization of patients with rhinitis is to educate them about the causes of their disease and relevant avoidance behaviors. The measures for mites, animal dander, and cockroaches will be described in detail.

VII. Dust Mite Control

Dust mites require a nest, a supply of food, warmth, and humidity. In most modern houses there is no shortage of carpets and upholstered furniture; human skin scales provide adequate food supply; and the temperature is maintained well within the range that is good for growth. Thus, the critical factor controlling mite growth is humidity. In the United States low humidity occurs for several reasons: in the mountain states, air is very dry year round due to altitude; in the northeast and northern Midwest the winters are very dry, because Arctic air is inherently dry and mites do not survive the winter; finally, apartments are drier than houses. In Boston, houses can have significant mite growth but apartments generally have very low levels.

In humid areas controlling mite growth is largely based on physical measures: encasing mattresses and pillows; decreasing carpets and upholstered furniture; decreasing humidity by using air conditioning as well as dehumidifiers in the basement; washing bedding in hot water weekly (53–56). Chemical measures are available for treating carpets but they only produce limited reductions in allergen and the changes are not maintained for more than 3 months (Table 3) (49,51,52). Air filtration with either electrostatic filters on the air conditioning or a HEPA room air cleaner may help any allergic patient. However, mite fecal particles fall rapidly after disturbance, so air filtration is not an important part of controlling exposure.

VIII. Cat or Dog Dander

Without doubt the most effective method for decreasing the concentration of cat allergen in a house is to relocate the animal. Following removal of the cat from a house the allergen levels fall slowly but steadily so that the concentration falls below 2 μg/g in 12–16 weeks (57,58). Reducing the allergen faster than this can only be achieved by removing carpets and washing down the walls (57). However, many cat-allergic patients are addicted to their animals and will not consider getting rid of them. Controlling cat allergen with the cat in the house requires considerable effort and is inevitably only partially effective.

Using an experimental room with a cat living in it, it was possible to demonstrate that the carpet accumulates allergen rapidly and the presence of this "reservoir" of Fel d 1 then makes it difficult to control airborne allergen by filtration (47). By contrast, in a room without a carpet, vacuum cleaning followed by use of a HEPA room air cleaner is effective in reducing allergens. In many parts of the United States it is normal practice to wash dogs regularly. For cats the procedure is less common. However, some interesting results suggested that washing the cat might be useful. Both Ohman and his colleagues and Glinert et al. found that the quantity of allergen coming off a cat was progressively reduced with repeated washing (59,60). Similarly, De Blay et al. reported that washing produced progressive decreases in the quantity of allergen coming off a cat (47). On the other hand, Klucka et al. found that repeated washing with 1 L of water did not reduce airborne allergen 1 week later (61). We have recently reexamined the issue in studies involving washing nine cats with several different techniques (48,62). The results allow several conclusions: (1) Washing cats in a bath can remove a large quantity of allergen, i.e., 2–20 mg Fel d 1. (2) Following washing, the allergen coming airborne off the cat is reduced by 70–90%. However, this reduction is not consistently maintained and in most cases the cat is shedding allergen again after 1 week. (3) Progressive reduction in the quantity of allergen coming off the cat is not a consistent phenomenon.

The conclusion is that although washing cats may be a useful way of decreasing allergen accumulating in a house, and an effective short-term method of decreasing allergen coming off the cat, the procedure would have to be repeated at least weekly to be effective. Interestingly, two controlled trials have been reported in which the combination of reducing furnishings, HEPA air filtration, and washing the cat significantly decreased cat allergen and symptoms of rhinitis (63,64). On the other hand, simply using a HEPA room air cleaner was not effective (65). Thus, it seems clear that allergen exposure can be reduced with the cat still in the house, but this requires aggressive measures that most patients will not be willing to carry out. In one study, encouraging patients to take the full control measures turned out to be an effective measure of persuading the family to remove cats from the house (63).

Although all published data on avoiding cat allergen has concerned houses with a cat, allergen is often present in houses without a cat (66,67). This allergen, which is presumed to be carried on clothing from other houses, can accumulate to concentrations as high as 80 µg/g and has been shown to become airborne in houses (68). Cat allergen can also become a problem in schools where, again, high concentrations have been reported. Providing accurate advice to a cat-allergic patient may require measuring the concentration of Fel d 1 in the house even if there is not a cat in the house.

IX. Cockroach

Cockroach avoidance measures are included here because many individuals are allergic to cockroaches and have blocked noses. However, almost all these patients present with asthma. In our experience perennial rhinitis without asthma is unusual in cockroach-allergic patients. Avoidance measures to reduce cockroach allergens are in their infancy. However, it is already clear that cockroach allergen becomes airborne only after disturbance (19–21). This is like mite allergen and suggests that avoidance measures would have to focus on controlling cockroaches. The current recommendations are for (1) obsessional enclosing of food in airtight containers or in a refrigerator; (2) careful cleaning to reduce food for the insects; (3) vacuuming to reduce quantities of allergen in the house; (4) controlling supplies of water (such as leaking taps, water pans in refrigerators); and (5) regular use of insecticides such as Hydramethylnon or Avermectin as bait. No controlled trials of cockroach avoidance have been reported.

X. Allergens Associated with Sinusitis

Most patients with chronic sinusitis whose symptoms are not related to any specific season or exposure have negative skin tests. In these patients it is difficult to make a case for the role of specific allergens even though the disease can have many of the hallmarks of a TH2 response, including eosinophilia, elevated IgG_4, and in some cases elevated serum IgE. However, some antigen-specific responses may be increased in patients with extensive sinus disease. These include IgE antibodies to dust mite, to the dermatophyte fungus, *Trichophyton*, and also to *Aspergillus* in children with cystic fibrosis (69–72). The direct relevance of these responses to chronic sinusitis is not clear. Allergic responses could contribute to the early phases where ostia become blocked and infection follows. Alternatively, the identified responses could simply be markers of the allergic diathesis since inhaled antigens are not a convincing cause of chronic sinusitis.

Sinusitis is almost universal among patients identified as having onychomycosis, *Trichophyton* sensitivity, and asthma (71). These patients, like almost all patients with the combination of sinusitis and steroid-dependent asthma, have eosinophilia. Recently, we have shown that they also have circulating T cells specific for *Trichophyton* proteins and that these cells will produce IL-5 in vitro (73). In addition, some of these patients report marked decrease in sinus symptoms while on treatment with the antifungal fluconazole (74). The question is whether there are other unusual allergens associated with sinusitis. Some of the more interesting candidates for this role are the yeast *Candida albicans*, food antigens, and the bacterial flora of the sinus tissue. However, these remain research issues because there is no convincing evidence about the immunochemistry of these antigens or immunology of the responses.

There is good evidence for the importance of diverse fungal allergens in the small subset of patients with allergic fungal sinusitis. In this disease patients have immediate hypersensitivity to a fungus growing in their sinuses associated with characteristic changes seen on computed tomographic scans of the sinuses.

XI. Conclusions

Any particle that becomes airborne and carries soluble protein will deliver proteins to the nasal mucosa. Given the known properties of allergens, it appears that almost any protein that is inhaled can become an allergen. Thus, the importance of each allergen source relates far more to the number and properties of the particles they release than to the chemical properties of the proteins. Starting with protein purification, leading to full sequence information, and most recently tertiary structure, it now appears unlikely that the inhaled proteins that induce IgE antibodies and are causes of allergic rhinitis have any special characteristics. They are all small, i.e., <50 kDa, freely soluble, released in large quantity, and immunologically foreign. Although many are enzymes, the evidence that this property is relevant to their allergenicity is not convincing. Indeed, the known allergens derive from a wide range of plant and animal species; in each case the key characteristic is whether the source is present (or abundant) in the environment of the patient.

The way in which allergens become airborne is also important in designing methods to control exposure. The animal danders that have been studied become airborne on particles that can ''float'' and thus remain airborne in relatively undisturbed conditions. By contrast, the allergens derived from mites and cockroaches are only airborne during and shortly after disturbance. For the former group air filtration may be helpful, while for the latter it plays very little role. However, in both cases effective avoidance measures require controlling the source as well as identifying and reducing the reservoirs in which allergen accumulates. As methods for controlling allergens have become better defined, they have also become progressively antigen-specific. Today the control measures recommended for mite, animal dander, and cockroach are quite distinct. This means that avoidance measures can only be recommended once the specific sensitivity of the patient is known. In some cases it would be better to know the quantities of allergen in the house before recommending avoidance. In many geographic areas it is difficult to predict the concentration of mite allergen in houses. Similarly, in inner-city areas where cockroach infestation is a major problem, there are very large differences between houses. For animal dander allergens it is clear that houses with a cat have high levels of allergen; however, in areas where there is a high prevalence of cats the quantity of allergen in houses without a cat cannot be predicted.

Given that the immune system sees the world only in terms of self or alien, it seems likely that any protein could become an allergen if delivered by the correct route. However, there are several ways in which allergens could be modified so that they could be used to therapeutically alter the type of immune response. These include the use of peptides reactive only with T cells; recombinant allergens with the amino acid sequence modified in such a way that they no longer bind IgE antibodies; and linking recombinant allergens to cytokines such as IL-12, which would favor a cell-mediated response, or to antibodies with isotypes other than IgE. Better understanding of allergens, including the ability to measure them accurately, has already improved the practice of allergy in standardization and in defining avoidance measures. Over the next few years the developments in the production of recombinant allergens and modified allergens will provide new approaches to immunotherapy that have the potential for greater safety and efficiency.

Acknowledgment

This work was supported by NIH Grants AI-20565 and AI-34607.

References

1. Blackley CH. Experimental Research in the Causes and Nature of Catarrhus Aestivus (Hay Fever or Hay Asthma). London: Bailliere Tindall & Cox, 1873. Reprinted by Dawson Publishing Co., London, 1959:57–58.
2. Wyman M. Autumnal Catarrh (Hay Fever). Cambridge, MA: Huro & Houghton, 1872.
3. Noon L. Prophylactic inoculation for hay fever. Lancet 1911; 1:1572.
4. Cooke RA. Allergy in Theory and Practice. Philadelphia: WB Saunders, 1947:130–158.
5. Voorhorst R, Spieksma FThM, Varekamp H, Leupen MJ, Lyklema AW. The house dust mite (*Dermatophagoides pteronyssinus*) and the allergens it produces: identity with the house dust allergen. J Allergy 1967; 39:325–339.
6. Platts-Mills TAE, Hayden ML, Chapman MD, Wilkins SR. Seasonal variation in dust mite and grass-pollen allergens in dust from the houses of patients with asthma. J Allergy Clin Immunol 1987; 79:781–791.
7. Platts-Mills TAE. Type I or immediate hypersensitivity: hay fever and asthma. In: Lachmann PJ, Peters DK, eds. Clinical Aspects of Immunology. Oxford: Blackford Publ., 1982:579–686.
8. Lewis WH, Vinay P, Zenger VE, eds. Airborne and Allergenic Pollen of North America. Baltimore: Johns Hopkins University Press, 1983.

9. Ishizaka K, Ishizaka T. Mechanisms of reaginic hypersensitivity and IgE antibody response. Immunol Rev 1978; 41:109.

10. Solomon WR, Platts-Mills TAE. Aerobiology and inhalant allergens. In: Middleton E, Reed CE, Ellis E, Adkinson NF, Yunginger JW, Busse WW, eds. Allergy Principles and Practice. St. Louis: CV Mosby, 1993:469–528.

11. Levetin E. Fungi. In: Bioaerosols. Burge HA, ed. Boca Raton, FL: Lewis Publishers, 1996:87–120.

12. Smith EG. Sampling and Identifying Allergenic Pollens and Molds. San Antonio: Bluestone Press, 1984.

13. Tovey ER, Chapman MD, Platts-Mills TAE. Mite faeces are a major source of house dust allergens. Nature 1981; 289:592–593.

14. Tovey ER, Chapman MD, Wells CW, Platts-Mills TAE. The distribution of dust mite allergen in the houses of patients with asthma. Am Rev Respir Dis 1981; 124: 630–635.

15. Platts-Mills TAE, Chapman MD. Dust mites: immunology, allergic disease, and environmental control. J Allergy Clin Immunol 1987; 80:755 (published erratum in J Allergy Clin Immunol 1988; 82:841.

16. Sieber K-P, Huber M, Kaslow D, Banks SM, Torii M, Aikawa M, Miller LH. The peritrophic membrane as a barrier: its penetration by *Plasmodium gallinaceum* and the effect of a monoclonal antibody to ookinetes. Exp Parasitol 1991; 72:145–156.

17. Luczynska CM, Yin L, Chapman MD, Platts-Mills TAE. Airborne concentrations and particle size distribution of allergen derived from domestic cats (*Felis domesticus*). Am Rev Respir Dis 1990; 41:361–367.

18. Findlay S, Stosky E, Lietermann K, Hemady Z, Ohman JL. Allergens detected in association with airborne particles capable of penetrating into the peripheral lung. Am Rev Respir Dis 1983; 128:1008–1012.

19. Mollet JA, Vailes LD, Avner DB, Perzanowski MS, Arruda LK, Chapman MD, Platts-Mills TAE. Evaluation of German cockroach (Orthoptera: Blattellidae) allergen and its seasonal variation in low-income housing. J Med Entomol 1997; 34: 307–311.

20. De Blay F, Kassel O, Chapman MD, Ott M, Verot A, Pauli G. Mise en evidence des allergenes majeurs des blattes par test ELISA dans la poussiere domestique. Presse Med 1992; 21:1685.

21. Sarpong SB, Hamilton RG, Eggleston PA, Atkinson NF. Socioeconomic status and race as risk factors for cockroach allergen exposure and sensitization in children with asthma. J Allergy Clin Immunol 1996; 97:1393–1401.

22. Darwin CE. The different forms of flowers on plants of the same species (1877). In: Ridley M, Ed. The Darwin Reader. New York: WW Norton, 1987.

23. Busse WW, Reed CE, Hoehne JH. Where is the allergic reaction in ragweed asthma? II. Demonstration of ragweed antigen in airborne particles smaller than pollen. J Allergy Clin Immunol 1972; 50:289.

24. Solomon WR. Uncovering the "fine details" of pollen allergen transport. J Allergy Clin Immunol 1984; 74:674.

25. Sporik RB, Arruda LK, Woodfolk J, Chapman MD, Platts-Mills TAE. Environmental exposure to *Aspergillus fumigatus* (Asp f I). Clin Exp Allergy 1993; 23:326–31.

26. Arruda LK, Platts-Mills TAE, Fox JW, Chapman MD. *Aspergillus fumigatus* Allergen I, a major IgE-binding protein, is a member of the mitogillin family of cytotoxins. J Exp Med 1990; 172:1529–1532.

27. Lehrer SR, Lopez M, Butcher BT, Olson J, Reed M, Salvaggio JE. Basidiomycete mycelia and spore-allergen extracts: skin test reactivity in adults with symptoms of respiratory allergy. J Allergy Clin Immunol 1986; 78:478–485.

28. Crenshaw R, Esch R, Portnoy J, Upadrasha B, Pacheco F, Barney C. Specific allergen content, enzymic profile and morphology of eleven strains of *Alternaria*. J Allergy Clin Immunol 1992; 89:242.

29. Bush RK. Aerobiology of pollen and fungal allergens. J Allergy Clin Immunol 1989; 84:1120–1123.

30. Stewart GA, Thompson PJ. The biochemistry of common aeroallergens. Clin Exp Allergy 1996; 26:1020–1044.

31. Chua KY, Steward GA, Thomas WR, Simpson RJ, Dilworth RJ, Plozza TM, Turner KJ. Sequence analysis of cDNA coding for a major house dust mite allergen, Der p I: Homology with cysteine proteases. J Exp Med 1988; 167:175–182.

32. Arruda LK, Vailes LD, Mann BJ, Shannon J, Fox JW, Vedvick TS, Hayden ML, Chapman MD. Molecular cloning of a major cockroach (*Blattella germanica*) allergen, Bla g 2: sequence homology to the aspartic proteases. J Biol Chem 1995; 270: 19563–19568.

33. Hewitt CRA, Brown AP, Hart BJ, Pritchard DI. A major house dust allergen disrupts the immunoglobulin E network by selectively cleaving CD23: innate protection by antiproteases. J Exp Med 1995; 182:1537–1544.

34. Heymann PW, Chapman MD, Aalberse RC, Fox JW, Platts-Mills TAE. Antigenic and structural analysis of group II allergens (Der f II and Der p II) from house dust mites (*Dermatophagoides* spp). J Allergy Clin Immunol 1989; 83:1055–1067.

35. Chua KY, Doyle CR, Simpson RJ, Turner KJ, Stewart GA, Thomas WR. Isolation of cDNA coding for the major mite allergen Der p II by IgE plaque immunoassay. Int Arch Allergy Appl Immunol 1990; 91:118–123.

36. Chapman MD, Aalberse RC, Brown MJ, Platts-Mills TAE. Monoclonal antibodies to the major feline allergen Fel d I. II. Single step affinity purification of Fel d I, N-terminal sequence analysis, and development of a sensitive two-site immunoassay to assess Fel d I exposure. J Immunol 1988; 140:812–818.

37. Morgenstern JP, Griffith IJ, Brauer AW, Rogers BL, Bond JF, Chapman MD, Kuo M. Amino acid sequence of Fel d I, the major allergen of the domestic cat: protein sequence analysis and cDNA cloning. Proc Natl Acad Sci USA 1991; 88:9690–9694.

38. Gajhede M, Osmark P, Poulsen FM, Ipsen H, Larsen JN, van Neerven RJJ, Schou C, Lowenstein H, Spangfort MD. X-ray and NMR structure of Bet v 1, the origina of birch pollen allergy. Nature Struct Biol 1996; 3:1040–1045.

39. Mueller G, Chapman M, Benjamin D, Smith AM. Structural and immunochemical comparison of native and recombinant Der p 2 in preparation. (in preparation).

40. Platts-Mills TAE. Allergens. In: Frank MM, Austen KF, Clamen HN, Unanue ER, eds. Samter's Immunologic diseases. Boston: Little, Brown, 1995:1231–1256.

41. Levine BB, Vaz NM. Effect of combinations of inbred strain, antigen, and antigen dose on immune responsiveness and reagin production in the mouse. A potential

mouse model for immune aspects of human atopic allergy. Int Arch Allergy Appl Immunol 1970; 39:156–171.

42. Esch RE, Klapper DG. Identification and localization of allergenic determinants on grass group I antigens using monoclonal antibodies. J Immunol 1989; 142:179–184.

43. Breteneder H, et al. The gene coding for the major birch pollen allergen, Bet v 1, is highly homologous to a pea disease resistance response gene. EMBO J 1989; 8: 1935–1938.

44. van Neerven RJ, van de Poll MM, van Milligan FJ, Jansen HM, Aallberse RC, Kapsenberg ML. Characterization of cat dander specific T lymphocytes from atopic patients. J Immunol 1994; 152:4203–4210.

45. Norman PS, Ohman JL, Long AA, Creticos PS, Gefter MA, Shaked Z, Wood RA, Eggleston PA, Hafner KB, Rao P, Lichtenstein LM, Jones NH, Nicodemus CF. Treatment of cat allergen with T-cell reactive peptides. Am J Respir Crit Care Med 1996; 154:1623–1628.

46. Smith AM, Chapman MD. Reduction in IgE binding to allergen variants generated by site-directed mutagenesis: contribution of disulfide bonds to the antigenic structure of the major house dust mite allergen Der p 2. Mol Immunol 1996; 33:399–405.

47. De Blay F, Chapman MD, Platts-Mills TAE. Airborne cat allergen (Fel d I): environmental control with the cat in situ. Am Rev Respir Dis 1991; 143:1334–1339.

48. Avner DB, Perzanowski MS, Platts-Mills TAE, Woodfolk JA. Evaluation of different techniques for washing cats: quantitation of allergen removed from the cat and the effect on airborne Fed d 1. J Allergy Clin Immunol 1997; 100:307–312.

49. Green WF, Nicholas NR, Salome CM, Woolcock AJ. Reduction of house dust mites and mite allergens: effects of spraying carpets and blankets with Allersearch DMS, an acaricide combined with an allergen reducing agent. Clin Exp Allergy 1989; 19: 203–207.

50. Bischoff E, Fischer A, Liebenberg B. Assessment and control of house dust mite infestation. Clin Ther 1990; 12:216–220.

51. Hayden ML, Rose G, Diduch KB, Domson P, Chapman MD, Heymann PW, Platts-Mills TAE. Benzyl benzoate moist powder: investigation of acarical activity in cultures and reduction of dust mite allergens in carpets. J Allergy Clin Immunol 1992; 89:536–545.

52. Woodfolk JA, Hayden ML, Couture N, Platts-Mills TAE. Chemical treatment of carpets to reduce allergen: comparison of the effects of tannic acid and other treatments on proteins derived from dust mites and cats. J Allergy Clin Immunol 1995; 96:325–333.

53. Ehnert B, Lau-Schadendorf S, Weber A, Buettner P, Schou C, Wahn U. Reducing domestic exposure to dust mite allergen reduces bronchial hypersensitivity in sensitive children with asthma. J Allergy Clin Immunol 1992; 90:135–138.

54. Murray AB, Ferguson AC. Dust-free bedrooms in the treatment of asthmatic children with house dust or house dust mite allergy: a controlled trial. Pediatrics 1983; 71: 418–422.

55. Owen S, Morganstern M, Hepworth J, Woodcock A. Control of house dust mite antigen in bedding. Lancet 1990; 335:396–397.

56. MacDonald L, Tovey E. The role of water temperature and laundry procedures in

reducing house dust mite populations and allergen content of bedding. J Allergy Clin Immunol 1992; 90:599–608.

57. Wood RA, Chapman MD, Adkinson NF Jr, Eggleston PA. The effect of cat removal on allergen content in household-dust samples. J Allergy Clin Immunol 1989; 83: 730–734.

58. Wood RA, Eggleston PA, Lind P, Ingemann L, Schwartz B, Graveson S, Terry D, Wheeler B, Adkinson NF Jr. Antigenic analysis of household dust samples. Am Rev Respir Dis 1988; 137:358–363.

59. Ohman JL, Baer H, Anderson MC, Leitermann K, Brown P. Surface washes of living cats: an improved method of obtaining clinically relevant allergen. J Allergy Clin Immunol 1983; 72:288–293.

60. Glinert R, Wilson P, Wedner HJ. Fel d I is markedly reduced following sequential washing of cats. J Allergy Clin Immunol 1990; 85:327 (abstract).

61. Klucka CV, Ownby DR, Green J, Zoratti E. Cat shedding of Fel d 1 is not reduced by washings, Allerpet-C spray, or acepromazine. J Allergy Clin Immunol 1995; 95(6):1164–1171.

62. Perzanowski M, Wheatley LM, Avner D, Woodfolk JA, Platts-Mills TAE. The effectiveness of Allergpet/c at reducing the cat allergen Fel d 1 on a cat. J Allergy Clin Immunol 1997; 100:428–430.

63. Juliusson S, Jakobinudottir S, Runarsdottir V, Blondal T, Gislason D, Bjornsdottir US. Environmental control (EC) can effectively reduce cat allergen (Fel d 1) in house dust samples without removal of the cat. J Allergy Clin Immunol 1997; 99:5388.

64. De Blay F, Soldatov D, Griess P, et al. Effects of environmental control measures on patient status and airborne Fel d 1 levels with a cat in situ. Allergy 1995; 50: 23–24.

65. Wood RA, Flanagan E, Van Natta M, Chen PH, Eggleston PA. The effect of a HEPA room air cleaner on cat-induced asthma and rhinitis. J Allergy Clin Immunol 1997; 99:5388.

66. Gelber LE, Seltzer LH, Bouzoukis JK, Pollart SM, Chapman MD, Platts-Mills TAE. Sensitization and exposure to indoor allergens as risk factors for asthma among patients presenting to hospital. Am Rev Respir Dis 1993; 147:573–578.

67. Sporik R, Ingram JM, Price W, Sussman JH, Honsinger RW, Platts-Mills TAE. Association of asthma with serum IgE and skin-test reactivity to allergens among children living at high altitude: tickling the dragon's breath. Am J Respir Crit Care Med 1995; 151:1388–1392.

68. Bollinger ME, Eggleston PA, Flanagan E, Wood RA. Cat antigen in homes with and without cats may induce allergic symptoms. J Allergy Clin Immunol 1996; 97: 907–914.

69. Freudenberger T, Grizzanti JN, Rosenstreich DL. Natural Immunity to dust mites in patients with chronic rhinosinusitis. J Allergy Clin Immunol 1988; 82:855–862.

70. Newman LJ, Platts-Mills TAE, Phillips CD, Hazen KC, Gross CW. Chronic sinusitis. Relationship of computed tomographic findings to allergy, asthma, and eosinophilia. JAMA 1994; 271:363–367.

71. Ward GW, Jr., Karlsson G, Rose G, Platts-Mills TAE. Trichophyton asthma: sensitization of bronchi and upper airways to dermatophyte antigen. Lancet 1989; 1:859–862.

72. El-dahr J, Fink R, Selden R, Arruda LK, Platts-Mills TAE, Heymann PW. Development of immune responses to *Aspergillus*, including Allergen Asp f I, at an early age in children with cystic fibrosis. Am Rev Respir Dis 1994; 150:1513–1518.
73. Slunt JB, Taketomi EA, Woodfolk JA, Hayden ML, Platts-Mills TAE. The immune response to *Trichophyton tonsurans*: distinct T cell cytokine profiles to a single protein among subjects with immediate and delayed hypersensitivity. J Immunol 1996; 157:5192–5197.
74. Ward GW, Hayden ML, Rose G, Call RS, Platts-Mills TAE. Trichophyton asthma: response to oral antifungal therapy with Fluconazole. J Allergy Clin Immunol 1993; 91:226 (abstract).

5

Occupational and Environmental Exposures and the Upper Respiratory Tract

REBECCA BASCOM

The Pennsylvania State College of
   Medicine and
Penn State Geisinger Health System
Hershey, Pennsylvania

DENNIS SHUSTERMAN

University of California
San Francisco, California

I. Introduction

A diverse group of occupational agents may cause upper respiratory tract symptoms and disease. Environmental exposures, too, may affect the upper respiratory tract. Symptoms include nasal irritation, rhinorrhea, nasal congestion, sneezing, throat irritation, hoarseness, and symptoms of upper airway obstruction. Diseases and syndromes include allergic and irritant rhinitis, laryngitis and laryngeal dysfunction, epithelial metaplasia, and upper airway neoplasms. Inflammatory responses of the upper airways resemble those of the lower airways, but changes in patency are effected primarily through changes in vascular tone rather than smooth muscle contraction.

Biological variability in the individual response to an environmental agent is well recognized. The presence of allergy can result in a marked upper airway inflammatory response to an allergen whereas a nonallergic individual will have no reaction. Some individuals with seasonal allergic disease report that their sensitivity to irritants increases during their allergen season. Healthy adults report variable sensitivity to common environmental irritants, independent of atopic status. Increased sensitivity to some irritants may be confirmed objectively in some individuals, but the response does not resemble the allergic response biochemically, nor does atopy predict the increased responsiveness. Human upper airway responses to many irritants (at doses found in workplaces) are notable for the absence of signs of increased vascular permeability; in contrast, rodent upper airways characteristically demonstrate irritant-induced vascular leak. Response mechanisms include both central (cholinergic) and local (axonal) neurogenic reflexes. Tissue remodeling from pseudostratified ciliated columnar epithelium to dysplasia or squamous metaplasia occurs in some individuals with some exposures, such as those with occupational wood dust exposure.

A careful history remains the best available clinical tool to identify work-related upper respiratory disease. Inadequate training in medical school in occupational medicine results in an imbalance between great skill in eliciting the clinical history, but little skill in eliciting a useful occupational history. Workers are an excellent source of useful information, however, and with practice, the clinician can learn quickly.

The advantage of asking about occupational exposures is that it enables the rational treatment of many upper respiratory tract disorders. Simple measures may markedly reduce workplace exposures and reduce risks of lower respiratory disease. Identification of causative agents and reduction of exposures that worsen the disease are cornerstones of modern allergy practice. The National Asthma Education and Prevention Guidelines encourage the identification and remediation of environmental stressors. The clinician is in an excellent position to alert employers about conditions that appear to be worsening an employee's health. Responses of the upper airways to occupational toxicants can be documented using objective, noninvasive methods such as rhinomanometry, analysis of nasal secretions, mucosal biopsy, and measures of mucociliary clearance. However, diagnostic tools that are practical for the primary care clinician are still lacking, particularly for symptoms of irritation.

Modification of environmental exposures is more difficult, because by definition these agents are present in the ambient air. Temporal and spatial variation in common pollutants does occur, and some clinical suggestions can be made to the individual interested in reducing exposures. Limited studies of the pharmacotherapy of pollutant effects also exist.

This chapter will identify agents encountered in occupational settings and in the ambient environment that have recognized effects on the upper respiratory tract. There is extensive discussion of the clinical approach to diagnosis and management of allergic and nonallergic rhinitis elsewhere in this book. Comments on clinical diagnosis and management will be limited to aspects of the evaluation that deserve particular emphasis.

II. Epidemiology

The second National Health and Nutrition Evaluation survey (NHANES, $n =$ 10,854) assessed upper respiratory symptoms and measured skin test reactivity

Table 1 Prevalence of Symptoms Associated with Common Indoor Exposures

	Never[a]	Rarely/sometimes	Often/always
Tobacco smoke	67–71	23–28	5–6
Fumes from copy machine	73–79	18–24	2–4
Fumes from printing process	90–92	7–9	0–1
Fumes from other chemicals	69–78	21–28	1–3
Fumes from pesticides	82–88	11–17	0–2
Fumes from new carpeting	62–78	20–31	2–7
Fumes from new drapes	78–86	13–19	1–4
Fumes from paint	62–78	19–34	4
Fumes from cleaning of carpets	75–79	19–22	2–3
Other fumes	85–94	5–8	3–8

[a]The percentage of individuals responding affirmatively is listed.

in a sample of the United States population from 1976 to 1980. Seasonal rhinitis was defined as the syndrome that occurred in persons who either reported a physician diagnosis of hay fever or complained of frequent eye/nasal symptoms that varied both by season and by pollen during the past 12 months, not counting colds or flu. Seasonal rhinitis was strongly associated with skin test reactivity at all ages.

Chronic rhinitis was defined as the syndrome that occurred in persons who complained of frequent nasal and/or eye symptoms that did not vary by both season and pollen during the past 12 months (not counting cold or flu), and did not have a physician diagnosis of hay fever. In the second NHANES survey, 15% of 12–24-year-olds reported chronic rhinitis, as did 15–20% of 25–49-year-olds and 20–30% of 50–74-years olds (1). In contrast with seasonal rhinitis, chronic rhinitis was not associated with skin test reactivity, suggesting that nonallergic factors or other antigens may be important in its pathogenesis.

Table 1 shows the percentage of office workers reporting eye, nose, throat, or respiratory irritation associated with identifiable office point sources, and the frequency of symptoms. No objective measures were performed in any of the subjects (3). Investigators lack objective methods for validating upper respiratory tract/mucous membrane irritant symptoms in population studies (2). As a result, few data exist on the prevalence of subjective sensitivity to common environmental irritants. An epidemiological study of U.S. office workers asked respondents, ''Do you consider yourself especially sensitive to any of the items'' in the following list?—tobacco smoke, fumes from photocopying machine, printing processes, other chemicals such as adhesives, glues, cleaners, liquid correction fluid, rubber cement; pesticides, new carpeting, new drapes, curtains, or furniture, paint, cleaning of carpets, drapes, or other furnishings (2). Twenty-nine to 32% responded that they were especially sensitive to these irritants. Subjects answering yes to that question were more likely to be women, and more likely to report mucosal symptoms.

An epidemiological study of 332 French men, aged 27–58, examined the prevalence of perceived nasal hyperresponsiveness, defined as sneezy or runny nose after specified stimuli. Subjects reported perceived hyperresponsiveness to hay (14%), cold air (14%), tobacco smoke (5%), and exercise (2%). Fifteen percent of men were atopic, defined as showing skin test reactivity to common allergens. Atopy was more common in subjects reporting hyperresponsiveness to one or more stimuli. Lifetime nonsmokers were more common among individuals reporting tobacco smoke rhinitis than among those who did not report tobacco rhinitis; usual rhinitis was more prevalent among ever-smokers. Peripheral basophil counts were significantly lower in those with usual rhinitis than those without (3), and peripheral eosinophilia was associated with an absence of nasal symptoms.

Occupational rhinitis is typically 2–5 times more prevalent than lower respiratory symptoms, and prevalence rates increase in work zones with increased agent exposure. A study of 218 dock workers showed that both dominant and contaminating allergens may contribute to symptoms, and that work-related symptoms may occur among some individuals without demonstrable allergy (4). The dock workers unloaded shipments of green coffee beans contained in sacks; 9.6% were sensitized by skin tests to either the green coffee beans, contaminating castor beans, or the sacks. Antigens from green coffee bean, castor bean, and chlorogenic acid are distinct and unrelated. Fourteen percent complained of allergic symptoms at work: oculorhinitis was most prevalent (9%), followed by oculorhinitis and asthma (4%) and asthma alone (1%). Eight of the nine people with both work-related oculorhinitis and asthma symptoms had skin tests positive for workplace allergens.

A cross-sectional study of workers exposed to phthalic anhydride showed symptoms of rhinitis in 40% of the heavily exposed workers and 20% of the low-exposure workers. Specific IgG antibodies were elevated in the former group. Rhinitis has been commonly reported among workers with exposure to Western red cedar, some of whom also have asthma (5). In a survey of 40 fur manufacturing workers and 31 controls, indices of work-related allergic rhinitis were present in 20–30% of the exposed group.

III. Agents with Recognized Effects on the Upper Airways

A. Allergens

Many allergens that cause occupational rhinitis are proteins, although some are chemicals of low molecular weight (i.e., <1000 daltons). Allergens range in size from large pollen grains of 10 μm or more, to cat allergen, which has a size range extending to <1 μm. The behavior of the allergen in the environment is

Table 2 Occupational Upper Respiratory Sensitizers

Protein allergens	Low-molecular-weight chemicals	Other agents
Latex	Western red cedar (pli-	Sodium iso-nonanyl
Laboratory animals	catic acid)	oxybenzene sulfonate
Guar gum	Trimellitic anhydride	Carbonless copy paper
(galactomannans)	Phthalic anhydride	Permanent wave solution
Psyllium	Isocyanates	
Coffee beans		
Grain mites		
Grain dust		
Flour dust		

highly variable (6); some allergens settle quickly to the ground, others remain suspended in the air, still others collect in reservoirs that may be disrupted with activities such as renovating or cleaning. Some data indicate that the structure and perhaps the allergenicity of the antigen may be altered by interaction with pollutants or by the adsorption of nonallergenic pollutants to the allergen surface. Examples include interactions of protein allergens with ozone, oxides of nitrogen, sulfur oxides, and diesel particles. Methods to assess total personal exposure to allergen have been lacking, but the flora and fauna of a particular microenvironment clearly influence an individual's allergen exposure profile.

The medical literature associates a wide range of allergens with occupational rhinitis (Table 2). In theory, any agent that causes occupational asthma could also cause rhinitis; long lists of agents causing occupational asthma (7,8) can be consulted for other possible causative agents. Rhinitis has been reported in association with exposure to protein allergens such as laboratory animal proteins, castor beans, and insect allergens. Low-molecular-weight materials such as the isocyanates and anhydrides have also been reported to cause rhinitis (9,10). In Finland where nasal provocation is routinely used in the diagnosis of rhinitis, 10% of 300–400 annual provocation tests demonstrate an occupational cause, principally flour dust.

Galactomannans are natural gums, high-polymer, water-soluble carbohydrates that are used as protective colloids and emulsifying agents in food products and pharmaceuticals and as sizing for textiles. Three cases of allergic rhinitis from vegetable gum–guar gum have been reported (11). Two were through exposure to a fine guar gum powder (an insulator in rubber cables) when opening cable in a power cable lab. After 1–2 years of exposure, these subjects developed rhinitis and nasal eosinophilia and were diagnosed with a positive scratch test, a nasal provocation test, and a positive RAST test. A third subject developed allergic rhinitis after 2 years of exposure in a paper factory. Exposure had not been especially heavy.

Schwartz et al. evaluated a nurse who reported symptoms of rhinitis and chest tightness after dispensing Metamucil in a skilled nursing facility (12). The authors documented a fivefold increase in nasal airway resistance immediately following exposure to psyllium dust in a laboratory setting; specific airways resistance and forced vital capacity, on the other hand, were only minimally affected. The patient's symptoms resolved and rhinomanometric findings normalized after institution of a cromolyn sodium nasal spray.

Niinimaki et al. studied a cosmetologist who experienced nasal itching, rhinorrhea, and conjunctival irritation when she mixed a papain-containing powder with an abrasive cream for purposes of a beauty treatment (13). Provocation testing with a papain-containing solution applied to the inferior turbinate by cotton pledget, but not with a saline control, produced acute rhinitis symptoms and a fourfold increase in nasal airway resistance. Symptoms resolved after the patient discontinued abrasive skin treatments on clients.

Eggleston et al. exposed 12 rat allergic volunteers and five allergic controls to a rat vivarium for 1 hr (14). Allergen concentrations ranged from <1.5 to 310 ng/m^3 and were highest during cage cleaning when compared to periods of quiet activity. All the rat-allergic subjects had an increase in nasal lavage TAME and histamine. TAME (tosyl-arginine methyl ester) is a radiochemical assay indicating the presence of either increased vascular permeability, glandular stimulation, or release of mast cell tryptase. Five of 12 volunteers had a FEV_1 decrement of >10%. Of the controls, 2/5 had a small TAME increase, and none had an FEV_1 response. Dose response occurred between the allergen concentration and the study endpoints.

Latex is increasingly recognized as an occupational allergen. Two mechanisms of sensitivity exist. Contact dermatitis associated with individual glove use involves sensitization to chemicals used in the rubber processing. More common since the introduction of universal precautions and the examination glove is IgE allergy to natural rubber latex allergens that become airborne during glove use. Two routes of exposure, dermal and respiratory, must now be considered and controlled. One study reported findings of 70 patients with hypersensitivity reactions caused by latex articles (15). All patients suffered from urticaria, 36 from rhinitis, 31 from conjunctivitis, 22 from dyspnea, and 17 from systemic reactions, and four patients developed severe systemic complications during surgery. Sodium dodecyl sulfate–polyacrylamide gel electrophoresis showed that the latex allergen was characterized as a mixture of proteins in a molecular weight range from 10 to 67 kDa. Inhalation challenge studies with powdered latex gloves showed that the cornstarch glove powder functioned as an airborne carrier for latex allergens. Five of 18 patients undergoing such challenge tests demonstrated a significant increase of specific airway resistance; 17 had acute rhinitis and/or conjunctivitis; and two had a systemic reaction. Sixty-two percent of the patients demonstrated specific IgE antibodies to natural latex, 58% to an irradiated, cross-linked, so-called, "hypoallergenic" latex preparation, and 46% to commercial-latex RAST disks (Pharmacia). No specific antibodies to cornstarch or a mixture of rubber chemicals were found. In a subgroup of 45 subjects, there was a good correlation (82%) between latex IgE RAST and latex skin prick test.

Exposure to common environmental allergens in the workplace may be responsible for work-associated rhinitis. In the workplace, the source of the allergen may be local point sources, or the worker as a vector, bringing in allergen from the outside. For example, offices in which cat-allergic workers had office-related symptoms have been shown to have cat allergen present. This is presumed to be due to adherence of cat protein to clothing in the home environment, and subsequent shedding of cat protein from clothing in the office environment. Fungal bioaerosols may develop in offices with a history of leaks, poorly functioning ventilation systems with fiberglass lining, or inadequate insulation of walls with significant thermal gradients. Fungal allergens are numerous and diverse, but purified antigens for use in diagnostic testing exist for only a few such as the *Aspergillus* species and *Aureobasidium pullulans*. Many others exist, and their role in human disease is unknown. There is a continuing need for the identification and purification of fungal allergens (6). Thin-walled bacteria, including thermophilic actinomycetes, *Micropolyspora faeni*, and *Thermoactinomycetes vulgaris*, have been found in some workplaces.

Outdoor workers are more heavily exposed during seasonal variation in the concentration of allergen dispersed in the air. For example, in the mid-Atlantic states there is an early spring allergen season as trees blossom and produce pollen. The late spring and early summer are characterized by rises in the concentration of grass allergens. Finally, the late summer and early fall are characterized by increases in ragweed concentrations. Even desert environments have clinically significant allergy seasons (e.g., juniper in the southwestern United States). Local patterns of allergens can be determined by consulting knowledgeable individuals such as community allergists. Some occupations may have a marked increase in exposure to common environmental allergens. One example was a young man with early summer rhinitis who developed severe rhinitis and asthma on the first day at a job in a grass seed factory.

B. Irritants

Definition

An irritant is defined as an agent that causes a condition of soreness or inflammation. Other chapters in this book and recent reviews summarize the anatomy, neurology, and pharmacology of the upper airway irritant response system in humans and animals (16–26).

Capsaicin

Capsaicin, the active ingredient in red pepper, directly stimulates the chemosensitive C-fiber afferent nerves. In animal models, capsaicin is used to study the irritant response in three different ways. A single dose in adult animals is used to induce and characterize the acute irritant response. Repeated local administration to adult animals, such as to an area of skin, will induce a transient local denervation of chemosensitive nerves. This approach is used to study the process of denervation and reinnervation. Neonatal administration of capsaicin intravenously will result in a permanent ablation of the C-fiber nerves. This approach is used to determine the contribution of the irritant nerves to processes as diverse as immediate hypersensitivity and acute irritant lung injury.

In humans, capsaicin has been used to characterize the response to irritants of subjects with and without upper airway symptoms. Bascom et al. intranasally challenged 10 historically environmental tobacco smoke (ETS)-sensitive and 11 ETS-nonsensitive subjects with increasing amounts of capsaicin (mixed with lactose powder) (27). ETS-sensitive subjects reported more capsaicin-related rhinorrhea, but showed no difference in nasal lavage histamine, albumin, or kinins compared to ETS-nonsensitive subjects. Approximately half of the subjects demonstrated elevations in TAME esterase activity, but this index of responsiveness was not related to historical ETS sensitivity. Given the apparent lack of capsaicin-induced mast cell activation (histamine or kinins) or vascular permeability changes (albumin or kinins), the TAME esterase response was thought to reflect glandular secretion in response to the capsaicin stimulus. There was an inverse relationship between the symptoms of burning and the increase in TAME-esterase activity.

Stjarne et al. examined the response to capsaicin and nicotine of normal subjects, subjects with vasomotor rhinitis (VMR), and those with VMR in whom sneezing and rhinorrhea were the dominant symptom (VMR-SR) (28). Capsaicin (3×10^{-6} to 3×10^{-3} M, dissolved in 70% ethanol and then diluted)), nicotine bitartrate (6.5×10^{-5} to 6.5×10^{-3} M diluted in saline), and methacholine bromide (5×10^{-6} to 5×10^{-2} M) were applied to the nasal surface. Perception of sensation was similar in the three groups; all reported irritation at the lower doses and increasingly severe pain at the higher doses. Secretion, quantified by the change in weight of a 5×50 mm preweighed piece of absorbent paper applied for 2 min to the septal wall, was increased from 50 to 200 mg in the VMR-SR group. The secretory response was blocked with a combination of ipratropium 0.25 mg/ml (200 µl sprayed 30 min in advance) and 0.5 mg atropine IM delivered via intramuscular injection. Other investigators were unable to block the secretory response to capsaicin with ipratropium alone (29).

The secretory response to capsaicin was blocked on the ipsilateral side with cotton strips soaked in a combination of lignocaine chloride (3.4%) and naphazoline (0.2 mg/ml), which were packed into the nasal cavity and left there for 15 min. Either the local anesthetic or the vasoconstrictor alone did not block the capsaicin-induced irritation or secretion although naphazoline did block basal secretion. Stjarne et al. state that the vasoconstrictor naphazoline served to improve the action of the local anesthetic (which did not alone block sensation). Capsaicin also caused contralateral secretion, which also was blocked by lignocaine and naphazoline combined (28).

More recent studies have demonstrated that capsaicin can increase vascular permeability in the nose, if given at sufficiently high concentrations, particularly in subjects with allergic disease. The relevance of this finding to the typical occupational setting is uncertain, as the dose used in these studies causes more subjective irritation than typically occurs in worksites.

Irritants In Industrial Occupational Settings

The work environment may cause exposure to a variety of reactive/irritant agents, including dusts, acid or caustic mists, solvent vapors, fumes, irritant gases, and combustion products. Nearly 40% of the compounds listed in the *NIOSH Guide to Chemical Hazards* are nasal irritants (30). Table 3 groups these chemicals according to permissible exposure limits. The limits reflect in part the irritant potential but may be lower if the chemical has also been listed as a carcinogen. Included in Table 3 are all substances listed in the *NIOSH Guide* as causing ''irritation: mucous membrane, pharyngeal or respiratory.''

A whole-animal bioassay using 50% inhibition of ventilation (RD50) as the endpoint is typically used to determine irritant potency and permissible exposure levels (28,29). The applicability of the animal assay for human toxicity has been assessed only to a limited degree using subjective irritation, not objective inflammation or mucosal injury. In animals, chronic irritant exposure results in focal upper airway injury occurs, but the site and nature of the injury clearly varies according to the toxicant. The interested reader is referred to excellent publications that summarize the animal toxicological literature (31,32).

Recent animal research has attempted to use two fundamental properties of a gas, reactivity and solubility, to predict the site and nature of the airway mucosal injury. More water-soluble materials, such as ammonia, would act on the proximal airways, while insoluble materials, such as ozone, would act on more distal structures. Reactive molecules would be more likely to exert a toxic effect than their nonreactive counterparts. Ozone, while initially expected to act primarily on the distal airways, has now been shown to act on the nose, and throughout the respiratory tract, a finding attributed to its high reactivity.

Human studies comparing the effects of gas reactivity and solubility on the upper respiratory response have not been performed systematically. However, some studies exist. Table 4 summarizes human studies of the acute effect of

Table 3 Occupational Respiratory Irritants

Levels <1 ppm	Levels <1 ppm, (cont.)	Levels 10–49 ppm	Levels 100–199 ppm
Acrolein	Ozone	Acetic acid	Acetaldehyde (NIOSH-Ca)
Antimony oxide	Paraquat	Ammonia	*n*-Amyl actate
Arsenic	Parathion	2-Butoxyethanol	sec-Amyl acetate
Azinphos-methyl	Pentachlorophenol	beta-Chloroprene	*n*-Butyl acetate
Barium compounds	Perchlorometylmercaptan	(NIOSH CA)	Dibromodifluoromethane
Benzene (NIOSH Ca)	Phosgene	Cyclohexanone	Dipropyleneglycolmonomethylether
Benzoyl peroxide	Phosphoric acid	Diethylamine	Ethylbenzene
Bromine	Phosphorus	2-Diethylaminothanol	Ethylformate
Bromoform	Phosphorus pentachloride	Diisobutylketone	Isoamylacetate
Tert-butyl chromate	Phosphorus pentasulfide	Dimethylamine	Isoamylalcohol
Cadmium	Phosphorus trichloride	Furfuryl alcohol	Isobutyl acetate
Calcium oxide	Pindone	Glycidol	Methyl (*n*-amyl ketone)
Camphor	Platinum	Hydrogen sulfide	Methyl formate
Chlorine	Selenium	Messityl oxide	Methyl methacrylate
Chlorine dioxide	Sulfur pentafluoride	Methyl acrylate	Naptha
Chlorine trifluoride	Terphenyls	Methylamine	*N*-Pentane
Chlorobenzylidene malonitrile	Thiram	Methylcellosolve acetate	2-Pentanone
bis-Chloromethyl ether	Organotins	5-methyl-3-heptanone	Turpentine
Chloromethyl methyl ether	Toluene 2,4-diisocyanate	Morpholine	Vinyl toluene
Chromic acid and chromates	Tributyl phosphate 2,4,6-Trinitrotoluene	Propylene oxide	Xylenes
Copper dusts, mists, and fume	Vanadium pentoxide	Tetrachloroethylene	
Cotton dust	Zinc chloride	(Perchloroethylene)	*At levels ≥200 ppm*
Demeton	Zirconium compounds	(NIOSH Ca)	1,3 Butadiene
Diazomethane		1,1,2 trichlorethane	(NIOSH-Ca)
1,2 Dibromo-3-chloropropane	*At levels 1–9 ppm*	(NIOSH Ca)	2-Butanone
(NIOSH Ca)	Acetic acid	Trichloroethylene	sec-Butyl acetate
Dibutyl phthalate	Acetylene	(NIOSH Ca) 1,2,3 trichloropropane	tert-Butyl acetate
33-		Triethylamine	Chlorobromomethane
		(NIOSH D)	Cyclohexane
			Cyclohexane

Source: This list is primarily drawn from the *NIOSH Pocket Guide to Chemical Hazards* (30) and includes all substances listed as causing "irritation, laryngeal, mucous membrane, pharyngeal, or respiratory." Compounds are grouped by the exposure limits (see text for explanation).
"NIOSH Ca" means the substance should be considered a possible carcinogen. See Acheson for additional discussion of upper airway carcinogens
"NIOSH D" indicates substances for which NIOSH has questioned whether the permissible exposure limits were adequate to protect workers from recognized health hazards.

Table 4 Human Provocation Studies Using Irritants

	Rhinomanometry	Nasal lavage	Mucociliary clearance	Mucosal blood flow	
Ozone	Blocks exercise de-congestion of nonallergics	Inc. PMNs (and eo-sinophils of aller-gic rhinitics)			Graham (1988) Koren et al. (1990) Bascom (1990)
Sulfur dioxide	Inc. NAR NC NAR		Dec. clearance		Andersen (1974) Tam (1988)
	Inc. NAR	NC histamine,			Bascom (1991)
ETS	Inc. NAR	NC albumin,			Willes (1992)
		NC kinins	NC Clearance Variable effects of MCC—some Inc., some NC, some Dec.		Corbo (1989) Nadarajah (1993)
VOCs		Inc. PMNs			Koren et al. (1992)
Carbonless copy paper	Inc. NAR				Morgan (1986)
Capsaicin	NC NAR	NC Histamine, albu-min, kinins some Inc. TAME			Bascom (1991) Rajakulasingam (1992) Stjarne (1989)

Source: Refs. 28, 48, 60, 76. Dec = decreased; Inc. = increased; NC = no change.

diverse irritants on the upper respiratory tract. McLean et al. (33) studied atopic and nonatopic subjects exposed to 100 ppm of ammonia gas insufflated passively into both nostrils for periods ranging from 5 to 20 sec. Although no differences were noted in the response of atopics and nonatopics, a clear dose-response relationship was apparent between duration of ammonia gas exposure and percent increase of nasal airway resistance over baseline. Preinstillation of atropine sulfate spray, but not chlorpheniramine spray, inhibited the response to ammonia in both atopics and nonatopics.

Lundqvist et al. (34) exposed seven normal volunteers to varying concentrations of diethylamine (DEA) and examined the sensory endpoints of olfaction, nasal and eye irritation, as well as changes in nasal airway resistance and nasal volume (as measured by acoustic rhinometry). A dose-response relationship was found for each of the three sensory endpoints with exposure to 0–12 ppm DEA in air. However, no group changes were observed in either nasal airway resistance or nasal volume after 15-min exposures to DEA at 25 ppm.

Petruson and Jarvholm (35) compared 18 workers exposed to dicumylperoxide at a chemical plant with a control group consisting of eight unexposed co-workers and 20 hospital workers; investigators examined a variety of self-reported symptoms and objective measures. The chemical plant workers reported more trouble with nasal crusting and nasal stuffiness—and were noted by examiners to have more nasal mucosal hyperemia, atrophy, and "visible blood vessels"—than did controls. Nasal peak airflow and mucociliary transport rate (as measured by the saccharine test) however, were no different between the two groups. Whether the changes observed were a specific chemical response—or were a nonspecific effect of dust exposure—remains to be determined.

Torjussen (36) compared 318 nickel refining workers with 57 age- and smoking-status-matched hospital controls. No significant differences were found between exposed and control groups for the symptoms of nasal obstruction, recurrent epistaxis, or persistent rhinorrhea, nor for roentgenographic changes. On physical examination, the finding of "hyperplastic rhinitis" was twice as frequent among nickel workers as among controls, as was the finding of nasal polyps; in two of 13 Ni-exposed workers, malignant changes were documented. On histological examination, epithelial dysplasia was significantly more prevalent among Ni-exposed workers than among controls. No physiological tests of nasal function (e.g., rhinomanometry or mucociliary clearance) were performed on this study population.

Ahman (37) compared 11 patients with complaints of work-related nasal congestion with 11 (hospital worker) controls. Identified precipitants included wood dust, paint, diesel exhaust, and paper dust. Over the course of their respective work weeks, patients showed significant decrements in nasal expiratory peak flow ($PEFR_N$) compared to controls.

Occupational Exposures in Nonindustrial Workplaces

Americans spend over 90% of their day indoors, and work increasingly in nonindustrial settings. Pollutants found in nonindustrial workplaces of the indoor environment are thus an important part of an individual's exposure profile (38,39). Irritants present in the indoor environment include combustion products (including environmental tobacco smoke, ETS) and volatile organic compounds (VOCs). A range of VOCs have been measured in indoor environments, often at concentrations much higher that those found in outside air (40). Carpets, upholstered furniture, pressed-wood products, and other interior furnishings/building materials emit a variety of VOCs into indoor air, particularly when new. Similarly, many cleaning products, including floor and furniture waxes, upholstery cleaners, rug shampoos, window cleaners, and tile cleaners, release VOCs into indoor air during normal use. Hydraulic fluid from a building's elevator system may also be a source (41). Examples of VOCs emitted include aliphatic hydrocarbons (hexane through undecane), aromatics (xylene, ethyl benzene), ketones (MEK), aldehydes (formaldehyde), alcohols (isopropanol, butanol), esters (*n*-butyl acetate), glycol ethers/esters (ethoxyethylacetate), and terpenes (a-pinene). VOCs are typically increased in indoor spaces that are newly constructed or recently renovated (42,43), but typically decrease in a logarithmic fashion once renovations are completed.

Despite such identifiable sources or risk factors as sealed windows, synthetic furnishings, ''smoking-permitted'' areas, and contaminated heating, ventilation, and air conditioning equipment, only a minority of problem building investigations have identified specific irritants or irritant sources as the cause of worker symptoms (44). It has been estimated that up to 20% of U.S. office workers consider their workplace to be a ''problem building''—i.e., one in which poor indoor air quality detracts from personal comfort and productivity (45). Typical symptoms reported by occupants of problem buildings include irritation of the eyes, nose, and throat, nasal stuffiness and rhinorrhea, and fatigue, headache, and dry skin (44).

Studies have examined the prevalence and determinants of upper airway symptoms in indoor office environments. Burge et al. surveyed 4373 office workers working in 42 office buildings with a total of 47 ventilation conditions (46). Eighty percent of the workers reported at least one work-related symptom, and more than 40% had work-related stuffy nose, dry throat, or headache. Questions had good short-term and long-term reproducibility. The average number of complaints ranged from 1.25 to 5.25 across the buildings with wide variation existing within each ventilation category. The experience of static electricity shocks was not associated with mucosal irritant complaints. Symptoms increased substantially in buildings in which the air supply was chilled or humidified. Although building-related chest tightness and difficulty breathing had low prevalence (9%),

                                                                Bascom and Shusterman

these symptoms were twice as frequent in buildings with, compared to those without, air chilling or humidification systems.

A brief clinical report entitled "Laser-Printer Rhinitis" described provocation testing performed on an office worker who complained of nasal congestion, headache, and skin burning after a laser printer was placed in his immediate work environment (47). When the patient handled laser-printed paper in a medical setting, the above symptoms were reproduced, along with a fourfold increase in nasal airway resistance. The authors speculated that pyrolized toner may have been a source of volatile irritants.

Morgan and Camp studied 30 office workers with a prior history of upper respiratory tract symptoms while using carbonless copy paper (48). Fifteen-minute controlled exposure to vapors from carbonless paper produced a significantly greater increase in nasal airway resistance than did exposure to filtered air. The magnitude of subjective symptom measures, however, did not correlate with these objective findings.

Theander and Bende (49) studied 15 subjects with a history of rhinitis symptoms from newsprint, and six asymptomatic volunteers. The patients with a history of vasomotor symptoms reported significantly increased nasal symptom scores after exposure to paper dust from newspapers, but not to printing ink vapor. Nasal airway resistance, on the other hand, did not change after either exposure.

Combustion occurs commonly in indoor environments. Tobacco products (cigarettes, cigars, pipes), gas stoves, kerosene space heaters, fireplaces, and malfunctioning furnaces and water heaters may emit carbon monoxide, particulate matter, and a variety of irritant gases. Irritant combustion products include oxides of nitrogen (NO, NO_2), aldehydes (acetaldehyde, formaldehyde, acrolein), pyridine (from cigarettes), sulfur dioxide, and ammonia. In addition, combustion products ("smoke") from outdoor sources (leaf burning, fireplace and wood stove chimneys) may infiltrate into adjacent homes and buildings, particularly when atmospheric inversions are present. ETS, defined as the smoke that non-smokers inhale, is one of the most prevalent indoor pollutants. ETS is a complex mixture of >3000 components. Vapors including carbon monoxide, aldehydes, oxides of nitrogen, nicotine and a semisolid particulate aerosol contain tar and metals. Active smokers reside in 40% of homes, and nearly 70% of adolescents have been exposed to residential ETS (50,51).

Acute symptoms of ETS exposure include eye and nasal irritation, and in some individuals, rhinitis symptoms including rhinorrhea and congestion. Subjects with a history of ETS rhinitis demonstrate increased nasal resistance with controlled exposure to brief high levels of smoke compared with subjects with no history of ETS rhinitis. Bascom et al. examined NAR and nasal lavage fluid before and after a 15-min challenge using sidestream tobacco smoke (45 ppm CO) as a surrogate for ETS (52). Ten historically ETS-sensitive subjects, on the average, reported more nasal symptoms, and experienced greater cross-exposure increases in NAR, than did 11 historically non-ETS-sensitive individuals. The biochemical profile of nasal lavage fluid was not characteristic of an allergic reaction. Specifically, the increased resistance is unassociated with increased vascular permeability or activation of mast cells (i.e., there was no increase in histamine, albumin, kinin, or TAME esterase activity postexposure). Thus while patients may report that they are "allergic to tobacco smoke," there is no evidence for an IgE-mediated allergic mechanism although there is objective evidence of altered reactivity. Additional studies demonstrate that both groups develop nasal congestion with prolonged exposure to moderate levels of ETS (53), but only subjects with a history of ETS rhinitis demonstrate increased congestion with exposure to moderate levels of the vapor phase of smoke. Increased congestion with intranasal substance P is also demonstrable in subjects with ETS-induced nasal congestion, but not in subjects without ETS-induced nasal congestion (54).

Exposure to ETS is associated with increased rates of middle ear effusions in children (50). Nasal mucociliary clearance times were determined in a randomly selected sample of schoolchildren (142 boys and 153 girls, age range 11–14 years). Nasal mucociliary clearance times showed a narrow coefficient of repeatability (6 min) in 50 subjects and there was substantial agreement between the two tests. Nasal mucociliary clearance time was less than 40 min in all the children. The authors were unable to show that passive smoking had any consistent effect on nasal mucociliary clearance. In controlled human exposure studies using adult volunteers, ETS has variable effects on nasal mucociliary clearance in human subjects (55). Some subjects demonstrate marked inhibition of mucociliary clearance following smoke exposure; others demonstrate acceleration of clearance. A history of tobacco smoke sensitivity may be related to an increased risk of decreased mucociliary clearance.

Formaldehyde is an aldehyde that is a common constituent at low levels in the indoor air. Sources of formaldehyde include insulation (no longer installed in residential dwellings) and finishes on fabrics used in furnishings. Acute symptoms of upper respiratory tract irritation occur with formaldehyde exposure. An epidemiological study compared several thousand Canadians living in homes insulated with urea formaldehyde foam insulation (UFFI) with those living in homes that were not insulated with UFFI. The study found a small excess of many symptoms among individuals living in the formaldehyde-insulated homes. Subjects who were intending to move or have the insulation removed had an increase in squamous metaplasia in nasal samples and a decrease in neutrophils (56). There was no difference in the nasal resistance, skin patch tests, or spirometric lung function in the two groups.

Toluene is a common workplace solvent. Andersen and colleagues (57) exposed 16 healthy volunteers for 6 hr to varying concentrations of toluene (0, 10, 40, and 100 ppm) in a climate-controlled chamber. A dose-response relationship was observed for odor intensity and deterioration of perceived air quality.

decongestion among healthy normal subjects, but decongests allergic subjects. Subjects with preexisting allergic rhinitis have a more complex cellular response to ozone and demonstrate an influx of neutrophils, eosinophils, and mononuclear cells in nasal lavage fluid (40).

Chronic exposure to ozone alters the nasal epithelium. Studies of Mexican military recruits show an increase in squamous metaplasia among those stationed in areas of urban pollution compared with recruits stationed in rural, low pollution areas (54). In studies of macaque primates who underwent exposure to O_3 for 6 or 90 days to 0.15 or 0.3 ppm, lesions consisted of ciliated cell necrosis, shortened cilia, and secretory cell hyperplasia. Inflammatory cell influx was present at 6 days of exposure but not at 90 days postexposure. Ultrastructural changes in goblet cells were evident at 90 days (55). Rodents also show the induction of focal epithelial changes in the anterior portion of the nasal passage. Studies using inbred strains of mice show that the presence of a neutrophil influx is genetically determined. Strains of mice that demonstrate the highest rates of neutrophil influx to the nasal mucosal surface show the lowest indices of epithelial injury.

The effect of ozone on primary allergic sensitization and secondary responses has been studied in a few protocols. Exposure to ozone at a concentration of 0.5 ppm for 4 hr did not increase the subsequent acute response to nasal challenge with allergen in subjects with a history of rhinitis (56). Alternating respiratory ozone and allergen exposure in guinea pigs resulted in increased rates of allergic sensitization, and clearance studies demonstrated reduced clearance of the antigen after ozone exposure (57–59). If the antigen was presented to the peritoneum alternating with respiratory ozone exposure, no increase in primary sensitization or in anaphylaxis occurred.

Particles, SO₂, and Acid Aerosols

Particles, SO_2, and acid aerosols are derived from combustion of fossil fuels. SO_2 is a highly soluble gas that is 99% absorbed by the upper airway under conditions of resting ventilation. Mouth breathing or rapid nasal breathing will result in delivery of some SO_2 to the lower airway (60). SO_2 exposure has been associated with an increased nasal work of breathing, an effect blocked by high-dose antihistamines (61,62). Andersen et al. (63) examined NAR and nasal mucus flow rate in 15 subjects before and after 3- and 6-hr exposures to SO_2 at 1, 5, and 25 ppm. A dose-response relationship was found for reduced nasal mucociliary clearance rate and increased NAR (expressed as effective cross-sectional nasal area), with the main response occurring between 1 and 5 ppm for NAR and between 5 and 25 ppm for mucociliary clearance rate. Six-hour exposures produced significantly greater changes in both NAR and mucus flow rates than did 3-hr exposures. Investigators noted anecdotally that subjects with lower baseline mucociliary clearance reported a greater intensity of irritation with SO_2 exposure.

Tam et al. examined nasal symptoms and NAR among 22 subjects with rhinitis and eight with both rhinitis and asthma (33). Exposure to SO_2 at up to 4 ppm times 10 min was compared with exposure to filtered air. In contrast to the Andersen study, no SO_2-related upper respiratory tract symptoms or NAR changes were observed after these relatively brief exposures, including among subjects with SO_2-induced pulmonary function changes.

Nitrogen Dioxide

Nitrogen dioxide (NO_2), a product of fossil fuel combustion, is present in outdoor air and indoor air (64,65). Animal studies indicate that NO_2 may alter host defense, particularly by increasing susceptibility to infection. The effect of NO_2 exposure on influenza viral infectivity was evaluated. While no statistically significant increase was demonstrated, high rates of baseline infectivity reduced the power of the study (66). Exposure of guinea pigs to alternating NO_2 and antigen exposure increases rates of primary sensitization.

Air Toxics

Ambient (outdoor) air pollution also includes a number of irritant compounds, and elevated levels of VOCs have been documented in ambient air near hazardous waste sites and near hazardous waste incinerators (67). Kharrazi et al. (68) reviewed telephone surveillance data for odor and symptom complaints near a hazardous waste site undergoing remedial action. Complaints of upper respiratory tract and eye irritation, in many cases without concurrently reported odors, peaked during a period that the site's air containment malfunctioned, at which time fence line measurements of volatile hydrocarbons also reached their highest levels (7–10 ppm).

Physical Stimuli

Exercise is associated with nasal decongestion (96). Exposure to cold air results in rhinitis in some, but not all, healthy normal subjects (97,98). Nasal challenge studies showed that subjects with a history of cold-induced rhinitis developed congestion and had elevations of nasal lavage epithelial cells and elevated concentrations of histamine, TAME-esterase activity, and albumin. Subjects without a history of cold-induced rhinitis showed no such changes. Exposure of either group of subjects to warm, moist air did not alter nasal patency, or cellular or mediator levels in lavage fluid.

A brief jet of air delivered to the anterior nasal surface will alter the nasal transepithelial potential difference of the anterior portion of the inferior turbinate but will not alter the potential difference of the vestibule or anterior septum (99). Inspection of the nasal mucosa following the stimulus will show no observable change although the subject reports focal irritation. This example illustrates the insensitivity of the physical examination in detecting altered nasal mucosal integrity.

Allergen exposure will alter the behavior of neural pathways. Allergic subjects out of their allergy season will demonstrate an ipsilateral inflammatory response to local application of intranasal kinins. Subjects currently symptomatic with seasonal allergic rhinitis will demonstrate both an ipsilateral and a contralateral response to local application of kinins. Animal studies indicate that allergen exposure of sensitized animals will increase the amplitude and prolong the duration of firing of autonomic ganglia (108).

D. Other Agents

Corrosives are defined as agents that provoke direct tissue injury. Chromium is one of the best-known corrosives, and exposed workers can develop nasal septal

Table 5 Miscellaneous Occupational Upper Respiratory Effects

Ulcers/perforated nasal septum
    Arsenic
    Calcium oxide
    Chromic acid and chromates
    Copper dusts and mists
Epistaxis
    Warfarin
    Pindone
Rhinorrhea (with miosis, lacrimation, salivation)
    Carbaryl
    EPN (*O*-Ethyl-*O*-*p*-nitrophenylbenzenephosphothioate)
    Malathion
    Parathion
    Phosdrin
    Pyrethrum
    TEDP (dithion)
    TEPP (ethylpyrophosphate)
Blue-gray nasal septum
    Silver
Numb mucous membrane
    Rotenone
    DDT
Edema on nasal folds
    Nitramine
Stomatitis
    Mercury vapor

Source: Data obtained from the *NIOSH Pocket Guide to Chemical Hazards*.

Table 6 Upper Respiratory Tract Exposures and Cancer: Upper Airway Carcinogens (possible or probable)

Ammonia	Upper airways
Arsenic	Upper airways/upper respiratory
Asbestos	Laryngeal
Benzene	Upper airways
Bis(-Ethylhexyl) phthalate	Upper respiratory
Cadmium	Upper airways, nasopharyngeal
Carbon black	Not specified
Chlorinated hydrocarbons	Upper airways
Chromium	Upper airways, upper respiratory
Chromic trioxide	Oral papillomas
Cutting oils	Respiratory
Diethyl sulfate	Laryngeal
Ethylbenzene	Upper respiratory
Isopropanol	Upper respiratory
Leather products	Type unknown, boot and shoe operatives and repairers
Mercury	Upper airways
Mineral fibers	Oral, pharyngeal
Mustard gas	Buccal, Pharynx, larynx
Nickel	Upper respiratory, nasal, sinus, and nasopharyngeal
Radium	Upper airway, mastoid, and paranasal sinuses
Silica	Upper respiratory
Sulfuric acid	Laryngeal, pharyngeal, sinuses
Tetrabromomethane	Upper respiratory
Vanadium	Upper airways
Wood dust	Nasal
Zinc	Sinus, nose, and throat

This list is based on one or more articles in the literature. It does not reflect the judgment of a regulatory or scientific review organization.

ulcers and septal perforation. Other occupational respiratory effects are also shown in Table 5. Upper airway neoplasms have been documented in some occupational groups; Table 6 lists implicated agents.

Regular contact with organic mixtures occurs in occupations such as farming, crop storage, and agriculture-based manufacturing. A current hypothesis receiving increasing experimental support is that contamination of the dust with endotoxin is the main cause of its toxicity (61–63).

Contamination of organic dusts with chemical irritants may cause toxicity that does not occur with the organic dust alone. Holmstrom et al. (64) compared workers exposed to dust from medium-density fiberboard (mdf) with workers exposed to other wood dust and to civil servants not exposed to dusts or irritants. Compared to both reference groups, mdf-exposed workers reported more symptoms of nasal and eye irritation, nasal congestion, and olfactory impairment. In addition, baseline NAR was higher, and decongestant-related changes in NAR were greater in the mdf-exposed group than in either reference group. Histological changes to the nasal mucosa were seen in the workers exposed to dust but not in the civil servants (65). Mdf exposure was thought secondary to the presence of formaldehyde as a component of the binder glue.

Wilmhelmsson and Drettner (66) surveyed 676 workers from 50 different wood furniture factories, comparing heavily exposed to minimally exposed individuals. The investigators found a significantly greater proportion of heavily exposed workers with self-reported nasal obstruction, rhinorrhea, and "frequent" (greater than twice-a-year) colds. In a subset of 61 intensively studied workers, heavily exposed workers tested during the work shift had greater decongestant-induced changes in nasal airway resistance than did less exposed controls. This finding indicated that vascular congestion was occurring in the heavily exposed workers. The heavily exposed workers also had a higher prevalence of delayed mucociliary clearance (cardiogreen and saccharine tests) than did controls. Industrial hygiene measurements documented between 0.3 and 5.1 mg/m^3 of wood dust in the air of the factories tested.

IV. Clinical Approach

A. Occupational History

Evaluation of a patient with a possible occupational rhinitis begins with a history of the present illness, with particular attention to temporal patterns of symptoms related to work exposures. Exacerbations on weekdays with improvement on weekends may suggest an occupational allergen or irritant. The dates of prolonged absences due to business travel or vacation should be ascertained, since some work-related problems improve only with prolonged absences. Workplace accidents or unusual incidents associated with disease onset should be reviewed and noted in the record. The use and type of respiratory protection should also be noted.

The occupational history consists of a complete, chronological list of all jobs. Providing the patient a questionnaire to complete in advance of the visit will save considerable time. For each job, the patient should list employer, job title, job description, duration of employment, reason for leaving, and any known exposures or health symptoms. With the initial questionnaire in hand, the physician can then obtain additional information as dictated by the history of the present illness. It is useful to determine whether workplace exposures are highly consistent from day to day or may vary tremendously. The identification of point sources, their disruption, transformation, and proximity to the patient all aid in the estimate of exposure intensity.

Worker "right-to-know" laws are well established in many countries. They state that the treating physician has a right to material safety data sheets (MSDS) that identify the composition and hazards of workplace substances. Many workplaces that have potential hazards have some kind of medical monitoring program for workers. Review of preplacement medical examinations can help determine antecedent symptoms.

Studies that may assist an occupational rhinitis evaluation include skin testing or RAST testing for allergens specific to the workplace and bulk dust sampling of the home and workplace. Completion of diaries to serial symptoms and lower airway function often contributes useful information about the temporal pattern of symptoms. Clinicians in some countries, such as Sweden, have experience with nasal peak flow meters, but these are not widely available at present. Nasal provocation is rarely used in the diagnosis of occupational rhinitis in the United States at present. However, allergists and occupational physicians in Finland routinely use nasal provocation testing for diagnosis. Generally speaking, the degree of skin test reactivity (measured by skin test wheal size) correlates with the nasal provocation response (quantified by posterior rhinomanometry and rhinitis symptoms) (67).

B. Clinical Syndromes

Allergic and Irritant Rhinitis

Exposure to allergens typically causes sneezing, itching, rhinorrhea, and congestion. In contrast, exposure to irritants rarely causes itching, but may cause acute symptoms of burning or irritation in addition to rhinorrhea and congestion. While avoidance is advised for both allergens and irritants (68), this may be difficult when the exposure is occupational in origin, or when the patient is not in control of the environment. Textbooks report that persistent irritation of the nasal mucosa may cause chronic rhinosinusitis, but the magnitude and time course of development are poorly understood (69). Allergen exposure will alter the behavior of neural pathways, and hence the response to irritants. Animal studies indicate that allergen exposure of sensitized animals will increase the amplitude and prolong the duration of firing of autonomic ganglia (70). Allergic subjects out of their allergy season will demonstrate an ipsilateral inflammatory response to local application of intranasal kinins. Subjects currently symptomatic with seasonal allergic rhinitis will demonstrate both an ipsilateral and a contralateral response to local application of kinins, indicating altered neural reflexes. These selected examples emphasize the likelihood of clinically important interactions, still poorly understood, between allergens and irritants.

The main clinical message from inhalation challenge studies is that the pathogenesis of allergic and irritant rhinitis is different. Also, the pathogenesis of different kinds of irritant rhinitis is different. A major clinical research challenge is to determine whether improved control of nonallergic rhinitis can be achieved by understanding and interrupting the responses to these common occupational irritants.

Epiglottic Dysfunction

Epiglottic dysfunction due to thermal and chemical burns may occur. Epiglottic dysfunction has been reported in association with isocyanate exposure (71). A 34-year-old, nonsmoking, nonatopic, previously healthy worker developed diaphoresis, nasal congestion, pleuritic chest pain, and a dry cough. He also had symptoms suggestive of aspiration. His job involved making award plaques using 65% methylene diisocyanate and 35% aromatic hydrocarbons. The epiglottic obstruction was demonstrated by barium contrast cineradiography and upper airway symptoms resolved with total epiglottectomy. Histology showed marked chronic submucosal inflammatory changes with focal fibrosis edema and reactive changes. Symptoms of asthma persisted.

Laryngeal Disease

Laryngeal symptoms are common among patients reporting symptoms of rhinosinusitis. Two symptoms are particularly troublesome. Hoarseness may interfere with a worker's ability to perform his or her tasks, if duties include verbal communication. A second symptom, far less common, is that of functional upper airway obstruction. Patients will report "laryngospasm" or a feeling that their airway is closing off. On examination the physician will observe the presence of stridor on inspiration during quiet breathing, with auscultation confirming the sound emanating from the region of the larynx. Patients are often markedly anxious and may be intubated by physicians fearing impending airway obstruction. Patients typically can speak normally, and the functional obstruction then recurs with quiet breathing. Visualization of the vocal cords during an episode of stridor shows paradoxical closure of the cords without edema or fixed obstruction. Symptomatic relief has been achieved in some cases with muscle relaxants and the use of a helium-oxygen mixture. Speech therapy may help to retrain patients to recognize and break the cycle. In some cases, this syndrome has begun after an occupational or environmental exposures. In one case, early closure of the inspiratory limb of flow volume loops was demonstrated. The pathogenesis of this syndrome is not well understood (72), nor is a single nomenclature widely accepted. We have used a clinical evaluation protocol, developed with a otolaryngologist and speech therapist, to evaluate patients for airways disease and dysfunction. In a pulmonary function laboratory, patients undergo methacholine challenge with speech evaluation and rhinolaryngoscopy pre- and postchallenge. With this approach, dignoses of hyperfunctional voice disorder, laryngeal dysfunction, and reactive airways are made in a high proportion of patients reporting work-associated symptoms.

Laryngeal obstruction can occur acutely as a sequel of an inhalation injury (73). The risk is related to the magnitude of the insult and the surface area that has been burned. An exception is facial burns, where delayed laryngeal edema has been observed. Ignition of hair grease is an example of an environmental exposure where upper airway injury is common (74).

Malignancy

Nasal blockage, developing in an adult, cannot be ascribed exclusively to septal deviation, unless the patient has had a traumatic fracture. Malignant tumors in the nose, paranasal sinuses, and nasopharynx usually start with uncharacteristic symptoms, although patients typically receive an initial diagnosis of perennial nonallergic rhinitis. Nasal endoscopy and imaging of paranasal sinuses are obligatory in patients with unilateral symptoms, hemorrhagic secretions, or pain (75).

V. Summary and Conclusions

Many agents encountered in the workplace may cause or worsen upper respiratory tract disease. These agents include allergens, irritants, corrosive agents, and carcinogens. Exposure to mixtures is common.

The approach to a patient with suspected occupational rhinitis begins with a clear definition of the problem. In addition, an occupational history focuses on the nature and magnitude of work site exposures and the temporal relationships between times at work and disease onset or exacerbation. Longitudinal evaluation will often be necessary to confirm the clinical history.

When occupational exposures are identified, the clinician may provide useful guidance to the employer about the nature and site of the exposure, the health risks, and necessary action. While the employer may need expert occupational and industrial hygiene assistance to address the problem, it is the treating physician who is often the first to diagnose the patient with occupational rhinitis.

References

1. Gergen PJ, Turkeltaub PC. The association of allergen skin test reactivity and respiratory disease among whites in the US population. Data from the second National Health and Nutrition Examination Survey, 1976–1980. Arch Intern Med 1991;151: 487–492.

2. Environmental Protection Agency. Indoor Air Quality and Work Environment Study: EPA Headquarters' Buildings. Vol 1: Employee Survey. EPA, 1989.

3. Kauffmann F, Neukirch F, Annesi I, Korobaeff M, Dore M-F, Lellouch J. Relation of perceived nasal and bronchial hyperresponsiveness to FEV_1, basophil counts, and methacholine response. Thorax 1988;43:456–461.

4. DeZotti R, Patussi V, Fiorito A, Larese F. Sensitization to green coffee bean (GCB) and castor bean (CB) allergens among dock workers. Int Arch Occup Environ Health 1988;61:7–12.

5. Chan-Yeung M, Barton G, MacLean L, Grzybowski S. Occupational asthma and rhinitis due to western red cedar. Am Rev Respir Dis 1973;1094–1102.

6. Pope AM, Patterson R, Burge H. Indoor allergens. Assessing and controlling adverse health effects. Committee on the Health Effects of Indoor Allergens (R. Bascom, committee member), Division of Health Promotion and Disease Prevention, Institute of Medicine, 1993:308.

7. Chan-Yeung (Chair) M, Brooks S, Alberts WM, Balmes JR, Barnhart S, Bascom R, Bernstein IL, Grammer LC, Harber P, Malo J-L, Rose C, Schawartz DA, Tarlo S, Utell MJ. ACCP Consensus Statement: Assessment of asthma in the workplace. Chest 1995;108:1084–1117.

8. Chan-Yeung M, Lam S. Occupational asthma: State of the Art. Am Rev Respir Dis 1986;133:686–703.

9. Venables KM. Low molecular weight chemicals, hypersensitivity, and direct toxicity: the acid anhydrides. Br J Indust Med 1989;46:222–232.

10. NIOSH. Criteria for a Recommended Standard. Occupational Exposure to Toluene Diisocyanate. NIOSH, 1973.

11. Kanerva DL, Tupasela O, Jolanki R, Vaheri E, Estlander U, Keskinen H. Occupational allergic rhinitis from guar gum. Clin Allergy 1988;18:245–252.

12. Schwartz H, Arnold J, Strohl K. Occupational allergic rhinitis reaction to psyllium. J Occup Med 1989;31:624–626.

13. Niinimaki A, RK,PT, and Am K. Papain-induced allergic rhinoconjunctivitis in a cosmetologist. J Allergy Clin Immunol 1993;92:492–493.

14. Eggleston PA, Ansari AA, Ziemann B, Adkinsor Jr NF, Corn M. Occupational challenge studies with laboratory workers allergic to rats. J Allergy Clin Immunol 1990; 86:63–72.

15. Jaeger D, Kleinhans D, Czuppon A, Baur X. Latex-specific proteins causing immediate-type cutaneous, nasal, bronchial, and systemic reactions. J Allergy Clin Immunol 1992;89:759–768.

16. Silver WL. Neural and pharmacological basis for nasal irritation. Ann NY Acad Sci 1992;641:152–163.

17. Bascom R. Differential responsiveness to irritant mixtures: possible mechanisms. Ann NY Acad Sci 1992;641:225–247.

18. Nielsen GD. Mechanisms of activation of the sensory irritant receptor by airbome chemicals. CRC Crit Rev Toxicol 1991;21:183–208.

19. Widdicombe J. Nasal pathophysiology. Respir Med 1990;84(Suppl A):3–9.

20. Cain WS. Perceptual characteristics of nasal irritation. In: Green BG, Mason JR, Kare MR, eds. Chemical Senses. Vol 2: Irritation. New York: Marcel Dekker, 1990: 43–60.

21. Baraniuk JN, Kaliner M. Neuropeptides and nasal secretion. Am J Physiol (Lung Cell Mol Physiol) 1991;261:L223–L235.

22. Barrow CS, Buckley LA, James RA, Steinhagen WH, Chang JCF. Sensory irritation: studies on correlation to pathology, structure-activity, tolerance development, and prediction of species differences to nasal injury. In: Barrow CS, ed. Toxicology of the Nasal Passages. Washington, DC: Hemisphere Publishing Corporation, 1986: 101–122.

23. Feron VJ, Woutersen RA, Spit BJ. 5. Pathology of chronic nasal toxic responses including cancer. In: Barrow CS, ed. Toxicology of the Nasal Passages. Washington DC: Hemisphere Publishing Corporation, 1986:67–89.

24. Jiang X-Z, Morgan KT, Beauchamp Jr RO. 4. Histopathology of acute and subacute nasal toxicity. In: Barrow CS, ed. Toxicology of the Nasal Passages. Washington, DC: Hemisphere Publishing Corporation, 1986:51–86.

25. Popp JA, Monteiro-Rivera NA, Martin JT. 3. Ultrastructure of the rat nasal mucosa. In: Barrow CS, ed. Toxicology of the Nasal Passages. Washington, DC: Hemisphere Publishing Corporation, 1986:37–49.

26. Schreider JP. 1. Comparative anatomy and function of the nasal passages. In: Barrow CS, ed. Toxicology of the Nasal Passages. Washington, DC: Hemisphere Publishing Corporation, 1986:1–25.

27. Bascom R, Kagey-Sobotka A, Proud D. Effect of intranasal capsaicin on symptoms and mediator release. J Pharmacol Exp Ther 1991;259:1323–1327.

28. Stjarne P, Lundblad L, Lundberg JM, Anggard A. Capsaicin and nicotine-sensitive afferent neurones and nasal secretion in healthy human volunteers and in patients with vasomotor rhinitis. Br J Pharmacol 1989;96:693–701.

29. Geppetti P, Fusco BM, Marabini S, Maggi CA, Fanciullacci M, Sicuteri F. Secretion, pain and sneezing induced by the application of capsaicin to the nasal mucosa in man. Br J Pharmacol 1988;93:509–514.

30. NIOSH Pocket Guide to Chemical Hazards. DHHS(NIOSH) Publication No. 1990; 90–117:245.

31. Barrow CS, ed. Toxicology of the Nasal Passages. Washington, DC: Hemisphere Publishing Corporation, 1986:317.

32. Kimbell JS, Morgan KT. Upper respiratory tract toxicology, airflow modeling, and supercomputers. CIIT Activ 1990;10:1–9.

33. McLean J, Mathews K, Solomon W, Brayton P, Bayne N. Effect of ammonia on nasal resistance in atopic and nonatopic subjects. Ann Otol Rhinol Laryngol 1979; 88:228–234.

34. Lundqvist G, Yamagiwa M, Pedersen O, Nielsen G. Inhalation of diethylamine— acute nasal effects and subjective response. Am Indust Hyg Assoc J 1992;53:181– 185.

35. Petruson B, Jarvholm B. Formation of new blood vessels in the nose after exposure to dicumylperoxide at a chemical plant. Acta Otolaryngol (Stockh) 1983;95:333–339.

36. Torjussen W. Rhinoscopical findings in nickel workers, with special emphasis on the influence of nickel exposure and smoking habits. Acta Otolaryngol 1979;88: 279–288.

37. Ahman M. Nasal peak flow rate records in work related nasal blockage. Acta Otolaryngol (Stockh) 1992;112:839–844.

38. Samet JM, Marbury MC, Spengler JD. Health effects and sources of indoor air pollution. Part I. Am Rev Respir Dis 1987;136:1486–1508.
39. Samet JM, Marbury MC, Spengler JD. Health effects and sources of indoor air pollution. Part II. Am Rev Respir Dis 1988;137:221–242.
40. Wallace L. The TEAM Study: Personal exposures to toxic substances in air, drinking water, and breath of 400 residents of New Jersey, North Carolina, and North Dakota. Environ Res 1987;43:290–307.
41. Weschler C, Shields H, Rainer D. Concentrations of volatile organic compounds at a building with health and comfort complaints. Am Indust Hyg Assoc J 1990;51:261–268.
42. Molhave L, Moller J. The atmospheric environment in modern Danish dwellings—measurements in 39 flats. In: Fanger PO, Valbjorn O, eds. Indoor Climate. Horsholm, Denmark: SBI, 1979:171–186.
43. Molhave L. Indoor air pollution due to organic gases and vapours of solvents in building materials. Environ Int 1982;8:117–127.
44. Kreiss K. The epidemiology of building-related complaints and illness. In: James MJH, Cone E, eds. Problem Buildings: Building-Associated Illness and the Sick Building Syndrome. Philadelphia: Hanley & Belfus, 1989:575–592.
45. Woods JE, Drewry GM, Moery PR. Office workers perceptions of indoor air quality effects on discomfort and performance. Indoor Air '87, Proceedings of the 4th International Conference on Indoor Air Quality and Climate, 1987.
46. Burge S, Hedge A, Wilson S, et al. Sick building syndrome: a study of 4373 office workers. Ann Occup Hyg 1987;31:493–504.
47. Skoner DP, Hodgson MJ, Doyle WJ. Laser-printer rhinitis. N Engl J Med 1990;322:1323 (letter).
48. Morgan MS, Camp JE. Upper respiratory irritation from controlled exposure to vapor from carbonless copy paper. J Occup Med 1986;1986:415–419.
49. Theander C, Bende M. Nasal hyperreactivity to newspapers. Clin Exp Allergy 1989;19:57–58.
50. The Health Consequences of Involuntary Smoking: A Report of the Surgeon General. Publication no. DHHS (CDC) 87-8398. 1986:227–260.
51. Weiss S, Tager I, Schenker M, Speizer F. State of the Art: The health effects of involuntary smoking. Am Rev Respir Dis 1983;128:933–942.
52. Bascom R, Kulle T, Kagey-Sobotka A, Proud D. Upper respiratory tract environmental tobacco smoke sensitivity. Am Rev Respir Dis 1991;143:1304–1311.
53. Bascom R, Fitzgerald TK, Permutt T, Sauder L, Nadarajah J, Swift DL. Response to environmental tobacco smoke: dose-response studies and the effect on acoustic rhinometry. Am Rev Respir Dis 1992;145:A92.
54. Leonard JF, Fitzgerald TK, Bascom R. Substance P nasal challenge in environmental tobacco smoke responsive subjects. Am Rev Respir Dis 1992;145:A87.
55. Bascom R, Kesavanathan J, Fitzgerald TK, Cheng K-H, Swift DL, Sidestream tobacco smoke exposure acutely alters human nasal mucociliary clearance. Environ Health Perspect 1995;103:1026–1030.
56. Broder I, Corey P, Cole P, Lipa M. Comparison of the health of occupants and characteristics of houses among control homes and homes insulated with urea form-

aldehyde foam. II. Initial health and house variables and exposure-response relationships. Environ Res 1988;45:156–178.

57. Andersen I, Lundqvist G, Molhave L, Pedersen O, Proctor D, Vaeth M, Wyon D. Human response to controlled levels of toluene in six-hour exposures. Scand J Work Environ Health 1983;9:405–418.

58. Molhave L, Bach B, Pedersen OF. Human reactions to low concentrations of volatile organic compounds. Environ Int 1986;12:167–175.

59. Hudnell H, Otto D, House D, Molhave L. Exposure of humans to a volatile organic mixture. II. Sensory. Arch Environ Health 1992;47:31–38.

60. Koren H, Graham D, Devlin R. Exposure of humans to a volatile organic mixture. III. Inflammatory response. Arch Environ Health 1992;47:39–44.

61. Rylander R, Haglind P, Lundholm M. Endotoxin in cotton dust and respiratory function decrement among cotton workers in an experimental cardroom. Am Rev Respir Dis 1985;131:209–213.

62. Rylander R, Burrell R. Endotoxins in inhalation research. Summary of conclusions of a workshop held at Clearwater, Florida, U.S.A., 28–30 September 1987. Ann Occup Hyg 1988;32:553–556.

63. Rylander R. Organic dusts—from knowledge to prevention. Scand J Work Environ Health 1994;20(spec no):116–122.

64. Holmstrom M, Rosen G, Wilhelmsson B. Symptoms, airway physiology and histology of workers exposed to medium-density fiber board. Scand J Work Environ Health 1991;17:409–413.

65. Holmstrom M, Wilhelmsson B, Hellquist H, Rosen G. Histological changes in the nasal mucosa in persons occupationally exposed to formaldehyde alone and in combination with wood dust. Acta Otolaryngol (Stockh) 1989;107:120–129.

66. Wilhelmsson B, Drettner B. Nasal problems in wood furniture workers. A study of symptoms and physiological variables. Acta Otolaryngol (Stockh) 1984;98:548–555.

67. Small P, Biskin N. Relationship between allergen-specific skin testing and nasal provocation in patients with perennial rhinitis. Ann Allergy 1992;68:331–333.

68. Meltzer EO, Schatz M, Zeiger RS. Allergic and Nonallergic rhinitis. In: Middleton Jr E, Reed CE, Ellis EF, Adkinson NF Jr, Yunginger JW, eds. Allergy Principles and Practice. Washington, II DC CV Mosby, 1988:1253–1289.

69. Gluckman JL, Stegmoyer R. Nonallergic rhinitis. In: Paparella MM, Shumrick DA, Gluckman JL, Meyerhoff WL, eds. Otolaryngology. Philadelphia: WB Saunders 1988;1889–1898.

70. Weinreich D, Undem BJ. Immunological regulation of synaptic transmission in isolated guinea pig autonomic ganglia. J Clin Invest 1987;79:1529–1532.

71. Sales JH, Kennedy K. Epiglottic dysfunction after isocyanate inhalation exposure. Arch Otolaryngol Head Neck Surg 1990;116:725–727.

72. Sim T, McClean S, Lee J, Naranjo M, Grant J. Functional laryngeal obstruction: a somatization disorder. Am J Med 1990;88:293–296.

73. Haponik E, Crapo R, Herndon D, Traber D, Hudson L, Moylan J. Smoke inhalation. Am Rev Respir Dis 1988;138:1060–1063.

74. Bascom R, Haponik E, Munster A. Inhalation injury related to the use of petrolatum-based hair grease. J Bum Care Rehabil 1984;5:327–330.

75. Mygind N, Naclerio RM. Definition, classification, terminology. In: Mygind N, Naclerio RM, eds. Allergic and Non-allergic Rhinitis. Copenhagen: Munksgaard, 1993;11–14.

76. Willes S, Raford P, Baroody F, Fitzgerald TK, Bascom R. Differential responses to ozone in allergic and non-allergic subjects. Am Rev Respir Dis 1991;143:A91.

77. Andersen I, Lundgvist GR, Jensen PL, Proctor DF. Human response to controlled levels of sulfur dioxide. Arch Environ Health 1974;28:31–39.

78. Tam EK, Liu J, Bigby BG, Boushey HA. Sulfur dioxide does not acutely increase nasal symptoms or nasal resistance in subjects with rhinitis or in subjects with bronchial responsiveness to sulfur dioxide. Am Rev Respir Dis 1988;138:1559–1564.

79. Willes S, Fitzgerald T., Bascom R. Nasal inhalation challenge studies with sidestream tobacco smoke. Arch Environ Health 1992;47:223–230.

80. Rajakulasingam K, Polosa R, Lau L, Church M, Holgate S, Howarth P. Nasal effects of bradykinin and capsaicin: influence on plasma protein leakage and role of sensory neurons. J Appl Physiol 1992;72:1418–1424.

81. Koren H, Hatch GE, Graham DE. Nasal lavage as a tool in assessing acute inflammation in response to inhaled pollutants. Toxicology 1990;60:15–25.

82. Graham D, Henderson F, House D. Neutrophil influx measured in nasal lavages of humans exposed to ozone. Arch Environ Health 1988;43:228–233.

83. Bascom R, Naclerio RM, Fitzgerald TK, Kagey-Sobotka A, Proud D. Effect of ozone inhalation on the response to nasal challenge with antigen of allergic subjects. Am Rev Respir Dis 1990;141:594–601.

84. Nadarajah J, Bascom R, Fitzgerald TK, Bickert M, Cheng K, Permutt T, Swift D. Sidestream tobacco smoke(SS) alters regional nasal mucociliary clearance: comparison of sensitive and nonsensitive subjects. Am Rev Respir Dis 1993;147:A216.

6

Food Allergy and Intolerance

HUGH A. SAMPSON

The Mount Sinai School of Medicine
New York, New York

PHILIPPE A. EIGENMANN

University of Geneva School of Medicine
Geneva, Switzerland

I. Introduction

In his "Discussion on Paroxysmal Rhinorrhea" to the Royal Society of Medicine in 1925, Freeman convincingly demonstrated that ingested food proteins could provoke nasal symptoms similar to those seen in grass pollenosis (1). On the morning of his lecture, Freeman passively sensitized the middle turbinate of a colleague's nose with serum from a grass-allergic patient and the middle turbinate of his own nose with serum from an egg-allergic patient. Prior to his lecture, Freeman's colleague inhaled a small amount of grass pollen and immediately developed sneezing, congestion, and rhinorrhea. Similarly, after Freeman ingested an "egg flip," he developed congestion and pruritus on the passively sensitized side of his nose. The nasal symptoms persisted for several hours. This demonstration clearly showed that ingested protein could reach the nasal mucosa and provoke classic allergic rhinitis symptoms in the sensitized host.

Adverse food reactions may result in a variety of symptoms involving the gastrointestinal tract, skin, respiratory tract, and cardiovascular system. The standardized definitions for food reactions recently adapted by the European Academy of Allergy and Clinical Immunology provide a mechanistic classification of these disorders (2). An *adverse food reaction* was defined as any aberrant reaction following the ingestion of a food or food additive. Adverse food reactions were divided into *toxic* and *nontoxic* food reactions. Toxic reactions may develop in anyone provided a sufficient dose is ingested. Nontoxic reactions depend on individual susceptibility and may be the result of immune mechanisms (*allergy* or *hypersensitivity*) or nonimmune mechanisms (*intolerances*). IgE-mediated food allergies have been most clearly delineated, but non-IgE-mediated immune reactions are being increasingly defined. Food intolerances probably account for the majority of adverse food reactions and may be due to *pharmacological* properties of the food (e.g., tyramine in aged cheeses, theobromine in chocolate), or unique susceptibilities of the host such as *metabolic* disorders (e.g., lactase deficiency) or *idiosyncratic* responses.

Adverse reactions to foods are more common in young children, which in part may relate to the immaturity of their gastrointestinal tract and immune system, and in part to the feeding practices of the population evaluated. In a survey of an American general pediatric practice 8% of the 480 infants followed for 3 years were found to have adverse reactions to foods (3). In four large prospective studies with appropriately performed milk challenges from four different countries, 2.2–2.5% of infants were found to have cow milk allergy in the first 1–2 years of life (3–6). In follow-up, nearly 85% of these milk-sensitive infants lost their reactivity by their third birthday (7). Adverse reactions to food additives also have been demonstrated in children. In a study of 4274 Dutch schoolchildren, results of double-blind, placebo-controlled food challenges (DBPCFCs) suggested a prevalence of about 1% (8). Children with atopic disorders tend to have a higher prevalence of food allergy. In children with moderate to severe atopic dermatitis, up to one-third have skin symptoms provoked by food hypersensitivity (9), and the more severe the atopic eczema, the more likely they are to have food allergy (10). Studies of asthmatic children attending general pulmonary clinics found that 6–8% of these patients have food-induced wheezing (11,12).

The prevalence of food hypersensitivity in adults also has been examined in the past several years. A recent survey in the United Kingdom found that approximately 20% of 7500 households reported a food intolerance (13). However, utilizing DBPCFC to confirm patients' reports, adverse food reactions were found in 1.4–1.8% of adults. A comparable study in the Netherlands concluded that about 2% of the adult Dutch population are affected by adverse food reactions (14). A second large population survey in the United Kingdom found the prevalence of adverse reactions to food additives in 0.01–0.23% of adults (15).

II. Food-Induced Nasal Symptoms

Adverse food reactions inducing isolated nasal symptoms appear to be uncommon. One form of food intolerance provoking nasal symptoms has been termed

Table 1 Prevalence of Milk-Induced Nasal Symptoms in the First Two Years of Life

Study	Total enrolled	Milk-reactive	Nasal symptoms	Pulmonary symptoms
Bock (3)	480	11 (2.3%)[a]	1 (9%)	0
Host (4)	1,749	39 (2.2%)	14 (36%)	17 (44%)
Schrander (5)	1,158	26 (2.2%)	1 (4%)	3 (12%)
Hill (19)	—	100	20 (20%)	12 (12%)

[a]Percent of total study group reactive to milk.

"gustatory rhinitis" (16). In a questionnaire survey of 60 adults, greater than 60% reported rhinorrhea following the ingestion of very spicy foods such as hot chili peppers, horseradish, hot-and-sour soup, etc. Unlike typical rhinitis, affected individuals do not develop sneezing, congestion, or pruritus. The spicy food elicits rhinorrhea within a few minutes of ingestion, which resolves almost immediately after the spicy food is eaten. The reaction results from the stimulation of atropine-inhibitable muscarinic receptors (16).

Several studies have identified patients who develop nasal symptoms due to IgE-mediated hypersensitivity. However, limited information is available on the prevalence of food-induced rhinitis. In a survey of 323 patients (aged 4 years and older) with chronic rhinitis attending an allergy clinic, 21 (6.5%) appeared to experience clearing of their nasal symptoms when placed on a strict milk-exclusion diet (17). However, only two of these 21 patients (0.6%) had nasal symptoms reproduced during two consecutive DBPCFCs. In a retrospective review of 25,000 patients presenting to an allergy clinic over 5 years, 400 were diagnosed by history and laboratory studies (18). Of 400 patients diagnosed with food allergy, 3% of subjects were diagnosed with food-induced nasal symptoms. This suggests that 0.05% of patients attending an allergy clinic had food-induced rhinitis. In three epidemiological surveys of infants through their first 3 years of life, milk-induced nasal symptoms were rare. Despite the notion that milk ingestion frequently leads to nasal congestion, 0.08–0.2% of infants were found to develop nasal symptoms following a milk challenge. As shown in Table 1, Host and Halken (4) found 14 of 39 milk-allergic infants (36%) developing nasal symptoms during oral milk challenges whereas Schrander et al. (5) found only one of 26 experiencing nasal symptoms following milk challenge (4%). In their study of 100 infants with milk allergy, Hill et al. (19) reported that 20 children (20%) developed rhinitis during oral milk challenges.

III. Nasal Symptoms in Patients Being Evaluated for Food Hypersensitivity

Children with atopic disorders and food allergy frequently experience nasal symptoms during DBPCFCs. Bock and Atkins reviewed their data on 480 children (age range: 9 months–19 years) referred for evaluation of adverse food reactions (20). Overall, 39% of the children experienced at least one positive DBPCFC. Respiratory symptoms (sneezing, rhinorrhea, nasal obstruction, wheezing, cough, ocular signs) were present in 39% of positive DBPCFCs. Isolated respiratory symptoms were seen in only 13 of 245 positive challenges (5%), whereas respiratory symptoms developed with other allergic symptoms in 82 of 245 positive challenges (30%). Overall the skin prick test was positive to the food precipitating a positive challenge in 98% of children 3 years of age and older, and in 91% of children less than 3 years of age (excluding non-IgE-mediated gastrointestinal reactions).

In our study of 320 children (age range: 4 months–19 years) referred for evaluation of atopic dermatitis and food hypersensitivity, 121 children (38%) were noted to develop respiratory symptoms during food challenges. Nasal symptoms occurred in about 25% of the group and included nasal congestion and pruritus, sneezing, rhinorrhea, and frequently periocular pruritus and conjunctivitis. Laryngeal symptoms consisted of a sensation of pruritus and/or tightness in the throat, dry "staccato" cough, and occasionally dysphonia and/or dysphagia. Pulmonary symptoms included a sensation of chest tightness or shortness of breath, deep cough, and/or wheezing. Overall, 263 positive DBPCFCs involved respiratory symptoms: nasal symptoms—166 (63%), laryngeal symptoms—114 (43%), and pulmonary symptoms—64 (24%). Skin prick tests were positive to over 95% of the foods provoking nasal symptoms. In both our study and the study by Bock and Atkins (20), egg, milk, peanut, and soy accounted for the majority of food hypersensitivity reactions.

Kivity et al. evaluated 112 patients with histories of adverse food reactions developing after 10 years of age (21). Unlike the onset of food allergy in the first several years of life, fruits and vegetables accounted for the majority of food allergy in this group. Seventy-one patients (age range: 10–48 years) were found to have positive food challenges; 36 (51%) had respiratory symptoms, predominantly nasal symptoms. Ten patients developed exercise-associated, food-induced nasal symptoms.

As shown in Table 2, several studies of food hypersensitivity in adults have noted the development of nasal symptoms during food challenges. Four of these studies were evaluating specific foods: shrimp (22), cow milk and egg (23), codfish (24), and cow milk (25). Except in the case of codfish allergy, patient histories of food sensitivity were verified in less than 50% of cases. Challenges with shrimp and fish generally provoked prompt reactions that rarely involved nasal symp-

Table 2 Nasal Symptoms in Adults Undergoing Food Challenges

Study	Number of patients	Positive reactions	Nasal symptoms	Pulmonary symptoms
Bernstein (44)	22	13	2	1
Atkins (45)[a]	25	10	7	0
Daul (22)	30	9	0	4
Pastorello (46)	23	10	8	4
Norgaard (23)	19	10	3	5
Hansen (24)	10	7	0	1
Stoger (25)[a,b]	34	34	23	22

[a]Challenges not performed in double-blind, placebo-controlled fashion.
[b]Retrospective experience over 10 years; challenges not performed in double-blind, placebo-controlled fashion.

toms. In other studies, the rate of nasal symptoms varied between 30% and 80% of positive challenges. Food dyes and preservatives are frequently implicated as a cause of respiratory symptoms in patients with asthma or rhinitis. However, performing 1868 DBPCFCs in 504 patients, Rosenhall could confirm positive reactions in only 2% of challenges to food preservatives and 3% of challenges to food dyes (26).

IV. Nasal Response During Food Challenges

As noted above, approximately 25% of children with atopic dermatitis being evaluated for food hypersensitivity were found to develop typical rhinitis symptoms during DBPCFCs. Symptoms typically developed within 15–90 min after initiation of the challenge and lasted 30–120 min. Nasal pruritus and periocular pruritus were generally the first symptoms noted, followed by rhinorrhea and nasal congestion. Prolonged bursts of sneezing, with up to 20 consecutive sneezes, and copious rhinorrhea were not infrequent. Nasal turbinates appeared markedly edematous and slightly pale upon inspection, and frequently required a nasal decongestant to restore airflow through the nose.

During allergic reactions, mediators are released by activated basophils, mast cells, and/or eosinophils, which can be measured in the serum after positive food challenges. Increased plasma histamine levels have been demonstrated in children with atopic dermatitis and food hypersensitivity following positive food challenges, suggesting degranulation of mast cells with release of histamine into the circulation in addition to localized tissues, provoking typical skin symptoms (27). Similarly, serum eosinophil cationic protein (ECP) concentrations have

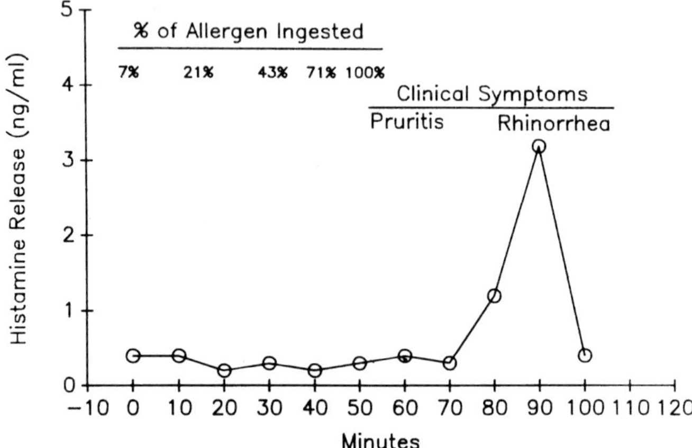

Figure 1   Nasal lavage histamine concentration in one patient experiencing nasal symptoms during a positive double-blind, placebo-controlled food challenge. (From Ref. 47.)

been measured in children undergoing food challenges (28,29). In a study of 16 children with atopic dermatitis, nasal lavage fluid histamine was evaluated (30). Thirty-one DBPCFCs were performed and 11 were positive. During positive food challenges, nasal lavage histamine increased significantly ($p < 0.01$) compared to negative or placebo challenges, increasing up to 10-fold in some children (Fig. 1). In a more recent preliminary study, nasal mediator release was evaluated in 13 patients with asthma and perennial rhinitis (10 males and three females; median age 10.8 years; range 6.6–16 years). Patients were challenged to suspected foods by DBPCFC as previously described (31). Briefly, challenges consisted of administering up to 10 g of dehydrated, powdered test food over a 60–90-min period, hidden in juices or solid foods known to be tolerated by the patient. Potential symptoms were recorded by an observer unaware of the challenge content on a standardized score sheet including skin, gastrointestinal, and respiratory symptoms (including upper respiratory symptoms such as nasal itchiness, sneezing, and/or rhinorrhea). All negative DBPCFCs were confirmed by subsequent open challenges.

Nasal secretions were collected with filter paper disks as described by Baroody et al (32). Prior to placement of the disk on the nasal mucosa, the patient was instructed to blow his/her nose to remove excessive secretions and mucus. A preweighed disk (8-mm-diameter disks from filter cards; Shandon Inc., Pittsburgh, PA) was then placed on the anterior wall of the septum under direct visualization using Duckbill forceps. Thirty seconds later, the disk was removed with

Table 3 Outcome of DBPCFC in 13 Patients with Asthma and Allergic Rhinitis

	Positive DBPCFC		Negative DBPCFC
Patient	Food	Symptoms	Food
1	Egg	C,L,W,N,S	
2	Egg	N,S	Oat
	Potato	S	
3	Egg	C,L,N,S	Turkey
			Pork
4			Milk
5	Soy	L,GI	
6	Egg	N,S	Pork
			Wheat
7	Egg	L,N	
8			Soy
9			Soy
10	Milk	L,S	
11			Egg
12			Pork
13			Pork
			Egg

L = laryngeal pruritus/edema; C = cough; W = wheeze; N = nasal syptoms; S = skin rash/pruritus; GI = vomiting/diarrhea.

the forceps, and immediately placed into the microtube and sealed to avoid evaporation. The amount of secretion collected was determined by measuring the total weight of the microtube and its content, and then subtracting the initial weight of the blank disk and the microtube. Next, 250 µl of normal saline solution was then added to the microtube, and absorbed secretions were expelled by compressing the disk against the bottom of the microtube. The samples were frozen at $-20°C$ and stored until assays were performed. Samples were obtained prior to the DBPCFC (time 0), and 30, 60, and 90 min after the first dose of the food challenge.

ECP concentrations in nasal secretions were measured using the FEIA CAP-RAST system (Pharmacia, Evansville, IL) and histamine levels in nasal secretions were determined using a sensitive radioenzymatic assay (33). The results are expressed as ECP and histamine concentrations divided by the weight of the sample collected on the disk to account for the volume of nasal secretions sampled.

Twenty DBPCFCs were performed; eight were positive (Table 3). Laryn-

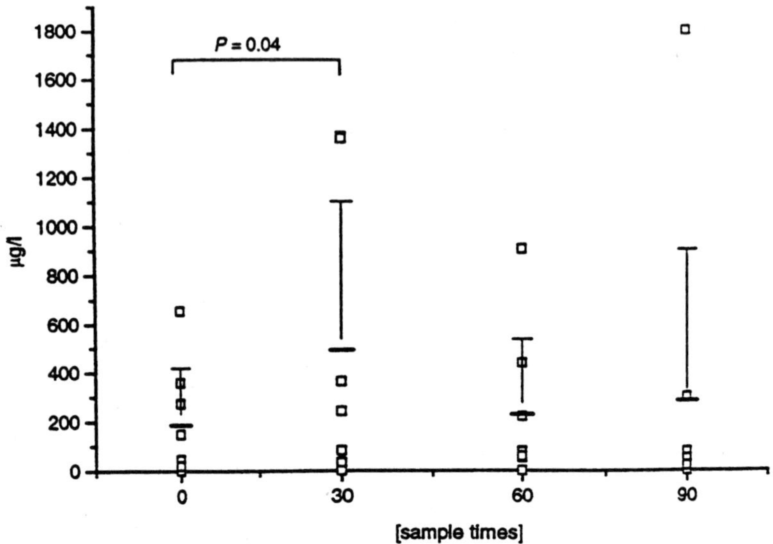

Figure 2 ECP values in nasal samples from asthmatic patients with positive (A) or negative (B) DBPCFC. Mean values are represented by bars ± SD.

geal symptoms were observed in five challenges, skin symptoms (hives or an erythematous morbilliform rash) in five challenges, chest symptoms (cough, chest tightness, and/or wheezing) in two challenges, and gastrointestinal symptoms in 1 challenge. Nasal symptoms (sneezing, itchiness, congestion, and/or rhinorrhea) developed in five challenges. All patients reacted within 30 min of initiation of the challenges.

Wide interpatient variation in nasal histamine concentration was observed at baseline (sample time 0) ranging from 0 to 1308 µg/ml (mean value ± SD: 424 µg/ml ± 491) in positive challenges, and from 0.3 to 957 µg/ml (mean value ± SD: 176 µg/ml ± 352) in negative challenges. The mean values then decreased at the 30-min sampling time in both positive and negative challenges (mean values ± SD: 162 µg/ml ± 145 in positive, 45 µg/ml ± 72 in negative). Mean histamine values remained below baseline at the 60- and 90-min sampling times in both positive and negative challenges and no significant differences in nasal histamine levels were observed between positive and negative challenges. The high baseline nasal histamine values probably obscured any real change in histamine secretion.

As seen with histamine, large interpatient variations were observed with ECP concentrations at all sampling times (Fig. 2). Baseline values varied between 0 and 656 µg/L in patients who experienced positive challenges (mean ±

SD: 188 µg/L ± 232), and between 0 and 1389 µg/L in negative challenges (mean ± SD: 255 µg/L ± 387). However, there was a statistically significant increase in ECP concentration in nasal secretions at the 30-min sampling point when compared to baseline in patients with a positive challenge (mean ± SD: 494 µg/L ± 609; $p = 0.04$; Wilcoxon signed-ranks test for paired data), whereas there was no significant change in patients with negative challenges (mean ± SD: 237 µg/L ± 245; p = n.s.). ECP values at 60 and 90 min reverted to baseline in positive challenges (mean value ± SD at 60 min: 229 µg/L ± 307, at 90 min: 283 µg/L ± 621; p = n.s.), and did not change significantly in negative challenges (mean value ± SD at 60 min: 235 µg/L ± 307, at 90 min: 265 µg/L ± 320; p = n.s.).

In this preliminary study, baseline histamine and ECP values in nasal secretions were highly variable, with no direct relationship to the extent of nasal symptoms at the sampling times. A significant increase in ECP levels was seen at the 30-min sampling time in positive DBPCFCs, but not in negative challenges. ECP levels then fell to baseline values at 60 and 90 min after the beginning of the challenges. Future studies should include saline lavages prior to obtaining baseline histamine and ECP values in order to remove residual mediators from nasal mucosa and to establish stable baseline values. Nevertheless, these findings do suggest that eosinophils are locally involved in the development of the early phase of a positive DBPCFC (i.e., less than 30 min after the first symptoms). Other investigators also have demonstrated an early-phase release of eosinophil mediators following exposure of the nasal mucosa to aeroallergens. Klementsson et al. observed an increased number of eosinophils in nasal lavage fluid from 60 min up to 24 hr after birch or grass pollen challenge, although an increase of ECP was seen as early as 30 min after the challenges with values returning to baseline after 120 min (34). In a study utilizing a similar design, Wang et al. found a progressive increase in both the eosinophil count and ECP in nasal secretions over a 24-hr period after the challenge (35).

V. Other Forms of Food-Induced Allergic Rhinitis

Most forms of food hypersensitivity follow sensitization and reaction to ingested food proteins. In some cases of occupational exposure, e.g., baker's asthma, sensitization and reaction to food allergens are the result of inhaled food proteins. Bakers develop IgE antibodies following inhalation of airborne flour dust in the workplace and with reexposure may develop rhinitis and asthma. A study of bakers' apprentices found that there was a progressive increase in positive skin tests to cereal flours, exceeding 20% by the fifth year of apprenticeship (36). In addition, 7% were found to develop rhinitis and wheezing in the work environment. More recent studies have reported skin test reactivity to cereal grains in up to 54% of established bakers and symptoms in about 20%, all with nasal symptoms and most with asthma (37). Similar symptoms have occurred with inhaled egg material in the confectionery industry where egg white is sprayed on rolls and various baked goods (38).

A rare cause of non-IgE-mediated, food-induced rhinitis is seen in patients with Heiner's syndrome. This is a pulmonary disease characterized by chronic rhinitis, pulmonary infiltrates and hemosiderosis, gastrointestinal blood loss, iron deficiency anemia, and failure to thrive (39). It is associated most often with a hypersensitivity to cow's milk, but reactivity to egg and pork has also been reported (40). Although peripheral blood eosinophilia and multiple serum precipitins to cow's milk are relatively constant features, the immunological mechanisms responsible for this disorder are not known. Avoidance of the precipitating allergen leads to resolution of symptoms, but the natural history of this disorder is not known.

VI. Diagnosing Food-Induced Rhinitis

The diagnosis food-induced rhinitis depends on a clinical test, the DBPCFC, which is the current "gold standard" for diagnosing food allergy (31,41). As with the evaluation of any adverse food reaction, the initial workup consists of a careful history and physical examination. The history should emphasize several points: whether any foods are suspected and the approximate quantity provoking symptoms, the time between the ingestion and development of symptoms, description of the symptoms, frequency and reproducibility of symptoms, the most recent occurrence, and whether other factors (e.g., exercise) are necessary to provoke the reaction. The physical examination should note any atopic features, which frequently are present in individuals with IgE-mediated food allergy.

Several laboratory tests have evolved for use in the diagnosis of IgE-mediated food hypersensitivity reactions and may be used in the initial screening of food-allergic complaints. If IgE-mediated hypersensitivity is suspected, skin tests with food extracts are used to demonstrate the presence of food-antigen-specific IgE antibodies on the surface of cutaneous mast cells, which are presumed to reflect the IgE present on mast cells in the nasal mucosa. When compared to DBPCFC, the negative puncture or prick skin test is extremely useful for excluding IgE-mediated food allergy, but inadequate for predicting the presence of clinical reactivity, i.e., low positive predictive accuracies (42). Intradermal skin tests are even less predictive than skin prick tests and are not recommended in the evaluation of IgE-mediated food allergy. Standard radioallergosorbent tests (RAST) or similar in vitro tests performed in a reliable laboratory provide predictive information that is similar to skin prick tests. Once suspected foods are identified by history and skin testing (or RAST), they are eliminated from the diet for 1–2 weeks. Single-blind challenges may be performed to rule out foods considered unlikely to provoke an allergic reaction. As described above, DBPCFC are then used to establish a diagnosis of food allergy (31). Although a DBPCFC is rarely equivocal when typical IgE-mediated symptoms are investigated, nasal lavage histamine, tryptase, and/or ECP concentrations may be used to provide objective measures of response. No satisfactory laboratory tests have emerged to assist in the diagnosis of non-IgE-mediated food allergic disorders, and because of pulmonary hemorrhage in Heiner's syndrome, challenges are not recommended where the diagnosis is likely.

VII. Conclusions

It has been clearly established that nasal symptoms may result from adverse food reactions. Rhinitis is often seen in patients experiencing IgE-mediated food hypersensitivity reactions, but is rarely seen as an isolated symptom. Skin prick tests are generally positive to the responsible food, but blinded food challenges are necessary to make the diagnosis since history is often unreliable and over 50% of positive skin tests are clinically "false positives." Treatment of food-induced rhinitis, like other forms of food allergy, consists of strict avoidance of the offending food (43) and symptomatic treatment with antihistamines and decongestants in case of accidental ingestion. In patients with food allergy and asthma, who are at higher risk for severe systemic reactions, epinephrine (e.g. Epi-Pen) also should be readily available. At present there is no evidence that immunotherapy is effective for treating food-allergic symptoms. In children and to a lesser extent in adults, food allergies are often "outgrown" (except to peanuts, nuts, and seafood), so symptoms may not be lifelong.

Acknowledgments

HAS is supported in part by NIH Grants AI 24439 and RR-00052, and the Allergy and Immunology Institute of the International Life Science Institute. PAE is supported by a grant from the Swiss National Research Foundation, the Eugenio Litta Foundation, and a Prize Award from Glaxo, Switzerland.

References

1. Freeman J. Discussion on paroxysmal rhinorrhea. Proc Roy Soc Med 1925; 18:29–32.
2. Bruijnzeel-Koomen C, Ortolani C, Aas K, Bindslev-Jensen C, Bjorksten B, Noneret-

Vautrin D, et al. Adverse reactions to food. Position paper. Allergy 1995; 50:623–635.

3. Bock SA. Prospective appraisal of complaints of adverse reactions to foods in children during the first 3 years of life. Pediatrics 1987; 79:683–688.

4. Host A, Halken S. A prospective study of cow milk allergy in Danish infants during the first 3 years of life. Allergy 1990; 45:587–596.

5. Schrander JJP, van den Bogart JPH, Forget PP, Schrander-Stumpel CTRM, Kuijten RH, Kester ADM. Cow's milk protein intolerance in infants under 1 year of age: a prospective epidemiological study. Eur J Pediatr 1993; 152:640–644.

6. Hide DW, Guyer BM. Cow milk intolerance in Isle of Wight infants. Br J Clin Pract 1983; 37:285–287.

7. Host A. Cow's milk protein allergy and intolerance in infancy. Pediatr Allergy Immunol 1994; 5:5–36.

8. Fuglsang G, Madsen C, Saval P, Osterballe O. Prevalence of intolerance to food additives among Danish school children. Pediatr Allergy Immunol 1993; 4:123–129.

9. Burks AW, Mallory SB, Williams LW, Shirrell MA. Atopic dermatitis: clinical relevance of food hypersensitivity reactions. J Pediatr 1988; 113:447–451.

10. Guillet G, Guillet MH. Natural history of sensitizations in atopic dermatitis. Arch Dermatol 1992; 128:187–192.

11. Novembre E, de Martino M, Vierucci A. Foods and respiratory allergy. J Allergy Clin Immunol 1988; 81:1059–1065.

12. Oehling A, Cagnani CEB. Food allergy and child asthma. Allergol Immunopathol 1980; 8:7–14.

13. Young E, Stoneham MD, Petruckevitch A, Barton J, Rona R. A population study of food intolerance. Lancet 1994; 343:1127–1130.

14. Niestijl Jansen JJ, Kardinaal AFM, Huijbers GH, Vlieg-Boerstra BJ, Martens BPM, Ockhuizen T. Prevalence of food allergy and intolerance in the adult Dutch population. J Allergy Clin Immunol 1994; 93:446–456.

15. Young E, Patel S, Stoneham MD, Rona R, Wilkinson JD. The prevalence of reactions to food additives in a survey population. J Roy Coll Phys Lond 1987; 21:241–271.

16. Raphael G, Raphael M, Kaliner M. Gustatory rhinitis: a syndrome of food-induced rhinorrhea. J Allergy Clin Immunol 1989; 83:110–115.

17. Simpson S, Somerfield S, Wilson J, Hillas J. A double-blind study for the diagnosis of cows' milk allergy. NZ Med J 1980; 92:457–459.

18. Oehling A, Garcia B, Santos F, Cordoba H, Dieguez, I, Fernandez M, et al. Food allergy as a cause of rhinitis and/or asthma. J Invest Allergol Clin Immunol 1992; 2:78–83.

19. Hill DJ, Firer MA, Shelton MJ, Hosking CS. Manifestations of milk allergy in infancy: clinical and immunological findings. J Pediatr 1986; 109:270–276.

20. Bock SA, Atkins FM. Patterns of food hypersensitivity during sixteen years of double-blind, placebo-controlled food challenges. J Pediatr 1990; 117:561–567.

21. Kivity S, Dunner K, Marian Y. The pattern of food hypersensitivity in patients with onset after 10 years of age. Clin Exp Allergy 1994; 24:19–22.

22. Daul C, Morgan JE, Hughes J, Lehrer S. Provocation-challenge studies in shrimp-sensitive individuals. J Allergy Clin Immunol 1988; 81:1180–1186.

23. Norgaard A, Bindslev-Jensen C. Egg and milk allergy in adults. Allergy 1992; 47: 503–509.

24. Hansen T, Bindslev-Jensen C. Codfish allergy in adults. Allergy 1992; 47:610–617.

25. Stoger P, Wüthrich B. Type I allergy to cow milk proteins in adults. Int Arch Allergy Appl Immunol 1993; 102:399–407.

26. Rosenhall L. Evaluation of intolerance to analgesics, preservatives and food colorants with challenge tests. Eur J Respir Dis 1982; 63:410–419.

27. Sampson HA, Jolie PL. Increased plasma histamine concentrations after food challenges in children with atopic dermatitis. N Engl J Med 1984; 311:372–376.

28. Suomalainen H, Soppi E, Isolauri E. Evidence for eosinophil activation in cow's milk allergy. Pediatr Allergy Immunol 1994; 5:27–31.

29. Niggemann B, Beyer K, Wahn U. The role of eosinophils and eosinophil cationic protein in monitoring oral challenge tests in children with food-sensitive atopic dermatitis. J Allergy Clin Immunol 1994; 94:963–971.

30. Silber G, Sampson H. Nasal mediator release following double-blind placebo-controlled oral food challenges. J Allergy Clin Immunol 1988; 81:185 (abstract).

31. Bock SA, Sampson HA, Atkins FM, Zeiger RS, Lehrer S, Sachs M, et al. Double-blind, placebo-controlled food challenge (DBPCFC) as an office procedure: a manual. J Allergy Clin Immunol 1988; 82:986–997.

32. Baroody F, Ford S, Lichtenstein L, Kagey-Sobotka A, Naclerio R. Physiologic responses and histamine release after nasal antigen challenge. Am J Respir Crit Care Med 1994; 149:1457–1465.

33. Sampson HA, Broadbent KR, Bernhisel-Broadbent J. Spontaneous release of histamine from basophils and histamine-releasing factor in patients with atopic dermatitis and food hypersensitivity. N Engl J Med 1989; 321:228–232.

34. Klementsson H, Venge P, Andersson M, Pipkorn U. Allergen-induced changes in nasal secretory responsiveness and eosinophil granulocytes. Acta Otolaryngol (Stockh) 1991; 111:776–784.

35. Wang D, Clement P, Smitz J, De Waele M, Derde M. Correlations between complaints, inflammatory cells and mediator concentrations in nasal secretions after nasal allergen challenge and during natural allergen exposure. Int Arch Allergy Appl Immunol 1995; 106:278–285.

36. Herxheimer H. The skin sensitivity to flour of Baker's apprentices. Acta Allergol 1973; 28:42–49.

37. Thiel H, Ulmer W. Baker's asthma: development and possibility for treatment. Chest 1980; 78:400–405.

38. Edwards J, McConnochie K, Trotman D, Collins G, Saunders M, Latham S. Allergy to inhaled egg material. Clin Allergy 1983; 13:427–432.

39. Heiner DC, Sears JW. Chronic respiratory disease associated with multiple circulating precipitins to cow's milk. Am J Dis Child 1960; 100:500–502.

40. Lee SK, Kniker WT, Cook CD, Heiner DC. Cow's milk–induced pulmonary disease in children. Adv Pediatr 1978; 25:39–57.

41. Sampson HA. Immunologically mediated food allergy: the importance of food challenge procedures. Ann Allergy 1988; 60:262–269.

42. Sampson HA, Albergo R. Comparison of results of skin tests, RAST, and double-

blind, placebo-controlled food challenges in children with atopic dermatitis. J Allergy Clin Immunol 1984; 74:26–33.

43. Barnes Koerner C, Sampson HA. Diets and nutrition. In: Metcalfe DD, Sampson HA, Simon RA, eds. Food Allergy: Adverse Reactions to Foods and Food Additives. Boston: Blackwell Scientific Publications, 1991:332–354.

44. Bernstein M, Day J, Welsh A. Double-blind food challenge in the diagnosis of food sensitivity in the adult. J Allergy Clin Immunol 1982; 70:205–210.

45. Atkins F, Steinberg S, Metcalfe D. Evaluation of immediate adverse reactions to foods in adult patients. II. A detailed analysis of reaction patterns during oral food challenge. J Allergy Clin Immunol 1985; 75:356–363.

46. Pastorello E, Stocchi L, Pravetonni V, Bigi A, Schilke M, Incorvaia C, et al. Role of the food elimination diet in adults with food allergy. J Allergy Clin Immunol 1989; 84:475–483.

47. Sampson HA, Metcalfe DD. Immediate reactions to foods. In: Metcalfe DD, Sampson HA, Simon RA, eds. Food Allergy: Adverse Reactions to Foods and Food Additives. Boston: Blackwell Scientific Publications, 1991:103.

7

Mucosal Inflammation and Allergic Rhinitis

PETER H. HOWARTH

University of Southampton
Southampton, England

I. Introduction

Allergic rhinitis is a clinical condition, associated with an excessive generation of specific IgE (1). It is characterized by the anterior nasal symptoms of pruritus, sneeze, discharge, and stuffiness, and in chronic or severe disease, there is often an associated loss of sense of smell and inability to taste. These symptoms may be present for part of the year (seasonal) or throughout the year (perennial), dependent upon the nature of the allergenic sensitivity. For seasonal disease the specific IgE is usually directed against outdoor allergens, such as tree, grass, or weed pollens, or fungal spores, as the atmospheric abundance of these allergens has a defined and limited periodicity (2). In contrast, perennial disease is usually associated with sensitivity against indoor allergens such as those related to house dust mites and animals (cats and dogs), although outdoor allergenic sensitivity may also give rise to symptoms all year in climates in which pollens and fungal spores have perennial characteristics. Allergy to food proteins can also give rise to rhinitis (3). This is, however, rare in adults in comparison to aeroallergen sensitivity and the rhinitic process is only one manifestation of this sensitivity, with other features often dominating.

For aeroallergen sensitivity the interaction between the environmental allergen and the specific IgE, bound to high-affinity receptors (FcεRI) on nasal mucosal mast cells, gives rise both to symptom expression, through release of preformed and newly generated mediators, and to the development of nasal mucosal inflammation, through release of cytokines (4). This mucosal inflammatory process is associated with endothelial cell activation and the tissue accumulation of eosinophils from the circulation, along with the epithelial localization of both mast cells and eosinophils. The expression of low-affinity IgE receptors (FcεRII) on other cell populations, such as eosinophils and lymphocytes, along with the nasal mucosal recruitment of basophils, which process high-affinity IgE receptors, expands the population of cells able to directly interact with the inducing allergen and modify the local cellular response through cytokine release. This process underlies the clinical experience of priming, a situation in which patients experience more symptoms for the same level of pollen exposure later in the season than at the beginning (5,6), as activation of basophils and eosinophils will elaborate the local generation of mediators. It is now also appreciated that epithelial cells are activated in allergic disease, and mediator release from this resident cell population contributes both to the generation of symptoms and to the epithelial cell accumulation through release of cytokines and, probably more importantly, chemokines.

It is thus apparent that there is a complex mucosal cellular response to environmental allergens in sensitized individuals and that this reaction, which forms the basis for the clinical disease expression, involves many cell populations (Fig. 1).

II. Mucosal Sensitization and IgE Production

It is now 30 years since the discovery of elevated IgE levels in the sera of ragweed-sensitive seasonal rhinitic subjects (7) and the elucidation that this was the previously uncharacterized ''reaginic antibody'' (8). Since then much has been learned about the regulation of IgE synthesis in allergic disease.

IgE is generated by B lymphocytes under the regulation of cytokines. Interleukin-4 (IL-4) was first implicated from in vitro studies as being critical for the isotype switching of immunoglobulin synthesis for IgE production (9,10). However, it is now appreciated that IL-4 alone is insufficient and that additional costimulatory signals are required for IgE synthesis to occur (11). In addition,

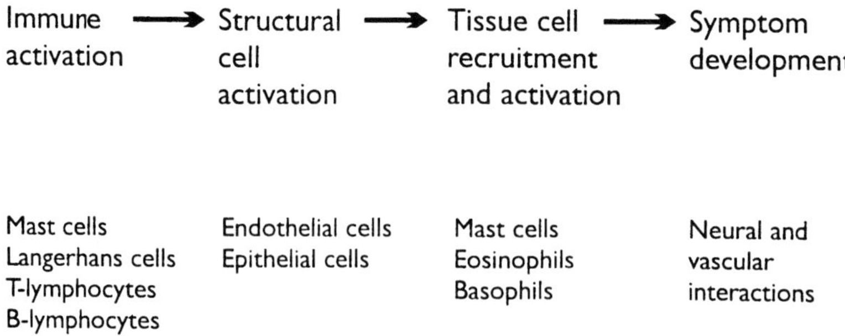

Figure 1   Flow chart of cellular involvement in the development of allergic rhinitis.

many of the functions of a more recently described cytokine, IL-13, are now also appreciated to overlap with those of IL-4 (12,13). In vitro studies have identified that IL-13 is able to support the synthesis of IgE by human and murine B lymphocytes (12). This effect is mediated through a discrete receptor that shares a signal-transducing component with the IL-4 receptor (14). Although in vitro this stimulatory effect of IL-13 is independent of IL-4, the independence of IL-13 as a stimulus in vivo is uncertain, as IL-4 "knockout" animals fail to synthesize IgE (15). This suggests that IL-13 alone is insufficient to support the process in vivo. Consistent with a critical role of IL-4, transgenic mice that overexpress the IL-4 gene develop high levels of circulating IgE as well as a severe chronic conjunctivitis (16). This conjunctivitis is characterized by mast cell, eosinophil, and mononuclear cell infiltration, cellular changes similar to those seen in allergic mucosal inflammation. IL-4, in addition to its effects on IgE-isotype switching, increases the expression of the low-affinity IgE receptor (CD23/FCεRII) and MHC class II antigen by B cells (17,18), actions opposed by interferon (IFN)-γ and IFN-α, cytokines that reduce the level of IL-4-induced IgE synthesis (9,10).

In addition to IL-4 or IL-13, the generation of IgE depends upon cell-cell contact, involving both cognate interactions between B-cell MHC class II antigen and the T-cell receptor/CD3 complex (19) and noncognate interactions between CD40 expressed on B cells and its complementary ligand expressed on activated T cells (20,21) and between B7 and CD28 receptor families (22). The requirement for T cells to interact with B cells to promote IgE synthesis can be replaced in vitro by the presence of anti-CD40 (23), and it is of interest in this respect that this CD40 ligand is also expressed on tissue mast cells and on basophils (24).

Within the nose, mRNA for IL-4 has been colocalized to both T lymphocytes and tissue mast cells (25) and the nasal mucosal mast cells have been shown to store IL-4 preformed in granules as well as expressing IL-4 in its activated form, presented in a cell-surface-associated fashion (26). For T-cell activation there has to be an interaction with antigen-presenting cells. Within the airways, the dendritic or Langerhans cell appears to be the capable antigen-presenting cell as this function is poorly served by macrophages. These cells form a dendritic network within the mucosa, and studies by Fokkens and colleagues have demonstrated a naturally occurring increase in mucosal Langerhans cells in seasonal rhinitis (27). This increase can be mimicked by repeated allergen challenge and is inhibited by the topical corticosteroid fluticasone propionate (28). Consistent with these seasonal findings, there is a seasonal increase in serum levels of IgE in allergic rhinitis (29,30). Although IgE synthesis has been considered to occur in draining lymph nodes, the recent identification of IgE mRNA expression in nasal mucosal biopsies following nasal allergen challenge (31) raises the potential that local mucosal synthesis of IgE can occur in rhinitis and provides a rationale for the binding of IgE to receptors on tissue cells participating in the mucosal inflammatory response.

III. Resident Tissue Cell Activation

In addition to tissue mast cell activation contributing to the rhinitic process, there is endothelial and epithelial cell activation.

A. Mast Cells

Mast cells are constitive cells of the normal nasal mucosa but are not found superficially within the airway epithelium. Immunohistochemical staining of nasal biopsies with monoclonal antibodies against mast cell tryptase identifies an increase in mast cells within the airway epithelium in both seasonal and perennial rhinitis, in comparison with biopsy findings in nonatopic, nonrhinitic subjects (31–33). One study using less specific immunohistochemical staining has reported, in addition, an increase in submucosal mast cells in seasonal rhinitis (34), but this could not be substantiated either in the tryptase immunohistochemical studies or in a detailed transmission electron microscopic analysis (35).

The epithelial mast cells are in an activated state in symptomatic rhinitis. Elevated levels of the mast cell mediators histamine and tryptase are evident in nasal lavage fluid and ultrastructural changes of degranulation are evident on electron microscopic examination of nasal biopsies (Fig. 2) (35–38). Crosslinking of IgE on the surface of mast cells by allergen leads to a series of intracellular events culminating in the release of preformed mediators from mast cells (histamine, tryptase, heparin) and the generation of lipid mediators, including prostaglandin D_2 (PGD_2) and the sulfidopeptide leukotrienes, leukotriene (LT) C_4 and its metabolites LTD_4 and LTE_4 (39). These released mediators induce the nasal symptoms of itch, sneeze, discharge, and blockage, through interactions with receptors present on both neural and vascular elements within the nasal mucosa (Table 1).

Histamine is prominent in this respect. Nasal challenge with histamine induces nasal pruritus, sneezing, discharge, and transient nasal blockage (40). The receptor specificity of these nasal actions has been explored by investigation of the effects of specific receptor antagonists. These studies identify that the nasal effects of histamine are primarily H_1-receptor mediated with respect to itch, sneeze, and nasal discharge (41,42). H_2-receptor blockade exerts a small and variable effect on rhinorrhea and nasal blockage consistent with H_2 receptors being located at vascular sites (42,43). The reduction in rhinorrhea may be related to a reduction in nasal vascular permeability rather than in glandular secretion, as both H_1- and H_2-receptor antagonists regulate mucosal blood flow following nasal allergen challenge. Neither H_1- nor H_2-receptor antagonists exert marked effects on induced nasal blockage (42–44). This raises the possibility of the involvement of a third histamine receptor, the H_3 receptor, in the genesis of histamine-induced nasal blockage. H_3 receptors have been identified on presynaptic, perivascular

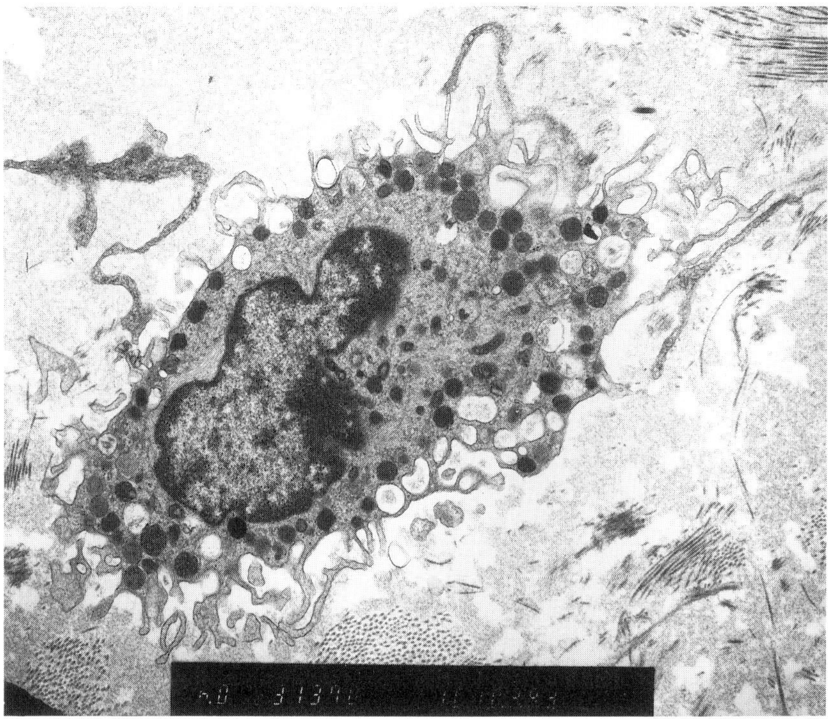

Figure 2 High-powered electron micrograph of a human nasal mast cell illustrating the presence of vacuolated granules consistent with degranulation.

nerve terminals where they regulate sympathetic tone (45). Stimulation of H_3 receptors would inhibit sympathetic tone and result in vascular engorgement and nasal blockage.

The lack of effect on nasal blockage with H_1-receptor antagonism in naturally occurring disease can also be explained by the redundancy within the system, as nasal blockage can be induced by kinins (46) as well as by lipid mediators, such as leukotrienes, prostaglandins, and platelet-activating factor (47). Leukotrienes appears to have a more prominent role than histamine in the genesis of nasal blockage, as 5-lipoxygenase inhibitors have been shown to inhibit acute allergen-induced nasal obstruction (48,49) and an LTD_4-receptor antagonist has been reported to prevent acute allergen-induced nasal obstruction in naturally occurring ragweed rhinitis (50). The contribution of prostaglandin D_2 and kinins to nasal obstruction has not been elucidated by specific receptor antagonism but has been clarified by nasal challenge studies using structural agonist analogs.

Table 1 Mediator Mechanisms of Rhinitis

Symptom	Mechanism	Mediator (receptor subtypes)
Nasal itch	Neural	Histamine (H_1)
		Endothelin (?)
Sneeze	Neural	Histamine (H_1)
		Endothelin (?)
Rhinorrhea	Neural	Histamine (H_1)
		Endothelin (?)
	Vascular	Histamine (H_1)
		Kinins (B_2)
		Leukotrienes (LTC_4/D_4)
Blockage	Vascular	Histamine ($H_1 + H_2 + ?H_3$)
		Kinins (B_2)
		Prostaglandin D_2 (DP)
		Leukotrienes (LTC_4/D_4)

These have demonstrated that the nasal obstructive effects of prostaglandin D_2 are mediated through the vascular DP receptor rather than the common TP receptor, as the PGD_2 metabolite, $9\alpha11\beta$ PGF_2, which is a TP but not a DP agonist (51), has no effect within the nose (52). Consistent with this, TP-receptor antagonism has no effect on PGD_2-induced nasal blockage (53). Comparable studies with bradykinin identify that its nasal effects are mediated through the bradykinin B_2 receptor, as the B_2 agonist kallidin, but not the B_1 agonist [des-arg[9]]-bradykinin, mimics the increase in nasal airways resistance and increase in plasma protein exudation induced by bradykinin (54,55).

In addition to the effects of acute mast cell degranulation on immediate symptom generation, mast cell degranulation will contribute to the eosinophilic mucosal inflammation that is evident in rhinitis. Mast cells within the nose have been demonstrated to contain preformed cytokines, in particular IL-4, IL-5, IL-6, and tumor necrosis factor (TNF)-alpha (32,56). Both IL-5 and $TNF\alpha$ have actions relevant to eosinophil activation and recruitment (57), while IL-4 will potentiate the effects of $TNF\alpha$ on the expression of VCAM-1 on the vascular endothelium (58). VCAM-1 is a leukocyte endothelial adhesion molecule relevant to tissue eosinophil recruitment through its interaction with the eosinophil ligand VLA-4 (vide infra). The immunoreactivity for IL-4 within nasal mucosal biopsies exists in two patterns when stained with different antibodies that recognize separate epitopes. One antibody 49D stains cytoplasmic IL-4 and this pattern is evident in both rhinitic and nonrhinitic biopsies, whereas the antibody 3H4 gives a peripheral ring staining to the cells and is considered to recognize a secretory form of IL-4. The IL-4 remains cell associated due to the limited diffusion of the exocytosed mast cell proteoglycan heparin. The 3H4 pattern of immunoreactivity is increased in seasonal and perennial rhinitis in comparison to the findings in the normal nose (32,33), indicative of ongoing cytokine secretion by mast cells in active disease.

B. Endothelial Cells

Endothelial cells are involved in allergic rhinitis not only as an end-organ, on which released inflammatory mediators act to induce plasma protein exudation (59), but these cells are also instrumental in inflammatory cell recruitment (60). The initial process of tissue leukocyte recruitment involves the adherence of circulating cells on the vascular endothelium prior to their diapedesis into the extravascular environment. This process involves the luminal expression on the vascular endothelium of leukocyte endothelial cell adhesion molecules (LECAMs) and their specific interaction with ligands expressed on the cell surface of leukocytes (60). Several LECAMs are considered to be involved in allergic inflammation, the selectins, P-selectin and E-selectin, along with ICAM-1 and VCAM-1, both members of the immunoglobulin supergene family. The initial phase of tissue leukocyte recruitment involves the mobilization of P-selectin onto the luminal surface from its preformed storage site in Wiebel-Palade bodies within the endothelial cell. This occurs under the influence of mediators such as histamine and PAF and will thus be the earliest vascular response to mast cell degranulation (61,62). P-selectin and the subsequent cytokine-dependent expression of E-selectin induces a rolling margination allowing the cells to subsequently adhere more firmly (Fig. 3). The endothelium expresses chemokines such as IL-8, MIP-1α, and RANTES. The exposure of the rolling leukocytes to these chemokines enhances cell surface ligand expression in an activated form and promotes firm cell adherence to the endothelium. This firmer adherence is regulated by LECAMs expressed following cytokine stimulation of the endothelial cells, in particular by the cytokines TNFα, IL-1β, and IFN-γ, with also a contribution from IL-4 with respect to VCAM-1 expression (58,63–65). This firm adherence has been linked to the later-appearing ICAM-1 and VCAM-1, predominately through the ligands LFA-1 and VLA-4, respectively (Fig. 4).

Immunohistochemical staining of nasal biopsies for the LECAMs and quantifying their expression in relationship to the total vascular component within biopsies has identified a seasonal increase in VCAM-1 in naturally occurring allergic rhinitis (66). VCAM-1 has very low or absent basal expression out of season, and the modest increase in season is associated with tissue eosinophil recruitment. An increased expression of VCAM-1 is also reported in nasal polyp tissue (67) and the extent of expression also related to tissue eosinophil accumulation in this study. VCAM-1 recognizes the ligand VLA-4, present on eosinophils, basophils, and T lymphocytes but not neutrophils (68). In contrast to other

LECAM-ligand interactions, VCAM-1–VLA-4 interactions confer some specificity with respect to tissue eosinophil accumulation. In perennial allergic disease, a condition that may be compounded by secondary infection and structural alterations, ICAM-1 has also been reported to have enhanced expression along with VCAM-1, when the findings are compared to those from nonrhinitic subjects (69). There is thus ongoing cell recruitment in active rhinitis, and consistent with this there is in perennial allergic disease, an increase in cells within the submucosa expressing LFA-1[+], a cell surface ligand for ICAM-1.

C. Epithelial Cells

The airway epithelium is now increasingly recognized as an active cell population involved in the inflammatory process. Upregulation of the epithelial expression of ICAM-1 is evident in both nasal smears (70) and nasal biopsies (71) in seasonal allergic rhinitis. Through its interaction with LFA-1 this may provide a mechanism for eosinophil retention at this site. The epithelium can also generate cytokines and chemokines relevant to tissue cell recruitment. Cultured human airway epithelial cells have been shown to synthesize GM-CSF, IL-6, IL-8, and RANTES (72,73), and the presence of enhanced IL-6, TNFα, IL-8, GM-CSG, and RANTES, immunoreactivity has been demonstrated with airway epithelium in nasal biopsies (74,75). These cytokines are regulated by the transcription factor NFkβ, and in concordance with this, the nasal airway epithelium also has the potential to generate nitric oxide (NO) and endothelin. There is enhanced expression of the inducible form of the enzyme NO synthase (iNOS) by the airway epithelium in allergic rhinitis. This enzyme generates NO, and consistent with these biopsy findings there are elevated levels of NO in exhaled air in rhinitis (Fig. 5) (76). NO is a vasodilator and its action in this respect may be opposed by the endothelins: a group of peptides with vasoconstrictor actions. The cytokines IL-1β, TNFα, and IFN-γ have been shown in in vitro epithelial culture systems to upregulate iNOS and endothelin (77). There is evidence of enhanced mRNA for endothelin in mucosal cells, vessels, and airway epithelium within the nose in allergic rhinitis (78). Endothelin has also been suggested to induce secondary mediator release (79), and although the evidence in this respect is conflicting (80), such an action may underlie the recent report that endothelin nasal challenge induces nasal itch, sneeze, and rhinorrhea (81). The local generation and release of endothelin by airway cells in rhinitis may thus contribute to the clinical disease expression.

IV. Cell Infiltration and Activation

Allergic rhinitis is also characterized by alterations in nonresident cell populations, not only with tissue eosinophil recruitment and activation but also with changes involving T lymphocytes and basophils.

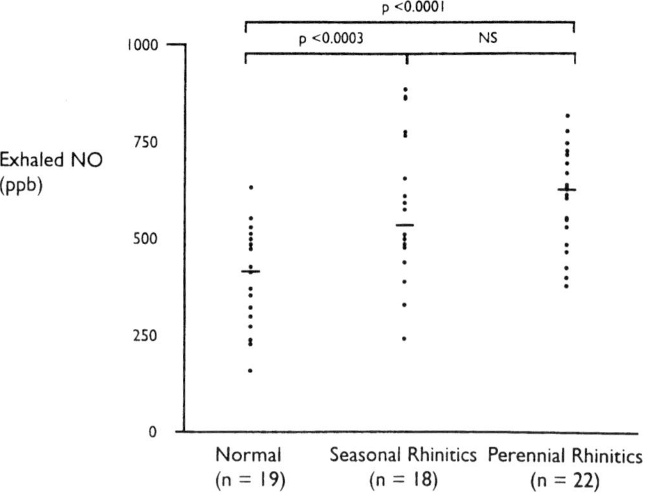

Figure 5 Measurements of NO in exhaled air by direct nasal sampling and chemiluminescence analysis in normal nonrhinitic subjects ($n = 19$), and patients with seasonal allergic ($n = 18$) and perennial allergic ($n = 22$) rhinitis, identifying significantly higher levels in the rhinitis patients than in the healthy subjects.

A. Eosinophils

Eosinophils are not a normal cellular constituent of the nose. Immunohistochemical staining of nasal mucosal biopsies identifies that eosinophils are evident in nasal mucosal biopsies within the submucosa and epithelium in active rhinitis (31–33) and their recovery is increased in nasal smear specimens (82,83). Transmission electron microscopy examination of nasal biopsies from patients with rhinitis reveals evidence of ultrastructural granular changes of eosinophil activation (Fig. 6). The normal eosinophil has granules that on electron microscopy have an electron-dense core surrounded by a less dense matrix. The electron-dense core is due to the presence of crystals of major basic protein (84), which comprise approximately 55% of the granular protein content. In addition to major basic protein (MBP), the eosinophil granules contain, within the matrix, eosinophil cationic protein (ECP), eosinophil-derived neurotoxin (EDN), and eosinophil peroxidase (EPX) as well as numerous enzymes such as ribonucleases and histaminase (85,86). Eosinophils in nasal biopsies in rhinitis have been demonstrated to also contain IL-5 (32). Eosinophil activation is associated both with the release of granule components and with the de novo generation of arachidonic acid products. The major lipoxygenase arachidonic acid cleavage product is LTC_4, and eosinophils, primed by chemotactic factors and cytokines such as IL-3, IL-5, and

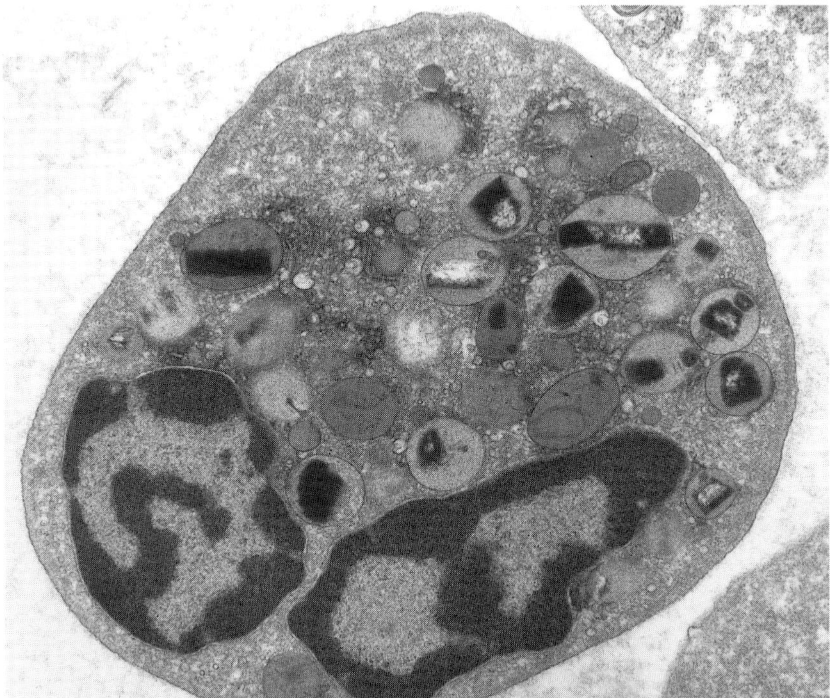

Figure 6 High-powered electron micrograph of a tissue eosinophil within the nasal mucosa illustrating the presence of granules within the cytoplasm and the loss of the electron-dense core to certain granules consistent with cell activation and degranulation.

GM-CSF, have an enhanced state of activation and exhibit exaggerated LTC_4 generation and release (87–89). The generation of LTC_4 by eosinophils may contribute to nasal obstruction and to rhinorrhea.

An elevation in immunoreactive LTC_4 is evident in nasal lavage fluid in seasonal allergic rhinitis (90). In addition to an eosinophil source, LTC_4 may also be derived following either mast cell or basophil activation (4). A marker that is more specific for eosinophil activation is ECP and an increase in nasal lavage ECP is evident in both seasonal and perennial allergic rhinitis (91,92).

B. Basophils

Basophils are evident in nasal smear samples in allergic rhinitis (93,94) and can be demonstrated to increase in asymptomatic seasonal rhinitic patients 24 hr following nasal allergen challenge (95). Basophils possesses fewer, larger granules and differ from the mast cell in that they contain less histamine. On immunological activation the basophil releases only 20–30% of the histamine released from a comparable number of mast cells. Basophils possess different proportions of proteoglycans, having predominantly chondroitin sulfate A and E rather than heparin, contain only 1–3% of the mast cell tryptase content, do not generate PGD_2, and, unlike the mast cell, store a small quantity of major basic protein (MBP) and eosinophil-derived neurotoxin (EDN) (96–98). The basophil does, however, generate a comparable amount of LTC_4 as the mast cell following immunological activation (60 ng/10^6 cells) (91).

Basophils, which, like mast cells, possess high-affinity IgE receptors, are also derived from CD34+ progenitor cells in the bone marrow (99). An increase in circulating basophils is described in rhinitis (100) consistent with stimulation of these progenitor cells. A number of cytokines have been reported to prime basophils in vitro for increased mediator release in response to subsequent stimulation. These stimuli include IL-1, IL-3, IL-5, and GM-CSF (101–103). Subsequently, studies have also identified that IL-1β, IL-3, GM-CSF, and TNFα are able to induce mediator release directly (104–107) although this has not been a consistent finding (108). A number of other cytokines have more recently been identified that may be of greater relevance to basophil activation in rhinitis as they are more potent and not solely restricted in their action to only a proportion of donors. These are "histamine-releasing factors" (HRFs), a term used to describe products released from activated mononuclear cells that are capable of inducing basophil histamine release (109,110). HRFs factors have been identified in nasal lavage (111). Several members of the chemokine family are now known to account for a proportion of this activity, including connective-tissue-activating peptide III (CTAP III) and its derivative neutrophil-activating peptide-2 (NAP-2 (112,113), MCP-1 (114), RANTES (115), and MIP-1α and MIP-1β (116). RANTES has been shown to be expressed within the airway epithelium and to be released following nasal allergen challenge (117), although levels of this chemokine are below the level of detection in lavage in the majority of patients with naturally occurring rhinitis (118). Elevated levels of MIP-1α and MCP-1 do, however, increase in nasal lavage in season during ragweed rhinitis (118), and there appears to be a reciprocal relationship between the level of these chemokines and IL-8, a chemokine that inhibits their HR activity on basophils. In addition, basophils themselves are now also appreciated to be capable of synthesizing the cytokines IL-4 and IL-8 (119,120). The relevance of this cell population to cytokine synthesis within the tissue is, however, uncertain as preformed IL-4 predominantly colocalizes to mast cells in nasal biopsies (32,33).

C. T Lymphocytes

The T lymphocyte represents a significant nonstructural cell within the nasal mucosa. An increase in certain T-cell populations has been described in nasal biopsy specimens in both seasonal (121–123) and perennial (121) rhinitic patients, although this is not a consistent finding (124). These cells have been reported to be activated (125) although IL-2 receptor expression is low and usually no different from that identified in normal controls (123,124) and there is no seasonal change within grass-pollen-sensitive subjects when symptomatic and nonsymptomatic periods are compared (121). Where there is a T-cell increase, it is largely related to an increase in the CD4 cell population, which has the potential to generate proinflammatory cytokines. Assessment of the cytokine profile may thus be a more accurate method of assessing relevant T-cell activation in rhinitis. T lymphocytes of the TH2 subpopulation can generate IL-3, IL-4, IL-5, GM-CSF, and TNF-α. Following nasal allergen challenge, an increase in IL-4, IL-5, and GM-CSF mRNA-positive cells has been described in association with a mucosal eosinophilia (126), and T-cell clones derived from nasal mucosa challenged with allergen in vivo have a cytokine profile comparable with a TH2-like population (127). These findings are consistent with allergen-related T-lymphocyte activation and cytokine secretion and, by inference, with a contribution by this cell population to tissue leukocyte cell recruitment. In chronic perennial allergic rhinitis there is an increase in T-cells expressing the $\delta\alpha$ T-cell receptor within the epithelium and these cells have an enhanced capacity to generate TH2-cytokines (128).

V. Inflammatory Model of Rhinitis

It is apparent that through their interaction with neural and vascular receptors, released mediators may induce the clinical features of rhinitis. Several cells are now appreciated to be involved in bringing about these end-organ responses, with mediator release from mast cells, basophils, eosinophils, and epithelial cells representing the effector function of this process (Fig. 7). The temporal interrelationship between these events has been studied by nasal allergen challenge using nasal lavage, nasal smear, and nasal biopsy techniques.

The immediate nasal response to allergen insufflation within the nose is nasal pruritus, sneezing, and anterior rhinorrhea followed by the development of nasal blockage. In association with symptom development, increased levels of histamine, tryptase, PGD_2, LTB_4, LTC_4, LTD_4, and kinins have been described in recovered nasal lavage fluid (129–136). These findings are indicative of acute mast cell degranulation. Consistent with this, analysis of nasal biopsies at this time reveals ultrastructural features of mast cell degranulation (137–139). The immediate response is followed by resolution of symptoms and a subsequent second increment in mediator levels (late response), which is characterized by elevations in lavage histamine but no increment in either PGD_2 or tryptase (128–

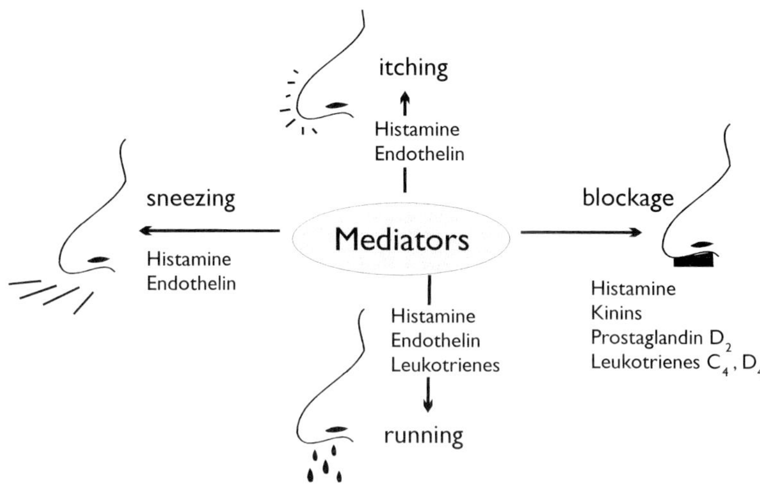

Figure 7   Mediators and symptom generation in allergic rhinitis.

134). This late increase in histamine, in the absence of PGD$_2$ or tryptase, is suggestive of basophil activation. Correspondingly, a late increase in basophil numbers has been identified in nasal cytospins following local allergen challenge (96). There is also evidence of a late accumulation of eosinophils in nasal smear and biopsy samples taken 24 hr post–allergen challenge (126,139,140) and of T-lymphocyte activation (25).

The initial phase of tissue cell recruitment is the upregulation of endothelial LECAMs (60). The first event in this process is mobilization of P-selectin onto the surface of the vascular endothelium from Wiebel-Palade bodies within the endothelial cells. This occurs in response to mediators, such as histamine, and will thus be related to mast cell degranulation (61). P-selectin interacts with carbohydrate moieties on leukocyte cell surfaces to induce a rolling leukocyte margination. Subsequently there is enhanced expression of endothelial expression of E-selectin and ICAM-1 followed by VCAM-1. These events are regulated by cytokines, in particular TNFα and IL-1β (150). IL-4 potentiates the effect of TNFα on VCAM-1 endothelial expression in vitro (58), and in animal models IL-4 antibodies substantially abrogate the expression of acute allergen-induced airway eosinophilia (141). A similar IL-4 dependency is evident in IL-4-deficient mice (142). Thus the release of cytokines from mast cells, as has been shown to occur within the nose following nasal allergen challenge (56), will substantially contribute to the events involved in acute allergen-induced tissue cell recruitment.

In accordance with this, an increase in E-selectin and ICAM-1 is evident in nasal biopsies within 6 hr of allergen challenge and this is associated within tissue accumulation of neutrophils, eosinophils, and T lymphocytes (143). The subsequent elaboration of cytokines from T lymphocytes will perpetuate this response. An increase in IL-4 and IL-5 mRNA-positive cells has been reported 24 hr following nasal allergen challenge (125), consistent with activation of a TH2-like population of cells.

The TH2-like cytokines, IL-3, IL-5, and GM-CSF have relevance for the tissue eosinophilia in allergic rhinitis (57) (Fig. 8). These cytokines stimulate progenitor cells from the marrow, enhance their maturation, exert weak chemotactic effects, prime the cells for activation, prolong survival and delay programmed cell death (144–160). Primed eosinophils have an enhanced LTC_4 generation (144,156,157) and also exhibit an exaggerated chemotactic response to stimuli, such as IL-8, to which they are relatively insensitive in the nonprimed state (151–154). The release of the chemokines IL-8 and RANTES from the airway epithelium will thus promote an eosinophil accumulation within an epithelial location (Fig. 9). IL-8 can be released from epithelial cells in vitro by mast cell tryptase (161), further linking mast cell activation with tissue leucocyte recruitment. Activated eosinophils can themselves generate cytokines and these cells have been shown to synthesize IL-3, IL-5, IL-6, IL-8, TNFα, MIP-1α, and GM-CSF (162), and in vivo both IL-4 and IL-5 have been colocalized in nasal biopsies to tissue eosinophils (32,33). The release of cytokines from activated eosinophils will serve an autocrine function, leading to their persistence at sites of allergic inflammation. In addition to an involvement in eosinophil recruitment, the epithelial generation and release of chemokines can also be related to the epithelial accumulation of mast cells in seasonal and perennial disease (32,33), as both IL-8 and RANTES have been reported recently to be mast cell chemoattractants (163,164).

The epithelium is increasingly recognized as an active cell population, and the recent identification that this cell population generates endothelin and that endothelin nasal insufflation induces nasal itch, sneeze, and rhinorrhea indicates that epithelial activation will significantly contribute to the clinical expression of rhinitis. The ability of endothelin to stimulate these responses also provides an explanation for the incomplete efficacy of H_1-antihistamines in alleviating nasal itch, sneeze, and rhinorrhea in allergic rhinitis, in particular at periods of high pollen exposure (41). The suggestion that epithelial cells may be able to directly interact with allergen would provide a mechanism for this release but this requires further verification within the nose.

In addition to these cellular events and their regulation, there is also neural involvement in the disease, not only as a component of the cholinergic rhinorrhea but also as a primary response. It is now appreciated that in addition to the autonomic regulation of glandular secretion and nasal vascular tone, there is also nonadrenergic, noncholinergic regulation within the nasal airways involving peptidergic nerves. Activation of sensory neurons by irritants and locally released mediators has been reported to induce vasodilation and enhance microvascular leakage through stimulation of local axonal reflexes and by modification of ganglionic neurotransmission (165,166). The neurotransmitters for the axon reflex include the sensory neuropeptides, substance P, neurokinin A, and calcitonin-gene-related peptide (CGRP) (167,168). Activation of the sensory nerves, in addition to simulating axonal reflexes, influences neural control of the vasculature via an action on the nerve cell bodies in the trigeminal and sphenopalatine ganglia. These reflexes seem to be mainly vasodilatory, causing nasal blockage through regulation of intrinsic sympathetic tone. Studies undertaken in humans have demonstrated the presence of receptors for substance P, neurokinin A, and CGRP in the nasal epithelium, venous blood vessels, arterial blood vessels, glands, and neural ganglia of the nasal mucosa (169,170). Both substance P and CGRP are released within 3 min of nasal allergen challenge (171), as evidenced by increased recovery of these neuropeptides in nasal lavage. Nasal challenge with substance P induces nasal blockage (172) and repeated application of substance P to the nose enhances vascular permeability (173). Thus substance P could be directly implicated in inducing nasal obstruction. The concentrations of substance P that induce nasal obstruction are, however, associated with noticeable facial flushing, raising the possibility that these nasal effects will occur only at supraphysiological concentrations. Counterbalancing this is the consideration that the local release of substance P from nerves in close proximity to the nasal vasculature may produce effects at local concentrations considerably less than that evidenced by nasal challenge studies. In addition to these considerations, substance P has the potential to indirectly influence nasal blockage, as it has been shown to induce eosinophil recruitment within the nose (174), and in human nasal explants substance P has been found to increase gene expression of cytokines that will prime eosinophils for enhanced activation (175). This effect on gene expression is more marked and more extensive in its profile in nasal tissue from patients with allergic rhinitis than in nasal tissue from healthy controls.

An understanding of the mechanisms of disease generation in rhinitis thus provides a framework for rational therapy for this disorder, which is important as allergic rhinitis is increasingly common.

References

1. Burrows B, Martinez FD, Halonen M, Barbee RA, Cline MG. Association of asthma with serum IgE levels and skin test reactivity to allergens. N Engl J Med 1989; 320:271–277.
2. Howarth PH. Allergic rhinitis: a rational choice of treatment. Respir Med 1989; 83:179–188.

3. Sampson HA. Immediate reactions to food. In: Metcalfe DD, Sampson HA, Simon RA, eds. Food Allergy: Adverse Reactions to Foods and Food Additives. Boston: Blackwell Scientific Publications, 1991:100–112.

4. Howarth PH. The cellular basis for allergic rhinitis. Allergy 1995; 50(Suppl 23): 6–10.

5. Connell JT. Quantitative intranasal pollen challenge. II. Effect of daily pollen challenge, environmental pollen exposure and placebo challenge on the nasal membrane. J Allergy 1968; 41:123–139.

6. Connell JT. Quantitative intranasal pollen challenge. III. The priming effect in allergic rhinitis. J Allergy 1969; 43:33–44.

7. Johansson SGO. Raised levels of a new immunoglobulin class (IgND) in asthma. Lancet 1967; 2:951–953.

8. Ishizaka K, Ishizaka T, Hornbrook MM. Physicochemical properties of human reaginic antibody. IV. Presence of a unique immunoglobulin as a carrier of reaginic activity. J Immunol 1986; 97:75–85.

9. Del Prete GF, Maggi E, Parronchi P, et al. IL-4 is an essential co-factor for the IgE synthesis induced in vitro by human T-cell clones and their supernatants. J Immunol 1988; 140:4193–4198.

10. Pene J, Rousset F, Briere F, Chretien I, Bonnefoy JY, Spits H, Yokota T, Arai N, Arai KI, Banchereau J, de Vries JE. IgE production by normal human lymphocytes is induced by interleukin-4 and suppressed by interferon γ and prostaglandin E2. Proc Natl Acad Sci USA 1988; 85:6880.

11. Gauchat J-F, Lebman DA, Coffman RL, Gascan H, de Vries JE. Structure and expression of germline ϵ transcripts in human B cells induced by interleukin 4 to switch to IgE production. J Exp Med 1990; 172:463–473.

12. Punnonen J, Aversa G, Cocks BG, McKenzie ANJ, Menon S, Zurawski G, de Waal Malefyt R, de Vries JE. Interleukin 13 induces interleukin 4-independent IgG4 and IgE synthesis and CD23 expression by human B cells. Proc Natl Acad Sci USA 1993; 90:3730.

13. Defrance T, Carayon P, Bilian G, Guillemot JC, Minty A, Caput D, Ferrara P. Interleukin 13 is a B cell stimulating factor. J Exp Med 1994; 179:135.

14. Zurawski SM, Vega F Jr, Huyghe B, Zurawski G. Receptors for interleukin 13 and interleukin 4 are complex and share a novel component that functions in signal transduction. EMBO J 1993; 12:2663–2670.

15. Kühn R, Rajewsky K, Müller W. Generation and analysis of IL-4 deficient mice. Science 1991; 254:707–710.

16. Tepper RI, Levinson, DA, Stanger BZ, Campos-Torres J, Abbas AK, Leder P. IL-4 induces allergic-like inflammatory disease and alters T cell development in transgenic mice. Cell 1990; 62:457.

17. Defrance T, Aubry JP, Rousset F, et al. Human recombinant interleukin 4 induces Fc_ϵ receptors (CD23) on normal human B lymphocytes. J Exp Med 1987; 165: 1459–1467.

18. Rousset F, de Waal Malefijt R, Slierendregt B, Aubrey J-P, Bonnefoy JY, Defrance T, Banchereau J, de Vries JE. Regulation of Fc receptor for IgE (CD23) and class II MHC antigen expression on Burkitt's lymphoma cell kines by human IL-4 and IFN-γ. J Immunol 1988; 140:2625.

19. Vercelli D, Jabara HH, Arai K, Geha RS. Induction of human IgE synthesis requires IL-4 and T/B cell interactions involving the T cell receptor/CD3 complex and MHC class II antigens. J Exp Med 1989; 169:1295–1307.

20. Spriggs MK, Armitage RJ, Strockbine L, Clifford KN, Macduff BM, Sato TA, Maliszewski CR, Fanslow WC. Recombinant human CD40 ligand stimulates B cell proliferation and immunoglobulin E synthesis. J Exp Med 1992; 176:1543.

21. Castle BE, Kishimoto K, Stearns C, Brown ML, Kehry MR. Regulation of expression of the ligand for CD40 on T helper lymphocytes. J Immunol 1993; 151:1777–1788.

22. June CH, Bluestone JA, Nadler LM, Thompson CB. The B7 and CD28 and receptor families. Immunol Today 1994; 15:321.

23. Zhang KE, Clark EA, Saxon A. CD40 stimulation provides an IFNγ-independent and IL-4-dependent differentiation signal directly to human B cells for IgE production. J Immunol 1991; 146:1836–1842.

24. Gauchet JF, Henchoz S, Mazzel G, Aubry JP, Brunner T, Blasey H, et al. Induction of human IgE synthesis in B cells by mast cells and basophils. Nature 1993; 365: 340–343.

25. Ying S, Durham SR, Jacobson MR, et al. T-lymphocytes and mast cells express messenger RNA for interleukin-4 in the nasal mucosa in allergen induced rhinitis. Immunology 1994; 82:200–206.

26. Bradding P, Feather IH, Wilson S, Bardin P, Holgate ST, Howarth PH. Immunolocalisation of cytokines in the nasal mucosa of normal and perennial rhinitis subjects: the mast cell as a source of IL-4, IL-5 and IL-6 in human allergic inflammation. J Immunol 1993; 151:3853–3865.

27. Fokkens WJ, Vroom T, Rijntes E, Mulder P. Fluctuation of the number of CD1a-positive dendritic cells, in the nasal mucosa of patients with isolated grass pollen allergy before, during and after the grass pollen season. J Allergy Clin Immunol 1989; 84:39–43.

28. Holm AF, Fokkens WJ, Godthelp T, Mulder PG, Vroom TM, Rijntjes E. Effect of 3 months steroid therapy on nasal T cells and Langerhans cells in patients suffering from allergic rhinitis. Allergy 1995; 50.204–209.

29. Lichtenstein LM, Ishizaka K, Norman PS, Sabotka AK, Hill BM. IgE antibody measurements in ragweed hay fever. J Clin Invest 1973; 52:472–482.

30. Naclerio RM, Atkinson NF, Creticos PS, Baroody FM, Hamilton RG, Norman PS. Intranasal steroids inhibit seasonal increases in ragweed specific immunoglobin E antibodies. J Allergy Clin Immunol 1993; 92:717–721.

31. Durham SR. Local IgE production in nasal allergy. Int Arch Allergy Appl Immunol 1998 (in press).

32. Bradding P, Feather IH, Wilson S, Bardin P, Holgate ST, Howarth PH. Immunolocalisation of cytokines in the nasal mucosa of normal and perennial rhinitis subjects: the mast cell as a source of IL-4, IL-5 and IL-6 in human allergic inflammation. J Immunol 1993; 151:3853–3865.

33. Bradding P, Feather IH, Wilson S, Holgate ST, Howarth PH. The effects of seasonal exposure to allergic nasal cytokine immunoreactivity and its modulation by fluticasone propionate. Thorax 1993; 48:1059.

34. Viegas M, Gomez E, Brooks J, Davies RJ. The effect of the pollen season on nasal mast cell numbers. Br Med J 1987; 294:414.

99. Kirschenbaum AS, Kessler SW, Gott JP, Metcalfe DD. Demonstration of the origin of human mast cells from CD34+ bone marrow progenitor cells. J Immunol 1991; 146:1410–1415.

100. Charance M, Herbeth B, Kauffman F. Seasonal patterns of circulating basophils. Int Arch Allergy Appl Immunol 1988; 86:462–464.

101. Massey WA, Randall J, Kagey-Sobotka A, Warner JA, MacDonald SM, Gillis S, Lichtenstein LM. Recombinant human IL-1α and IL-1β potentiate IgE dependent basophil histamine release. J Immunol 1989; 143:1875–1880.

102. Bischoff SC, De Weck AL, Dahinden CA. Interleukin-3 and granulocyte/macrophage-colony-stimulating factor render human basophils responsive to low concentrations of complement component C3a. Proc Natl Acad Sci USA 1990; 87: 6813–6817.

103. Bischoff SC, Brunner T, De Weck AL, Dahinden CA. Interleukin 5 modifies histamine release and leukotriene generation by human basophils in response to diverse agonists. J Exp Med 1990; 172:1577–1582.

104. Haak-Frendscho M, Arai N, Arai K, Baeza ML, Finn A, Kaplan AP. Human recombinant granulocyte-macrophage colony-stimulating factor and interleukin 3 cause basophil histamine release. J Clin Invest 1988; 82:17–20.

105. MacDonald SM, Schleimer RP, Kagey-Sobotka A, Gillis S, Lichtenstein LM. Recombinant IL-3 induces histamine release from human basophils. J Immunol 1989; 142:3527–3532.

106. Haak-Frendscho M, Dinarell C, Kaplan AP. Recombinant human interleukin-1 beta causes histamine release from human basophils. J Allergy Clin Immunol 1988; 82: 218–223.

107. Subramanian N, Bray MA. Interleukin 1 release histamine from human basophils and mast cells in vitro. J Immunol 1987; 138:271–275.

108. Alam R, Wetter JB, Forsythe PA, Lett-Brown MA, Grant JA. Comparative effects of recombinant IL-1, -2, -3, -4 and -6, IFN-γ, granulocyte-macrophage colony stimulating factor, tumour necrosis factor-α and histamine releasing factors on the secretion of histamine from basophils. J Immunol 1989; 142:3431–3435.

109. Thueson DO, Speck LS, Lett-Brown MA, Grant JA. Histamine-releasing activity (HRA). 1. Production of a histamine releasing lymphokine by mitogen or antigen stimulated human mononuclear cells. J Immunol 1979; 123:623–632.

110. Thueson DO, Speck LS, Lett-Brown MA, Grant JA. Histamine-releasing activity (HRA). II. Interaction with basophils and physicochemical characterisation. J Immunol 1997; 123:633–639.

111. Sim TC, Hilsmeier KA, Alam R, Allan RK, Lett-Brown MA, Grant JA. Effect of topical corticosteroids on the recovery of histamine releasing factors in nasal washings of patients with allergic rhinitis. Am Rev Respir Dis 1992; 145:1316–1320.

112. Baeza ML, Riddigari SR, Kornfield D, Ramani N, Smith E, Hossler PA, Fischer T, Castor CW, Gorevic PG, Kaplan AP. Relationship of one form of human histamine-releasing factor to connective tissue activating peptide-III. J Clin Invest 1990; 85: 1516–1521.

113. Reddigari SR, Kuna P, Miraliotta GF, Kornfield D, Baeza ML, Castor CW, Kaplan AP. Connective tissue-activating peptide-III and its derivative, neutrophil-activat-

ing peptide-2, release histamine from human basophils. J Allergy Clin Immunol 1992; 89:666–672.

114. Kuna P, Reddigari SR, Racinski D, Oppenheim JJ, Kaplan AP. Monocyte chemotactic and activating factor is a potent histamine-releasing factor for human basophils. J Exp Med 1992; 175:489–493.

115. Kuna P, Reddigari SR, Schall TJ, Rucinski D, Viksman MY, Kaplan AP. RANTES, a monocyte and T-lymphocyte chemotactic cytokine, releases histamine from human basophils. J Immunol 1992; 149:636–642.

116. Kuna P, Reddigari SR,Schall TJ, Rucinski D, Sadick M, Kaplan AP. Characterization of the human basophil response to cytokines, growth factors, and histamine releasing factors of the intercrine/chemokine family. J Immunol 1993; 150:1932–1943.

117. Rajakulasingam K, Hamid Q, O'Brien M, et al. Increases in RANTES messenger RNA and protein in the nasal mucosa and nasal secretions in hayfever patients after allergen challenge. J Allergy Clin Immunol 1996; 97:43.

118. Kuna P, Lazarorich M, Kaplan AP. Chemokines in seasonal allergic rhinitis. J Allergy Clin Immunol 1996; 97:104–112.

119. Brunner T, Hausser CH, Dahinden CA. Human peripheral blood basophils primed by interleukin-3 (IL-3) produce IL-4 in response to immunoglobulin E receptor stimulation. J Exp Med 1993; 177:605–611.

120. Elmedal B, Bjerke T, Rendiger N, Markvardsen P, Nielsen S, Schiotz PO. IL-8 is produced and prestored in human blood basophils. Allergy 1993; 16:2861 (abstract).

121. Calderon MA, Lozewicz S, Prior A, Jordan S, Trigg CJ, Davies RJ. Lymphocyte infiltration and thickness of the nasal mucus membrane in perennial and seasonal allergic rhinitis. J Allergy Clin Immunol 1994; 93:635–643.

122. Saito H, Asakura K, Kataura A. Studies on the properties of infiltrating T-lymphocytes and ICAM-1 expression in allergic nasal mucosa. Acta Otolaryngol (Stockh) 1994; 114:315–323.

123. Karlsson MG, Davidsson A, Hellquist HB. Increase in CD4+ and CD45Ro+ memory T-cells in the nasal mucosal of allergic patients. APMIS 1994; 102:753–758.

124. Fokkens WJ, Holm AF, Rijntes E, Mulder PS, Vroom TM. Characterisation and quantification of cellular infiltrates in nasal mucosa of patients with grass pollen allergy, nonallergic patients and controls. Int Arch Allergy Immunol 1990; 93:66–72.

125. Okuda M, Pawankar R. Flow cytokine analysis of intraepithelial lymphocytes in the human nasal mucosa. Allergy 1992; 47:255–259.

126. Durham SR, Ying S, Varney VA, Jacobson MR, Sudderick RM, Mackay IS, Kay AB, Hamid QA. Cytokine messenger RNA expression of IL-3, IL-4, IL-5 and granulocyte/macrophage colony-stimulating factor in the nasal mucosa after local allergen provocation: relationship to tissue eosinophilia. J Immunol 1992; 148:2390–2394.

127. Del-Prete GF, De Cari M, D'Elios MM, Maestrelli P, Ricci M, Fabbri L, Romagnani S. Allergen exposure induces the activation of allergen-specific Th2 cells in the airway mucosa of patients with allergic respiratory disorders. Eur J Immunol 1993; 23:1445–1449.

128. Pawankar R, Okuda M, Suzuki Ki K, Okumara K, Ra-C. Phenotypic and molecular characteristics of nasal mucosal gamma delta T cells in allergic and infectious rhinitis. Am J Resp 1996; 153:1655–1665.

129. Raphael GD, Igrashi Y, White MV, Kaliner MA. The pathophysiology of rhinitis. V. Sources of protein in allergen-induced nasal secretions. J Allergy Clin Immunol 1991; 88:33–42.

130. Nacleiro RM, Proud D, Togias AG, et al. Inflammatory mediators in late antigen-induced rhinitis. N Engl J Med 1985; 313:65–70.

131. Castells M, Schwartz LB. Tryptase levels in nasal-lavage fluid as an indicator of the immediate allergic response. J Allergy Clin Immunol 1988; 82:348–355.

132. Proud D, Bailey GS, Naclerio RN, et al. Tryptase and histamine as markers to evaluate mast cell activation during the responses to nasal challenge with allergen, cold, dry air, and hyperosmolar solutions. J Allergy Clin Immunol 1992; 89:1098–1110.

133. Proud D, Togias A, Naclerio RM, Crush SA, Norman PS, Lichtenstein LM. Kinins are generated in vivo following nasal airway challenge of allergic individuals with allergen. J Clin Invest 1983; 72:1678–1685.

134. Creticos PS, Peters SP, Adkinson Jr NF, et al. Peptide leukotriene release after antigen challenge in patients sensitive to ragweed. N Engl J Med 1984; 310:1626–1630.

135. Freeland HS, Pipkorn U, Schleimer RP, et al. Leukotriene B_4 as a mediator of early and late reactions to antigen in humans. The effect of systemic glucocorticoid treatments in vivo. J Allergy Clin Immunol 1989; 83:634–642.

136. Kawabori S, Unno T. Degranulation of nasal epithelial mast cells after challenge of allergen. J Submicrosc Cytol Pathol 1983; 15:823–832.

137. Kawabori S, Okuda M, Unno T. Mast cells in allergic nasal epithelium and lamina propria before and after provocation. Clin Allergy 1983; 13:181–189.

138. Gomez E, Corrado OJ, Baldwin DL, Swanston AR, Davies RJ. Direct in vivo evidence for mast cell degranulation during allergen induced reactions in man. J Allergy Clin Immunol 1986; 78:637–645.

139. Bascom R, Pipkorn U, Lichtenstein LM, Naclerio RM. The influx of inflammatory cells into nasal washings during the late response to antigen challenge. Am Rev Respir Dis 1988; 138:406–412.

140. Klementsson H, Andersson M, Baumgarten CR, Venge P, Pipkorn U. Change in non-specific nasal reactivity and eosinophil influx and activation after allergen challenge. Clin Exp Allergy 1990; 20:539–549.

141. Lukas NW, Strieter RM, Chensue SW, Kunkel SL. Interleukin-4-dependent pulmonary eosinophil infiltration in a murine model of asthma. Am J Respir Cell Mol Biol 1994; 10:526–532.

142. Bruselle GG, Kips JC, Travernier JH, Van der Heyden JG, Cavelier CA, Pauwels RA, Bluethmann H. Alteration of allergic airway inflammation in IL-4 deficient mice. Clin Exp Allergy 1994; 24:73–80.

143. Feather IH, Montefort S, Hibbert J, Wilson S, Howarth PH. The influence of allergen challenge on cell accumulation and leucocyte endothelial cell adhesion molecule (CAM) expression within the nasal mucosa in rhinitis. Eur Respir J 1994; 7(Suppl 18):1605.

144. Lopez AF, Williamson DW, Gamble JR, et al. Recombinant human granulocyte-macrophage colony-stimulating factor stimulates in vitro mature human neutrophil and eosinophil function, surface receptor expression, and survival. J Clin Invest 1986; 78:1220–1228.

145. Campbell HD, Tucker WQJ, Hort Y, et al. Molecular cloning, nucleotide sequence, and expression of the gene encoding human eosinophil differentiation factor (interleukin 5). Proc Natl Acad Sci USA 1987; 84:6629–6633.

146. Clutterbuck EJ, Shields JG, Gordon J, et al. Recombinant human interleukin 5 is an eosinophil differentiation factor but has no activity in standard human B cell growth factor assays. Eur J Immunol 1987; 17:1743–1750.

147. Clutterbuck E, Hirst EMA, Sanderson CJ. Human interleukin-5 (IL-5) regulates the production of eosinophils in human bone marrow cultures: comparison and interaction with IL-1, IL-3, IL-6, and GM-CSF. Blood 1989; 73:1504–1512.

148. Saito H, Hatake K, Dvorak AM, et al. Selective differentiation and proliferation of haemopoietic cells induced by recombinant interleukins. Proc Natl Acad Sci USA 1988; 85:2288–2292.

149. Clutterbuck EJ, Sanderson CJ. Regulation of human eosinophil precursor production by cytokines: a comparison of recombinant human interleukin-1 (rhIL-1), rhIL-3, rhIL-5, rhIL-6 and rh granulocyte-macrophage colony-stimulating factor. Blood 1990; 75:1774–1779.

150. Wang JM, Rimaldi A, Biondi A, Chen ZG, Sanderson CJ, Mantovani A. Recombinant human interleukin 5 is a selective eosinophil chemoattractant. Eur J Immunol 1989; 19:701–705.

151. Warringa RAJ, Koenderman L, Kok PTM, Kreukniet J, Bruijnzeel PLB. Modulation and induction of eosinophil chemotaxis by granulocyte-macrophage colony-stimulating factor and interleukin-3. Blood 1991; 77:2694–2700.

152. Sehmi R, Wardlaw AJ, Cromwell O, Kurihara K, Waltmann P, Kay AB. Interleukin-5 selectively enhances the chemotactic response of eosinophils obtained from normal but not eosinophilic subjects. Blood 1992; 79:2952–2959.

153. Warringa RAJ, Mengelers HJJ, Kuijper PHM, Raaijmakers JAM, Bruijnzeel PLB, Koenderman L. In vivo priming of platelet-activating factor-induced eosinophil chemotaxis in allergic asthmatic individuals. Blood 1992; 79:1836–1841.

154. Warringa RAJ, Schweizer RC, Maikoe T, Kuijper PHM, Bruijnzeel PLB, Koenderman L. Modulation of eosinophil chemotaxis by interleukin-5. Am J Respir Cell Mol Biol 1992; 7:631–636.

155. Schweizer R-C, Welmers BAC, Raaijmakers JAM, Zanen P, Lammers J-W, Koenderman L. RANTES- and interleukin-8-induced responses in normal human eosinophils: effect of priming with interleukin-5. Blood 1994; 83:3697–3704.

156. Owen Jr WF, Rothenberg ME, Silberstein DS, Gasson JC, Stevens RL, Austen KF, Soberman RJ. Regulation of human eosinophil viability, density and function by granulocyte/macrophage colony-stimulating factor in the presence of 3T3 fibroblasts. J Exp Med 1987; 166:129–141.

157. Rotheburg ME, Owen Jr WF, Silberstein DS, Woods J, Soberman RJ, Austen KF, Stevens RL. Human eosinophils have prolonged survival, enhanced functional properties, and become hypodense when exposed to human interleukin 3. J Clin Invest 1988; 81:1986–1992.

158. Tai P-C, Sun L, Spry CJF. Effects of IL-5, granulocyte/macrophage colony-stimulating factor (GM-CSF) and IL-3 on the survival of human blood eosinophils in vitro. Clin Exp Immunol 1991; 85:312–316.

159. Valerius T, Repp R, Kalden JR, Platzer E. Effects of IFN on human eosinophils

in comparison with other cytokines: a novel class of eosinophil activators with delayed onset of action. J Immunol 1990; 145:2950–2958.

160. Stern M, Meagher L, Savill J, Haslett C. Apoptosis in human eosinophils: programmed cell death in the eosinophil leads to phagocytosis by macrophages and is modulated by IL-5. J Immunol 1992; 148:3543.

161. Walls A, He S, Teran L, et al. Granulocyte recruitment by human mast cell tryptase. Int Arch Allergy Appl Immunol 1995; 107:372–373.

162. Moqbel R, Levi-Schaffer F, Kay AB. Cytokine generation by eosinophils. J Allergy Clin Immunol 1994; 94:1183–1189.

163. Hartman K, Zuberbier T, Lippert U, Czarinelaki DM. In vitro migratory response of human mast cells towards zymosan-activated serum and interleukins. J Invest Dermatol 1994; 718:618A.

164. Mattoli S, Ackerman V, Vi Hori E, Marini M. Mast cell chemotactic activity of RANTES. Biochem Biophys Res Commun 1995; 209:316–321.

165. Lunblad L, Saria A, Lundberg JM, Änggard A. Increased vascular permeability in rat nasal mucosa induced by substance P and stimulation of capsaicin sensitive trigeminal neurons. Acta Otolaryngol (Stockh) 1983; 96:479–484.

166. Lunblad L, Lundberg JM, Änggard A. Local and systemic capsaicin pretreatment inhibits sneezing and the increase in nasal vascular permeability induced by certain chemical irritants. Neuntyn Schmiedebergs Arch Pharmacol 1984; 326:254–261.

167. Uddman R, Änggard A, Widdicombe JG. Nerves and neurotransmitters in the nose. In: Mygind N, Pipkorn U, eds. Allergic and Vasomotor Rhinitis: Pathophysiological Aspects. Copenhagen: Munksgaard 1987:50–62.

168. Uddman R, Sundler F. Innervation of the upper airways. Clin Chest Med 1966; 7:201–209.

169. Baraniuk JN, Lundgren JD, Okayama M, et al. Substance P and neurokinin A (NKA) in human nasal mucosa. Am J Respir Cell Mol Biol 1991; 4:228–236.

170. Baraniuk JN, Lundgren JD, Goff J, et al. Calcitonin gene related peptide (CGRP) in human nasal mucosa. Am J Physiol 1990; 258:L81–L88.

171. Mossiman BL, White MV, Hohman RJ, Golovich MS, Kaulbach HC, Kaliner MA. Substance P, calcitonin-gene related peptide and vasoactive intestinal peptide increases in nasal secretions after allergen challenge in atopic patients. J Allergy Clin Immunol 1993; 92:95–104.

172. Devillier P, Dessanges JK, Rakatosihanaka JF, et al. Nasal response to substance P and methacholine in subjects with and without allergic rhinitis. Eur Respir J 1988; 1:356–361.

173. Brannstein G, Fajac I, Lacronique J, Frossard N. Clinical and inflammatory responses to exogenous tachykinins in allergic rhinitis. Am Rev Respir Dis 1991; 144:630–636.

174. Fajac I, Braunstein G, Ickovic MR, Lacronique J, Frossard N. Selective recruitment of eosinophils by substance P after repeated allergen exposure in allergic rhinitis. Allergy 1995; 50:970–975.

175. Okamoto Y, Shirotori K, Kudo K, et al. Cytokine expression after the topical administration of substance P to human nasal mucosa: the role of substance P in nasal allergy. J Immunol 1993; 151:4391–4398.

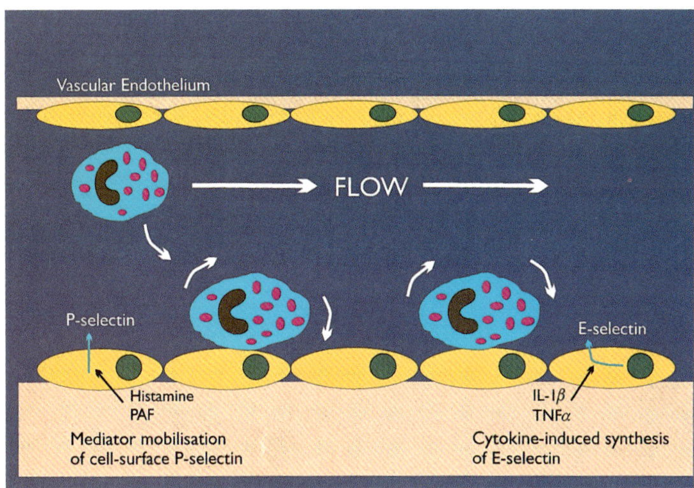

Figure 3 Rolling leucocyte endothelial adherence under the influence of P-selectin, mobilized in a preformed state from Wiebel-Palade bodies within endothelial cells, and E-selectin synthesized by cytokines as IL-1β and TNFα.

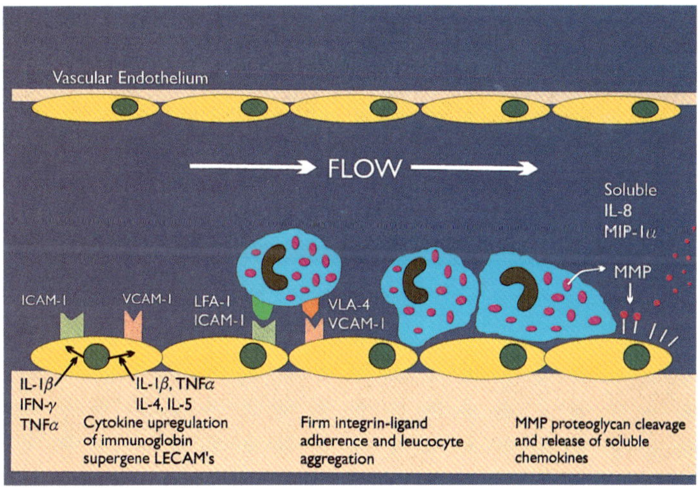

Figure 4 Firm leucocyte endothelial adherence under the influence of the immunoglobulin supergene family ICAM-1 and VCAM-1 through specific interactions with the leucocyte cell surface expressed ligands LFA-1 and VLA-4.

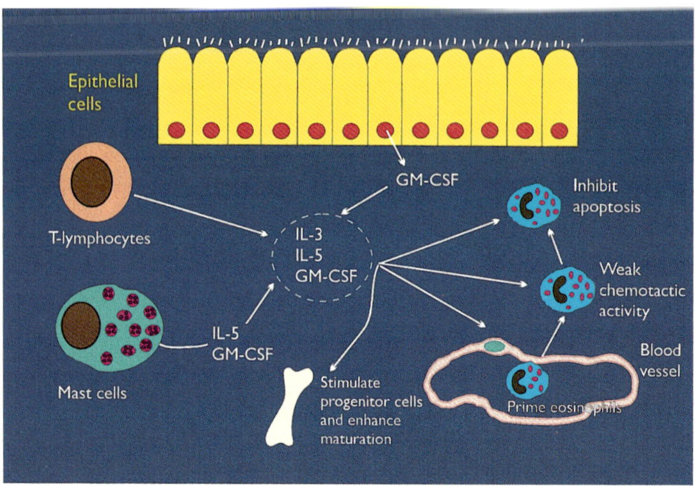

Figure 8   IL-5 cytokine cluster and their involvement in tissue eonsinophilia.

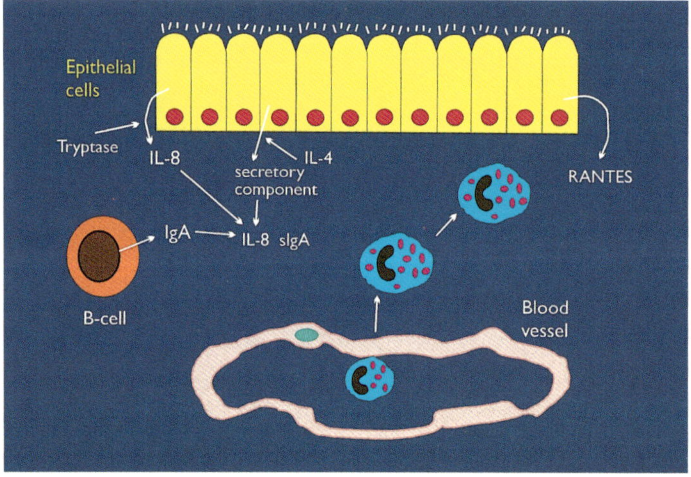

Figure 9   Epithelial chemokine synthesis and release in relationship to airway eosinophil recruitment, reflecting the eosinophil chemoattractant and activator properties of both RANTES and IL-8 when complexed with secretory IgA. Mast cell activation can be linked to the epithelial generation of IL-8 and secretory component through the release of tryptase and IL-4 respectively.

8

Health-Related Quality of Life in Rhinitis

ELIZABETH F. JUNIPER

McMaster University Medical Centre
Hamilton, Ontario, Canada

I. Introduction

Over the last 10 years, there has been an increasing awareness of the importance of including health-related quality of life (HRQL) in clinical assessments. For many clinicians HRQL is a new term, not a new concept. This chapter addresses some of the questions most commonly asked about the assessment of HRQL in patients with rhinitis and contains a discussion on the role of HRQL assessments in both clinical trials and clinical practice.

II. What Is HRQL?

''Quality of life'' is a rather nebulous expression often meaning different things to different people and this has made defining it very difficult. However, most clinicians agree that many factors, such as finances, spirituality, and health, contribute to quality of life and also affect each other. Simply, HRQL is the component of overall quality of life that is determined primarily by the person's health and that can be influenced by clinical interventions. For simplicity and focus, the definition by Schipper and colleagues (1)—''the functional effects of an illness and its consequent therapy upon a patient, as perceived by the patient''—is preferred. The final phrase is important because it emphasizes that these are the impairments that the patients consider important.

III. Why Is HRQL Important in Rhinitis?

If one accepts the three reasons for treating patients: to prevent mortality, to reduce the probability of future morbidity, and to improve patient well-being (2), it is apparent that for the majority of rhinitis patients, and especially for those with seasonal allergic rhinitis, improving patient well-being or, in other words, improving the HRQL is the primary goal of treatment.

Clinicians use a range of measures to assess the clinical status of the nose. These measures include such indices as nasal symptom severity, rhinomanometry, cytology, and nasal hyperreactivity (3,4). Certainly, these measures are important, but there is growing evidence suggesting that correlations between the markers of nasal inflammation and the patient's rhinitis-specific quality of life are only weak to moderate (4,5). Therefore, if one wants to know how impaired a patient is in daily functioning as a result of rhinitis and whether treatment produces an improvement, then HRQL has to be measured directly. Why should this relationship be so weak? Let us take as an example two hypothetical patients with identical clinical rhinitis. The first patient is really bothered by the symptoms themselves. In addition, she is a light sleeper and finds that her rhinitis prevents her getting a good night's sleep, so she feels tired during the day. She is susceptible to headaches. She is a model and her appearance prevents her from working. She is an ''uptight'' person and her rhinitis tends to make her feel irritable. The second patient ignores her symptoms and is a sound sleeper. She rarely gets a headache and cares little about her looks. She is a laid-back person. Although these two patients have identical clinical rhinitis, HRQL in the former patient is more impaired than in the latter. Furthermore, if we treat both patients with an identical medication that produces an identical improvement in clinical rhinitis, the improvement in HRQL is likely to be greater in the former patient than in the latter because the former's symptoms are less troublesome, she sleeps well, and she functions normally at work.

There has been a tendency among clinicians to underestimate the problems that patients with rhinitis experience. Recent work by Bousquet and colleagues has shown convincingly that rhinitis can be troublesome to patients and cause quite severe impairment of HRQL (6). They examined the burden of illness experienced by a sample of asthma patients, with a full range of asthma severity (7), and a sample of patients with perennial rhinitis (6). Using the generic health profile, the SF-36, they showed that in seven of the nine domains, quality of life tended to be worse in the rhinitis patients than in the asthma patients.

IV. What Problems Are Most Troublesome to Patients with Rhinitis?

Although some studies on the functional status of patients with rhinitis exist, the outcomes were chosen by clinicians and there is inadequate evidence that these outcomes are actually important to the patients themselves (8,9). When we developed a disease-specific HRQL questionnaire for adults and children with rhinitis (5,10,11), we asked the patients themselves to describe the impaired functions that bothered them most in their day-to-day lives. Problems that were identified most frequently and that scored the highest in importance (1 = not important, 5 = very important) can be summarized in six domains: sleep problems, nonnasal symptoms, nasal symptoms, practical problems, activity limitations, and emotional problems.

Adults with rhinitis are certainly bothered by the symptoms themselves, particularly a stuffy/blocked nose, a runny nose, and sneezing. They are bothered by not being able to sleep well at night and often feel tired and worn out during the day. They experience nonnasal symptoms that are troublesome, such as thirst, poor concentration, and headache. They find practical problems annoying such as having to carry tissues and always having to blow their nose, they are limited in their daily activities, and they feel frustrated and irritable (5).

Adolescents (aged 12–17 years) with rhinitis experience similar problems to adults except that they do not have the sleeping problems but they have more problems with concentration, particularly with school work (10).

Younger children (aged 6–12 years) present a slightly different picture (11). They are certainly bothered by their symptoms and the practical problems of carrying tissues and taking medications, but they experience minimal interference with their normal daily activities and do not have the emotional dysfunction experienced by adults and adolescents. We observed that parents were more bothered by their child's rhinitis than the child. This observation is consistent with other conditions where parents appear to have a poor perception of their child's HRQL (12).

V. Selecting a Quality-of-Life Instrument

We now have a range of valid instruments for measuring HRQL in patients with rhinitis. There is no best instrument. Each has been developed for a different purpose and has different measurement properties.

A. Generic Versus Specific (Table 1)

There are two types of HRQL questionnaires, generic and specific. Generic instruments are designed to be applicable to patients with all medical conditions.

Table 1 Types of Health-Related Quality of Life Instruments

Instrument type	Strengths	Weaknesses
Health profiles	Comparison across conditions possible	Do not focus adequately on areas of interest May not be responsive
Utilities	Single number representing quality of life Cost-utility analysis possible	Do not allow examination of different aspects of quality of life May not be responsive
Disease-specific	Clinically sensible More responsive	Comparison across conditions not possible

Source: From Juniper EF. Assessment of asthma control: quality of life. In: Thomson NC, O'Byrne PM, eds. Manual of Asthma Control. London: WB Saunders, 1995.

The most commonly used and the best validated are the Sickness Impact Profile (SIP) (13), the Medical Outcomes Survey Short Form 36 (SF-36) (14), the Nottingham Health Profile (15), and the McMaster Health Index Questionnaire (16). Although each profile attempts to measure all important aspects of health-related function, they achieve this in different ways. For instance, the SF-36 contains nine domains, which can be combined into two primary functions, mental and physical. In contrast, the SIP has two major domains, physical and psychosocial, which combine to give one overall score.

The great advantage of generic instruments is that the burden of illness can be compared across different medical conditions. For instance, one can compare the burden of illness experienced by patients with rhinitis, asthma, inflammatory bowel disease, and rheumatoid arthritis. However, because these instruments are comprehensive, they have little depth and, as a result, impairments that are important to patients with a specific condition may be excluded. Consequently, in many conditions including rhinitis, generic instruments are often unresponsive to small, but important changes in HRQL (17–19). Therefore, the use of generic instruments in clinical trials and clinical practice, where one wants to examine the effect of treatment within individuals or groups of patients, is limited.

This lack of depth of focus of the generic instruments has led to the development of specific instruments. These instruments may be specific for a group of patients (e.g., the elderly), a particular function (e.g., pain, sexual function), or a disease. Disease-specific instruments are developed by asking the patients themselves about the impairments that are most important to them, and therefore these instruments focus on the problems that are the targets for interventions. As a result, disease-specific instruments are more likely to detect small, but clinically important changes in the patient's problems.

B. Utilities

Utilities measure the value that either the patient or society places on various health states. They are very popular with health economists not only because they provide a single number representing HRQL from 0 = death to 1 = perfect health, but because the majority of instruments meet the assumptions for utility theory. For measuring the value that patients themselves place on their own health state, the most common instruments are the Standard Gamble (20), the Time Trade Off (20), and the Feeling Thermometer (20). For measuring the value that society places on various health states, there are the Quality of Well-Being Scale (21), the Multiattribute Health Utilities Index (22), and the EuroQol (23). For a long time, these instruments were used only in generic form, i.e., to be applicable in all medical conditions, and in this form they have the same weakness as the generic health profiles—they are less responsive to disease-specific change (17,18). Recently, the Standard Gamble and the Feeling Thermometer have been modified for use as disease-specific instruments for children with asthma and appear to have improved measurement properties (18). There have been no evaluations of these instruments in rhinitis.

C. Measurement Properties

Face and Content Validity

When selecting an instrument, one first ensures that it has face and content validity; i.e., the instrument appears to measure what it purports to measure (face validity) and the items in a questionnaire have been selected using recognized procedures that ensure that they capture all the areas of function that are considered important by patients (content validity). Feinstein has called these properties ''sensibility'' (24). Questionnaires in which items have been selected by clinicians rarely meet this criterion because some impairments that patients themselves consider important may have been omitted.

Evaluation Versus Discrimination (Table 2)

Instruments used in cross-sectional studies (e.g., screening and surveys) are known as discriminative instruments because they discriminate between different levels of patient impairment. Instruments used in longitudinal studies (clinical trials and clinical practice) are called evaluative instruments because they evaluate change in impairment over time. The two types of instruments require different measurement properties, although some well-constructed instruments are capable of both functions.

Discriminative Properties

An instrument used to distinguish between individuals or groups of patients at a single point in time, e.g., between individuals who do or do not have impaired

Table 2 Measurement Properties Necessary for Evaluative and Discriminative Instruments

	Discrimination	Evaluation
Signal	Between-subject differences	Within-subject differences related to true within-subject change
Noise	Within-subject differences	Within-subject differences unrelated to true within-subject change
Signal-to-noise ratio: descriptive term	Reliability	Responsiveness
Construct validity	Cross-sectional	Longitudinal

Source: From Juniper EF. Assessment of asthma control: quality of life. In: Thomson NC, O'Byrne PM, eds. Manual of Asthma Control. London: WB Saunders, 1995.

HRQL, or, within rhinitis patients, between those who have mild, moderate, or severe impairment, requires reliability and cross-sectional construct validity (25).

Reliability is the ability of the instrument to measure differences between patients at a single point in time. The test statistic usually used to express reliability is the intraclass correlation coefficient (ICC), which relates the between-subject variance to the total variance (Cronbach's alpha, which measures the internal consistency, does not give an indication of this property).

When there is no gold standard against which to demonstrate that the instrument is actually measuring what it purports to measure, the developer puts forward hypotheses or constructs, which, if they are met, provide evidence that the instrument is valid (construct validity). The approach frequently used is to demonstrate that the various domains of the new HRQL instrument correlate in a predicted manner with other indices of rhinitis severity and with other HRQL instruments.

Evaluative Properties

An instrument that is to be used to measure longitudinal change within an individual or group of patients must have good responsiveness and longitudinal validity (25). Responsiveness is the ability of the instrument to respond to small, but clinically important changes that occur either spontaneously or as the result of an intervention. The signal is the true within-subject change over time and the noise is the within-subject variance unrelated to the true within-subject change; the relationship between the two is known as the responsiveness index (26). If a formal estimate of the responsiveness index is not available, an instrument that has already performed well in a clinical trial will probably have acceptable responsiveness.

Evaluative instruments also require longitudinal validity. When there is a change in score, this must reflect a true change in rhinitis HRQL. Longitudinal validity is usually demonstrated by showing that changes in the various domains of the new HRQL instrument correlate in a predicted manner with changes in other outcome measures, such as clinical rhinitis severity and generic HRQL.

Most developers publish reliability and cross-sectional validity data and, good as these may be, they do not guarantee that the instrument will be capable of performing well in a clinical trial. There are now a number of studies in which patients experienced clinically important changes in the HRQL but which instruments, with good reliability and cross-sectional validity, failed to detect (17–19).

VI. Interpreting Quality-of-Life Data

Repeated experience with a wide variety of physiological measures allows clinicians to make meaningful interpretation of results. For instance, the experienced clinician will have little difficulty in interpreting a 0.5-L increase in forced expiratory volume in 1 sec (FEV_1). In contrast, the meaning of a change in score of 1.0 on a HRQL instrument is less intuitively obvious, not only because there are no units but also because health professionals seldom, as yet, use HRQL measures in clinical practice and each instrument has its own scoring system. Two approaches have been suggested for the interpretation of HRQL data (27). The first, "distribution-based," is based entirely on the statistical distribution of the results, the most commonly used being the effect size, which is derived from the magnitude of change and the variability in stable subjects. The problem with this approach is that there is still no indication as to whether the effect is important to the patient. The second approach, which is the one we use and which has been used for the St. George Respiratory Questionnaire, is referred to as "anchor-based," where the changes in HRQL measures are compared, or anchored, to other clinically meaningful outcomes. For our instruments, we have calculated the minimal important difference (MID) (defined as "the smallest difference in score in the domain of interest which patients perceive as beneficial and would mandate, in the absence of troublesome side-effects and excessive cost, a change in the patient's management"), using patients' global rating of change (28). For the Rhinoconjunctivitis Quality of Life Questionnaire, we have found the MID to be a change in mean score of 0.5 (29). Other developers have determined the MID from patient-perceived benefits during clinical trials (30) and patients' perception of their own illness relative to other patients (31).

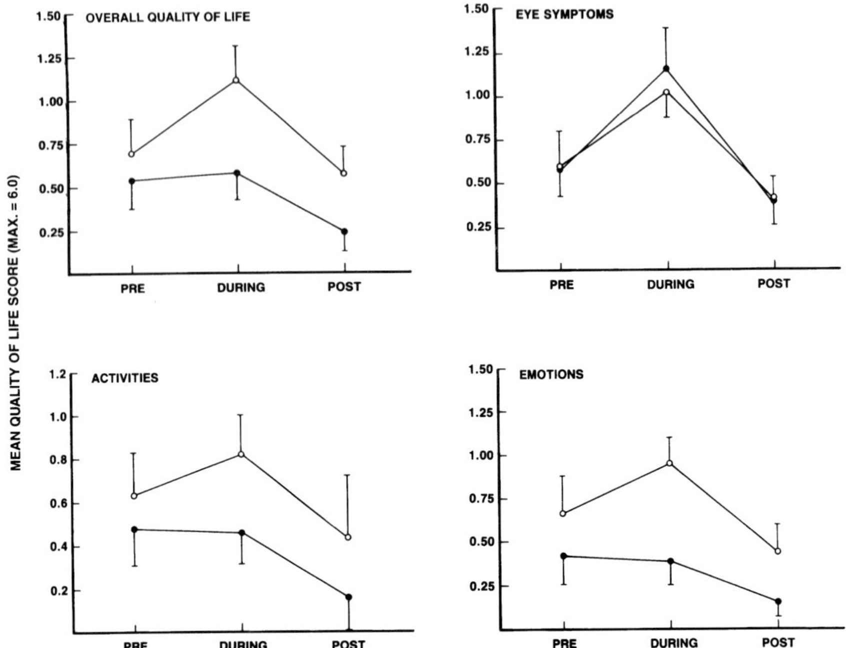

Figure 1 HRQL results from a clinical trial that compared regular (closed circles) versus prn (open circles) beclomethasone dipropionate (bdp) nasal spray in the treatment of ragweed-pollen-induced rhinoconjunctivitis (32). In these patients with moderate to severe rhinoconjunctivitis, there was minimal impairment of quality of life at the height of the ragweed season (1 = hardly troubled at all). Differences between the two treatment groups were statistically significant for all but the eye symptom and activities domain. However, in none of the domains was the mean difference in score greater than 0.5 (the MID) at the height of the ragweed season. This strongly suggests that very few patients will experience better HRQL if they use bdp regularly compared with if they use it only when needed.

VII. The Place of HRQL Assessments in Clinical Trials and Clinical Practice

The recognition of the importance of HRQL, the poor correlation between the conventional clinical indices of nasal impairment and HRQL, and the development of HRQL instruments with strong measurement properties have already led to a number of rhinitis clinical trials including an assessment of HRQL as one of the primary end-points (Fig. 1). These instruments are short, easily understood, and usually self-administered, making completion little burden to either the inves-

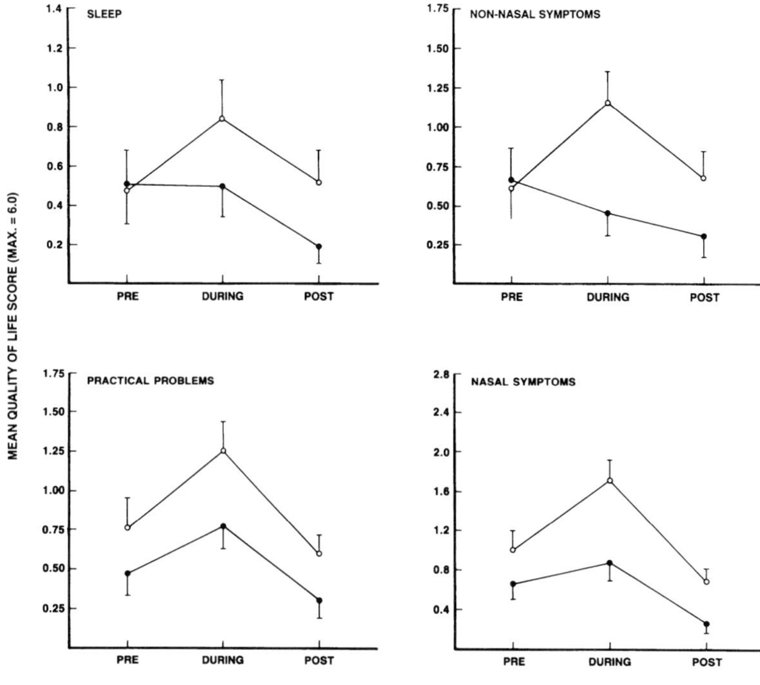

Figure 1 Continued.

tigator or the patient. We have found that patients enjoy completing HRQL questionnaires because they relate to the questions and they know that the things that are important to them are being taken into consideration. In addition, it is likely that national pharmaceutical regulatory agencies maybe soon ask for HRQL data for new product submissions.

The role of HRQL instruments in clinical practice is not clear. There is no doubt that a growing number of clinicians are now measuring HRQL during routine assessments. A disease-specific quality-of-life questionnaire is a formalized and quantified method for taking a simple patient history. The advantages are that the patient can complete the questionnaire while sitting in the waiting room and a quick scan of the responses will save consultation time. The clinician does not have to remember all the important questions and can quickly focus on areas of particular impairment to the patient. The questionnaires often reveal problems not spontaneously volunteered by patients, particularly children. In addition, responses at each clinic visit can be compared to determine whether interventions have been beneficial. However, all these benefits are at present conjectural and need to be confirmed in properly designed clinical trials.

VIII. Conclusions

Many clinicians now recognize the importance of incorporating an assessment of HRQL into their clinical evaluations. Conventional clinical measures provide valuable information about the status of the affected organ system but they rarely capture the functional impairments (physical, social, and emotional) that are important to patients in their everyday lives. Patients with rhinitis are not only distressed by nasal symptoms, such as sneezing, stuffy nose, and runny nose, they have problems with nonnasal symptoms, such as headache and tiredness. They are limited in their daily activities and have difficulty sleeping. They have to deal with practical problems, such as carrying tissues. Often they feel frustrated and irritable and their appearance and behavior (sneezing and blowing their noses) cause them embarrassment. Disease-specific quality-of-life questionnaires have been developed for adults, adolescents, and children with rhinitis. These questionnaires have good measurement properties and validity, and can be used both in clinical trials and in clinical practice to assess the impact of rhinitis on a patient's life. Since one of the aims of treatment in rhinitis must be to ensure patient benefit, an essential component of clinical assessment in these patients should be the evaluation of HRQL.

References

1. Schipper H, Clinch J, Powell V. Definitions and conceptual issues. In: Spilker B, ed. Quality of Life Assessment in Clinical Trials. New York: Raven Press, 1990: 11–24.
2. Guyatt GH, Naylor CD, Juniper EF, Heyland DK, Jaeschke R, Cook DJ, for the Evidence-Based Medicine Working Group. Users' guides to the medical literature. XII. How to use articles about health-related quality of life. JAMA 1997; 277:1232–1237.
3. Meltzer EO, Orgel HA, Bronsky EA, et al. A dose ranging study of fluticasone propionate nasal spray for seasonal allergic rhinitis assessed by symptoms, rhinomanometry and nasal cytology. J Allergy Clin Immunol 1990; 86:221–230.
4. De Graaf-in 't Veld T, Koenders S, Garrelds IM, Gerth van Wijk R. Relationship between nasal hyperreactivity, quality of life and nasal symptoms in perennial rhinitis. J Allergy Clin Immunol 1996; 98:508–513.
5. Juniper EF, Guyatt GH. Development and testing of a new measure of health status for clinical trials in rhinoconjunctivitis. Clin Exp Allergy 1991; 21:77–83.
6. Bousquet J, Bullinger M, Fayol C, Marquis P, Valentin B, Burtin B. Assessment of quality of life in patients with perennial rhinitis with the French version of the SF-36 health status questionnaire. J Allergy Clin Immunol 1994; 94:182–188.
7. Bousquet J, Knani J, Dhivert H, Richard A, Chicoye A, Ware JE, Michel FB. Quality of life in asthma. 1. Internal consistency and validity of the SF-36 questionnaire. Am J Respir Crit Care Med 1994; 149:371–375.

8. Marshall PS, Colon EA. Effects of allergy season on mood and cognitive function. Ann Allergy 1993; 71:251–258.

9. Gauci M, King MG, Saxarra H, Tulloch BJ, Husband AJ. A Minnesota Multiphasic Personality Inventory Profile of a woman with allergic rhinitis. Psychosom Med 1993; 55:533–540.

10. Juniper EF, Guyatt GH, Dolovich J. Assessment of quality of life in adolescents with allergic rhinoconjunctivitis: development and testing of a questionnaire for clinical trials. J Allergy Clin Immunol 1994; 93:413–423.

11. Juniper EF, Howland WC, Roberts NB, Thompson AK, King DR. Measuring quality of life in children with rhinoconjunctivitis. J Allergy Clin Immunol (submitted).

12. Guyatt GH, Juniper EF, Feeny DH, Griffith LE. Children and adult perceptions of childhood asthma. Pediatrics 1997; 99:165–168.

13. Bergner M, Bobbitt RA, Carter WB, Gilson BS. The Sickness Impact Profile; development and final revision of a health status measure. Med Care 1981; 19:787–805.

14. Stewart AL, Hays R, Ware JE. The MOS Short-Form General Health Survey. Reliability and validity in a patient population. Med Care 1988; 26:724–732.

15. Hunt SM, McKenna SP, McEwen J, Backett EM, Williams J, Papp E. A quantitative approach to perceived health status; a validation study. J Epidemiol Commun Health 1980; 34:281–286.

16. Sackett DL, Chambers LW, MacPherson AS, Goldsmith CH, McAuley RG. The development and application of indices of health; general methods and summary of results. Am J Public Health 1977; 67:423–428.

17. Rutten-van Molken MPMH, Clusters F, Van Doorslaer EKA, Jansen CCM, Heurman L, Maesen FPV, Smeets JJ, Bommer AM, Raaijmakers JAM. Comparison of performance of four instruments in evaluating the effects of salmeterol on asthma quality of life. Eur Respir J 1995; 8:888–898.

18. Juniper EF, Guyatt GH, Feeny DH, Griffith LE, Ferrie PJ. Minimum skills required by children to complete health-related quality of life instruments: comparison of instruments for measuring asthma-specific quality of life. Eur Respir J (in press).

19. Juniper EF, Guyatt GH, Griffith LE, Ferrie PJ. A generic versus a disease-specific quality of life questionnaire for rhinoconjunctivitis clinical trials? (submitted).

20. Torrance GW. Measurement of health state utilities for economic appraisal. J Health Econ 1986; 5:1–30.

21. Kaplan RM, Anderson JP, Wu AW, Matthews WC, Kozin F, Orenstein D. The Quality of Well-Being Scale: application in AIDS, cystic fibrosis and arthritis. Med Care 1989; 27:S27–43.

22. Feeny D, Furlong W, Barr RD, Torrance GW, Rosenbaum P, Weitzman S. A comprehensive multi-attribute system for classifying the health status of survivors or childhood cancer. J Clin Oncol 1992; 10:923–928.

23. The EuroQol Group. A new facility for the measurement of health-related quality of life. Health Policy 1990; 16:199–208.

24. Feinstein A. The theory and evaluation of sensibility. In: Feinstein A. Clinimetrics. New Haven: Yale University Press, 1987:141–166.

25. Guyatt GH, Kirshner B, Jaeschke R. Measuring health status: what are the necessary measurement properties? J Clin Epidemiol 1992; 45:1341–1345.

26. Guyatt GH, Walter S, Norman G. Measuring change over time: assessing the usefulness of evaluative instruments. J Chronic Dis 1987; 40:171–178.
27. Lydick E, Epstein RS. Interpretation of quality of life changes. Qual Life Res 1993; 2:221–226.
28. Juniper EF, Guyatt GH, Willan A, Griffith LE. Determining a minimal important change in a disease-specific quality of life questionnaire. J Clin Epidemiol 1994; 47: 81–87.
29. Juniper EF, Guyatt GH, Griffith LE, Ferrie PJ. Interpretation of Rhinoconjunctivitis Quality of Life Questionnaire data. J Allergy Clin Immunol 1996; 98:843–845.
30. Jones PW, Lasserson D. Relationship between change in St. George's Respiratory Questionnaire score and patients' perception of treatment efficacy after one year of therapy with nedocromil sodium. Am J Respir Crit Care Med 1994; 149:A211.
31. Wells GA, Tugwell P, Kraag GR, Baker PRA, Groh J, Redelmeier DA. Minimum important difference between patients with rheumatoid arthritis: the patient's perspective. J Rheumatol 1993; 20:557–560.
32. Juniper EF, Guyatt GH, O'Byrne PM, Viveiros M. Aqueous beclomethasone dipropionate nasal spray: regular versus ''as required'' use in the treatment of seasonal allergic rhinitis. J Allergy Clin Immunol 1990; 86:380–386.

9

Allergy Diagnosis

STEPHEN R. DURHAM

Imperial College School of Medicine at the
   National Heart and Lung Institute
London, England

I. Introduction

In clinical terms rhinitis may be defined as symptoms of nasal discharge, blockage, and itch/sneezing (two of three symptoms) occurring for more than 1 hr on most days either seasonally or throughout the year (1,2). Allergy is an important cause of rhinitis symptoms particularly in the young and middle-aged. Recently published guidelines emphasize a practical approach to rhinitis diagnosis and management in which four main causes of rhinitis symptoms are considered: allergy, infection, structural, and ''other'' (1). The latter refers to a heterogeneous group of disorders including nasal hyperreactivity (i.e., an exaggerated response to nonspecific triggers including changes in temperature, strong smell, and environmental pollutants) (Fig. 1). Frequently more than one cause for rhinitis symptoms may coexist in the same individual. Their relative frequency will depend upon the population studied. For example, the percentage of rhinitis patients with allergies in a pediatric or allergy clinic population is likely to be very high whereas in general practice the proportion of patients presenting with nasal symptoms for which an allergic cause can be found is likely to be lower (3).

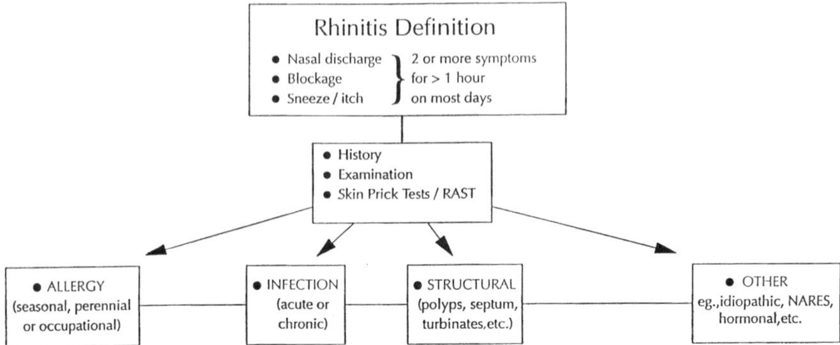

Figure 1 Differential diagnosis of allergy and other causes of rhinitis symptoms. (Reproduced with permission from Ref. 1.)

II. Sensitization

The basis of allergy diagnosis is the patient's clinical history (4,5). Objective tests such as skin prick tests or in vitro IgE measurements provide helpful, but only supportive, objective information, which must be interpreted with the clinical history (3). In this chapter ''atopy'' refers to a tendency to develop exaggerated IgE responses and is defined by a positive skin prick test (3 mm > negative control) to one or more common inhaled allergens; i.e., atopy refers to a predisposition to develop allergy. Allergy, by contrast, refers to the clinical expression of allergic symptoms within atopic individuals, the common manifestations being rhinitis, asthma, eczema, and, less commonly, food allergy and IgE-mediated anaphylaxis. There is considerable overlap between the presence of rhinitis symptoms and the atopic and nonatopic state. For example, atopic individuals may have rhinitis due to a cause independent of their atopic status. Skin prick tests or IgE measurements identify sensitization and cannot alone define whether there is clinically relevant allergy to the corresponding allergen (Fig. 2). Sensitization depends upon repeated exposure to the relevant allergen, generally over a period of months or several years before clinical manifestations develop (if at all). The time course of evolution of allergic manifestations differs according to the target organ (Fig. 3) and in a large proportion of subjects may be followed by the development of tolerance as shown by the reduction in clinical symptoms with age in a proportion of individuals. For example, allergy to milk and egg may appear during infancy and early childhood following high exposure and frequently resolves by 4–8 years. In contrast, eczema peaks in late childhood.

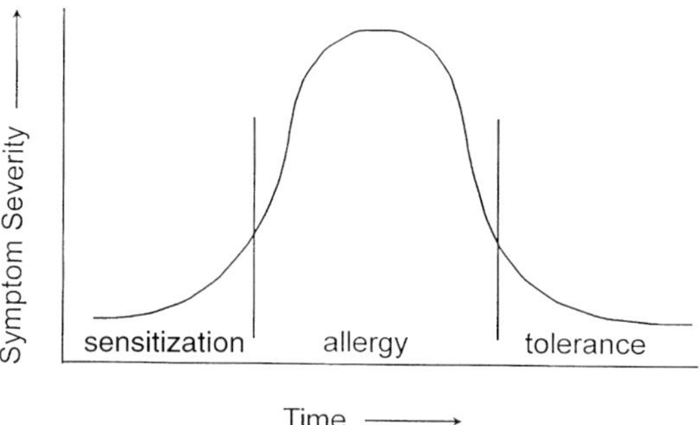

Figure 2 Positive skin prick tests or positive allergen-specific IgE to common allergens may represent atopy (sensitization only), allergy (clinical symptoms on exposure to the relevant allergen), or tolerance (previous history of symptoms on exposure to allergen, now resolved).

Asthma often has a biphasic time course with a decrease in symptoms or resolution in teenage, only to recur in adult life. In contrast, rhinitis typically peaks in teenage and early adulthood. However, allergy may occur for the first time in later years depending on various factors, mainly the level of allergen exposure and predisposition by other factors such as viral infections.

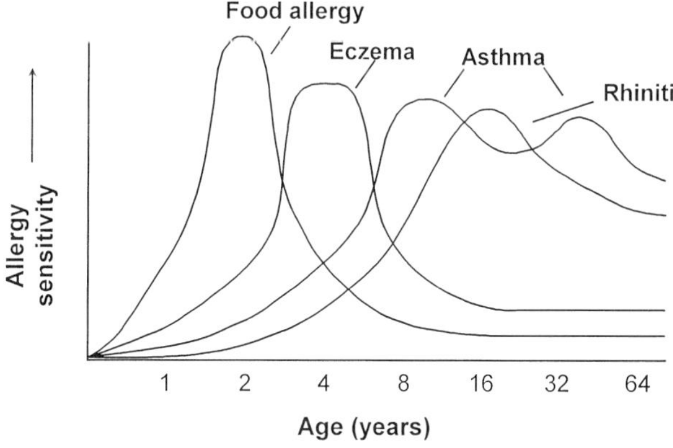

Figure 3 Schematic representation of time course of different organ-specific allergies in relation to symptom severity and age.

III. Allergy History

The clinical history should focus on the following questions:

1. Is the patient atopic? (requires confirmatory skin testing)
2. Does allergy contribute to the patient's symptoms?
3. Which are the clinically relevant allergens?

Taking a comprehensive clinical history requires experience, time, and patience. The first priority is to put the patient at ease with a personal welcome. This involves avoiding telephones ringing or completing case notes from a previous interview when the patient arrives for consultation. A professional but friendly manner and frequent eye contact are also important. The patient should then be allowed to give his own account of the symptoms in his own time. This is followed by structured prompts/questions to covers those points listed in Table 1. The seasonality (or lack of seasonality) of symptoms and the dominant symptom should be identified. Itching/sneezing, watery discharge, and associated eye symptoms may suggest an allergic cause. The frequency, severity, and duration

Table 1 Allergy History

Welcome!
Patient's account of symptoms
Impact on life-style
Frequency/severity
Work/school
Leisure time
Sleep
Seasonal/perennial
Trigger factors
Allergic
Nonallergic
Occupation/hobbies
Allergens in the home
Asthma, eczema, rhinitis, drug allergy,
food allergy
Family history
Treatment
Compliance
Efficacy
Side effects
What is your main symptom?

of symptoms should be noted. Importantly, their impact on the individual's life-style should be assessed in terms of impairment of school/work performance and time missed (6,7), interference with leisure activities, and any sleep disturbance.

A history of potential allergic triggers (pets, pollen, house dust mite, or occupational causes) should be recorded. Patients with mite sensitivity may complain of immediate symptoms during activities such as bed making, dusting, and vacuum cleaning. Symptoms are frequently worse on entering damp, older buildings. Are symptoms worse on exposure to pets? The absence of known contact with pets does not exclude animal sensitization/allergy. A recent study in Sweden confirmed high levels of the major allergens of cat and dog (Fel d 1, Can f 1) in schools on chairs and desks but not on the floor, suggesting contamination from the clothes of children who own pets (8). Seasonal pollinosis is usually evident from the clinical history and is based on the timing and geographic location of symptoms and a knowledge of the dominant local flora. In Scandinavia tree pollinosis is dominant in February–May whereas in the United Kingdom grass-pollen-induced symptoms peak in June–July. Weed pollens (ragweed in the United States, mugwort in Europe) peak in late summer (August–September) whereas mould spores (*Alternaria*, *Cladosporium*, and *Aspergillus*) have a longer season throughout the summer, peaking during autumn months.

Patients with inhalant allergy frequently exhibit cross-reactions with certain food allergens taken by mouth (9–15). The commonest example is the association between springtime allergy to birch pollen and itching/lip swelling and buccal discomfort after eating apples, stone fruits, and nuts (Table 2). The higher the sensitivity to birch pollen on skin prick testing, the more frequent the association (16).

Patients with rhinitis from whatever cause may develop "hyperreactivity" with symptoms following irritant exposures. Certain features in the history may point to either an allergic or nonallergic trigger (Fig. 4). In general, allergen-induced symptoms require a prior period of sensitization (latency), affect only a minority of subjects, and may occur in response to very low allergen exposures. Patients may develop both early (0–1 hr) and late (6–24 hr) symptoms following either natural or experimental allergen exposure (17,18). In contrast, irritant triggers may provoke symptoms on first exposure, generally in high-exposure concentrations, and may affect the majority of exposed subjects to a lesser or greater extent. Also irritant-induced symptoms tend only to be immediate with resolution within minutes or hours. However, these distinctions should only be regarded as a guide, since there is considerable overlap and exceptions occur. For example, a particular problem may be that continuous exposure to allergens, especially perennial allergens, may result in repeated early and late symptoms in addition to an increase in nasal hyperresponsiveness with heightened sensitivity to nonspecific triggers (19). In these circumstances, symptoms may become continuous

Table 2 Some Cross-Reactions Between Inhalant
Allergens and Food Allergens

Inhalant allergy	Food allergy
Birch pollen	Nuts, apple, pear, peach, plum, cherry, carrot
Ragweed pollen	Melon, banana
Mugwort pollen	Celery, carrot, parsley, spices (fennel, coriander, aniseed, cumin)
Grass pollen	Tomato, peanut, pea, wheat, rye
Latex	Banana, chestnut, kiwi, avocado
Chironomids	Crustaceans

Source: Reproduced from Ref. 4 with kind permission of
Dr. N. Eriksson.

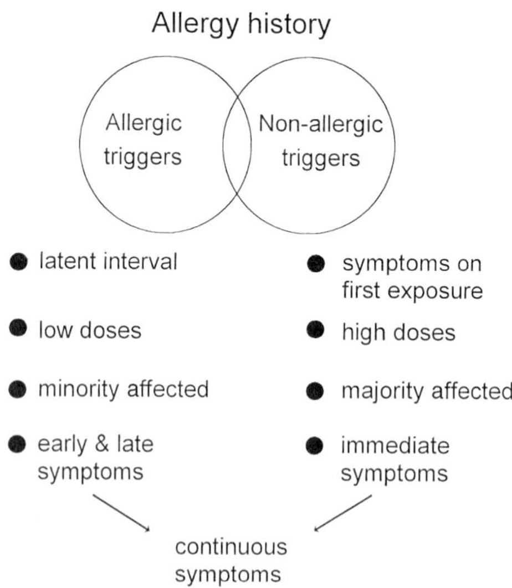

Figure 4 Relationship between allergic and nonallergic triggers of rhinitis. Prolonged
exposure, particularly to perennial allergens, may result in continuous symptoms with no
apparent relation to provoking allergen.

such that a causal relationship between allergen exposure and symptoms may not be evident to either the patient or the physician.

An occupational history should be obtained. In contrast to occupational asthma, occupational rhinitis is less well documented although likely to be very common, with or without associated asthma. Common examples include exposure to laboratory animals (20,21) (scientists, animal house technicians), flour (bakers), latex (health workers), and certain low-molecular-weight chemicals including isocyanates {two-part paint systems, resins, and printing (particularly flexible packaging)}, colophony (solderers in the electronics industry), and antibiotics such as penicillin and streptomycin (manufacturers and health workers). A knowledge of potential occupational causes is important. Symptoms generally occur within the workplace or during the evening following work. Symptoms tend to improve on weekends and during periods of vacation. In occupational asthma symptoms may persist in up to 50% of workers following termination of exposure and it is likely that the same may apply for rhinitis symptoms (22,23). For this reason it may be important to take a history of all occupations since leaving school, if the critical timing of exposure to a potential occupational sensitizer is not to be missed.

The effect of previous attempts at allergen avoidance may be obtained from the history, bearing in mind that several months of vigorous environmental control/avoidance or respiratory protection may be required before any improvement may be apparent. Similarly, the response to any pharmacological treatment should be assessed in terms of improvement in symptoms and any potential side effects of drugs taken. The patients' knowledge and potential fears about their condition should be explored. Compliance with medication should be carefully assessed in every case, particularly where there has been an apparent poor response to treatment. Finally, at the end of the interview it may be helpful to ask the patients to recap their main symptom and whether they have any particular worries relating to their treatment (particularly side effects of treatment such as corticosteroids) or any other specific questions.

IV. Examination

Physical examination is required for all patients although the extent will clearly be guided by the history.

When rash is a presenting symptom, then the entire skin, including hair and nails, should be examined. Eczema and urticaria are common associated skin manifestations that may occur in patients presenting with rhinitis symptoms. Eczema during infancy may be prominent over the face and trunk, whereas later in childhood and adulthood, eczema characteristically affects the flexural areas (neck, wrists, ankles, and flexures of knees and elbows). Urticaria takes the form of itchy, raised, pale irregular wheals on reddened skin, which may occur anywhere over the body. Individual lesions may coalesce and characteristically last several hours (generally less than 24 hr). Urticarial lesions that remain fixed, persist for longer than 24–48 hr, or leave a residual bruise should raise the possibility of an underlying vasculitic cause. Dermographism may confound interpretation of skin prick tests, although it will usually be apparent by inspection of the negative (allergen, diluent) control skin test which will be "false positive."

External examination of the nose may occasionally reveal a transverse skin crease in allergic rhinitis sufferers due to constant rubbing because of itchiness (the "allergic salute"). Profuse watery rhinorrhea may occasionally cause nasal soreness and tenderness of the skin around the nasal vestibule, with or without secondary infection. The nasal mucosa should be examined, ideally by use of a head mirror and speculum or a flexible or rigid endoscope, although inspection with the largest auroscope attachment using an ophthalmoscope will do. The nasal mucosa may appear normal, particularly if the patient is asymptomatic at the time of examination. However, *current symptomatic allergic rhinitis* is usually associated with a typical blue or pale "boggy," swollen appearance of the nasal mucosa with asymmetrical (nasal cycle) enlargement of the inferior turbinates, which shrink following topical decongestion. Thick yellow/brown inspissated mucus may be a manifestation of allergic fungal sinusitis (24).

Incidental findings including septal deflections, nasal polyps, and presence/ absence of nasal septal perforation should be documented. Oropharyngeal candidiasis may be evident in patients on inhaled (but not nasal) corticosteroids. The larynx should be examined in occasional cases with associated hoarseness of the voice, although this will usually be due to concomitant inhaled corticosteroid therapy for asthma. Typically the larynx may appear normal although occasionally a "midline chink" on voluntary adduction of the vocal cords will be evident.

Rhinitis is not uncommonly associated with asthma. Conversely, approximately 80% of asthmatics will have concomitant rhinitis. Recent studies have shown that treatment of rhinitis with nasal corticosteroids may improve asthma and reduce airway hyperresponsiveness (25). If asthma is suspected from the history, examination of the chest may elicit signs of hyperinflation and expiratory wheeze. Peak expiratory flow and/or 1-sec forced expiratory volume (FEV_1) may be diminished with reversibility demonstrable following inhalation of a short-acting beta-sympathomimetic agonist. If the history is suggestive but simple lung function tests are normal, a period of peak flow monitoring may show diurnal variation and/or exercise-induced asthma. Alternatively, airway hyperresponsiveness may be recorded by inhalation testing with histamine or methacholine solutions (26).

Rarely, both allergic asthma and/or rhinitis may be manifestations of underlying systemic disease. In Churg-Strauss syndrome additional clinical features may include vasculitis, rash, purpura, cardiomegaly, and/or pericardial rub, peripheral neuropathy, and proteinuria/hematuria. These are generally accompanied by a considerably raised erythrocyte sedimentation rate, leukocytosis, and markedly high eosinophil count.

V. Diagnostic Tests

A. Skin Prick Tests

Skin prick tests provide important objective information although results must always be interpreted in light of the clinical findings (27,28). As mentioned above, skin prick tests may confirm or exclude atopy and identify sensitization to particular allergens although they cannot predict their clinical relevance independent of the history (4,5). Their potential value is also dependent upon the quality of the allergen extracts used and the technical performance of the test, including the experience of the operator. The reliability of a particular skin prick test extract will depend upon the presence of all major allergenic determinants in sufficient concentrations (28). Extracts should be biologically standardized with low batch-to-batch variation. Solutions should be made up with preservative and generally stored in a refrigerator at $+4°C$. Attention should be paid to the manufacturers recommendations regarding shelf life. In general, skin prick tests are more sensitive than in vitro determinations of allergen-specific IgE. They are essential when avoidance measures or allergen-specific immunotherapy is being considered. They are also of educational value and provide a visual illustration that may serve to reinforce verbal advice (29) (Table 3). They should not be performed in patients on antihistamines or in the presence of severe eczema or dermographism (Table 4).

The size of the skin wheal is often regarded as a measure of degree of sensitivity to the allergen. However, a rather flat dose-response curve results in poor repeatability from one test to another even in the same individual by the same operator (3,30). This may be improved by expressing immediate cutaneous allergen sensitivity as the provocation concentration of allergen to cause a skin

Table 3 Usefulness of Skin Prick Tests

Diagnosis (or exclusion) of atopy—the underlying predisposition to allergic disease
Supportive evidence (positive or negative) for the clinical history
Essential when expensive or time-consuming avoidance measures (house dust mite) or
   removal of a family pet or consideration for immunotherapy is involved
Educational value, providing a clear illustration to the patient that may reinforce verbal
   advice

Table 4 Skin Prick Tests: Practice Points

Always check that patient is not on antihistamines before performing skin prick tests.
Always include positive (histamine) and negative (allergen diluent) control tests.
A positive test is (arbitrarily) 2 mm or more greater than the negative control.
Skin prick tests should be performed on the flexor aspect of the forearm using a sterile lancet (a 25-gauge orange needle will do). The procedure should be nonpainful and not draw blood.
Oral corticosteroids do not (significantly) inhibit allergen skin prick tests.
Dermographism may confound results (although it is evident as a positive response at the negative control site).
Skin prick tests should not be performed in the presence of severe eczema.
Measurement of allergen-specific IgE concentrations (RAST) is an alternative if skin prick tests cannot be performed.

wheal of predetermined size, generally 5 or 6 mm (Fig. 5). The mean value is recorded as the average of the longest diameter and the diameter at right angles to its midpoint. This value is chosen because 5 or 6 mm identifies the linear part of the log dose allergen–skin wheal diameter response curve. Changes in immediate cutaneous sensitivity may then be expressed as a shift in the dose-response curve, for example to the left during natural seasonal exposure (representing increased sensitivity) and to the right following treatment, e.g., following treatment with allergen injection immunotherapy (representing decreased sensitivity) (3,31). However, such precision is not normally required for routine clinical use. Similarly, the late cutaneous response at 6–24 hr that occurs following intradermal allergen challenge (and uncommonly following skin prick tests in sensitive subjects) is only of pathophysiological significance. However, intradermal tests are cumbersome to perform, not without risk, and their precise clinical relevance has not been determined. However, the late response is markedly inhibited by immunotherapy (32) and by corticosteroids. It remains to be determined whether the late response might predict response to immunotherapy or whether its inhibition correlates closely with clinical improvement in allergic symptoms (as opposed to reduced allergen sensitivity alone).

B. Serum Total and Allergen-Specific IgE

Total IgE levels have been used to diagnose atopy. However, total IgE levels vary with gender and age and are increased in smokers. There is marked overlap between normal subjects and allergy sufferers, particularly in monosensitive patients. For these reasons the test lacks precision. However, it is of interest that the prevalence of asthma adjusted for age and gender is linearly related to total

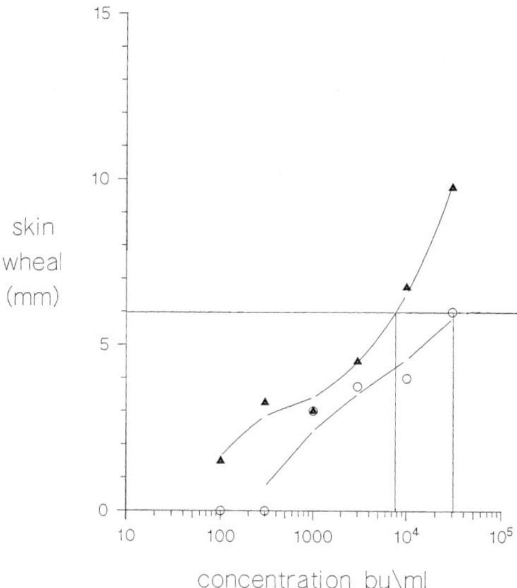

Figure 5   Relationship between allergen dose and skin wheal size. Immediate allergen sensitivity may be expressed as a provocation concentration of allergen that causes a 5 or 6 mm skin wheal (for research and evaluation of pharmacotherapy, immunotherapy in controlled trials).

IgE levels (33). Moreover, recent data have shown that total IgE levels may correlate with asthma severity and increase during asthma exacerbations (34). For these reasons total IgE may have more clinical value in individual patients than previously recognized, but further prospective studies are required.

In vitro allergen-specific IgE provides essentially the same information as skin prick tests. In general, skin prick tests are more sensitive whereas allergen-specific IgE tends to be more specific (35). A number of well-validated clinical IgE assay kits are available. Examples are shown in Table 5 (4,36). In general, purified allergen extracts containing the principal allergenic determinants are absorbed onto a solid phase such as a paper disk. The patient's diluted serum is added and incubated for a defined period. After washing a radiolabeled (RAST) or enzyme-linked (ELISA) anti-human IgE is added. After washing, radioactivity is counted, or after addition of enzyme substrate, a color reaction is monitored photometrically and the results compared against known IgE standards.

There is a moderate correlation between skin tests and RAST tests. The important point is that for clinical purposes the test must be interpreted in the context of the patient's symptoms.

Table 5 Some Test Systems for In Vitro Determination of Specific IgE

Company	System
Abbot Diagnostics	MATRIX
ALK	Magic Lite
Bioallergy	ENEA
Diagnostic Prod. Corp (DPC)	AlaSTAT
Kallestad	EAST (enzyme allergosorbent test)
MAST Immuno System	MAST CLA (multiple antigen simultaneous test)
Pharmacia	Phadebas RAST, Phadezym RAST, CAP RAST
Quidel	Quidel allergen screening
Ventrex	Modified RAST
Whittaker Diagnostics	FAST (fluorescent allergosorbent test)

Source: Reproduced from Ref. 4 with kind permission of Dr. N. Eriksson.

C. Provocation Tests

Provocation tests, at least in the United Kingdom, are not widely used for routine diagnosis. They confirm allergen sensitivity in the target organ. Thus nasal provocation using allergen extract applied as a nasal spray or on filter paper disks inserted into the nose provokes symptoms of itch/sneezing within seconds followed by nasal discharge and congestion, which is maximal at 15–30 min. Late responses are less prominent in the nose, occurring in less than 50% of individuals, and manifest largely as nasal congestion/obstruction (17,18). Nasal provocation tests are less well standardized than skin or bronchial provocation tests. They may be helpful when the diagnosis remains in doubt despite the above methods. A simpler alternative is the conjunctival provocation test, which involves applying drops of allergen solution of increasing concentration to the alternate eye at 10-min intervals (37). A positive reaction includes itching, redness, swelling, and tears. In general, there is good correlation between conjunctival and nasal provocation tests in the same subject.

VI. Diagnostic Approach

Allergy diagnosis depends upon the clinical history. This requires time and skill. The history should be supplemented by a physical examination and objective measures of IgE sensitivity, either skin prick tests or/and serum IgE measurements. Eriksson compared the values of case histories and combinations of case histories, skin tests, and the RAST test compared with provocation tests (38). The RAST score, skin test, and case history score were graded on a scale of 0–3, giving a total possible score of 9. Scores obtained for each patient and allergen

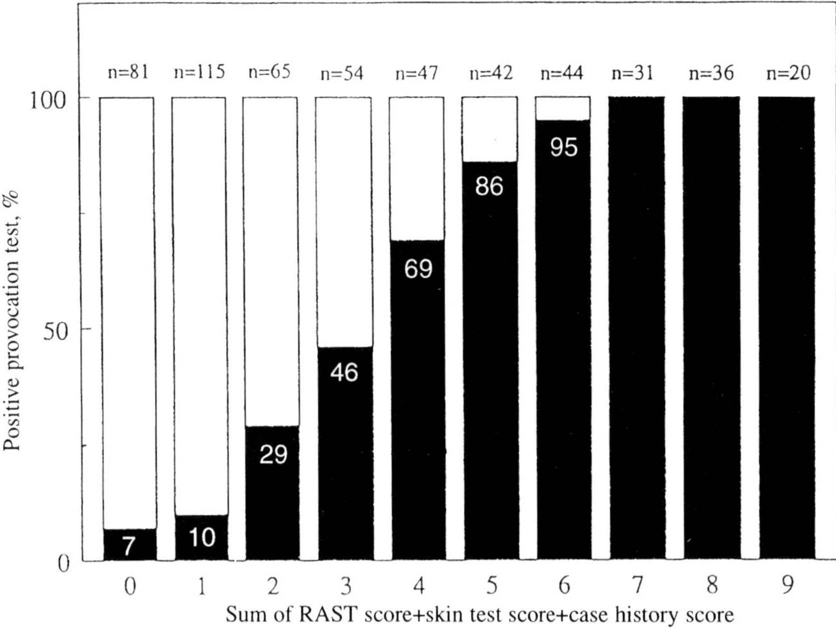

Figure 6   Relationships among a positive nasal allergen provocation test and the sum of scores (0–3) for the patient's case history, skin test, and RAST. (Reproduced from Ref. 4 by kind permission of Dr. N. Eriksson.)

were compared with the outcome of a provocation test with the corresponding allergen. The results are shown in Figure 6. The higher the score, the more likely a positive provocation test result. More refined IgE measurements may relate more closely to clinical symptoms to the relevant allergen, as suggested in a recent study from Italy (39).

Eriksson (4) recently discussed the value of various diagnostic tests in terms of their sensitivity, specificity, and predictive value of negative or positive tests (Table 6). In general, no test, even combined with a careful history, will confirm or exclude relevant allergy in every individual case. Dreborg commented on the relative lack of prospective studies that examine the efficiency of various tests and pointed out the importance of studying defined populations (28). For example, the false positive and false negative rates for a particular test will vary according to the prevalence of allergy in the population studied (e.g., specialist allergy clinic vs. unselected patient group in a primary care setting).

A simple diagnostic approach is suggested in Figure 7. There should be a

Table 6 Definition of Test Characteristics

Patient group	Diagnostic test positive	Diagnostic test negative	Total
Allergics	True positive (TP)	False negative (FN)	TP + FN
Nonallergics	False positive (FP)	True negative (TN)	FP + TN
Total	TP + FP	FN + TN	

Sensitivity: TP/(TP + FN).
Specificity: TN/(FP + TN).
Predictive value of negative test (Pv_{neg}): TN(FN + TN).
Predictive value of positive test (Pv_{pos}): TP(TP + FP).
Source: Reproduced from Ref. 4 with kind permission of Dr. N. Eriksson.

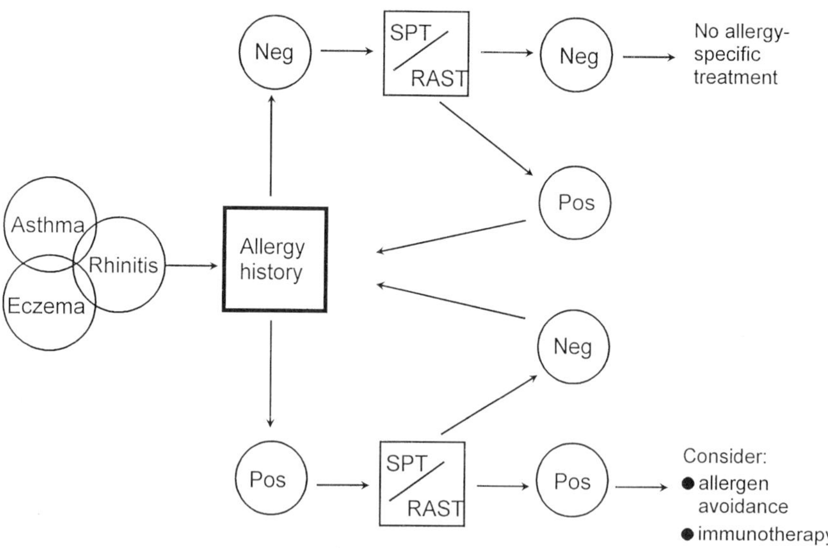

Figure 7 Where there is discordance between the patient's symptoms and test results, the first requirement is reevaluation of the history and, if indicated, repeat skin tests and consideration for nasal provocation testing.

high index of suspicion for allergy in all patients presenting with rhinitis symptoms, particularly if there is an associated personal or family history of other atopic disease. Whether or not allergy is suspected on the basis of the initial history, it is the author's view that skin prick tests and/or RAST tests to several common aeroallergens should be performed in the majority of patients presenting with rhinitis symptoms. Physical examination should also be included. When both the history and test are negative, one can exclude allergy with a high degree of confidence and no specific treatment is indicated. Similarly, when the history and test are both positive, then allergen avoidance measures, and in selective cases immunotherapy, should be carefully considered for each individual patient. When there is disagreement between the history examination findings and test results, then, above all, a careful reevaluation of the history is required. Specialist referral and, occasionally, specific provocation tests may be required. The threshold when to intervene with potentially time-consuming and expensive avoidance measures or removal of a family pet, particularly when the specific allergy diagnosis is not clear cut, will depend upon the patient's disease severity, requirement for pharmacotherapy, the likelihood of successful avoidance measures, and the motivation of the patient.

A major advance has been the characterization and cloning of the major allergenic determinants of common perennial aeroallergens including house dust mite (Der p 1, Der p 2) cats (Fel d 1), and dog (Can f 1) (8,40). Routine quantification of allergen exposure in the patient's home/work/school environment will greatly assist both allergy diagnosis and the efficiency of environmental control measures in reducing allergen load (40). Computer-assisted diagnosis may more effectively intercollate the history and diagnostic tests (although I doubt it). Whether computer assisted or not, a structured approach is required with the consent, active participation, and understanding of the patient at each step. Very often, at the end of the consultation the patient's response to the question "What do you think is your major problem?" will confirm/reinforce the relevant diagnosis and approach to therapy.

References

1. International Rhinitis Management Working Group. International consensus report on the diagnosis and management of rhinitis. Allergy 1994; 49 (Suppl 19):1–34.
2. Durham SR. Medical approach to rhinitis. Br J Hosp Med 1993; 50:458–462.
3. Dreborg S. The skin prick test. Methodological studies and clinical implications. Linkoping University Medical Dissertations No 239, 1987:1–148.
4. Eriksson NE. Diagnosis of IgE mediated allergy in clinical practice. Allergol Immunopathol 1994; 22:139–151.
5. Mygind N, Dahl R, Pedersen S, Kristian Thestrup-Pedersen. Diagnosis of allergy. In: Essential Allergy, 2nd ed. Oxford: Blackwell Science, 1996: 109–128.

6. Juniper EF, Guyatt GH. Development and testing of a new measure of health status for clinical trials in rhinoconjunctivitis. Clin Exp Allergy 1991; 2:77–83.

7. Juniper EF, Guyatt GH, Dolovich J. Assessment of quality of life in adolescents with allergic rhinoconjunctivitis: development and testing of a questionnaire for clinical trials. J Allergy Clin Immunol 1994; 93:413–423.

8. Munir AKM, Einarsson R, Schou C, Dreborg SKG. Allergens in school dust. I. The amount of the major cat (Fel d 1) and dog (Can f 1) allergens in dust from Swedish schools is high enough to probably cause perennial symptoms in most children with asthma who are sensitised to cat and dog. J Allergy Clin Immunol 1993; 91:1067–1074.

9. Eriksson NE, Formgren H, Svenonius E. Food hypersensitivity in patients with pollen allergy. Allergy 1992; 37:347–443.

10. Eriksson NE, Wihl JA, Arrendal H. Birch pollen-related food hypersensitivity: Influence of total and specific IgE levels. Allergy 1983; 38:353–357.

11. Anderson BL, Dreyfuss EM, Logan J, Johnstone DE, Glaser J. Melon and banana sensitivity coincident with ragweed pollinosis. J Allergy 1969; 45:310–319.

12. Wurthrich B, Dietschi R. Das sellerie-karotten-beifuss-gewurz-syndrom hauttest und RAST ergebnisse. Schweiz Med Wochenschr 1985; 115:358–364.

13. De Martino M, Novembre E, Cossa G, De Marco A, Bonazza A, Vierucci A. Sensitivity to tomato and peanut allergens in children monosensitised to grass pollen. Allergy 1988; 43:206–213.

14. Rodriguez M, Vega F, Garcia M, Panizo C, Laffon E, Montalvo A, Cuevas M. Hypersensitivity to latex, chestnut and banana. Ann Allergy 1993; 70:31–34.

15. Eriksson NE, Ryden B, Jonsson P. Hypersensitivity to larvae of chironomids (nonbiting midges). Allergy 1989; 44:305–313.

16. Eriksson NE, Wihl JA, Arrendal H, Strandhede SO. Tree pollen allergy. III. Cross reactions based on results from skin prick tests and the RAST in hay fever patients. A multi-centre study. Allergy 1987; 42:205–214.

17. Gronborg J, Bisgaard H, Romeling F, Mygind N. Early and late nasal symptom response to allergen challenge. Allergy 1993; 48:87–93.

18. Rak S, Jacobson MR, Sudderick RM, Masuyama K, Kay AB, Hamid Q, Lowhagen O, Durham SR. Influence of prolonged treatment with topical corticosteroid (fluticasone propionate) on early and late phase nasal responses and cellular infiltration in the nasal mucosa after allergen challenge. Clin Exp Allergy 1994; 24:930–939.

19. Cockcroft DW. Mechanism of perennial allergic asthma. Lancet 1983; 2:253–256.

20. Cockcroft A, Edwards J, McCarthy P, Andersson N. Allergy in laboratory animal workers. Lancet 1981; 1:827.

21. Platts Mills TAE, Longbottom J, Edwards J, Cockcroft A, Wilkins S. Occupational asthma and rhinitis related to laboratory rats: serum IgG and IgE antibodies to the rat urinary allergen. J Allergy Clin Immunol 1987; 79:505–515.

22. Malo JC, Cartier A, Ghezzo H, Lafrance M, Cante M, Lehrer SB. Patterns of improvement in spirometry, bronchial hyperresponsiveness and specific IgE antibody levels after cessation of exposure in occupational asthma caused by snowcrab processing. Am Rev Respir Dis 1988; 138:807–812.

23. Venables KM, Topping MD, Nunn AJ, Howe W, Newman Taylor AJ. Immunologic and functional consequences of chemical (tetrachlorophthalic anhydride) induced asthma after four years of avoidance of exposure. J Allergy Clin Immunol 1987; 80: 212–218.

24. DeShazo RD, Kimberle C, Swain RE. Fungal sinusitis. N Engl J Med 1997; 337: 254–259.

25. Welsh PW, Stricker WE, Chu Pin C, et al. Efficacy of beclomethasone nasal solution, flunisolide and cromolyn in relieving symptoms of ragweed allergy. Mayo Clin Proc 1987; 62:125–134.

26. Juniper EF, Frith PA, Hargreave FE. Airway responsiveness to histamine and methacholine: relationship to minimum treatment to control symptoms. Thorax 1981; 36: 575.

27. Frew A, Dreborg S. Position paper: Allergen standardisation and skin tests. Allergy 1993; 48(Suppl 14):49–82.

28. Dreborg S. Allergy diagnosis. In: Mygind N, Naclerio RM, eds. Allergic and Nonallergic Rhinitis: Clinical Aspects. Copenhagen: Munksgaard, 1993: 82–94.

29. Sibbald B, Barnes G, Durham SR. Skin prick testing in general practice: a pilot study. J Adv Nurs 1997; 26:537–542.

30. Dreborg S, Basomba A, Belin L et al. Biological equilibration of allergenic preparations. Methodological aspects and reproducibility. Clin Allergy 1987; 17:537–550.

31. Walker S, Varney V, Jacobson MR, Durham SR. Grass pollen immunotherapy: efficacy and safety during a four year follow-up study. Allergy 1995; 50:405–413.

32. Varney VA, Hamid QA, Gaga M, Sun Ying, Jacobson M, Frew AJ, Kay AB, Durham SR. Influence of grass pollen immunotherapy on cellular infiltration and cytokine mRNA expression during allergen-induced late-phase cutaneous responses. J Clin Invest 1993; 92:644–651.

33. Burrows B, Martinez FD, Halonen M, Barbee RA, Cline MG. Association of asthma with serum IgE levels and skin-test reactivity to allergen. N Engl J Med 1989; 320: 271–277.

34. Kerstjens HAM, Schouten JP, Brand PLP, Schoonbrood DFME, Sterk PJ, Postma DS, and the Dutch CNSLD Study Group. Importance of total serum IgE for improvement in airways hyperresponsiveness with inhaled corticosteroids in asthma and chronic pulmonary disease. Am J Respir Crit Care Med 1995; 151:360–368.

35. Zetterstrom O, Osterman K, Axelsson G. Differential diagnosis of atopic allergy in asthma and rhinitis with an improved technology applying the Phadiatop principle. In: Johansson SGO, ed. Clinical workshop, IgE-antibodies and the Pharmacia CAP system in allergy diagnosis. A report of an international workshop, June 23, 1988, Pharmacia, Uppsala, Sweden.

36. Emanuel A. A comparison of in vitro allergy diagnostic assays. Ear Nose Throat J 1990; 69:27–41.

37. Dreborg S. Conjunctival provocation test. Allergy 1985; 40(Suppl 4):66–67.

38. Eriksson NE. Diagnosis of reaginic allergy with house dust, animal dander and pollen allergens in adult patients. III. Case histories and combinations of case histories, skin tests and the radioallergosorbent test, RAST, compared with provocation tests. Int Arch Allergy Appl Immunol 1977; 53:441–449.

39. Pastorello EA, Incorvaia C, Pravettoni V, Bonini S, Canonica GW, Ortolani C, Romagnani S, Tursi A, Zanussi C. A multicentre study on sensitivity and specificity of a new in vitro test for measurement of IgE antibodies. Ann Allergy 1991; 67: 365–370.
40. Colloff MJ, Ayres J, Carswell F, et al. The control of allergens of dust mites and domestic pets: a position paper. Clin Exp Allergy 1992; 22(Suppl 2):1–28.

10

Rhinoscopy: Endoscopic Diagnosis

HEINZ R. STAMMBERGER

ENT—Hospital University Medical School
Graz, Austria

I. Allergic Rhinitis

From a rhinoscopist's view, the "truly" allergic nose is very boring, especially when dealing with a seasonal allergy. If not exposed to allergens, the mucosa usually cannot be differentiated from a healthy, nonallergic individual's nose. In case of allergen exposure, little else but watery secretions and a swollen mucosa with increased vascularity, sometimes presenting with a purplish color, can be noted. At the extreme, the nose is totally blocked, allowing no visibility at all (Fig. 1).

But even in an allergic nose, factors predisposing to early manifestations of allergic symptoms can be identified and differential diagnoses ruled out endoscopically, as will be described below.

II. Nonallergic Rhinitis

Nonallergic rhinosinusitis, in contrast, is a demanding challenge for the nasal endoscopist. Using rigid endoscopes for diagnosis, it becomes evident that anterior and/or posterior rhinoscopy with speculum and mirror provide very limited information, not enough in any case to understand the pathophysiology of the nose and its sinuses. Augmented by modern imaging techniques like computed-tomography (CT) scan, the endoscope may help the diagnostician, the surgeon, and the scientific researcher and thus serve the patient.

III. Infectious Rhinosinusitis

Endoscopic investigations of the lateral nasal wall over the last decades have demonstrated that most infections of the larger sinuses are rhinogenic: disease spreads from the nose to the paranasal sinuses. At the beginning of a nonallergic inflammatory process, the nasal mucosa usually is affected in a very limited and circumscribed area: at the entrance of the middle nasal meatus, where the clefts of the anterior ethmoidal labyrinth form a complex system of cells and pathways, through which frontal and maxillary sinuses are ventilated and drained. It is here that changes occur first, making it evident that the nasal mucosa does not react uniformly as an entity but that there are predilection sites from which disease spreads through the nose and eventually to the larger sinuses.

The normally very narrow clefts of the anterior ethmoid hold the key position for normal function and the pathophysiology of the larger sinuses. These clefts can be seen as prechambers, on which frontal and maxillary sinuses are dependent. Many anatomical variants can here obstruct these clefts and the prechambers even more and thus predispose this area to recurring and persistent infections (1).

The space between the middle turbinate and the lamina papyracea is very limited. An anatomical variation of one of the structures hidden underneath the middle turbinate may constrict or completely block another physiologically important cleft in the vicinity, or at least bring opposing mucosal areas in close proximity. Here, a minimal mucosal swelling—whatever the underlying cause may be—can bring opposing mucosal areas into contact and their ciliary activity can be impeded. The secretion between such contact areas cannot be transported away, and lesions—caused by allergens, noxious substances, bacteria, viruses, or other immunologically active agents—are prone to start here. Under certain conditions infection can spread to adjacent sites, affecting the entire lateral nasal wall and eventually the dependent larger sinuses.

Even a relatively limited disease in the ethmoidal infundibulum—the prechamber to the maxillary sinus—or the frontal recess—the prechamber to the frontal sinus—may severely affect the respective sinus. This may result in retention of secretions, poor ventilation of the sinus, and inflammation if superinfection occurs. The symptoms of this diseased sinus may dominate the clinical picture. The underlying cause of the disease, however, in most cases will be found in the lateral nasal wall and not in the sinus itself.

The patient can have massive symptoms long before diseased mucosa or free polyps appear in the common nasal meatus protruding out of the ethmoid. The key symptom of even mild ethmoiditis is nasal obstruction (2) (Figs. 2–6).

The preferred areas of contact sites in the nose—apart from septal deviations—include the frontal recess and the ethmoidal infundibulum, the cleft between the uncinate process and the middle turbinate, between the ethmoidal bulla

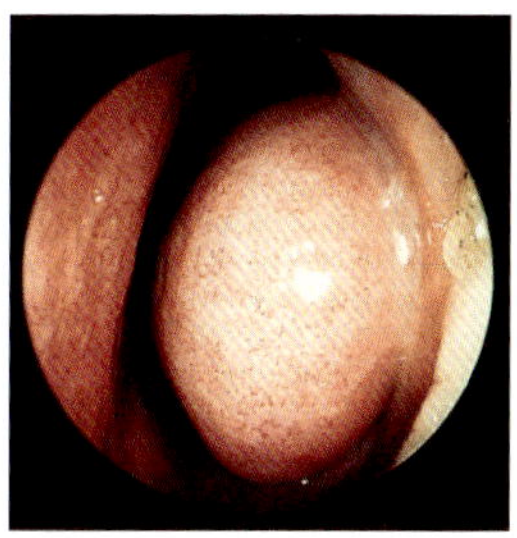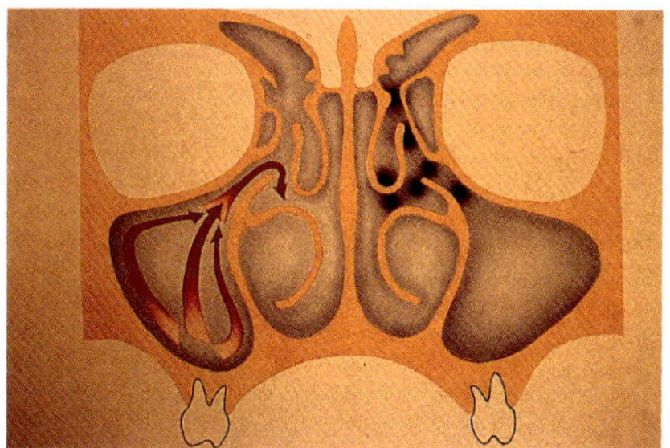

Figure 1 *(left)*   Endoscopic view onto the inferior turbinate (left) side in an allergic patient during acute symptoms. The turbinate mucosa presents with typical purplish color and hypersecretion and is massively swollen.

Figure 2 *(right)*   Drawing of mucus transport out of the maxillary sinus through the ostium and the ethmoidal infundibulum into the middle meatus (red arrows). On the other side, predilection sites for a mucosal swelling and interference with ventilation and drainage in the ostiomeatal complex are indicated.

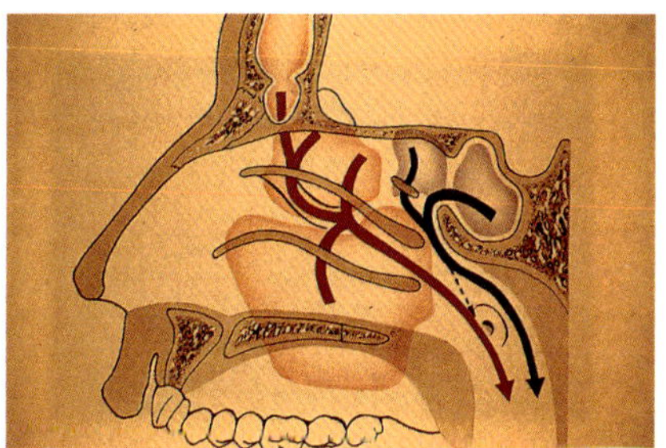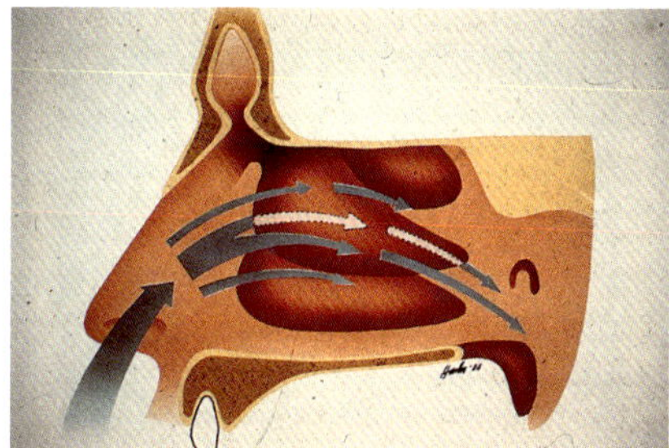

Figure 3 *(left)*   Active secretion transportation routes through lateral nasal wall. Red = mucus transport out of frontal, anterior ethmoidal, and maxillary sinuses. Blue = mucus transport out of posterior ethmoidal and sphenoidal sinus.

Figure 4 *(right)*   Schematic drawing of airflow through the nose.

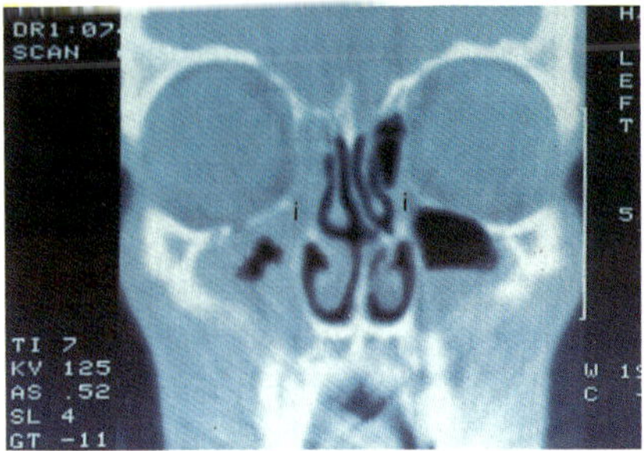
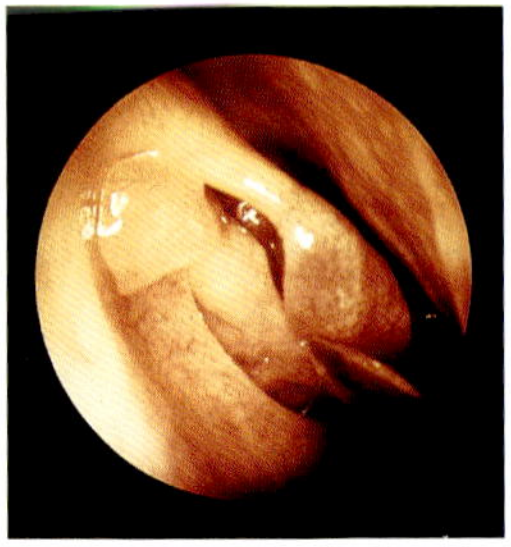

Figure 5 *(left)*   Coronal CT-scan of bilateral nonallergic rhinosinusitis. On anterior rhinoscopy, the nose was unremarkable except for the septal spur (left). Endoscopically the disease in the anterior ethmoids on both sides could be identified. Both sides present with disease in the maxillary sinus due to blockage of the ethmoidal infundibulum (i). This patient responded to functional endoscopic sinus surgery and required no further medication.

Figure 6 *(right)*   The entrance to the middle nasal meatus (right). The middle turbinate is pushed medially with Freer's instrument (4 o'clock). Polyps can be seen originating from the anterior face of the bulla, between the bulla and the middle turbinate, and between the bulla and the free posterior margin of the uncinate process.

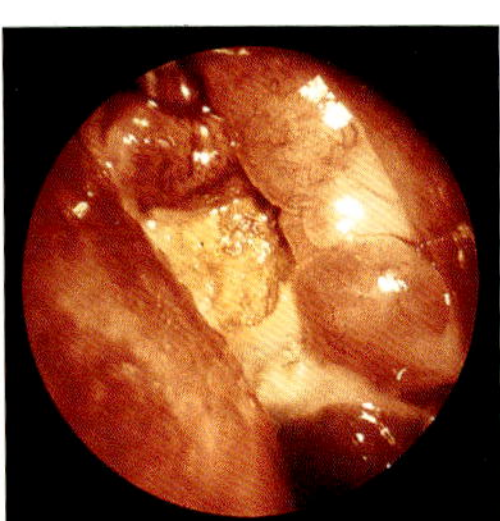
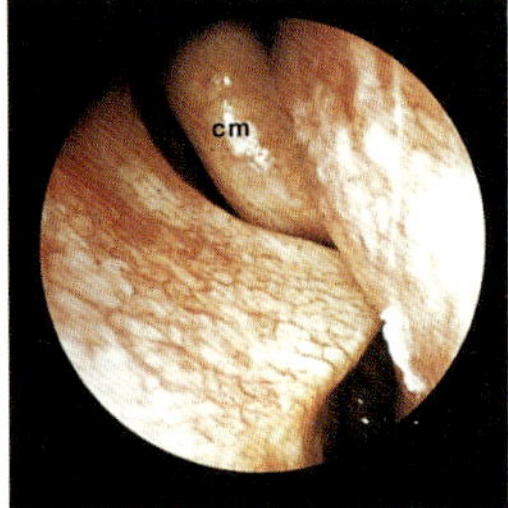

Figure 7 *(left)*   Right middle meatus: An adenocarcinoma in a wood worker. The disease started where the carcinogens had been deposited with the airflow; in the most anterior portion of the middle meatus and the anterior ethmoid.

Figure 8 *(right)*   Endoscopic view of the patient in Figure 5. The septal spur can be identified piercing into the inferior turbinate. The nasal mucosa appears normal despite the presence of considerable disease in the lateral nasal wall (cm = middle turbinate).

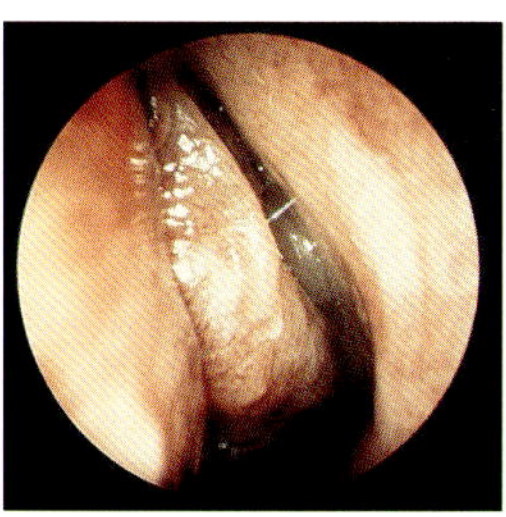

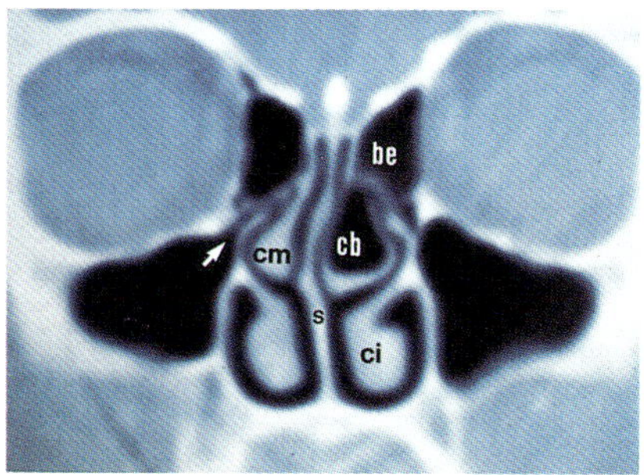

Figure 9 *(left)* Only the endoscope revealed this allegedly minimal polyp between a concha bullosa of the middle turbinate and the lateral nasal wall. During surgery considerable amounts of polyps could be removed from the anterior ethmoid, proving that the visible polyp was just "the tip of the iceberg."

Figure 10 *(right)* Coronal CT-scan of a patient with nasal obstruction. The pneumatization of the middle turbinate on the patient's left side can be seen. There is contact between the concha bullosa (cb) and the septum medially and with the ethmoidal bulla (be) lateral superiorly (s = septum, ci = inferior turbinate, arrow = ethmoidal infundibulum).

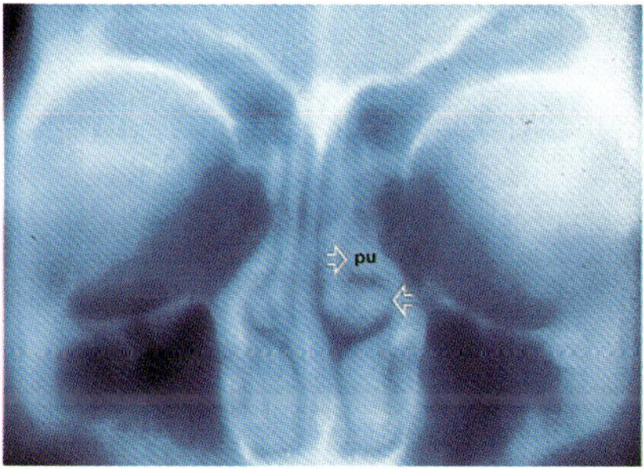

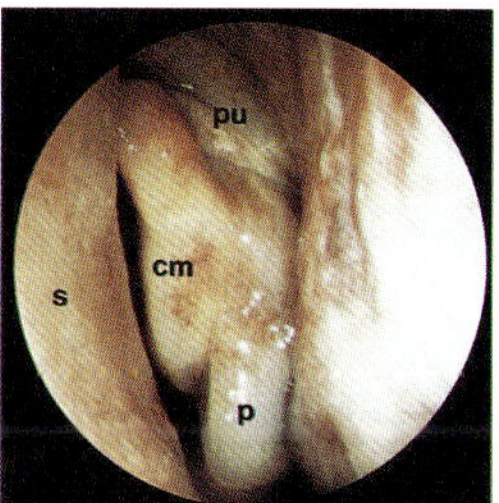

Figure 11 *(left)* Conventional tomography demonstrates an uncinate process (pu) which as an anatomical variant is curved medially, creating two areas of contact with the middle turbinate (arrows). The patient suffered from nasal obstruction, a feeling of fullness, postnasal discharge, and episodes of sneezing. After resection of the uncinate process and the diseased ethmoidal bulla (not visible) the symptoms disappeared.

Figure 12 *(right)* Large polyps protrude from the middle meatus of the left nose. The uncinate process is bent medially and curved anteriorly (doubled middle turbinate). The polyps originate from the contact area between uncinate process, anterior face of the ethmoidal bulla, and the middle turbinate. (s = septum, cm = middle turbinate, p = polyp, pu = uncinate process.)

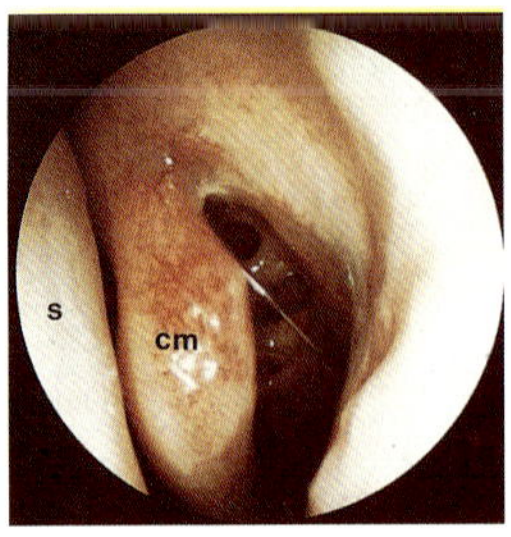

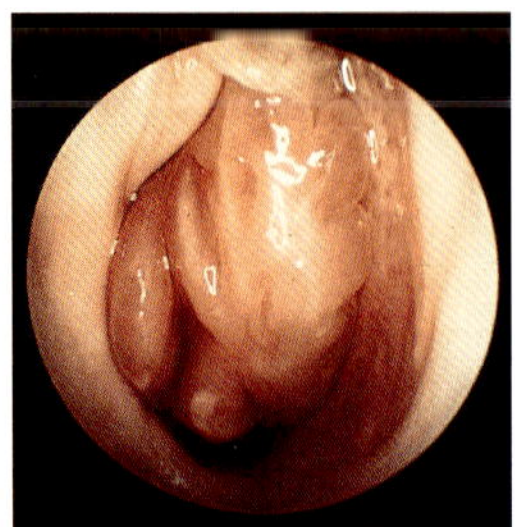

Figure 13 *(left)*   A few weeks after endoscopic surgery. There is free passage into the middle meatus, the ethmoidal mucosa has normalized after resection of the uncinate process and most of the ethmoidal bulla. (s = septum, cm = middle turbinate.)

Figure 14 *(right)*   Right side: Diffuse polyposis filling the choana in a patient with allergic fungal sinusitis.

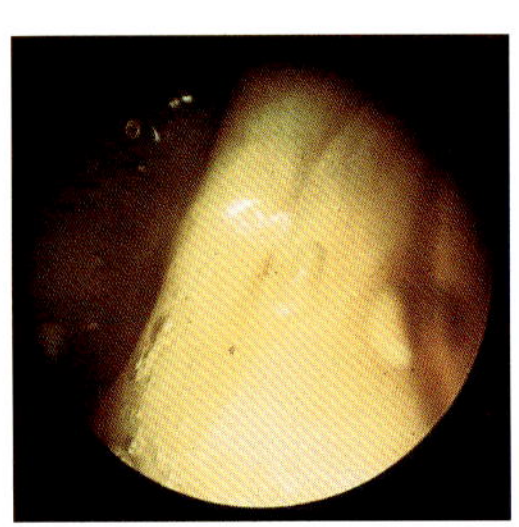

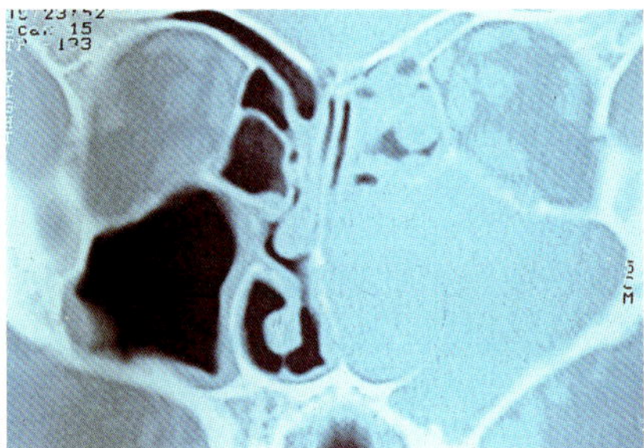

Figure 15 *(left)*   "Peanut butter-like" mucus in a patient with allergic fungal sinusitis.

Figure 16 *(right)*   CT-finding of an antrochoanal polyp. A large cystic portion fills the maxillary sinus, the solid portion has eroded the lateral nasal wall (= medial maxillary sinus wall) and fills the middle and common nasal meatus. The solid portion reached as far back as the nasopharynx. The opacification of the ethmoids was secondary to the blockage by this lesion.

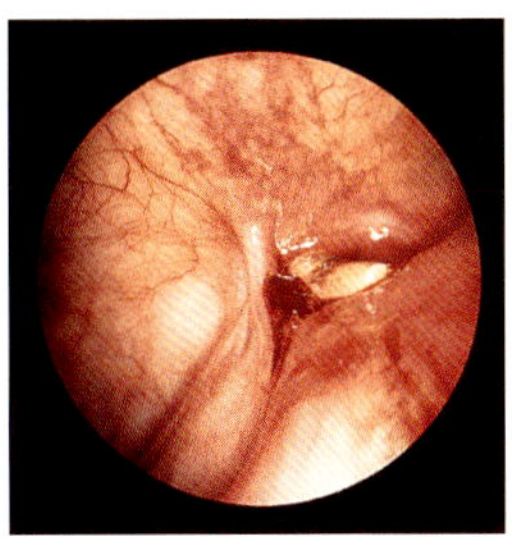 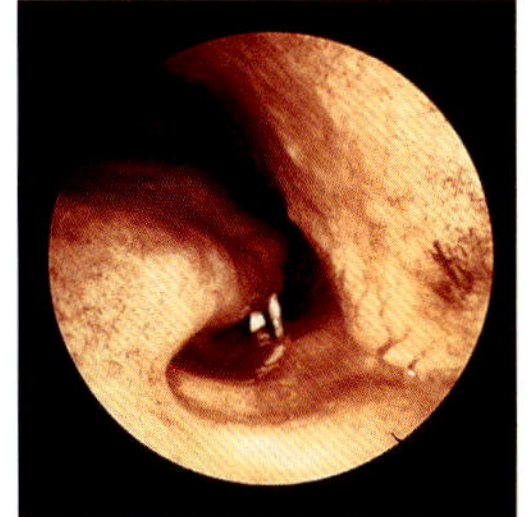 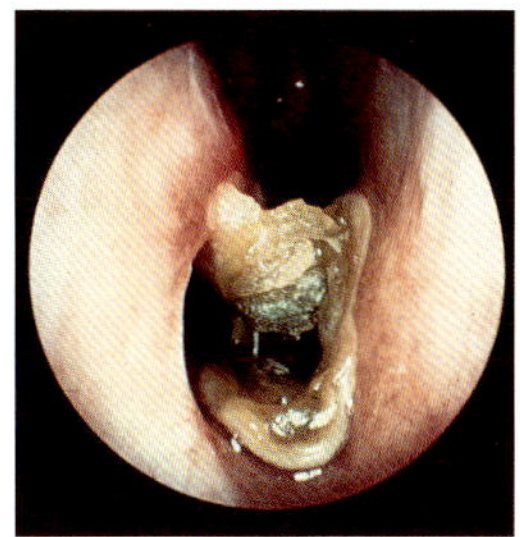

Figure 17 *(left)*   Foreign body "trapped" in a maxillary sinus ostium (left). This dental root filling material had gone astray and was too large to be transported through the natural ostium. 30° lens, view via canina fossa.

Figure 18 *(center)*   Foreign body. This patient's rhinorrhea and sneezing attacks were due to the "roots" of this dental implant, which penetrated through the nasal floor and into the inferior turbinate (right).

Figure 19 *(right)*   Foreign body. Hard crusts formed and a rhinolith was developing around a fragment from a plastic toy, which this 2-year-old patient had implanted into the right nose. The watery secretions on the floor of the nose were the only symptom.

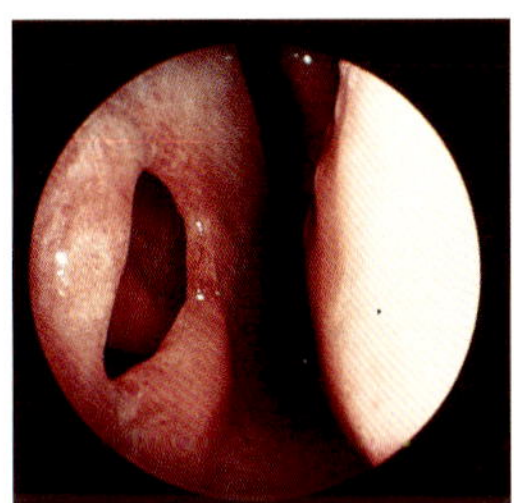 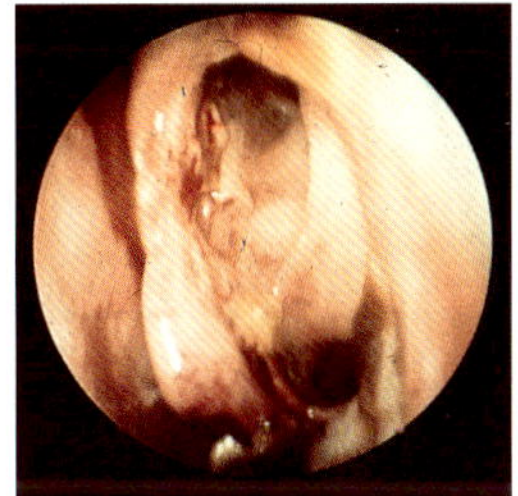 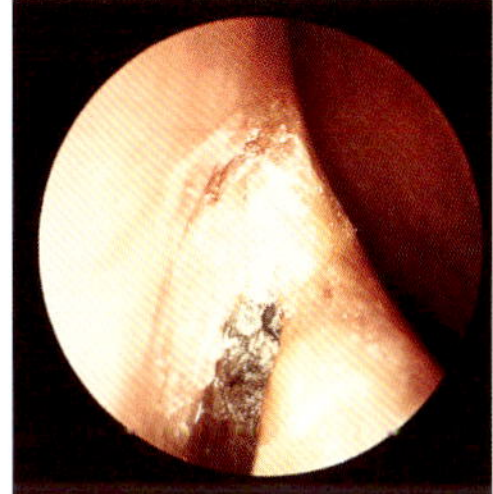

Figure 20 *(left)*   Septal perforation (left) following frequent packing and cautery after epistaxis. Clinical symptoms were watery running nose; feeling of nasal obstruction.

Figure 21 *(center)*   Result of insufficient surgery on a patient's left side. Significant scar formation between the bulla and the middle turbinate, the bulla is still diseased and the symptoms (nasal obstruction, rhinorrhea, occasional sneezing) persist.

Figure 22 *(right)*   Crust formation at the insertion of the middle turbinate on the right in a patient using long-term topical corticosteroid therapy. The fungal growth on the crusts was identified as *Candida*.

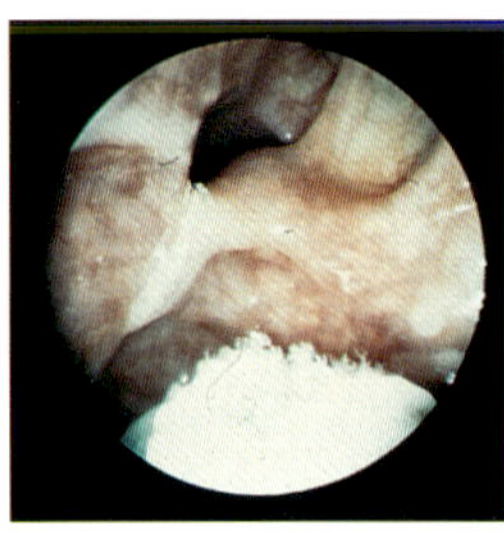 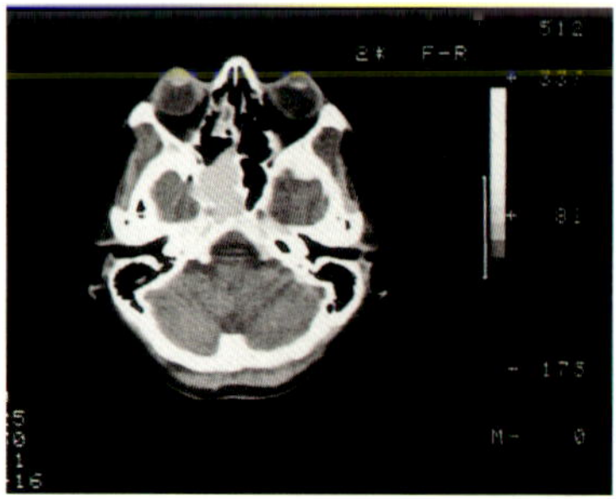

Figure 23 *(left)*   Maxillary sinoscopy (left). A cherry-size fungus ball (*Aspergillus fumigatus*) can be found on the floor of the sinus. The fungal colonies on its surface are visible. Fungal concrements can even be seen in the mucus, transported towards the natural ostium.

Figure 24 *(right)*   CT-scan finding of noninvasive *Aspergillus* fungus ball in a sphenoid sinus. Note high and low density areas within the opacification.

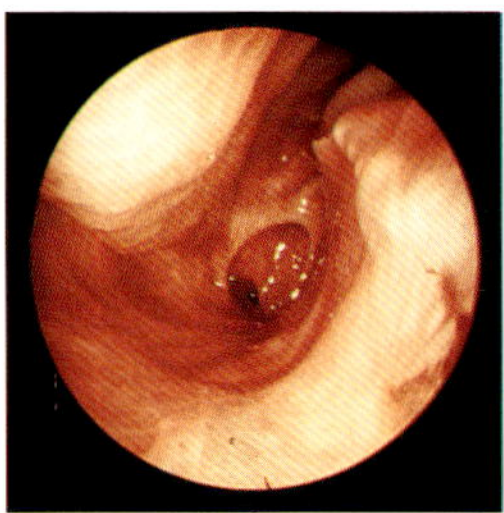 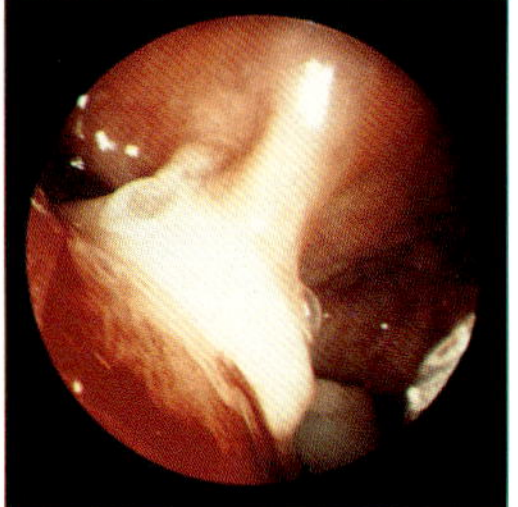 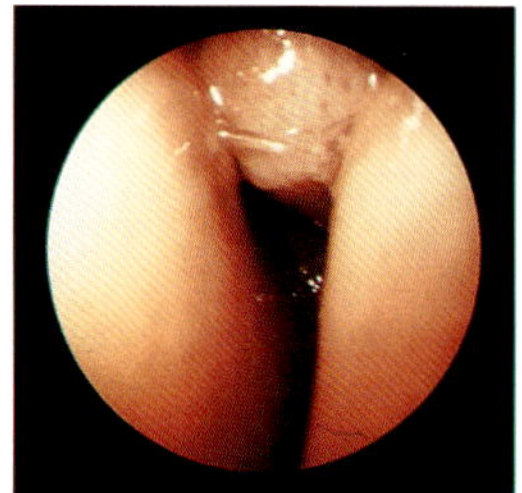

Figure 25 *(left)*   After aspiration of thickened and retained mucus, a bilateral choanal stenosis was identified in this 11-year-old boy. The stenotic choana was blocked by adenoids protruding through the latter (right).

Figure 26 *(center)*   "Circular transport" of mucopus into the maxillary sinus (6 o'clock) through an accessory ostium in the posterior fontanelle, and out of the sinus (10 o'clock) through the natural ostium.

Figure 27 *(right)*   A small "polyp" is visible between the middle turbinate and the septum. This innocent looking lesion proved to be esthioneuroblastoma.

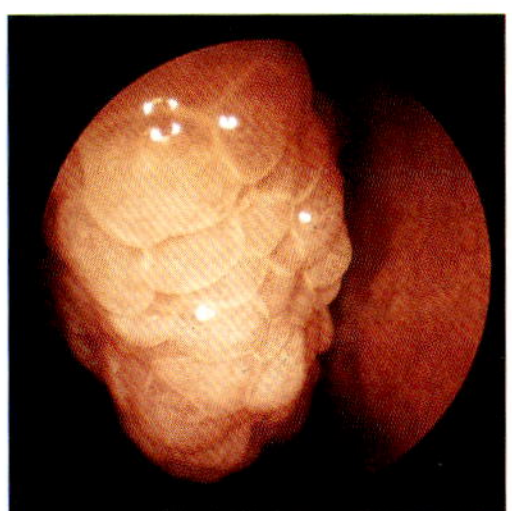 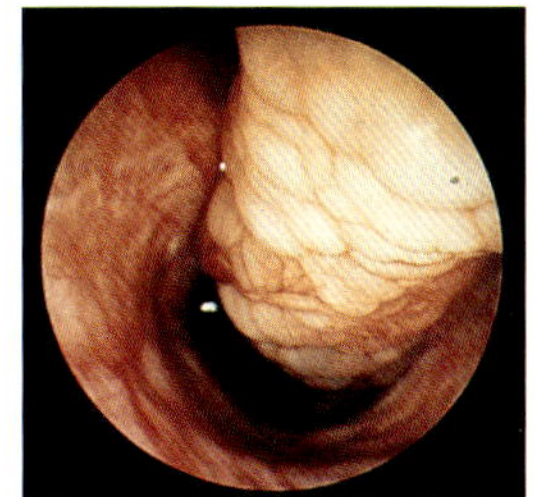 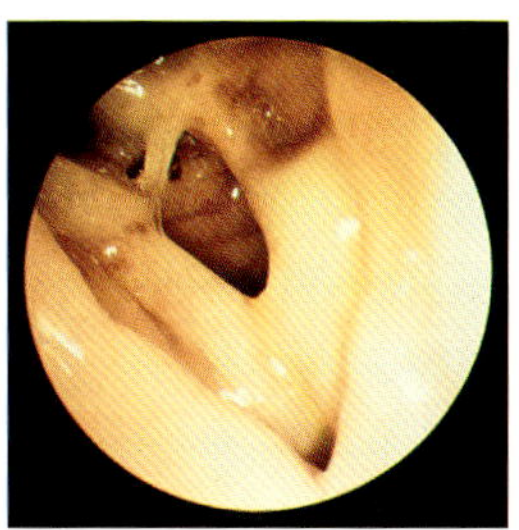

Figure 28 *(left)*   On biopsy, this "cobble-stone aspect" of mucosa on an inferior turbinate on the right proved to be a sarcoidosis.

Figure 29 *(center)*   Inferior nasal turbinate (left). This lesion was not a harmless hypertrophy of the mucosa, but tuberculosis. The disease was identified after the nasal diagnosis, as it had been asymptomatic so far.

Figure 30 *(right)*   Endoscopic view into a sphenoid sinus (left) in a patient with watery secretion from the nose. There is some mucus from the central opening (6 o'clock).

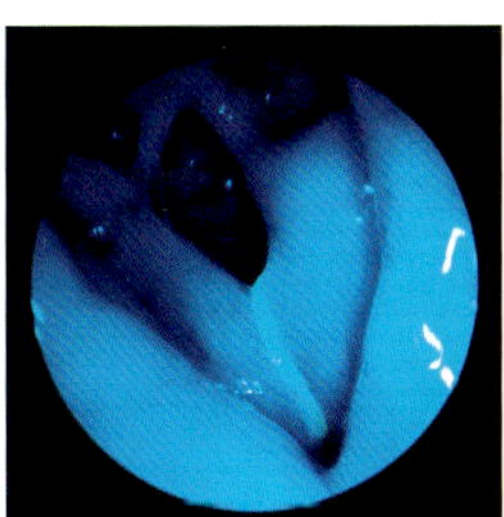 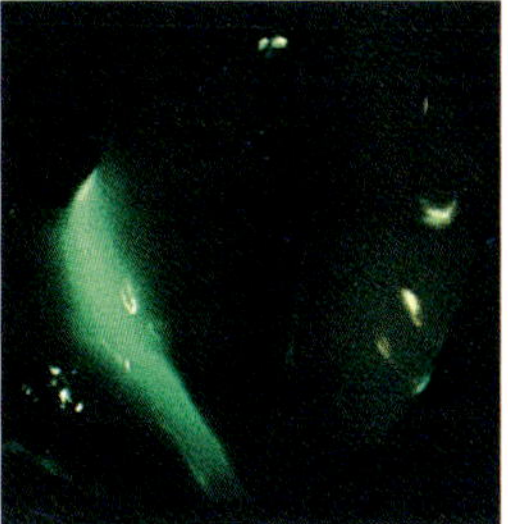 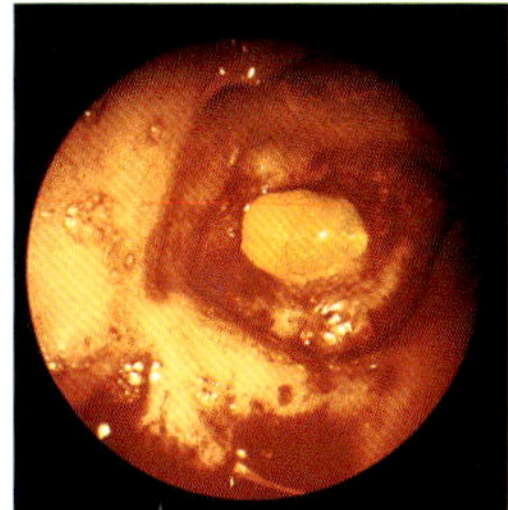

Figure 31 *(left)*   After fluorescein had been injected intrathecally, the greenish color of mucus can be identified.

Figure 32 *(center)*   With an orange blocking filter, all visible light is blocked except the fluorescence from the stained cerebrospinal fluid. Thus the diagnosis of a CSF-leak can be confirmed.

Figure 33 *(right)*   The fluorescein technique was used to identify this meningoen-cephalocele through the posterior wall of the sphenoid (right), which could be closed successfully via this endoscopic approach.

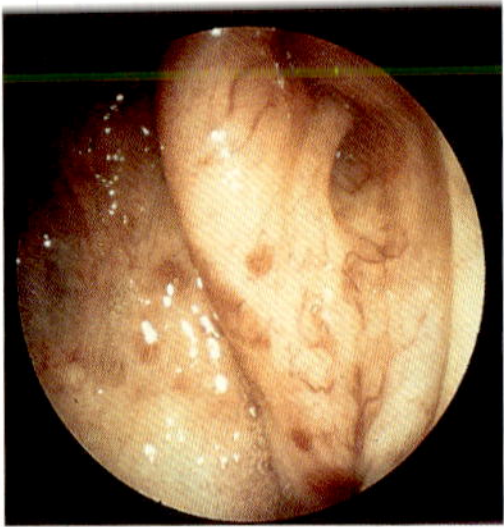 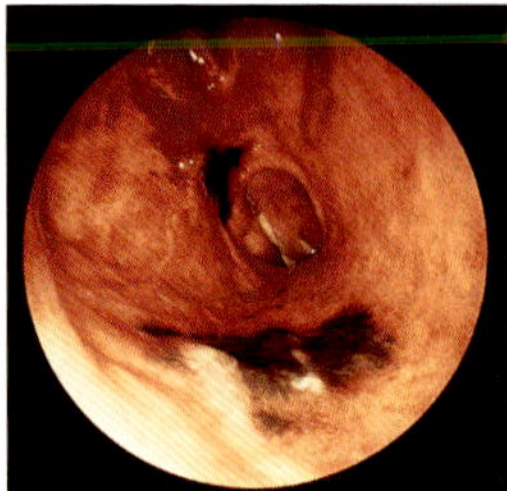

Figure 34 *(left)*   Tiny vascular patches on the tubal lip and in Rosenmüller's fossa (left) of a young hemophiliac turned out to be early stages of Kaposi's sarcoma.

Figure 35 *(right)*   The metastatic spread of a malignant melanoma can be seen on the nasal floor and the nasopharynx on this right side.

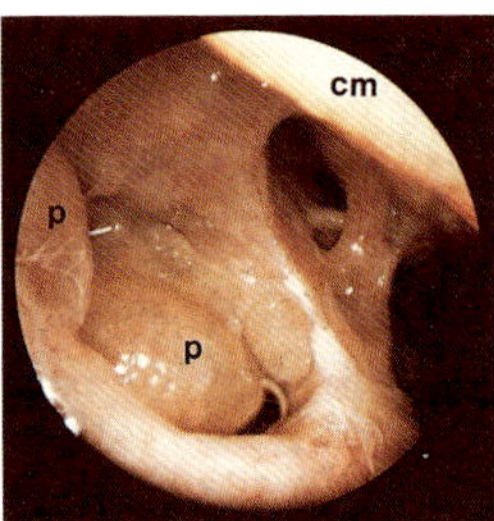 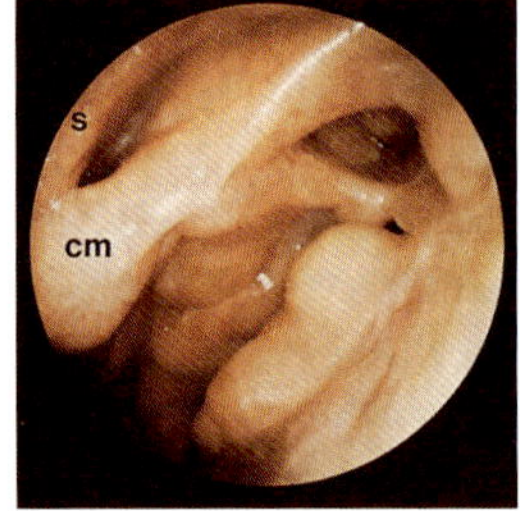

Figure 36 *(left)*   Polyp recurrence in the maxillary sinus ostium on the right side of a patient 6 months after endoscopic surgery. Topical corticosteroid therapy was applied and the mucosa almost normalized after three weeks. The patient continued topical therapy to prevent regrowth of polyps. Whenever topical corticosteroids were discontinued polyps reappeared. This was an eosinophil dominated polyposis in a patient with asthma and aspirin intolerance (cm = middle turbinate, p = recurring polyps).

Figure 37 *(right)*   Eosinophil dominated polyposis. View into the middle nasal meatus on the left side, following numerous surgical procedures, including radical ethmoidectomy, for a diffuse polypoid disease. The symptoms had improved; the mucosa is far from normal. Despite topical and interval systemic corticosteroid therapy this was the best condition achieved (s = septum, cm = middle turbinate).

and the middle turbinate, and the supra- and retrobullar recess above and behind the ethmoidal bulla. Many anatomical variants of these structures and the clefts between them may constrict the pathways of mucociliary transport even more, thus apparently predisposing patients to recurring disease, especially if combinations of the anatomical variations exist. Table 1 lists some of the more frequent anatomical variants that we have encountered in patients with chronic or recurrent rhinosinusitis.

Once a localized problem is established in one of these clefts, a cascade effect may start: the hiatus semilunaris can be affected from an infected area between the uncinate process and the middle turbinate. This in turn may lead to inflammation of the infundibulum and/or the frontal recess from which maxillary or frontal sinuses may be affected (Fig. 5).

IV. Nasal Polyps

The endoscope furthermore reveals that nasal polyps usually do *not* start *inside* the sinuses or cells, but from contact areas in ethmoidal clefts in the middle meatus.

Table 2 lists the findings from our study of 200 consecutive patients during endoscopic examination or surgery. The majority of polyps originated in the anterior ethmoid, the most frequent sites being contact areas of the uncinate process

Table 1 Frequent Anatomical Variations to Acute and Recurrent Rhinosinusitis

Variants	Clinical significance
Septal deviation/spurs	Narrowing middle common nasal meatus, contact areas
Agger nasi cells	Large, narrowing frontal recess
Uncinate process	Medially bent, laterally bent, curved anteriorly (''double middle turbinate''), fractures (trauma, iatrogenic), contacting turbinate, pneumatized
Middle turbinate	Concha bullosa, paradoxically bent, narrowing lateral nasal wall
Ethmoidal bulla	Large, filling middle nasal meatus, contact areas, anterior growth, overlapping hiatus semilunaris, protruding out of middle meatus
Orbitoethmoidal cells (Haller cells)	Narrowing maxillary ostium/ethmoidal infundibulum
Accessory ostia in fontanelles	Circular transport of mucus, infection of secondary sinuses
Combinations of all the above	

Table 2 Origin of Polyps in 200 Consecutive Patients

Site of origin	Percent of patients
Uncinate, turbinate, infundibulum	80
Face of bulla, hiatus semilunaris, infundibulum	65
Frontal recess	48
Between bulla and middle turbinate	42
Inside bulla	30
Supra- and retrobullar recess	28
Posterior ethmoid (superior meatus)	27
Middle turbinate	15
Secondary sinuses affected	
Maxillary sinus (mucosal swelling)	65
Frontal sinus (mucosal swelling)	23
Sphenoid sinus	8

and the middle turbinate and the ethmoidal infundibulum as well as the ethmoidal bulla and its vicinity in almost two-thirds of our patients. From here polyps obstructed the hiatus semilunaris, invaded the ethmoidal infundibulum, or protruded anteriorly between the middle turbinate and the uncinate process into the middle meatus (Fig. 6).

In about 50% of all patients, polyps were found in the frontal recess. This is particularly of interest since in this area polyps may not be visible in many cases, even through the endoscope. In this situation the combination of endoscopy and tomography is particularly valuable (Fig. 5). Less than one-third of the patients had their posterior ethmoid affected and less than 8% had polyps or mucosal thickening in the sphenoid sinus. Though this study was performed over 8 years ago, the findings are confirmed again and again in our everyday routine examinations.

The airflow through the nose apparently plays an important role. Due to the direction of the nasal valve, it is aimed at the head of the middle turbinate. When passing through the middle meatus, the airstream here meets frontally with structures like the uncinate process, the anterior face of the ethmoidal bulla; particles and inhaled other matter preferably are deposited here (Fig. 4). It is not by chance that the adenocarcinoma of woodworkers starts in this part of the anterior ethmoid, as it is here that the carcinogens are deposited by the airstream (Fig. 7). Contact areas apparently allow noxious substances to adhere longer locally and thus develop their potentially irritating, noxious, allergic, or immunological activity, resulting in mucosal irritation and/or lesions or triggering other cascade effects (Fig. 8) (3).

V. Treatment

It is fascinating to see polyps rise from contact areas (Figs. 4, 5, and 9). They are easily detectable at the entrance of the middle meatus or—more challenging for the endoscopist—hidden in the narrow clefts of the ethmoid. Those changes cannot be detected with the microscope, let alone the unaided eye. But "hidden" lesions may irritate the nasal function, give the patient the feeling of nasal obstruction, and even mimic allergic symptoms (Figs. 10 and 11). With the identification of this kind of "hidden disease," functional endoscopic sinus surgery concept can achieve a sometimes dramatic improvement of a patient's symptoms (Figs. 12 and 13).

The endoscope is of great value in the medical as well as the surgical approach. In patients who are treated medically we now are able to better evaluate the efficacy of our therapy as we can actually watch the response of the nasal mucosa. This is especially true for the response of polypoid changes to either systemic or topical steroid therapy. We no longer have to rely on the patient's symptoms alone or on the results of rhinomanometry/rhinometry. *The endoscope therefore is the tool that helps to avoid unnecessary surgery by allowing for better diagnosis and therapeutic evaluation.*

If, in an otherwise typical allergic rhinitis patient, antiallergic and/or immunotherapy does not improve the nasal symptoms as expected, an endoscopic approach may help to identify an anatomical variation in the lateral nasal wall, such as a concha bullosa, an overpneumatized ethmoidal bulla, or a deflected uncinate process (Figs. 9–13). Surgical correction of these variations usually is a minimal procedure with little risk in the hands of an experienced surgeon. Of course, an IgE-mediated allergy cannot be cured by surgery. But in the situation mentioned above, a functional endoscopic approach can be a helpful adjunctive therapy by eliminating contact areas and stenotic clefts, where, under allergen exposure, symptoms would occur first. Thus, a better threshold may be reached when the mucosa is exposed to allergens. We have found that antiallergic medication could significantly be reduced or fully omitted after such therapy in selected cases (4).

VI. Differential Diagnosis

Differential diagnosis should not be forgotten: not infrequently, malignant diseases of the nose present rhinitis symptoms as their only manifestation for a considerable period and/or such disease may be hidden behind reactive polyps. In particular, unilateral disease should always be investigated with this possibility in mind.

With the exception of the "allergic fungal sinusitis," which presents to the endoscopist as diffuse polyposis (Figs. 14 and 15), no allergic disease is present unilaterally. Sometimes intensive mucosal contact, in cases of septal spurs or other contact areas in the lateral nasal wall that have anatomical variants, may interfere with rapid transport of allergens deposited here. These may therefore deploy their activities and the allergic cascade may have a unilateral dominance. Factors like the ones mentioned should carefully be ruled out, before a diagnosis of allergy is made in a patient with unilateral symptoms.

To be excluded are "harmless" lesions such as antrochoanal polyp (Fig. 16), foreign bodies (Figs. 17–19), scars or other processes following previous surgery or other intranasal manipulations like intubations and packings (for instance for epistaxis) (Figs. 20 and 21), as well as noninvasive mycotic disease. The latter can be present as saprophytic fungi on crusts, sometimes even in patients who use topical corticosteroids for long periods (Fig. 22). So-called "fungus balls" in predominantly maxillary, but rarely ethmoidal, frontal, and sphenoidal, sinuses (Figs. 23 and 24) can cause sinusitis-like symptoms and nasal irritation, mimicking allergic symptoms. These are rare cases, where diagnostic maxillary sinoscopy via the inferior nasal meatus or the canine fossa may be indicated. In doubtful cases, CT scans should be performed rather than starting symptomatic therapy.

In the 11-year-old patient shown in Figure 25, bilateral rhinorrhea, nasal obstruction, and occasional sneezing were noted. An allergy test was positive for pollen. Endoscopically, however, a choanal stenosis with mild hypertrophy of the adenoids was identified. After surgical correction, the patient was free of symptoms (Fig. 25).

Accessory ostia—usually those in the posterior nasal fontanelles—may cause a circular transport of mucus. Through the accessory ostium, mucus is actively transported *into* the maxillary sinus, where it follows the genetically determined pathways of transport up toward the natural ostium of the maxillary sinus. From here it passes through the ethmoidal infundibulum, only to reach the region of the posterior nasal fontanelle again. Thus a circular transport results, during which the mucus usually is considerably thickened. This may not only irritate the patient and cause rhinitis symptoms, but frequently gives the feeling of nasal obstruction and annoying postnasal discharge. This mechanism is one of the ways that pathogens can actively be transported into an otherwise healthy maxillary sinus and cause symptoms there (Fig. 26).

Not all unilateral "polyps" are harmless. The lesion shown in Figure 27 proved to be a highly malignant esthesioneuroblastoma. Figure 7 depicts an adenocarcinoma in a woodworker, the early symptoms of which were mild, sometimes intermittent nasal obstruction, watery secretions, and sneezing.

Inverting papillomas of the nose and the sinuses may look like polyps, but in 16–30% of cases they may represent malignant degeneration, according to the literature. Hemangiomatous lesions usually can easily be identified as such, as long as they are clearly visible in the nose and its meatus. Specific diseases such as sarcoidosis (Fig. 28) have been mentioned, as they tend to present with the same—usually minimal—symptoms with which unspecific rhinitis starts.

Increasing numbers of patients have been seen with tuberculosis of the nasal mucosa, the unspecific symptoms of which are the same as those of a mild rhinosinusitis. Once identified by nasal endoscopy, the mucosal areas can easily be biopsied and the diagnosis be established. In the case shown in Figure 29 this led to the discovery of pulmonary tuberculosis previously unknown to the patient.

Though usually associated with a different case history, a cerebrospinal fluid (CSF) rhinorrhea in some cases should be considered for differential diagnosis. Figures 30–33 demonstrate the possibilities afforded by endoscopy with blue light and the use of intrathecal fluorescein in those cases. In a patient with watery rhinorrhea and mild "rhinitis" some discrete "mucus" was identified endoscopically from the sphenoid sinus (Fig. 30). The patient received 0.7 ml of 5% sodium fluorescein solution intrathecally; after this, endoscopy was repeated with blue light (Fig. 31). The "mucus" then showed a greenish fluorescence. After a blocking (complementary orange) filter was added, all visible light was blocked with the exception of the light from fluorescein-containing areas (Fig. 32). The picture then appeared almost black, but the trays of fluorescein-stained CSF could clearly be seen. The diagnosis of CSF leak of the anterior skull base therefore could be established with absolute certainty in this case (Fig. 33).

Figure 34 demonstrates minor vascular patches over the eustachian tube orifice of a young hemophiliac, who was seen for "rhinitis." These proved to be early stages of Kaposi's sarcoma as the patient had acquired AIDS via a blood transfusion. Finally, Figure 35 shows with frightening clarity the metastatic spread of a malignant melanoma over the floor of the nose.

VII. Future Research

The endoscopic findings should provide a new stimulus to researchers. What goes wrong in those contact areas? What lesions do occur here? What triggers the cascade of disease spreading into the surroundings? How can such small lesions interfere with the nasal cycle and the nasal function?

Clinical experience has shown that after relatively limited removal of such contact areas and diseased clefts, patients can be cured and nasal function as well as the appearance of the mucosa can be completely normalized. We still do not, however, know and understand how we achieve what we are achieving: what pathophysiological spiral are we able to break by surgical intervention and why does it not work to the same degree in all syndromes?

Apparently we are facing several entirely different groups of "nasal polyposis," one of which is extremely therapy-resistant, frequently requires long-term corticosteroid therapy, and, despite this, accounts for the majority of surgical failures. Are there criteria to differentiate different kinds of nasal polyps before choosing a therapy, thus limiting our frequency of indication for surgery (5–11) (Figs. 36 and 37)? There are many more questions than we can answer at present. The use of diagnostic endoscopy may help in several respects.

The endoscope might be a tool to bring closer together the two groups of people who ''work'' in the nose, but have communicated so little to each other: allergologists/immunologists and surgeons. For the latter group this could mean being more selective with their indications of surgery by trying to exclude those cases that could better be approached with antiallergic or immunotherapy. Immunologists should consider the fact that the mucosa is not lining a simple box with plane walls in the nose with allergic/immunological reactions taking place anywhere, but that the ethmoidal labyrinth in the lateral nasal wall holds a key position, with its clefts, meatus, and cells. Here, mechanistic (anatomical variations causing stenosis and contact areas) and aerodynamic principles must be considered as well. In a multifactorial disease complex, a closer cooperation between those involved in research and those in therapy is required to meet the challenge of the present and the future.

VIII. Conclusions

1.   There is more in the allergic and nonallergic nose than can be seen with the speculum, the unaided eye, and standard X-rays. Especially in chronic and/or therapy-resistant cases, anterior and posterior rhinoscopy simply are not sufficient means to evaluate a nose.

2.   In addition to evaluating the patient's symptomatic improvement under a given therapy, the endoscope allows for visual evaluation of mucosal changes in areas otherwise hidden from the unaided eye and even from the microscope.

3.   The endoscope may help to direct the researcher's interest to the sites where the problems (and most of the polyps) start. Biopsies of those areas might provide useful additional information that may not be present in biopsies or smears from mucosal areas that are only secondarily involved, such as the inferior turbinate or the maxillary sinus.

4.   When discussing the problem of ''nasal polyposis'' we should be aware that we are not talking about one disease entity, but apparently are dealing with a mucosal reaction to various, apparently quite different stimuli, which may well require different therapeutic approaches.

5.   Differential diagnosis should not be forgotten. Frequently, the unaided eye is simply not enough to identify the problems with anterior and/or posterior rhinoscopy. In many instances, even the microscope and the endoscope are not sufficient to explore the remotest corners of this complex system. Even in allegedly classic straightforward symptoms, a rational degree of suspicion should be

maintained. The level of suspicion must significantly increase when dealing with unilateral symptoms. In all those cases other causes must be ruled out prior to initiation of therapy.

References

1. Messerklinger W. Endoscopy of the Nose. Baltimore: Urban & Schwarzenberg, 1978.
2. Stammberger H. Functional Endoscopic Sinus Surgery. Philadelphia: BC Decker–Mosby Year Book, 1991.
3. Kleinsasser O, Schroeder H-G. Adenocarcinomas of the inner nose after exposure to wood dust. Arch Oto-Rhino-Laryngol 1988; 245:1–15.
4. Posawetz W, Stammberger H. Chirurgische Massnahmen im Rahmen einer Inhalationsallergie. Allergologie 1991; 14:440–445.
5. Ogava H. Atopic aspect of eosinophilic nasal polyposis and a possible mechanism of eosinophil accumulation. Acta Oto-Laryngol (Stockh) 1986; (Suppl 430):12–7.
6. Ogino S, Harada T, Okawachi I, Irifune M, Matunaga T, Nagano T. Aspirin induced asthma and nasal polyps. Acta Oto-Laryngol (Stockh) 1986; (Suppl 430):21–27.
7. Hsieh V. Nonallergic rhinitis with eosinophilia (NARES) a precursor of the triad nasal polyposis—intrinsic asthma intolerance to aspirin. Rhinology 1988; (Supp 1): 129.
8. Barnes PJ. Asthma as an axon reflex. Lancet 1986; 1:242–245.
9. Mygind N, Winter B. Immunological barriers in the nose and paranasal sinuses. Acta Oto-Laryngol (Stockh) 1987; 103:363–368.
10. Amr Ali Sbieh. Endoscopic study and surgery of paranasal sinus disease in asthmatic patients. Thesis, Cairo, Egypt: Alahzar University Press, 1990.
11. Wolf G, Saria A, Gamse R. Neue Aspekte zur autonomen Innovation der menschlichen Schleimhaut. Laryngol Rhinol Otol 1987; 66:149–151.
12. Stammberger H, Hawke M. Essentials of Functional Endoscopic Sinus Surgery. St Louis: Mosby–Year Book, 1993.
13. Mygind N, Lildholdt T, eds. Nasal Polyposis: An Inflammatory Disease and Its Treatment. Copenhagen: Munksgaard, 1997.
14. Setipane GA, Lund VJ, Bernstein JM, Tos M, eds. Nasal Polyps: Epidemiology, Pathogenis and Treatment. Providence, RI: Ocean Side Publications, 1997.
15. Anderhuber W, Walch C, Braun H. Die Sarkoidose der Nasennebenhöhlen als Ursache einer therapieresistenten Dacryozystitis. Laryngol-Rhinol-Otol 1997; 76:315–317.

11

Nasal Cytology

ELI O. MELTZER, H. ALICE ORGEL, and ALFREDO A. JALOWAYSKI

University of California
San Diego, California

I. Introduction

A series of diagnostic modalities can help to classify nasal disorders (Table 1) (1). These include history, physical examination, rhinoscopy, rhinomanometry, provocation challenges, biochemical determinations, immunological studies, in vivo and in vitro testing for specific IgE, imaging, blood flow, and ciliary function analyses, and examination of nasal cytology.

This chapter focuses on nasal cytology and presents (1) techniques for obtaining, processing, and interpreting cytological specimens, (2) findings in various rhinopathies, and (3) findings in the nasal cytology consequent to various therapeutic agents. This review documents that evaluating nasal cytology can assist in: (1) distinguishing inflammatory from noninflammatory rhinopathies; (2) distinguishing between allergic, nonallergic, and infectious rhinitis; (3) distinguishing between viral and bacterial infections; (4) classifying the cellular response to an infection; (5) following the course of a disease; and (6) following the response to treatment. Morphological changes in the nasal mucosa may reflect reactions that are also valid for other parts of the airways.

Table 1 Classification of Chronic Rhinopathies

Inflammatory rhinitis
  Allergic rhinitis
    Seasonal
    Perennial
  Eosinophilic nonallergic rhinitis
  Basophilic nonallergic rhinitis
  Infectious rhinitis
    Viral
    Bacterial
    Fungal
  Nasal polyposis
  Atrophic rhinitis
Noninflammatory rhinitis
  Vasomotor rhinitis, e.g., physical, chemical stimuli
    Autonomic dysfunction, idiopathic rhinitis
    Associated with systemic conditions, e.g., pregnancy or thyroid disease
  Rhinitis medicamentosa
    Local sympathomimetic overuse
    Systemic medications, e.g., antihypertensives, contraceptives, NSAIDs
Structure-related rhinitis
  Anatomical deformities, e.g., septal deviations, ciliary disorders, choanal
    atresia, cerebrospinal rhinorrhea
  Obstruction, e.g., adenoidal hypertrophy, foreign body, tumor, granuloma

---

II. Methods

Various techniques have been used for obtaining, processing, evaluating, and interpreting nasal cytology specimens (2).

A. Sampling Methods

The selection of a sampling method depends on the requirements of the specimen. Considerations include the age of the patient, the need for repeated sampling, the site, depth, and thickness of the nasal mucosa, and the requirement for simultaneous biochemical studies.

Blown Secretions

In this method, secretions in the nasal airways are blown onto wax paper or a plastic wrap and then placed onto a glass slide (3,4). The cells originate from the secretions and may thus reflect a different population from that collected from the epithelium. A disadvantage is that many children and patients with some nasal disorders cannot produce an adequate secretion specimen. A microsuction technique to aspirate nasal secretions is more likely to provide adequate specimens for cytological analysis (5,6).

Smears Taken with Cotton Wool Swabs

This is a simple procedure for obtaining cells from the adherent secretions and epithelial layer. As with blown specimens, the cell count varies considerably. However, this method can be used to determine the presence or absence of a specific cell population in terms of a relative proportion (7).

Imprints

These involve the use of thin plastic strips painted with 1% albumin to produce a sticky surface. The strips are gently pressed onto the mucosal surface, usually the septum. A reasonably good cell yield is obtained and the number of specific cell types counted. Disadvantages of this method include the need to be manually dexterous and the presence of a considerable quantity of secretions on the strip (8).

Brush Method

This technique employs small plastic-coated, steel-wire brushes with nylon bristles. The brush is placed between the septum and inferior turbinate and rotated while being removed. The total number of cells can be estimated, as the volume in which the cells are suspended is known. The cells obtained include those from secretions and those from the epithelial surface layer (9). Local discomfort is a disadvantage.

Nasal Scraping

A nasal specimen of both the secretions and surface epithelium can, with minimal trauma, be easily obtained by scraping the surface in the middle third of the inferior turbinate. After excess secretions are cleared, the more patent side is sampled using a plastic curette (Rhino-Probe, ASI, Arlington, TX) under direct visual inspection (10,11). The cells harvested from the epithelial lining are well preserved and permit differential evaluation of specific cell elements. Advantages of this method include specificity of sampling site, minimal trauma with no need for anesthesia, ease of repetition, and adequacy of specimens at any age in all nasal conditions. Cell samples can also be used for rapid viral and bacterial diagnostic studies as well as biochemical analysis (12). The main disadvantage is that the superficial quality of the specimen does not permit evaluation of changes in the deeper mucosal layers.

The sampling methods of nose blowing and mucosal scraping have been compared in several studies in adults and children (13–15). In adults with allergic rhinitis, a specimen adequate for microscopic grading could be obtained 100% of the time by the scraped technique, but in only 60–66% of the patients by the blown method. In children and in patients with rhinopathies not characterized by an increase in anterior discharge, the yield of evaluable specimens is even lower with the nose-blowing technique. There was no difference between the two techniques as to the presence of neutrophils, and the concordance for the presence of eosinophils was fair (67%). However, eosinophils were found more often in the nasal-scraping sample when they were absent in the blown secretion than vice versa (28% vs. 5%). Basophils/mast cells were much more frequently noted in the scrapings than in the blown specimens (70% vs. 4%).

Nasal Lavage

This is performed by introducing saline solution in each nasal cavity with the patient's head bent backward during closure of the soft palate. The volume of the return lavage fluid is known and the total number of cells harvested can be calculated. The cells are counted in a hemocytometer and the cell differential determined on a cytospin slide (16).

The cytological findings from nasal mucosal scrapings and nasal lavages have been studied to examine their correlation (17). In patients with allergic rhinitis challenged with relevant allergens, scrapings and lavages correlated for increased eosinophil number and percentage and for increased neutrophil count and percentage. In nonallergic patients or allergic rhinitis patients provoked by an irrelevant allergen, the correlation was not good, although the neutrophils increased in response to the nonspecific stimulus. These data indicate that there tends to be a positive correlation between mucosal scrapings and lavages for cell number and percentage.

Biopsy

The most common site of biopsy is the lower edge of the inferior turbinate. It is important to know the site of the biopsy since the mucosal lining changes from the squamous type anteriorly to the ciliated, columnar epithelium in the middle and posterior parts of the nasal cavities. Anesthesia is necessary and a vasoconstrictor agent is often required. A disadvantage of the biopsy procedure is that it is too traumatic to repeat in a serial fashion. The major advantage is that it allows examination of not only the superficial epithelium, but also the basement membrane and the submucosal components.

The leukocytes found in nasal lavage fluid have been compared to those in biopsies following antigen challenge. In allergic patients after challenge, in both the lavage fluid and the biopsy tissue, eosinophils and mononuclear cells increased although the cell counts did not correlate. Neutrophils increased more in the lavage samples than in mucosal biopsies in both allergic and nonallergic subjects, possibly reflecting nonspecific irritation (18).

B. Processing Methods

The specimen is transferred to a slide. In the case of the Rhino-Probe specimen, the cupped tip is tilted onto the glass and the wet contents of the sample spread over a small area. The specimen should be visible to the naked eye on the microscope slide.

Fixatives for the specimen on the slide include: air drying—not recommended: acetone; unscented hair sprays; Mota's basic lead acetate; buffered formalin; methyl alcohol; ether–95% ethyl alcohol (1:1); and 95% ethyl alcohol. The latter preparation gives excellent results.

Histological stains have variable advantages: Hansel's—eosinophils; Wright's—basophils; Wright-Giemsa—eosinophils, neutrophils, and basophils/mast cells; Papanicolaou—epithelial cells, nuclear and cytoplasmic changes; toluidine blue—basophils/mast cells; Leishman's—eosinophils; alcian yellow—mast cells; Randolph's—eosinophils; alcian blue—basophils/mast cells; May-Grunwald—neutrophils.

Staining may be achieved with the Wright-Giemsa dip method as follows: (1) Remove the slide(s) from the jar containing 95% ethyl alcohol and drain the excess alcohol. Do not allow the cells to air dry; (2) dip the slide(s) in Wright-Giemsa (Volu-Sol) stain for 10–15 sec; (3) drain the excess stain, then dip the slide(s) in Volu-Sol buffer for 10–30 sec; (4) drain the excess buffer, then dip the slide(s) in Volu-Sol hematology rinse for 4–5 sec, using quick dips, or flood slides with rinse contained in a squeeze bottle; (5) drain the excess rinse and air-dry the specimens.

C. Modes of Evaluation

Light Microscopy

Add a drop of immersion oil to the specimen and scan at low power ($\times 100$) to determine whether the specimen has an adequate number of nonsquamous epithelial cells and a good-quality stain. The nasal cytogram should then be viewed at high power (oil immersion, $\times 1000$). The various cell types seen in the stained specimen are listed in Table 2.

Two evaluation methods of the cytogram can be used. One is a quantitative or semiquantitative assessment of the specimen, graded as a mean of cells per 10 high-power fields, or qualitatively on a scale of 0–4+ as suggested in Table 2. The other method involves making a percentage calculation of specific leukocytes, e.g., 10% eosinophils. The finding of 10% eosinophils in blown secretions

Table 2 A Guide for Grading Nasal Cytograms

Quantitative analysis	Semiquantitative analysis	Grade
Epithelial cells		
N/A	Normal morphology	N
N/A	Abnormal morphology	A
N/A	Ciliocytophthoria	CCP
Eosinophils, neutrophils		
0^a	None	0
$0.1–1.0^a$	Occasional cells	1/2+
$1.1–5.0^a$	Few scattered cells or small clumps	1+
$6.0–15.0^a$	Moderate number of cells and larger lumps	2+
$16.0–20.0^a$	Larger clumps of cells that do not cover the entire field	3+
$>20^a$	Larger clumps of cells covering the entire field	4+
Basophilic cells		
0^a	None	0
$0.1–0.3^a$	Occasional cells	1/2+
$0.4–1.0^a$	Few scattered cells	1+
$1.1–3.0^a$	Moderate number of cells	2+
$3.1–6.0^a$	Many cells easily seen	3+
$>6.0^a$	Large number of cells, as many as 25 per high-power field	4+
Bacteria[b]		
N/A	None seen	0
N/A	Occasional clumps	1+
N/A	Moderate number	2+
N/A	Many easily seen	3+
N/A	Large numbers covering the entire field	4+
Goblet cells[c]		
0	None	0
1–24%	Occasional to few cells	1+
25–49%	Moderate number	2+
50–74%	Many easily seen	3+
75–100%	Large number, may cover the entire field	4+

N = normal; A = abnormal; CCP = ciliocytophthoria.
[a]Mean of cells per 10 high-power fields ($\times 1000$).
[b]Note presence of intracellular bacteria.
[c]Ratio of goblet cells to epithelia cells, expressed as percentage.

Table 3 A Guide for Interpreting the Nasal Cytogram

Cellular type	Diagnostic classification
Increased eosinophils (1–4+)	Allergy
	Nonallergic rhinitis with eosinophilia
	Aspirin sensitivity
Increased basophilic cells (1–4+)	Allergy
	Nonallergic rhinitis with eosinophilia
	Aspirin sensitivity
	Nonallergic rhinitis with basophilia
Increased neutrophils (2–4+)	
With intracellular bacteria	Nasopharyngitis or sinusitis
With ciliocytophthoria	Viral upper respiratory infection
With fungi	Fungal upper respiratory infection
With no bacteria	Irritant reaction
Bacteria (2–4+)	
(diagnostic if intracellular)	Nasopharyngitis or sinusitis

generally corresponds to a 1+ grading seen in the nasal-scraping cytogram. However, as previously stated, inadequate specimens for microscopic evaluation are often obtained by the blown method. The quantitative or semiquantitative method is generally more informative.

A guide for interpreting the nasal cytogram is presented in Table 3 (11).

III. Cytology Findings in Clinical Conditions

A. Normal Subjects

The normal nasal mucosal cytology of infants, children, and adults consists of numerous epithelial cells including ciliated columnar, nonciliated columnar, goblet, and basal cells. An adequately sampled specimen will always contain some ciliated cells and goblet cells. There are usually no eosinophils or basophilic cells (<1+) within the superficial layer above the basement membrane. A moderate number of neutrophils (≤2+) and a few bacteria (≤1+) can be seen, especially if the specimen is taken from the anterior portion of the inferior turbinate (19–24).

B. Allergic Rhinitis

In allergic rhinitis, after allergen exposure, some of the antigen is bound by antigen-presenting cells. In the airways, these cells appear to be dendritic or Langerhans cells. They are increased in the nasal epithelium and lamina propria following allergen challenge and with natural allergen exposure (25).

Following antigen challenge and in seasonal and perennial allergic rhinitis there is a slight increase in the total number of T cells (CD3+), T-helper cells (CD4+), and activated T cells (CD25+) but there is a considerable overlap with normal controls (26,27).

The immunologically sensitized patient develops an immediate nasal response, and in over 50% of patients, a late-phase response with allergen provocation. Pelikan and Pelikan-Filipek (28) studied the cytology of these responses. The cells seen in the blown secretions of 102 patients were evaluated for their immediate nasal response as defined by a period of 0–120 min after allergen challenge. The positive symptom responses were accompanied by significant changes in the count of eosinophils (increase followed by decrease) in 67%, of basophilic cells (decrease) in 13%, and of neutrophils (decrease followed by increase) in 40%. No significant changes in the count of individual cell types in nasal secretions were found during most cases of 68 negative immediate nasal responses, or during any of the 102 saline control challenges. Increase in eosinophils immediately following allergen challenge has also been described by other investigators (29,30).

The cells of nasal secretion were also examined 4–12 hr following antigen challenges in 164 allergic rhinitis patients for their late nasal response. The 104 positive late nasal responses were accompanied by significant changes in the count of eosinophils in 58% of the cases (increase immediately before and decrease during appearance of the late response), in basophils in 8% (slight increase during appearance of the late response), and in neutrophils in 84% (increase immediately before and decrease during appearance of the late response and increase again during resolution of the late response). Most of the 60 cases of negative allergen response were not accompanied by significant changes in the count of individual cell types and no changes were recorded during saline-control challenges (31).

Nasal lavage studies have also confirmed the changes of inflammatory cells during the late-phase reaction. The pattern of influx varied among individuals, but in general eosinophils increased within 1–2 hr after challenge and peaked (in contrast to Pelikan's work) at 7–10 hr, neutrophils increased somewhat later than eosinophils and represented the greatest number of infiltrating cells in the late response, and basophilic cells also increased significantly but did not exceed 1% of the total cells (32).

Natural Allergen Exposure

The cellular response of the allergic mucosa to natural allergen exposure has also been studied. During a symptom-free period, patients with sensitization to mites and a detectable level of dust mite allergen present were evaluated and compared to healthy volunteers. All allergic patients showed a wide infiltration of inflammatory cells in the nasal mucosa, especially neutrophils, but also eosinophils and metachromatic cells. This suggests that with low-level allergen exposure, a subclinical minimal persistent inflammation is induced, even during clinical latency (33).

Pipkorn and co-workers (34) studied 10 patients with isolated birch-pollen allergy from a symptom-free state before, and then in the symptomatic state during, the birch-pollen season. As the birch pollen increased, and the symptoms increased, the percentage and total number of eosinophils from the nasal lavages increased. The number of eosinophils increased 20-fold. The total number of basophilic cells found imprinted on plastic strips also significantly increased during the pollen season, but did not start to appear after until 4–5 days of pollen exposure. A tendency toward an increase in the number of neutrophils was noted at the peak of the pollen season (Fig. 1).

In contrast to Pelikan's challenge data, Karlsson and Pipkorn (35) have noted no change following natural pollen allergen exposure in the number of goblet cells in the nasal mucosa.

Clinical Findings

Increased numbers of eosinophils are found in the nasal mucosa in active allergic disease (3,20,21). In university students, schoolchildren, and infants, a highly significant correlation has been shown with nasal secretion eosinophilia and evidence of allergy such as nose rubbing, sneezing, sniffing, runny nose, and wet and swollen turbinates (36,37). The degree of nasal eosinophilia appears to correlate with the extent of allergen exposure and with symptoms in allergic rhinitis (38). In particular, the increase in eosinophils generally correlates well with the symptom of nasal obstruction as measured by rhinomanometry (39). The presence of eosinophilia also correlates with the presence of positive allergy skin tests and, along with basophilic cells, with the serum IgE level (24,40,41).

Regional differences in the presence of eosinophils in the nose have been observed following antigen provocation of allergic rhinitis patients with significant increases occurring only at the site of challenge (42). Gristwood (43) noted eosinophils in 100% of adult patients with perennial allergic rhinitis in specimens from both the middle and inferior turbinates. However, more cells were found in the middle turbinate specimens. Adult allergic rhinitis patients in another study had eosinophils in 90% of the specimens obtained from the ethmoid region and maxillar sinus mucosa, 80% and 40% of specimens from the middle and inferior turbinates, respectively, and 50% of nasal secretions (44).

Surveying for possible variability of eosinophil detection from each nostril in clinically symptomatic patients, Kaufman et al. (45) found a concordance be-

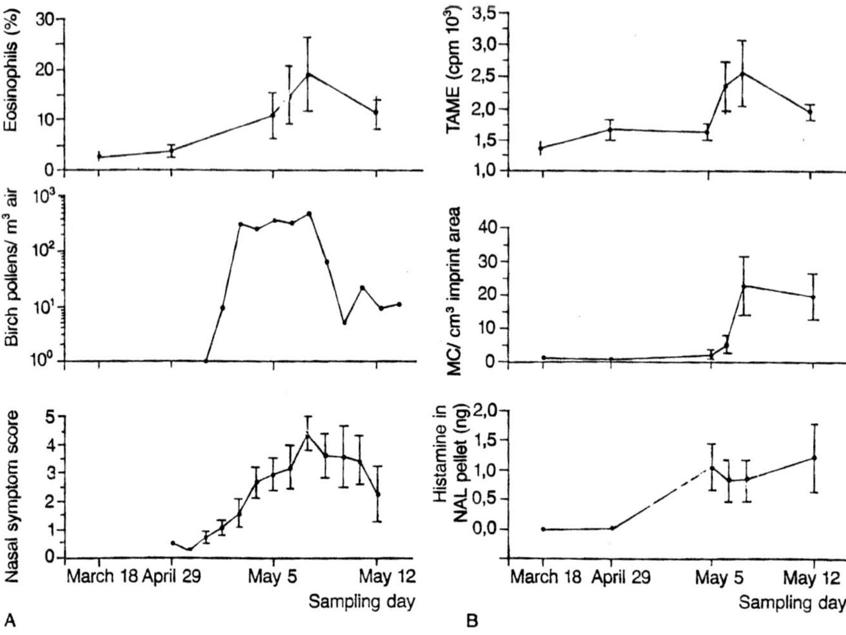

Figure 1 Natural allergen exposure. (A) Mean percentage of eosinophils found in the nasal lavages. Birch-pollen counts expressed as pollen grains per cubic meter of filtered air, and the nasal symptoms experienced by the patients. (B) TAME-esterase levels in the nasal lavages, the mean number of mast cells per square centimeter imprint area, and the histamine content of the lavage cell pellet. Mean values and standard errors are indicated by vertical bars. Significance levels denote changes in relation to preseasonal values. (From Ref. 34.)

tween nostrils for the absence or presence ($>8\%$) of nasal secretion eosinophils in 90% and 80%, respectively, but with an overall detection rate for eosinophils $>90\%$.

Eosinophils are found in allergic disease at all ages. In 186 children under 6 years of age referred to a group of pediatric allergists, 42% of blown secretions were positive ($>10\%$ of leukocytes). Ninety-five percent of the positive nasal smears were obtained in children determined to be atopic, 5% in an undecided group, and none in the nonatopic group (40).

In a prospective study of infants with a strong family history of allergic disease, it has been shown that both eosinophils and basophilic cells increase in number in nasal scrapings of allergic children between birth and 4 years of age but are uncommon in children with no allergic disease (46). Fifty children, aged

Table 4 Nasal Cytology[a]

	Seasonal allergic rhinitis ($n = 210$)	Perennial allergic rhinitis ($n = 88$)	Nonallergic rhinitis ($n = 78$)	Chronic sinusitis ($n = 51$)
Eosinophils	81%	89%	25%	78%
Basophilic cells	42%	31%	9%	41%
Neutrophils	64%	67%	47%	90%
Bacteria	28%	29%	10%	24%

[a]Percent of patients with specific cell type present in nasal scraping.

2–7 years, were categorized into five groups of 10 subjects as normal, allergic rhinitis, nonallergic rhinitis, allergic with otitis media, and nonallergic with otitis media by history, physical examination, allergy skin testing, and tympanometry. Adequate cytological samples were obtained from all subjects via the Rhino-Probe. Allergic groups had significantly more eosinophils than other groups. Basophilic cells were also increased in the allergic children compared to nonallergic children but the difference was significant only in those with allergic rhinitis (47).

Miller et al. (23) confirmed the diagnostic usefulness of the nasal smear for eosinophilia in 177 children aged 4–15 years. Significant nasal smear eosinophilia ($\geq 4\%$) was observed by either nose-blowing or scraping techniques in 69% of children with seasonal allergic rhinitis ($n = 65$) and 12% with nonallergic rhinitis ($n = 70$). In their study, although the nose-blowing and scraping techniques evidenced an equal sensitivity of 70% and specificity of 94%, almost 40% of children could not provide blown specimens.

In a study of adults, 19–72 years of age, Lans and co-workers (24) reported that with Rhino-Probe scrapings 43% of patients with allergic rhinitis had over 20% of sampled cells that were eosinophils. No nasal eosinophilia of this magnitude was seen in a control population or in patients with nonallergic rhinitis. Thus, in their study, the sensitivity of finding increased eosinophils in allergic rhinitis was 43%; the specificity was 100%. In another study of 210 adults with seasonal allergic rhinitis using the Rhino-Probe scraping technique, eosinophils were present in 81%, basophilic cells in 42%, neutrophils in 64%, and bacteria in 28% with at least 1+ grading (48) (Table 4). The frequency of neutrophil-positive and bacteria-positive specimens in patients with allergy is noteworthy, although this no doubt represents noninfectious inflammation; whether there is any presence of infectious inflammation requires further investigation.

Lim, Taylor, and Naclerio (42) performed nasal lavages to study the cytology in the secretions of normal subjects, perennially allergic subjects, and seasonally allergic subjects asymptomatic and out of season and after an allergen challenge. The predominant leukocyte in all subjects was the neutrophil ($73 \pm 10\%$). Perennially allergic subjects' specimens contained significantly more total cells, neutrophils, and eosinophils than specimens from the normal subjects. Seasonally allergic subjects at baseline had significantly more total cells and neutrophils than normal subjects and perennially allergic subjects. After an antigen challenge, the normal subjects did not have a significant change in their cell number or pattern. In contrast, the seasonally allergic subjects showed a significant increase in the number of lavage eosinophils. Although the total number of cells and number of neutrophils increased following challenge, the change did not reach statistical significance.

Biopsy specimens from these groups of subjects revealed that the predominant leukocyte in the tissue was not the neutrophil but the mononuclear cell (most likely lymphocytes). Following antigen provocation, seasonally allergic subjects showed significant changes in the tissue subepithelial inflammatory cells including increases in total cells, neutrophils, eosinophils, and mononuclear cells. Goblet cells did not differ among groups at baseline or after antigen challenge (42).

The normal basophilic cell content of the nose is about 200–400 cells/mm^3 of mucosa (49). The great majority of these cells are located in the lamina propria. Some patients with chronic rhinitis have more than 2000 basophilic cells/mm^3 as the only histological abnormality. They have been referred to as having ''nasal mastocytosis'' (50).

There are three populations of basophilic, metachromatic cells in the nose: basophil leukocytes and two histochemically distinct populations of mast cells. The basophils are recognized by their small size (5–6.5 µm), limited number of granules of different size, lobed nucleus that tends to be located at one edge of the cell, and peripherally condensed chromatin. Mast cells range from 5 to 12 µm in diameter. They have an abundance of small granules, which often obscure an oval nucleus that is generally centrally located within the cell.

Basophilic cells have been identified as being biologically active in allergic reactions. As the number of basophilic cells increases, the nasal symptoms become more severe and provocative challenge response usually becomes stronger (51). However, nasal reactivity to allergen challenge can also increase without a concomitant increase in the number of surface basophilic cells (52). The number of basophilic cells also correlates with nasal eosinophilia in allergic rhinitis (53). The finding of these cells and/or eosinophils increases the sensitivity of the test for confirming an allergic diagnosis to nearly 80% (54).

Some workers have found that, in allergic rhinitis, basophils are the predominant basophilic cell in nasal secretions and ''connective tissue mast cells'' (MC$_{CT}$) are the most abundant basophilic cell in the submucosa. They also have determined that ''mucosal mast cells'' (MC$_T$) are the major cell type in nasal scrapings in the epithelium and lamina propria of patients with allergic rhinitis (55).

In contrast, other researchers have asserted that basophil leukocytes, not "mucosal mast cells," constitute the majority of the basophilic cells in mucosal scrapings and nasal lavages. In studies using either a specific staining procedure (naphthol-ASD-chloroacetate esterase reaction) (56) or by direct morphological examination (57), it was found that only 6–8% of the metachromatic cells are mast cells.

In Bascom's study (57) of allergic rhinitis patients, allergen challenge produced a 12-fold increase in the number and a threefold increase in the percentage of basophilic cells in nasal lavage fluid during the late-phase response. At least two-thirds of these cells were observed to be basophils.

In biopsies of nasal mucous membranes from eight patients with allergic rhinitis both during and after a pollen season there was an eightfold increase in the number of basophilic cells seen in the superficial epithelium and deeper lamina propria during the pollen season. In the surface epithelial layer, counts increased from almost totally absent out of season to between 2000 and 28,000/mm^3 in season (58).

C. Nonallergic Rhinitis

In patients undergoing evaluation for chronic perennial rhinitis, approximately 50% have history and skin reactivity consistent with allergic rhinitis. In the remaining 50%, who are nonallergic, over two-thirds are characterized by the absence of eosinophils on nasal smear. They have been classified as having vasomotor rhinitis. This term is used to describe a nonimmunological, noninfectious, chronic rhinopathy. There is a history of nasal congestion and/or rhinorrhea with no history of allergen exacerbation and with negative skin tests. The majority of these patients identify physical irritants and climatic changes as precipitants (59). In addition to the scarcity of eosinophils in patients with vasomotor rhinitis, there is also no increase in basophilic cells or plasma cells (60).

About one-fourth of nonallergic patients with chronic rhinitis have eosinophilic nonallergic rhinitis or the nonallergic rhinitis with eosinophilia syndrome (NARES) (Table 4). Nonallergic rhinitis with eosinophilia can present at any age and symptoms are similar to those of patients with allergic rhinitis and vasomotor rhinitis. As with allergic rhinitis, nasal cytology during symptomatic periods shows marked eosinophilia. In Jacobs' study (61), eosinophil percentages varied from 19% to 66% in spontaneously collected nasal secretions and from 7% to 74% in nasal wash specimens. According to Mullarkey and co-workers (59), sinusitis and nasal polyps are more common in this rhinopathy than in allergic rhinitis or vasomotor rhinitis. This may be the result of damage to the mucosal epithelium induced by eosinophils and their products (62). A subset of patients with increased nasal eosinophils also have increased blood eosinophils (63).

Another form of nonallergic rhinitis is the rhinitis of pregnancy. Studies suggest that estrogen and progesterone cause both an increased activity of nasal mucosal glands and mucosal swelling. Increased circulating blood volume probably leads to increased airway resistance (64). Unless there is an associated allergic rhinitis or bacterial rhinosinusitis, nasal cytology is normal.

D. Irritant Rhinitis

Nasal cytology has been studied following exposure to various intranasal stimuli. Saline ($n = 7$) causes no change in number or types of cells in nasal lavage fluid; similarly distilled water ($n = 7$) causes no change in number or types of cells in nasal lavage fluid (65). Formaldehyde exposure occasionally causes epithelial metaplasia and dysplasia (66), while cigarette smoke causes metaplasia and frequent dysplasia (correlating with pack-years) (67). Cold-air exposure causes no change in number or types of cells in nasal lavage fluid (68). Excessive alpha-adrenergic agents result in rhinitis medicamentosa, but no change in number or types of cells in nasal lavage fluid. Nonatopic or atopic individuals receiving irrelevant allergen challenge had an increased number of neutrophils possibly induced by repeated scraped nasal infectious rhinitis sampling (17).

E. Infectious Rhinitis

Upper respiratory tract infections are frequently observed in children and less often in adults. With bacterial infections such as rhinosinusitis, especially if they have been recurrent, a number of histopathological abnormalities have been noted, including: (1) fewer and abnormal ciliated cells causing decreased mucus transport; (2) disruption of epithelial lining; (3) thickened basement membrane; (4) increased inflammatory cells such as lymphocytes and plasma cells; (5) increased microabscesses with bacteria and leukocytes; and (6) increased number of mast cells (69).

Nasal cytology is also useful in evaluating patients for bacterial infections. In a study of acute and chronic sinusitis, Wilson et al. (70) compared cytograms with radiological findings. A nasal scraping, obtained by the Rhino-Probe, was considered positive if there was greater than 1.1 neutrophils per high-power field (HPF) ($\geq 1+$) with bacteria present. An X-ray was positive if the radiologist reported asymmetry, mucoperiosteal thickening, opacification, or air-fluid levels.

Correlation between the nasal cytology and the sinus X-rays was 79%. Ninety percent of the sinus X-rays were positive in those patients with 2+ or greater neutrophils and bacteria present on nasal cytograms. Unfortunately, no asymptomatic control patients were included in this study.

In children with nonallergic rhinitis and nonallergic otitis, neutrophils increased in the cytogram in comparison with normal children. Bacteria are more commonly seen in these groups compared to normal and allergic children. These findings suggest the presence of infectious disease (47). Although small numbers of bacteria and of neutrophils may be normal, large numbers of bacteria, especially intracellular bacteria, support the diagnosis of infections.

Two other studies have shown nasal cytology to be informative in the diagnosis of sinusitis. Using a wax paper blow for specimen collection, Gill and Neiburger (71) found in their study of 300 children and adults that sinus radiographs were significantly more likely to be positive when there were >5 neutrophils/HPF ($\geq$2+). The presence of >5 neutrophils/HPF was 86% sensitive and 40% specific in predicting radiographic pathology. When the Rhino-Probe scraping technique was used, the results in 20 children showed that >5 neutrophils/HPF correlated with radiographic sinusitis to a greater degree. The sensitivity and specificity were 100% and 53%, respectively. Counts of other nasal cells, such as eosinophils, epithelial cells, and bacteria, did not yield significant correlations with radiographic sinusitis. The test's high sensitivity suggests that if no neutrophils are found in cytology, the chance of the patient having occult chronic sinusitis is low. Due to the low specificity of the Rhino-Probe in diagnosing chronic sinusitis, confirmation via radiographs is still necessary if neutrophils are present on the Rhino-Probe cytology (72).

The observations made in another study are not as conclusive as to the usefulness of nasal cytology as an aid in the diagnosis of bacterial infections. Nasal cytology was evaluated in 51 patients, 14 years of age and older, with sinusitis. The diagnosis was defined by symptoms and an X-ray demonstrating at least 6 mm of maxillary mucosal thickening, opacification, or an air-fluid level. In this population of patients, culled from an allergy medical practice, nasal-scraping specimens revealed eosinophils in 78%, basophilic cells in 41%, neutrophils in 90%, and bacteria in 24% of the patients. The eosinophil, basophilic cell, and bacteria percentages noted were similar to those observed in studies of patients with both seasonal and perennial allergic rhinitis (48) (Table 4). Only the frequency of neutrophils seen in these sinusitis patients (90%) was different from the percentages usually seen in allergic rhinitis (60–70%).

Although not all the study patients were allergic, many were, and this may account for the high incidence of eosinophils and basophils. Increased eosinophilia has also been seen in surgical sinus mucosal specimens from patients with nonallergic, chronic sinusitis. Certainly the high frequency of eosinophils in our sinusitis patients' nasal cytology is in contrast to previous observations that, in the presence of infection and increased numbers of neutrophils, eosinophils decreased (3,36). Basophilic cells have not been shown to increase in infectious rhinosinusitis (73). Neutrophils have been shown to be increased in the nasal cytology of patients with allergic rhinitis and from nonspecific stimulation (17). Because of these findings, the previously described relationship between increased neutrophils and sinusitis may be clouded in the individual patient who has allergic rhinitis and/or irritant-exposure rhinitis. It is also clear that many patients with clinical and radiologically confirmed sinusitis do not have bacteria in their nasal mucosal specimen (74).

In viral nasal infections, ciliated epithelial cells undergo destructive changes termed ''ciliocytophthoria.'' The features of the cytopathic effects of the viruses include clumping of the nuclear chromatin material, margination of the pyknotic chromatin mass attached to inclusion material within the nucleus, halo formation around the nucleus, increased granulation of the cytoplasm, constriction of the ciliated cell, and finally separation of the nucleus-containing basal portion from the ciliated apical portion (75). After the considerable fall in the number of ciliated cells due to the viral infection, regeneration is usually slow (76). This may produce long-lasting impairment of nasal mucociliary clearance function.

F. Nasal Polyps

In comparison to healthy nasal and sinus mucosa and mucosa of patients with chronic sinusitis, polyps show a statistically significant increase in the number of eosinophils. Patients with nasal polyps had up to 10 times more eosinophils per surface unit than patients with sinusitis or healthy mucosa (77). In patients with nasal polyps, basophilic cells were also more numerous. They were found in 65% of these patients as compared with 5% of normal controls, 14% of patients with chronic sinusitis, and 91% of patients with nasal allergy (78).

G. Atrophic Rhinitis

Atrophic rhinitis on cytological examination shows epithelial squamous metaplasia and a chronic inflammatory cell infiltrate (79).

Table 5 summarizes the current data on nasal cytology findings in various clinical conditions.

IV. Cytology Findings Consequent to Therapeutic Agents

A. Saline and Distilled Water

Exposure causes no change in the number or types of cells in nasal lavage fluid (65).

B. Propylene and Polyethylene-Glycyl

These agents tend to cause a decrease in eosinophils seen on nasal smear (80).

C. Antihistamines

Oral antihistamines, such as terfenadine and cetirizine given prior to an allergen challenge, have no significant effect on the increase in the number of percentage

Table 5 Nasal Cytology in Various Clinical Conditions

	Eosinophils	Basophilic cells	Neutrophils	Bacteria	Ciliated cells
Normal	0	0	0–1+	0	N
Allergic rhinitis	1–4+	1–4+	1–4+	0	N
Vasomotor rhinitis	0	0	0–1+	0	N
NARES	1–4+	1–4+	?	0	N
Pregnancy	0	0	0–1+	0	N
Rhinitis medicamentosa	0	0	0–1+	0	N
Irritants	0	0	1–4+	0	N
Bacterial rhinosinusitis	0	0	1–4+	1–4+[a]	N
Viral rhinitis	0	0	1–4+	0	Decreased[b]
Polyps	1–4+	0–4+	?	?	Decreased
Atrophic rhinitis	0	0	1–4+	0	Decreased[c]

N = normal.
[a] Bacteria may be intracellular.
[b] Ciliacytophthoria.
[c] Squamous metaplasia.

of eosinophils after allergen challenge (81). In one clinical trial, cetirizine showed no effect in preventing an increased percentage (10%) and number (67 cells/mm^2) of eosinophils in smears and biopsies of patients with seasonal allergic rhinitis compared with placebo (8%, 12 cells/mm^2) (82). In another clinical trial, following terfenadine 60 mg BID for 4 weeks, there was no significant change in the presence of eosinophils, basophilic cells, or neutrophils (83).

Topical application of an antihistamine, e.g., azelastine, also does not reduce the percentage of eosinophils or neutrophils in patients with allergic rhinitis (84).

D. Decongestants

Data are available on oral and intermittent topical use. Rhinitis medicamentosa due to intranasal alpha-adrenergic agents appears to cause no significant change in nasal cytology.

E. Anticholinergic Agents

Ipratropium bromide has been studied extensively as treatment for both allergic rhinitis and perennial nonallergic rhinitis (9). No significant change in the percentage of eosinophils, basophilic cells, neutrophils, or bacteria found in nasal scrapings has been noted following ipratropium therapy for either of these rhinopathies (85,86).

F. Cromolyn Sodium

Patients with allergic rhinitis have increased inflammatory cells in blown secretions. In preliminary reports by Pelikan-Filipek and Pelikan (87,88), the response to allergen challenge was examined in 12 patients with and without pretreatment with intranasal cromolyn sodium (sodium cromoglycate). They found that the immediate nasal response without pretreatment was accompanied by changes in the count of eosinophils in 66%, basophilic cells in 8%, and neutrophils in 42% of challenges. No significant changes in the counts of these cells were recorded during the immediate nasal response after pretreatment with cromolyn sodium. In the late nasal response, the nonpretreated patients developed changes of eosinophils in 58%, basophilic cells in 8%, and neutrophils in 75% of challenges. The changes in those pretreated with cromolyn sodium were less pronounced for the eosinophils and neutrophils.

In a clinical study by Orgel et al. (83) there was a statistically significant decrease in eosinophils, but not basophilic cells or neutrophils, in patients treated with intranasal cromolyn 4%, 4 times a day for 4 weeks. In Okuda's study (89), nasal basophilic cells did not decrease after 2 weeks of intranasal cromolyn.

G. Topical Corticosteroids

Intranasal corticosteroids are highly effective in reducing allergic symptomatology. Their effect on nasal cytology has been evaluated in a number of studies. Treatment with topical corticosteroids markedly reduces the number of Langerhans cells in biopsies of the nasal mucosa in both the epithelium and the lamina propria in perennial allergic rhinitis (90). This, no doubt, reduces antigen presentation and partly explains the anti-inflammatory effect of this therapy. Treatment with topical glucocorticoids prior to allergen challenge significantly decreases the total number of T cells (CD3+), and subsets of CD4+, CD8+, and activated T cells (CD25+). These reductions are more pronounced in the nasal surface epithelium than in the lamina propia (91). Holm and co-workers found no such effect in the biopsies after 3 months of glucocorticoid (fluticasone propionate) treatment of patients with perennial allergic rhinitis (90).

With allergen challenges, the immediate nasal response in the number of eosinophils and neutrophils in nasal secretions was not affected by pretreatment with the topical glucocorticoid budesonide (87). In the late nasal response to allergen challenge (88), however, budesonide lowered the number of eosinophils and neutrophils in secretions. Topical steroid pretreatment with flunisolide for 1 week before allergen challenge blocked the influx of eosinophils, neutrophils, and basophilic cells (68% identified as basophils) in the late-phase response examined in nasal washings (57).

In clinical studies, nasal secretion eosinophilia has been decreased after beclomethasone dipropionate in both seasonal and perennial rhinitis patients as compared to placebo (92). A decrease in eosinophils after treatment by beclomethasone dipropionate has also been observed in nasal scrapings. This occurred with both the aerosol and the aqueous formulations in patients with allergic rhinitis in doses as low as 42 µg per nostril twice a day (93). Another topical corticosteroid, flunisolide, has been shown after 4 weeks of twice-a-day treatment to decrease the number of allergic rhinitis patients with nasal eosinophilia (94).

Beclomethasone has been shown to inhibit the increase in density of basophilic cells that occurs in the nasal mucosa during the pollen season. Gomez et al. (95) studied allergic rhinitis patients by biopsy at the start and after 3 months of a pollen season. Significantly fewer basophilic cells were seen in the corticosteroid-treated group than in those receiving placebo. Okuda and co-workers (89) studied nasal surface basophilic metachromatic cells in epithelia scrapings from symptomatic allergic rhinitis patients before and after 2 weeks of treatment with beclomethasone. The number of basophilic cells was significantly reduced in the beclomethasone group (64%) as compared with the controls (20%). The mean number was 647 cells/mm^2 before and 205 cells/mm^2 after beclomethasone; it was 708 cells/mm^2 before treatment with placebo. Otsuka et al. (96) reported formalin-sensitive mast cells found in the layers were more susceptible to the effects of corticosteroids than formalin-resistant mast cells. Pipkorn (97,98) also saw no quantitative effect of budesonide on subepithelial mast cells in biopsy specimens taken either out of season or in season from patients with allergic rhinitis.

Examination of nasal-scraping specimens of allergic rhinitis patients treated with fluticasone propionate has revealed a significant decrease on the scores for eosinophils and basophilic cells in multiple reports. In one study in which symptomatic patients received one of three doses of fluticasone propionate (25, 200, or 400 µg twice daily) or placebo, over 80% had nasal eosinophilia before treatment. The graded eosinophil score decreased in 50–70% of patients treated with fluticasone propionate for 2 weeks and in only 20% of placebo-treated patients. Forty-two percent of the patients had basophilia before treatment. After treatment with fluticasone propionate, basophil numbers decreased in a significantly greater number of patients (35–45%) compared to after placebo (15%) (48) (Fig. 2).

Fewer patients had neutrophils after treatment with fluticasone, but in most studies, the difference from placebo was not statistically significant. Approximately 30% of the studied patients had bacteria noted in their nasal mucosal specimens at baseline. There was no significant change in the percentage after any treatment regimen. All patients had similar numbers of goblet cells before and after treatment (99).

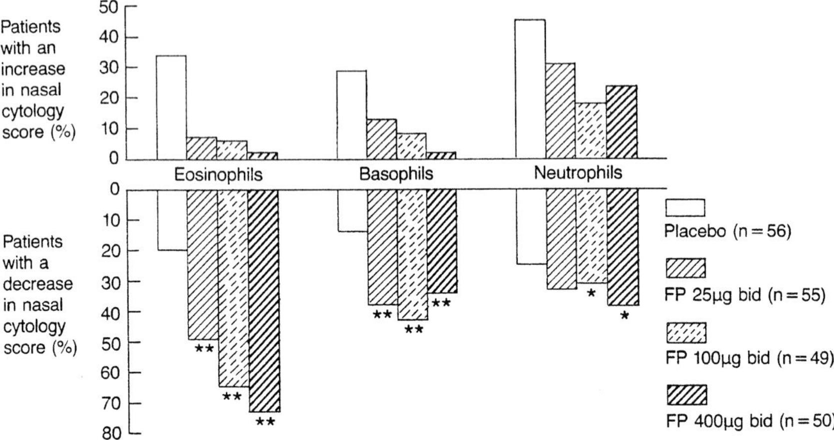

Figure 2   Percent of patients demonstrating increases or decreases in eosinophils, basophils, and neutrophils among patients with evaluable nasal mucosal specimens on both days 1 and 15. $*p < 0.05$; $**p < 0.003$: fluticasone propionate aqueous nasal spray-treated patients by comparison with placebo. (From Ref. 48.)

The response to topical steroids of nasal mucosal cells obtained by biopsy has confirmed the absence of atrophy or other steroid damage (100,101).

In a study in which biopsy specimens were examined by light microscopy after 1 year of intranasal treatment with fluocortin butyl, special attention was paid to the surface epithelium. The results showed that long-term topical therapy with this glucocorticoid led to a change from squamous metaplasia to normal columnar epithelium in some patients. Nasal biopsies also showed decreases in mucosal eosinophils, basophilic cells, and neutrophils as has been shown to occur in nasal secretions and mucosal scrapings after treatment with topical corticosteroids. A number of patients had an increase in intact mast cells, suggesting that long-term therapy may inhibit degranulation (102).

In summary, the effects of corticosteroids in allergic rhinitis include: (1) improvement of the epithelial barrier, (2) inhibition of eosinophil influx and reduction of numbers present, (3) inhibition of basophilic cell influx and reduction of numbers present, (4) inhibition of neutrophil influx and modest reduction of numbers present, (5) no change in numbers of submucosal masts and reduction in secondary monocyte influx.

H.   Oral Corticosteroids

Oral prednisone effect on the late nasal response to allergen challenge was studied by Bascom and colleagues (103,104). They demonstrated that pretreatment for

2 days with prednisone blocked the influx of eosinophils but not of neutrophils or mononuclear cells.

I. Immunotherapy

Nasal allergen challenges induces an influx of eosinophils, basophilic cells, and neutrophils in sensitive subjects. The effects of immunotherapy on this influx have been evaluated. In a study by Iliopoulos and colleagues (105) there was no significant difference in the number of eosinophils, basophilic cells, neutrophils, and mononuclear cells prior to a ragweed allergen challenge in two groups of ragweed-sensitive hay fever patients. One of the groups ($n = 20$) was treated for 8 months with placebo and the other ($n = 21$) with a low dose of ragweed antigen extract. Following challenge, the increase in eosinophils, basophilic cells, and neutrophils was not significantly different between the groups. Further work from this group showed that higher immunotherapy doses can decrease the eosinophil influx (106).

In Otsuka's clinical study (107) evaluating the nasal cytological changes due to immunotherapy, 25 patients with perennial allergic rhinitis were divided into two groups. Eleven served as controls and 14 underwent allergen injection treatments. At the initiation of the study, the number of basophilic cells in nasal mucosal scrapings was not significantly different between groups. Following 3 and 6 months of immunotherapy, nasal symptom scores, nasal provocation sensitivity, and the number of basophilic cells were significantly reduced ($p < 0.05$) in the antigen immunotherapy group, but unchanged in the control group compared to pretreatment values.

J. Antibiotics

In a study of 51 patients with documented sinusitis, 46 (90%) had neutrophils noted on the initial scraped nasal mucosal specimen. Forty-four had adequate specimens for evaluation both prior to and following a course of amoxicillin/clavulanate potassium (Augmentin) 500 mg, given 3 times a day for 3 weeks. Of these 44 patients, 39 (89%) had neutrophils present at the first visit and 37 (84%) had neutrophils noted after the Augmentin. Following the antibiotic treatment, 11 of 44 (25%) had an increase in the neutrophil grade, 18 of 44 (41%) had a decrease in the neutrophil grade, and 15 of 44 (34%) showed no change. Thus antibiotic intervention in documented sinusitis did not have a predictable effect on the numbers of neutrophils in the nasal cytogram.

Twelve of the 51 sinusitis patients (24%) had bacteria observed in the initial nasal scrapings. Of the 11 patients with evaluable samples both before and after antibiotic therapy, four had bacteria still present (36%), and seven of 11 had no bacteria observed (64%). Thus the trend with antibiotic treatment was to reduce the bacteria seen in the nasal cytograms (74).

V. Conclusions

Interest in nasal cytology as a method for evaluating disease and treatment has progressed. Several factors have, in the past, diminished its usefulness: (1) the inability to procure adequate samples consistently and with minimal discomfort, (2) the limited use of Hansel's stain, (3) the variety of methods for grading results, (4) the fact that eosinophils are not pathognomonic for allergy, (5) the lack of available data on how to interpret findings, and (6) the assumption that the procedure was not cost-effective. This review has demonstrated that techniques for obtaining, staining, and interpreting nasal cytology specimens are improving. These have contributed to the ability to differentiate the chronic rhinopathies, monitor their course, and develop meaningful therapies. The prospect of greater satisfaction for both clinicians and the patients they serve is advanced by this scientific understanding (33).

References

1. Meltzer EO. Evaluating rhinitis: clinical rhinomanometric and cytologic assessments. J Allergy Clin Immunol 1988; 82:900–908.
2. Meltzer EO, Schatz M, Zeiger RS. Allergic and non-allergic rhinitis. In: Middleton E Jr, Reed CE, Ellis EF, eds. Allergy: Principles and Practice, 3rd ed. St Louis: CV Mosby, 1988: 1253–1289.
3. Hansel FK. Observation on the cytology of the secretions in allergy of the nose and paranasal sinuses. J Allergy 1934; 5:357–366.
4. Hastie R, Heroy JH, Levy DA. Basophil leukocytes and mast cells in human nasal secretions and scrapings studied by light microscopy. Lab Invest 1979; 49:541–554.
5. Biewenga J, Stoop AE, Baker HE, et al. Nasal secretions from patients with polyps and healthy individuals, collected with a new aspiration system: evaluation of total protein and immunoglobulin concentrations. Ann Clin Biochem 1991; 28: 260–266.
6. Wang D, Clement P, Smitz J, et al. Monitoring nasal allergic inflammation by measuring the concentration of eosinophil cationic protein and eosinophils in nasal secretions. Allergy 1995; 50:147–151.
7. Bryan WTK, Bryan MT. Cytologic diagnosis in otolaryngology. Trans Am Acad Ophthalmol Otolaryngol 1959; 63:597–611.
8. Pipkorn U, Karlsson C. Methods for obtaining specimens from the nasal mucosa for morphological and biochemical analysis. Eur Respir J 1988; 1:856–862.
9. Pipkorn U, Karlsson G, Enerback L. A brush method to harvest cells from the nasal mucosa for microscopic and biochemical analysis. J Immunol Meth 1988; 112:37–42.
10. Jalowayski AA, Zeiger RS. Examination of nasal or conjunctival epithelial speci-

mens. In: Lawlor GJ Jr, Fischer TJ, eds. Manual of Allergy and Immunology, 2nd ed. Boston: Little, Brown, 1988; 432–434.

11. Meltzer EO, Jalowayski AA. Nasal cytology in clinical practice. Am J Rhinol 1988; 2:47–54.

12. Jalowayski AA, Meltzer EO, Orgel HA, et al. Nasal histamine levels in young children with allergic and non-allergic rhinitis and chronic otitis. J Allergy Clin Immunol 1991; 87:146.

13. Welch MJ, Meltzer EO, Kemp JP, et al. Comparison of two different techniques for obtaining specimens for nasal cytology. Nose-blowing vs. nasal mucosal scraping. J Allergy Clin Immunol 1991; 87:144.

14. Galindo C, Jalowayski A, Meltzer E. Correlation between nasal cytogram and blown technique for the diagnosis of allergic rhinitis. Ann Allergy 1991; 66:86.

15. Angel-Solano G, Shturman R. Comparative cytology of nasal secretions and nasal mucosa in allergic rhinitis. Ann Allergy 1986; 56:521.

16. Naclerio RM, Meier HL, Kagey-Sobotka A, et al. Mediator release after nasal airway challenge with allergen. Am Rev Respir Dis 1983; 128:597–602.

17. Piancentini GL, Kaulbach HC, Scott T, et al. Correlation between inflammatory cell responses in nasal mucosal scrapings and lavages after allergen challenge. J Allergy Clin Immunol 1991; 87:145.

18. Brown M, Lim M, Furin M, et al. A comparison between antigen-induced leukocyte populations in the nasal mucosa and nasal secretions. J Allergy Clin Immunol 1991; 87:145.

19. Cohen GA, MacPherson GA, Golembesky HE, et al. Normal nasal cytology in infancy. Ann Allergy 1985; 54:112–24.

20. Bryan MP, Bryan WTK. Cytologic diagnosis in allergic disorders. Otolaryngol Clin North Am 1974; 7:637–666.

21. Bickmore JT. Nasal cytology in allergy and infection. Otorhinolaryngology Allergy 1978; 40:39–46.

22. Ohtsuka H, Okuda M. Important factors in the nasal manifestations of allergy. Arch Otorhinolaryngol 1981; 233:227–235.

23. Miller RE, Paradise JL, Friday GA, et al. The nasal smear for eosinophils. Am J Dis Child 1982; 136:1009–1011.

24. Lans DM, Alfano N, Rocklin R. Nasal eosinophilia in allergic and non-allergic rhinitis: Usefulness of the nasal smear in the diagnosis of allergic rhinitis. Allergy Proc 1989; 10:275–280.

25. Fokkens WJ, Rijntjes E, Vroom TM, Mulder PGH. Fluctuation of the number of the CD-1 positive dendritic cells, presumably Langerhans cells, in the nasal mucosal of patients with an isolated grass-pollen allergy before, during and after the grass pollen season. J Allergy Clin Immunol 1989; 84:39–43.

26. Varney VA, Jacobson MR, Sudderick RM, et al. Immunohistology of the nasal mucosa following allergen-induced rhinitis. Am Rev Respir Dis 1992; 146:170–176.

27. Calderon MA, Lozewicz S, Prior A, et al. Lymphocyte infiltration and thickness of the nasal mucous membrane in perennial and seasonal allergic rhinitis. Immunology 1994; 93:635–643.

28. Pelikan Z, Pelikan-Filipek M. Cytologic changes in the nasal secretions during the immediate nasal response. J Allergy Clin Immunol 1988; 82:1103–1112.

29. Klementsson H, Andersson M, Baumgarten CR, et al. Changes in non-specific nasal reactivity and eosinophil influx and activation after allergen challenge. Clin Exp Allergy 1990; 20:539–547.

30. Pipkorn U, Karlsson G, Enerback L. Nasal mucosal response to repeated challenges with pollen allergen. Am Rev Respir Dis 1989; 140:729–736.

31. Pelikan Z, Pelikan-Filipek M. Cytologic changes in the nasal secretions during the late nasal response. J Allergy Clin Immunol 1989; 83:1068–1079.

32. Togias A, Naclerio RM, Proud D, et al. Studies on the allergic and non-allergic inflammation. J Allergy Clin Immunol 1988; 81:782–790.

33. Ciprandi G, Buscaglia S, Pesce G, et al. Minimal persistent inflammation is present at mucosal level in patients with asymptomatic rhinitis and mite allergy. J Allergy Clin Immunol 1995; 96:971–979.

34. Pipkorn U, Karlsson G, Enerback L. The cellular response of the human allergic mucosa to natural allergen exposure. J Allergy Clin Immunol 1988; 82:1046–1054.

35. Karlsson G, Pipkorn U. Natural allergen exposure does not influence the density of goblet cells in the nasal mucosa of patients with seasonal allergic rhinitis. J Otorhinolaryngol 1989; 51:171–174.

36. Malmberg H. Symptoms of chronic and allergic rhinitis and occurrence of nasal secretion granulocytes in university students, school children and infants. Allergy 1979; 34:389–394.

37. Murray AB, Anderson DO. The epidemiologic relationship of clinical nasal allergy to eosinophils and to goblet cells in nasal smear. J Allergy 1969; 43:1.

38. Hansel FK. Cytologic diagnosis in respiratory allergy and infection. Ann Allergy 1966; 24:564–569.

39. Wang D, Clement P, DeWaele M, Derde M-P. Study of nasal cytology in atopic patients after nasal allergen challenge. Rhinology 1995; 33:78–81.

40. Orgel HA, Kemp JP, Meltzer EO, et al. Atopy and IgE in a pediatric allergy practice. Ann Allergy 1977; 39:161–168.

41. Salas A, Wilson N, Hamburger RN. Relation of serum IgE level to the cells observed in the nasal cytograms. Ann Allergy 1988; 60:175.

42. Lim MC, Taylor RM, Naclerio RM. The histology of allergic rhinitis and its comparison to cellular changes in nasal lavage. Am J Respir Crit Care Med 1995; 151:136–144.

43. Gristwood RE. Observations on the histopathology of allergic rhinitis: regional differences in mucosal cosinophilia. J Laryngol Otol 1982; 49:270.

44. Vaheri E. Nasal allergy with special reference to eosinophilia and histopathology. Acta Allergol 1956; 10:203–211.

45. Kaufman HS, Rosen I, Shaposhnikov N, et al. Nasal eosinophilia. Ann Allergy 1982; 49:270–271.

46. Zeiger S, Heller S. Development of nasal basophilic cells and nasal eosinophils from ages 4 months through 4 years in children of atopic parents. J Allergy Clin Immunol 1993; 91:723–734.

47. Meltzer EO, Orgel HA, Jalowayski AA. Histamine levels and nasal cytology in

children with chronic otitis media and rhinitis. Ann Allergy Asthma Immunol 1995; 74:406–410.

48. Meltzer EO, Orgel HA, Bronsky EA, et al. A dose-ranging study of fluticasone propionate aqueous nasal spray for seasonal allergic rhinitis assessed by symptoms, rhinomanometry and nasal cytology. J Allergy Clin Immunol 1990; 86:221–230.

49. Connell JT. Nasal disease: mechanisms and classification. Ann Allergy 1983; 50: 227–235.

50. Connell JT. Nasal mastocytosis. J Allergy 1969; 43:182.

51. Borres MP, Irander K, Bjorksten B. Metachromatic cells in nasal mucosa after allergen challenge. Allergy 1990; 45:98–103.

52. Wihl J-Å, Brofeldt S, Gronborg H, Mygind N. Blind study of basophilic cells in nasal smears from patients with grass pollen hayfever. Eur J Respir Dis 1983; 64 (Suppl 128):383–386.

53. Okuda M, Otsuka H. Basophilic cells in allergic nasal secretions. Arch Otorhino-laryngol 1977; 214:283–289.

54. Lang DM, Howland WC, Stevenson DD. Sensitivity and features of nasal cytology in diagnosis of allergic (IgE mediated) rhinitis. Ann Allergy 1988; 60:176.

55. Otsuka H, Denburg J, Dolovich J, et al. Heterogeneity of metachromatic cells in human nose: significance of mucosal mast cells. J Allergy Clin Immunol 1985; 76: 695–702.

56. Jalowayski AA, Maes TW, Wasserman SI, et al. Histochemical differentiation of the human nasal mucosa mast cells from basophil leukocytes. J Allergy Clin Immunol 1983; 71:89.

57. Bascom R, Waschs M, Naclerio RM, et al. Basophil influx occurs after nasal antigen challenge: effects of topical corticosteroid pretreatment. J Allergy Clin Immunol 1988; 81:580–589.

58. Viegas M, Gomez E, Brooks J, et al. Changes in nasal mast cell numbers in and out of pollen season. Int Arch Allergy Appl Immunol 1987; 82:275–276.

59. Mullarkey MF, Hill JS, Webb DR. Allergic and non-allergic rhinitis: their characterization with attention to the meaning of nasal eosinophilia. J Allergy Clin Immunol 1980; 65:122–126.

60. Elwany S, Bumsted R. Ultrastructural observations on vasomotor rhinitis. J Oto-Rhino-Laryngol 1987; 49:199–205.

61. Jacobs RL, Freedman PM, Boswell RN. Nonallergic rhinitis with eosinophils (NARES syndrome). J Allergy Clin Immunol 1981; 67:253–262.

62. Davidson AE, Miller SD, Settipane RJ, et al. Delayed nasal mucociliary clearance in patients with nonallergic rhinitis and nasal eosinophilia. Allergy Proc 1992; 13: 81–84.

63. Settipane GA, Klein DE. Non-allergic rhinitis: demography of eosinophils in nasal smear, blood total eosinophil counts and IgE levels. Allergy Proc 1985; 6:363–366.

64. Schatz M, Zeiger RS. Diagnosis and management of rhinitis during pregnancy. Allergy Proc 1988; 9:545–554.

65. Meslier N, Braunstein G, Lacronique J, et al. Local cellular and humoral responses to antigenic and distilled water challenge in subjects with allergic rhinitis. Am Rev Respir Dis 1988; 137:617–624.

66. Boysen M, Zadig E, Digernes V, et al. Nasal mucosa in workers exposed to formaldehyde: a pilot study. Br J Indust Med 1990; 47:116–121.

67. Gluck U, Gebbers JO. Cytopathology of the nasal mucosa in smokers: a possible biomarker of air pollution? Am J Rhinol 1996; 10:55–57.

68. Togias A. Unpublished data.

69. Petruson B, Hansson HA. Nasal mucosal changes in children with frequent infections. Arch Otolaryngol Head Neck Surg 1987; 113:1294–1300.

70. Wilson NW, Jalowayski AA, Hamburger RN. A comparison of nasal cytology with sinus X-rays for the diagnosis of sinusitis. Am J Rhinol 1988; 2:55–59.

71. Gill FF, Neiburger JB. The role of nasal cytology in the diagnosis of chronic sinusitis. Am J Rhinol 1989; 3:13–15.

72. Jong CN, Olson NY, Nadel GL, et al. Use of nasal cytology in the diagnosis of occult chronic sinusitis in asthmatic children. Ann Allergy 1994; 73:509–514.

73. Melen I, Pipkorn S, Pipkorn U. Mast cells on the surface of the mucous membrane—a general feature of inflammatory reactions in the nose? Rhinology 1985; 23:187–190.

74. Meltzer EO, Orgel HA, Backhaus JW, et al. Intranasal flunisolide spray as an adjunct to oral antibiotic therapy for sinusitis. J Allergy Clin Immunol 1993; 92:812–823.

75. Bryan WTK, Bryan MP, Smith CA. Human ciliated epithelial cells in nasal secretions. Morphologic and histochemical aspects. Ann Otol Rhinol Laryngol 1964; 73:474.

76. Pedersen M, Sakakura Y, Winther B, Mygind N, et al. Nasal mucociliary transport, number of ciliated cells, and beating pattern in naturally acquired common colds. Eur J Respir Dis 1983; 64 (Suppl 128):355–365.

77. Jankowski R, Bene MC, Moneret-Vautrin AD, et al. Immunohistological characteristics of nasal polyps. A comparison with healthy mucosa and chronic sinusitis. Rhinology 1989; 8:51–58.

78. Sakaguchi K, Okuda M, Ushijima K, et al. Study of nasal surface basophilic cells in patients with nasal polyps. Acta Oto-Laryngol (Stockh) 1986; 430:28–33.

79. Abdel-Latif SM, Baheeg SS, Aglan YI, et al. Chronic atrophic rhinitis with fetor (ozena): a histopathologic treatise. Rhinology 1987; 25:117–120.

80. Spector SL, Toshener D, Gay I, et al. Beneficial effects of propylene and polyethylene glycol and saline in the treatment of perennial rhinitis. Clin Allergy 1982; 12:187–196.

81. Klementsson H, Andersson M, Pipkorn U. Allergen-induced increase in nonspecific nasal reactivity is blocked by antihistamines without a clear-cut relationship to eosinophil influx. J Allergy Clin Immunol 1990; 86:466–472.

82. Howarth PH, Wilson SJ, Brewster H. The influence of cetirizine on symptom generation and nasal eosinophilia in seasonal allergic rhinitis. J Allergy Clin Immunol 1991; 87:151.

83. Orgel HA, Meltzer EO, Kemp JP, et al. Comparison of intranasal cromolyn sodium, 4%, and oral terfenadine for allergic rhinitis: Symptoms, nasal cytology, nasal clearance, and rhinomanometry. Ann Allergy 1991; 66:237–244.

84. Pelucchi A, Chiapparino A, Mastropasque B, et al. Effect of intranasal azelastine and beclomethasone dipropionate on nasal symptoms, nasal cytology and bronchial

responsiveness to methacholine in allergic rhinitis in response to grass pollens. J Allergy Clin Immunol 1995; 95:515–523.

85. Meltzer EO, Orgel HA, Bronsky EA, et al. Ipratropium bromide aqueous nasal spray for patients with perennial allergic rhinitis: a study of its effect on their symptoms, quality of life and nasal cytology. J Allergy Clin Immunol 1992; 90:242–249.

86. Bronsky EA, Druce H, Findlay SR, et al. A clinical trial of ipratropium bromide nasal spray in patients with perennial nonallergic rhinitis. J Allergy Clin Immunol 1995; 95:1117–1122.

87. Pelikan-Filipek M, Pelikan Z. Nasal secretions cytology during the immediate nasal response pretreated with disodium cromoglycate and budesonide. J Allergy Clin Immunol 1991; 87:144.

88. Pelikan Z, Pelikan-Filipek M. Cytologic changes in nasal secretions during the late nasal response pretreated with disodium cromoglycate and beclomethasone dipropionate or budesonide. J Allergy Clin Immunol 1991; 87:281.

89. Okuda M, Otsuka H, Sakaguchi K, et al. Effect of antiallergic treatment on nasal surface basophilic metachromatic cells in allergic rhinitis. Allergy Proc 1989; 10:23–26.

90. Holm AF, Fokkens WJ, Godthelp T, et al. Effect of 3 months' nasal steroid therapy on nasal T cells and Langerhans cells in patients suffering from allergic rhinitis. Allergy 1995; 50:204–209.

91. Rak S, Jacobson MR, Sudderick RM, et al. Influence of prolonged treatment with topical corticosteroid (fluticasone propionate) on early and late phase responses and cellular infiltration in the nasal mucosa after allergen challenge. Clin Exp Allergy 1994; 24:930–939.

92. Holopainen E, Malmberg H, Tarkiainen E. Experiences of treating allergic rhinitis with intra-nasal beclomethasone dipropionate. Acta Allergol 1977; 32:263–277.

93. Orgel HA, Meltzer EO, Kemp JP, et al. Clinical, rhinomanometric, and cytologic evaluation of seasonal allergic rhinitis treated with beclomethasone dipropionate as aqueous nasal spray or pressurized aerosol. J Allergy Clin Immunol 1986; 77:858–864.

94. Meltzer EO, Orgel HA, Bush RK, et al. Evaluation of symptom relief, nasal airflow, nasal cytology, and acceptability of two formulations of flunisolide nasal spray in patients with perennial allergic rhinitis. Ann Allergy 1990; 64:536–540.

95. Gomez E, Claque JE, Gatland D, et al. Effect of topical corticosteroids on seasonally induced increases in nasal mast cells. Br Med J 1988; 296:1572–1573.

96. Otsuka H, Denburg JA, Befus AD, et al. Effect of beclomethasone dipropionate on nasal metachromatic cell subpopulations. Clin Allergy 1986; 16:589–595.

97. Pipkorn U. Effect of topical glucocorticoid treatment on nasal mucosal mast cells in allergic rhinitis. Allergy 1983; 38:125–129.

98. Pipkorn U, Enerback L. Nasal mucosal mast cells and histamine in hayfever. Int Arch Allergy Appl Immunol 1987; 84:123–128.

99. Meltzer EO, Orgel HA, Rogenes PR, Field EA. Nasal cytology in patients with allergic rhinitis: effects of intranasal fluticasone propionate. J Allergy Clin Immunol 1994; 94:708–715.

100. Holopainen E, Malmberg H, Binder E. Longterm follow-up of intranasal beclo-

methasone treatment. A clinical and histologic study. Acta Otolaryngol (Stockh) 1982; 386:270–275.

101. Pipkorn U, Pukander J, Suonpaa J, et al. Long-term safety of budesonide nasal aerosol: a 5.5 year follow-up study. Clin Allergy 1988; 18:253–259.

102. Orgel HA, Meltzer EO, Bierman CW, et al. Intranasal fluocortin butyl in patients with perennial rhinitis: a twelve-month efficacy and safety study including nasal biopsy. J Allergy Clin Immunol 1991; 88:257–264.

103. Bascom R, Pipkorn U, Gleich G, et al. Effect of systemic steroids on eosinophils and major basic protein during nasal antigen challenge. J Allergy Clin Immunol 1986; 77:246.

104. Bascom R, Pipkorn U, Lichtenstein LM, et al. The influx of inflammatory cells into nasal washings during the late response to antigen challenge. Effect of systemic steroid pretreatment. Am Rev Respir Dis 1988; 138:406–412.

105. Iliopoulos O, Proud D, Adkinson NF Jr, et al. Effects of immunotherapy on the early, late, and rechallenge nasal reaction to provocation with allergen: changes in inflammatory mediators and cells. J Allergy Clin Immunol 1991; 87:855–866.

106. Furin MJ, Norman PS, Creticos PS, et al. Immunotherapy decreases antigen-induced eosinophil cell migration into the nasal cavity. J Allergy Clin Immunol 1991; 88:27–32.

107. Otsuka H, Mezawa A, Ohnishi M, et al. Changes in nasal metachromatic cells during allergen immunotherapy. Clin Exp Allergy 1991; 21:115–119.

12

Radiographic Evaluation of the Nasal Cavity and Paranasal Sinuses

S. JAMES ZINREICH

The Johns Hopkins University
Baltimore, Maryland

I. Introduction

Inflammatory sinus disease is a serious health problem, which affects an estimated 30–50 million people in the United States alone (1). Because the history and physical examination can be nonspecific in these patients, radiological evaluation is essential in the diagnosis of paranasal sinus pathology. Traditionally, conventional radiography was the modality of choice in the evaluation of the paranasal sinuses. Clinically and radiographically the emphasis was primarily on the maxillary and frontal sinuses. In recent years, however, due to technological advancements in imaging and a change in the therapeutic approach, computed tomography (CT) has supplanted conventional radiography as the primary diagnostic modality.

While most patients are initially treated medically, medical therapy alone may not resolve the problem. In addition, there is a crucial need to develop a clear understanding of sinus anatomy because of the implications of previous surgery and resultant surgical complications on anatomical structures. Surgical treatment of refractory inflammatory sinus disease has undergone revolutionary change in the past decade. These advances are due to several factors: (1) an improved understanding of the mucociliary clearance pathways in the nasal cavity

"

and paranasal sinuses; (2) improved endoscopes that afford direct access to nasal cavity and ethmoid sinus drainage portals; (3) the availability of high-resolution coronal CT images that provide an accurate display of the regional anatomy. CT is also valuable in the staging of sinus pathology with regard to therapeutic management and outcomes research.

II. Normal Anatomy and Anatomical Variations

A. Mucociliary Clearance

For a clear understanding of the regional anatomy and the importance of the anterior ethmoid sinus structures, it is critical that one understand the flow pattern of the mucous blanket coating the major sinuses (mucociliary clearance). Further one must be acquainted with the concept that inflammatory sinus disease is largely the result of compromise of the drainage portals (osteomeatal channels) of the individual sinus cavities.

The mucosal lining of the paranasal sinuses is made up of a ciliated cuboidal epithelium. In turn, a mucous blanket is found on the surface. The cilia are in constant motion and act in concert to propel the mucus in a specific direction. The pattern of flow is specific for each sinus and will persist even if alternative openings are surgically created in the sinus (2–6). Therefore, functional endoscopic sinus surgery (FESS) has gained widespread acceptance because its goal is to restore drainage of the sinuses via their anatomical drainage pathways.

In the maxillary sinus, the mucous flow originates in the antral floor with the flow directed centripetally toward the primary ostium. The mucus is then transported through the infundibulum to the hiatus semilunaris, from where it is passed into the middle meatus and ultimately the nasopharynx. This pattern of mucus movement persists even after a nasal antrostomy is created (2–8).

In the frontal sinus the mucous flow is up along the medial wall, laterally across the roof, and medially along the floor. As the flow approaches the medial aspect of the floor, some is directed into the primary ostium while the remainder is recirculated. The cleared mucus travels down the frontal recess, and then on into the middle meatus, where it joins the flow from the ipsilateral maxillary sinus (2–8).

The posterior ethmoid and sphenoid sinus clear their mucus into the sphenoethmoidal recess. The flow then enters the superior meatus and subsequently the nasopharynx.

Thus, there are two main osteomeatal channels. The anterior osteomeatal unit includes the frontal sinus ostium, frontal recess, maxillary sinus ostium, infundibulum, and middle meatus. These channels provide communication between the ipsilateral frontal, anterior ethmoid, and maxillary sinuses. The posterior osteomeatal unit consists of the sphenoid sinus ostium, sphenoethmoidal recess, and the superior meatus. The radiological representation of the anatomy should stress display of these osteomeatal channels.

B. Normal Anatomy

An understanding of the anatomy of the lateral nasal wall and its relationship to adjacent structures is essential (9,10). The lateral nasal wall contains three bulbous projections: the superior, middle, and inferior turbinates (conchae). The turbinates serve to divide the nasal cavity into three distinct air passages: the superior, middle, and inferior meati. The superior meatus drains the posterior ethmoid air cells and, more posteriorly, the sphenoid sinus (via the sphenoethmoidal recess). The middle meatus receives drainage from the frontal sinus (via the nasofrontal recess), maxillary sinus (via the maxillary ostium and subsequently the ethmoidal infundibulum), and the anterior ethmoid air cells (via the ethmoid cell ostia). The inferior meatus receives drainage from the nasolacrimal duct, a structure usually identifiable on coronal sections.

On CT scanning, the first coronal images display the outline of the frontal sinuses. The frontal sinuses are funnel shaped. Their aeration varies from patient to patient. They can be small and occupy only the diploic space of the medial frontal bone or they can be large enough to extend through the floor of the entire anterior cranial fossa posteriorly to the planum sphenoidale. In general, a central septation separates the left and right sides; however, often there may be several septations. The floor of the frontal sinus slopes inferiorly toward the midline.

Close to the midline, the primary ostium is located in a depression in the floor. The frontal recess is an hourglass-like narrowing between the frontal sinus and the anterior middle meatus through which the frontal sinus drains (11) (Fig. 1). It is not a tubular structure, as the term ''nasofrontal duct'' might imply, and therefore the term ''recess'' is preferred.

Anterior, lateral, and inferior to the frontal recess is the agger nasi cell. This cell is a remnant ethmoid turbinal, which in our experience is present in nearly all patients. It is aerated and represents the most anterior ethmoid air cell. It usually borders the primary ostium/floor of the frontal sinus, and thus its size may directly influence the patency of the frontal recess and the anterior middle meatus. The frontal recesses are the narrowest anterior air channels and are common sites of inflammation. Their obstruction subsequently results in loss of ventilation and mucociliary clearance of the frontal sinus.

The uncinate process is a superior extension of the lateral nasal wall (medial wall of the maxillary sinus) (11,12). Anteriorly, the uncinate process fuses with the posteromedial wall of the agar nasi cell and the posteromedial wall of the nasolacrimal duct. The uncinate process has a ''free'' (unattached) superoposterior edge. Laterally this free edge defines the infundibulum (Fig. 2). The infundibulum is the air passage that connects the maxillary sinus ostium to the middle

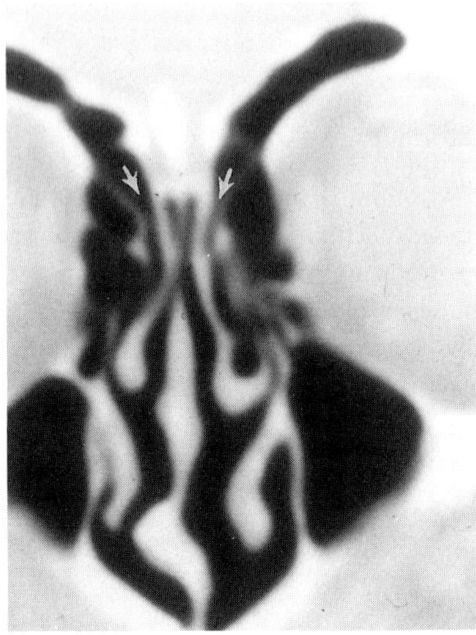

Figure 1 Coronal CT image of the frontal recess. White arrows show the point of communication between the frontal sinus and middle meatus.

meatus. Posterior to the uncinate is the ethmoid bulla, usually the largest of the anterior ethmoid cells. The uncinate process usually courses medial and inferior to the ethmoid bulla. The ethmoid bulla is enclosed laterally by the lamina papyracea.

The gap between the ethmoid bulla and the "free" edge of the uncinate process defines the hiatus semilunaris. Medially, the hiatus semilunaris communicates with the middle meatus, the air space lateral to the middle turbinate (13,14). Laterally and inferiorly, the hiatus semilunaris communicates with the infundibulum, the air channel between the uncinate process and the inferomedial border of the orbit. The infundibulum serves as the primary drainage pathway from the maxillary sinus (12,13).

The structure medial to the ethmoid bulla and the uncinate process is the middle turbinate. Anteriorly, it attaches to the medial wall of the agger nasi cell and the superior edge of the uncinate process. Superiorly, the middle turbinate adheres to the cribriform plate. As it extends posteriorly, the middle turbinate emits a laterally coursing bony structure, the basal or grand lamella, that fuses with the lamina papyracea just posterior to the ethmoid bulla. The basal lamella demarcates the anterior ethmoid sinus from the posterior ethmoid sinus.

In most patients, the posterior wall of the ethmoid bulla is intact, and an

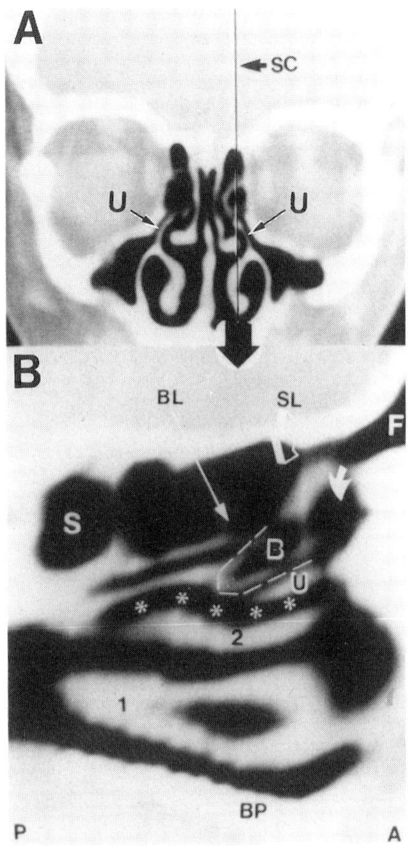

Figure 2 (A and B) CT of the uncinate process. Direct coronal CT image (A) reveals the uncinate process (U). A sagittally reconstructed plane (SC) (Fig. 3) through the middle of the ethmoid bulla (B) and uncinate process. Note the relationship between the uncinate process (U), and the middle meatus (asterisk), the hiatus semilunaris (dashed lines), and ethmoid bulla (B), sphenoid sinus (S), basal lamella (BL), sinus lateralis (SL), frontal recess (white arrow), frontal sinus (F), middle turbinate (2), inferior turbinate (1), bony palate, anterior (A) and posterior (P).

air space is usually found between the basal lamella and the ethmoid bulla. This air space, the sinus lateralis, may extend superior to the ethmoid bulla and communicate with the frontal recess. A dehiscence or total absence of the posterior wall of the ethmoid bulla is common and may provide communication between these two usually separated air spaces.

The posterior ethmoid sinus consists of air cells between the basal lamella and the sphenoid sinus. The number, shape, and size of these air cells vary significantly from person to person (11,13–15).

The sphenoid sinus is the most posterior sinus. It is usually embedded into the clivus and bordered superoposteriorly by the sella turcica. Its ostium is located medially in the anterosuperior portion of the anterior sinus wall, which in turn communicates with the sphenoethmoidal recess into the posterior aspect of the superior meatus. The sphenoethmoidal recess lies just lateral to the nasal septum and can sometimes be seen on coronal images, but is best displayed in the sagittal and axial planes (11,12,14) (Fig. 3).

The relationship between the aerated portion of the sphenoid sinus and the posterior ethmoid sinus needs to be accurately represented so the surgeon can avoid operative complications (Fig. 4). Usually in the paramedian sagittal plane, the sphenoid sinus is the most superior and posterior air space. More laterally (1–1.5 cm), the sphenoid sinus is located more inferiorly, and the posterior ethmoid air cells become the most superior and posterior air space. This relationship is well demonstrated on axial and sagittal images. The number and position of the septations of the sphenoid sinus are quite variable. Some of these septations can adhere to the bony wall covering the internal carotid artery, which can frequently penetrate into the sphenoid sinus.

Anatomically, the paranasal sinuses are in close proximity to the anterior cranial fossa, cribriform plate, internal carotid arteries, cavernous sinuses, the orbits and their contents, and the optic nerves as they exit the orbits (16–20). The surgeon must be cautious when maneuvering instrumentation in the posterior direction, to avoid inadvertent penetration and drainage of these structures (7,13,18,19).

C. Anatomical Variations and Congenital Abnormalities

Even though the nasal anatomy varies significantly from patient to patient, certain anatomical variations are observed commonly in the general population and are often seen more frequently in patients with chronic inflammatory disease (7,8,11,12,14,21). The significance of a particular anatomical variant is deter-

---

Figure 3 (A–C) Sphenoethmoid recess. Direct coronal CT data (A) are used to sagitally reconstruct (SC) a plane through the sphenoethmoid recess (curved white arrow). Sphenoid sinus (S), frontal sinus (F), frontal recess (dotted arrow), middle meatus (asterisk), middle turbinate (2), bony palate (BP), anterior (A) and posterior (P). Axial image (C) shows the position of sphenoethmoid recesses (arrows); mucoperiosteal thickening (asterisk) is present within the left anterior and posterior ethmoid sinus.

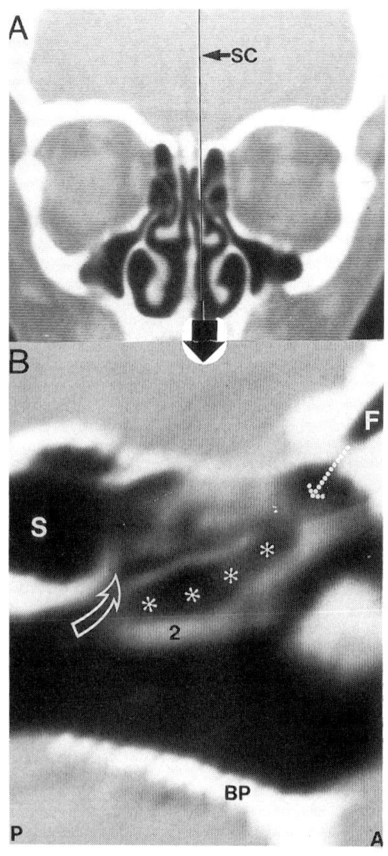

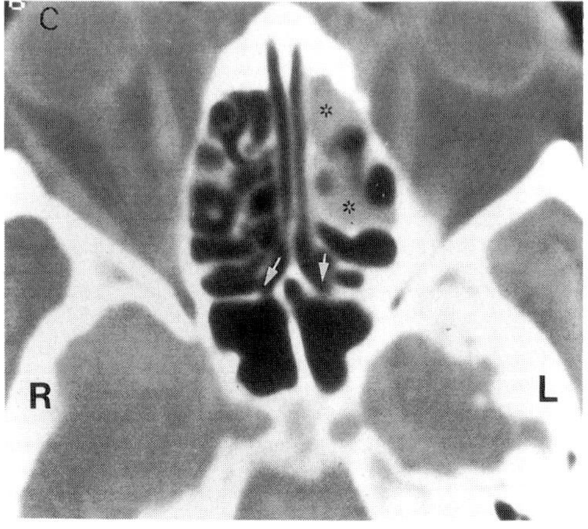

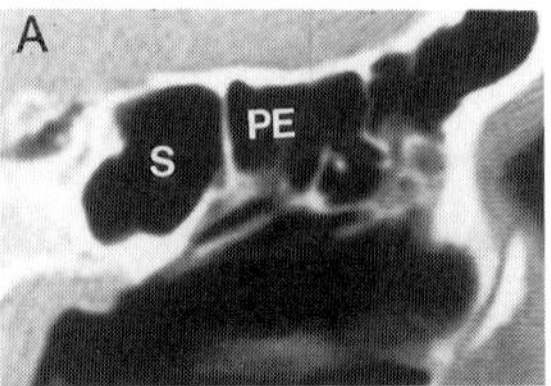

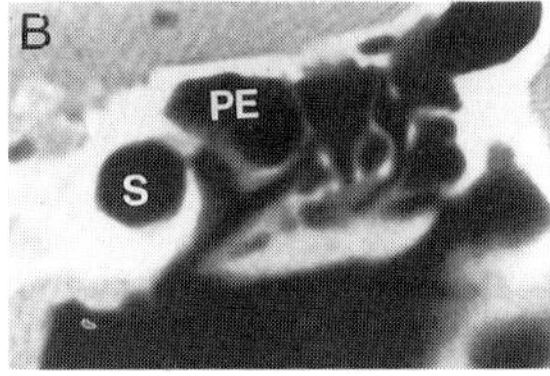

Figure 4 (A and B) Relationship between sphenoid sinus and posterior ethmoid sinus. Paramedian sagittal CT scan (A) shows that the sphenoid sinus (S) is the most superoposterior air space. It is located posterior to the posterior ethmoid sinus (PE). Sagittal CT image approximately 1–1.5 cm lateral to the nasal septum (B) shows the posterior ethmoid sinus (PE) to be above the sphenoid sinus (S).

mined by its relationship with the osteomeatal channels and nasal air passages. The ability of the variation to obstruct the air passages implies a role in the recurrence of sinusitis. In our experience, the most common variations are as follows (7,8,11,12,14,22–24).

Concha Bullosa

A concha bullosa is defined as an aeration in a middle turbinate (Fig. 5). It may be unilateral or bilateral. Less frequently, aeration of the superior turbinate may occur, while aeration of the inferior turbinate is infrequent. A concha bullosa in the middle turbinate may enlarge to obstruct the middle meatus or the infundibulum. The air cavity in a concha bullosa is lined with the same epithelium as the rest of the nasal cavity, and thus these cells can undergo the same inflammatory disorders experienced in the paranasal sinuses. Obstruction of the drainage of a concha can lead to mucocele formation.

Nasal Septal Deviation

This is an asymmetrical bowing of the nasal septum that may compress the middle turbinate laterally, narrowing the middle meatus. Bony spurs are often associated with septal deviation, and this may further compromise the osteomeatal unit.

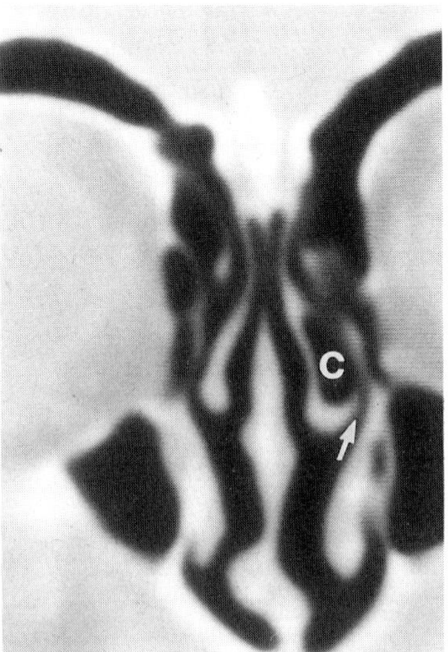

Figure 5 Concha bullosa. Coronal CT image shows a concha bullosa (C) and minimally narrowed middle meatus (arrow).

Nasal septal deviation is usually congenital, though it may be a posttraumatic finding in some patients.

Paradoxic Middle Turbinate

The middle turbinate usually curves medially toward the nasal septum. However, its major curvature can project laterally, and thus narrow the middle meatus and infundibulum. Such a variant is called a "paradoxical middle turbinate." The inferior edge of the middle meatus may assume various shapes with excessive curvature, which in turn may obstruct the nasal cavity, infundibulum, and middle meatus.

Variations in the Uncinate Process

The course of the "free edge" of the uncinate process has several variations. In most cases, it either extends slightly obliquely toward the nasal septum with the free edge surrounding the inferior/anterior surface of the ethmoid bulla or extends more medially to the medial surface of the ethmoid bulla.

Sometimes, the free edge of the uncinate is noted to adhere to the orbital floor/inferior aspect of the lamina papyracea. This is referred to as an "atelectatic uncinate process." This variant is usually associated with a hypoplastic, and often opacified, ipsilateral maxillary sinus due to closure of the infundibulum. It is important to note this variant for surgical planning, as the ipsilateral orbital floor will be low-lying due to the hypoplastic maxillary sinus. This increases the risk of inadvertent penetration of the orbit during surgery.

An additional variation of the uncinate is its extension superiorly to the roof of the anterior ethmoid sinus, thus causing the superior infundibulum to end as a "blind pouch," and is referred to as the lamina terminalis. Here, the infundibulum drains via the posterior aspect of the middle meatus.

If the free edge of the uncinate deviates laterally, there can be obstruction of the infundibulum. Less frequently, we have encountered "medial curling" of the uncinate, which will encroach upon the middle meatus.

Aeration of the Uncinate

This anomaly expands the width of the uncinate, thus potentially compromising the infundibulum. Functionally, it acts like a concha bullosa or an enlarged ethmoid bulla. In our experience it occurs infrequently.

Haller Cells

These are ethmoid air cells that extend along the medial roof of the maxillary sinus. They can have a variable appearance and size. They may cause narrowing of the infundibulum when they are large. Haller cells may exist as discrete cells or they may open into the maxillary sinus or infundibulum.

Onodi Cells

These are lateral and posterior extensions of the posterior ethmoid air cells. They extend the paranasal sinus cavity to a very close proximity to the optic nerves as they exit the orbits. These "cells" may surround the optic nerve tract and put the nerve at risk during surgery. In our experience, Onodi cells are rare.

Giant Ethmoid Bulla

The largest of the ethmoid air cells, the ethmoid bulla, may enlarge to narrow or obstruct the middle meatus and infundibulum.

Extensive Pneumatization of the Sphenoid Sinus

Pneumatization of the sphenoid sinus can extend into the anterior clinoids and clivus, surrounding the optic nerves. When this occurs, the optic nerves are at increased risk of being damaged during surgical exploration.

Medial Deviation and/or Dehiscence of the Lamina Papyracea

This may be a congenital finding or can be the result of prior facial trauma. In either case, the intraorbital contents are at risk during surgery due to the common dehiscences in the area as well as the ease of confusing this "medial bulge" with the ethmoid bulla. Excessive medial deviation and bony dehiscence both tend to occur most often at the site of the insertion of the basal lamella into the lamina papyracea, thus rendering this portion of the laminal papyracea to be most delicate.

Aerated Crista Galli

Aeration of this normally bony structure can occur. When aerated, these cells may communicate with the frontal recess. Obstruction of this ostium can lead to chronic sinusitis and mucocele formation. It is important to recognize this entity preoperatively and to differentiate it from an ethmoid air cell to avoid extension of surgery into the cranial vault.

Cephalocele

Preoperative CT scanning is useful to assess for congenital abnormalities, such as cephaloceles (25) (Fig. 6). These may be spontaneously present or may occur as a result of previous ethmoid/sphenoid sinus surgery. Their presence needs to be considered when dealing with an isolated soft tissue mass adjacent to the ethmoid or sphenoid roof, especially if complimented with adjacent bone erosion. The differential diagnosis includes mucocele, neoplasm, cephalocele, and, less likely, a polyp associated with an adjacent bony dehiscence. Coronal CT scanning will best display the extent of bony erosion and sagittal and coronal MRI images will be very helpful in narrowing the differential diagnosis.

Posterior Septal Air Cell

Air cells are commonly found within the posterior-superior portion of the nasal septum. When present, the communication is with the sphenoid sinus. They also may be affected with mucosal inflammation like any other air cell within the paranasal sinuses. Such inflammatory disease may obliterate this cell. In such cases, these may resemble a cephalocele. CT and magnetic resonance imaging (MRI) scanning may be beneficial in defining the involved pathology.

Asymmetry in Ethmoid Roof Height

It is important to make note of any asymmetry in height of the ethmoid roof. There is a higher incidence of intracranial penetration during FESS when this

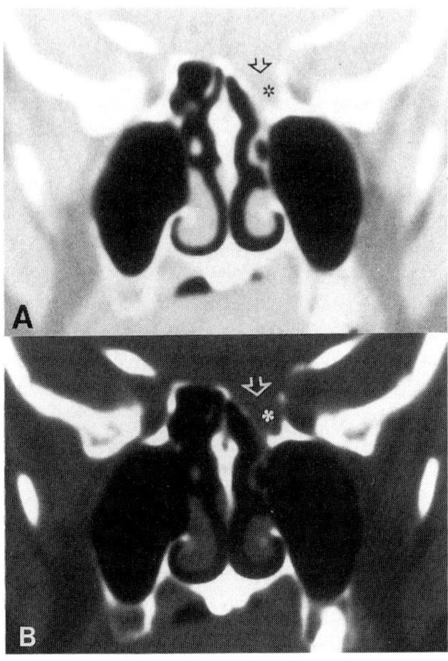

Figure 6 (A and B) Coronal CT images with soft tissue windowing (A) and bony windowing (B) show an encephaloceal penetrating into the sphenoid sinus (open arrow, and asterisk).

anatomical variation occurs. The intracranial penetration is more likely to occur on the side where the position of the roof is lower (26).

III. Methods of Evaluation

The primary purpose of the radiological evaluation of the paranasal sinuses and related structures is to provide an accurate display of the regional anatomy, and to establish the extent of disease. Although standard roentgenograms can depict the changes of acute sinusitis in the maxillary, frontal, and sphenoid sinuses, they cannot delineate the status of the individual ethmoid air cells or osteomeatal complexes, nor can conventional radiograms accurately evaluate the extent of inflammatory disease in these patients (11–13).

CT is currently the modality of choice in the evaluation of the paranasal sinuses and adjacent structures (13). Its ability to optimally display bone, soft tissue, and air facilitates accurate depiction of anatomy and extent of disease in and around the paranasal sinuses (7,12,13). The cross-sectional plane that most closely correlates with the surgical approach is the coronal plane. This plane also shows the osteomeatal channels, the relationship of the brain and fovea ethmoidalis to the ethmoid sinus, and it depicts the relationship of the orbits to the paranasal sinuses (7,12). The anatomy is best displayed when the amount of inflammation is optimally controlled by medications prior to imaging.

In evaluating the sinuses, we position the patient in a prone position with the chin hyperextended on the bed of the CT scanner. The scanner gantry is angled to be as perpendicular as possible to the hard palate. Scanning is performed from the anterior frontal sinus posteriorly through the sphenoid sinus. Contiguous 3-mm images are obtained. Scans should overlap if thicker slices are used so that multiplanar reconstructions can still be performed. The field of view is adjusted to include only the areas of interest. This helps reduce artifact from the teeth and associated metallic restorations as well as magnify the small structures of the nasal cavity and adjacent paranasal sinuses (12,13). Windows are chosen to accentuate the air passages, the bony detail, and the soft tissues. Our experience shows that a window width of $+2000$ with a level of -200 is the best starting point. The potentiometers can then be manually manipulated to optimally display the anatomical detail of the uncinate process and ethmoid bulla. This same setting is then used to film the entire study (11).

Sagittal reconstructions can be obtained for a morphological orientation. Various distances and angles can be measured to aid in the passage of instruments during surgery on these views. Axial reconstructions can be helpful in displaying the position of the internal carotid arteries with respect to the bony margins of the sphenoid sinus.

MRI provides better visualization of soft tissue than CT (12), but is not well suited for routine evaluation of the paranasal sinuses (11,12). Cortical bone and air yield no MR signal and thus are not depicted on the images. Furthermore, the signal intensity of the mucosal lining during the edematous phase of the nasal cycle is similar to the appearance of mucosal inflammation. The nasal cycle is a physiological phenomenon in which the nasal mucosa undergoes alternating cycles of left- and right-sided mucosal swelling. The cycle varies from 20 min to 6 hr. Although inflammation of the mucosa gives very bright signal intensity on T2-weighted images, neoplastic processes usually are of intermediate increased signal intensity on T2-weighted images. Fungal concretions have a very low signal intensity on T2-weighted images (12).

IV. Complications of Endoscopic Sinus Surgery

Although FESS is a popular surgical treatment modality in chronic sinusitis, there are inherent complications that must be recognized. CT is of value in this regard, particularly in preoperative imaging and staging of disease.

The rate of complications from the procedure is related to the instrumentation, the patient's underlying anatomy, the overall health of the patient, and the extent of disease (18–29).

The field of view available to the surgeon during FESS is quite small. Variant anatomy can make surgical landmarks difficult to identify. The surgeon's view is limited to the surface mucosa; he/she cannot see beyond the mucosa directly in view. The presence of various anatomical variants can contribute to surgical complications if not noted prospectively (17). With regard to orbital complications, the most notable of these include loss of integrity of the lamina papyracea, Onodi cells, and pneumatization of the anterior clinoid processes of sphenoid bones (17). Due to the need for an accurate surgical road map, all patients scheduled to undergo FESS should have a preoperative high-resolution CT scan preferably in the coronal plane. This plane is best as it simulates the surgeon's working plane afforded by the endoscope (11).

Further, brisk bleeding in the operative field as well as extensive nasal polyposis can hinder visibility and predispose the patient to operative complications (17). Standard surgical techniques and microscope-assisted surgery are adjuncts that can be used when the aforementioned problems arise. They, however, are fraught with the same orbital complications.

In general, complications can be either minor or major (18,19,28,29). Minor complications include periorbital emphysema, epistaxis, postoperative nasal synechiae, and tooth pain. Although these all can commonly occur, they are usually self-limited and do not require postoperative radiological evaluation. Major complications are rarer but can be severely devastating or even fatal (19). Preoperatively, if the lamina papyracea is discontinuous due to prior trauma or erosion from chronic sinus disease, intraorbital fat can herniate into the ethmoid sinuses. Intraoperatively, it is difficult to discern between abnormal mucosa and this herniated intraorbital hemorrhage and emphysema (27). If intraorbital and intraocular pressure builds up due to an expanding hematoma or due to air being forced into the orbit from the nasal cavity, then visual impairment or blindness secondary to ischemia can result (27).

Direct damage to the medial rectus muscle or superior oblique muscle can occur if there is preexisting or intraoperative disruption of the lamina papyracea (27). This will result in postoperative diplopia. The etiology of the diplopia can be from muscle entrapment among bone fragments, direct muscle laceration, or be secondary to nerve injury. Thin-section axial and coronal CT can be of benefit in evaluation. Clinically, subconjunctival hemorrhage is often associated with extracelluar muscle damage (27).

Blindness, temporary or permanent, due to injury of the optic nerve itself can occur during posterior ethmoidectomy if the bony limit of the sinus is violated (18,19,27,29). Trauma to the vascular supply to the optic nerve can also result in visual loss. This is why preoperative observation of aeration of the anterior clinoid should be noted. Thin section in two planes can be used to study the optic canal postoperatively in such cases (17).

Injury to the lacrimal duct can result during anterior enlargement of the maxillary ostium in the middle meatus. Injury to the membranous portion of the duct may be self-limited and remit by spontaneous fistulization into the middle meatus. Total occlusion of the nasolacrimal duct can result from more severe injury (27).

Postoperative cerebrospinal fluid (CSF) leak is another possible major complication of FESS (19,30). Inadvertent penetration of the dura of the cranium can occur at several sites during FESS. Perforation of the cribriform plate, fovea ethmoidalis, anterior cranial fossa, as well as the skull base have all been reported. The CSF leak may not become clinically apparent for up to 2 years after surgery (17,18). These CSF leaks will often close spontaneously with conservative measures (i.e., lumbar drain) (17,18). However, if they persist, radiological workup with CT-cisternogram can be done. Secondary nasal encephalocele or deep penetration of the cerebrum can be seen following violation of the cranial vault (17).

Massive hemorrhage from direct injury to major vessels can occur. Laceration of the internal carotid artery has been reported and indeed is not uncommonly a fatal complication (18,19). Emergent angiography with balloon occlusion of the lacerated artery has been performed. Patients who report severe postoperative headache, photophobia, or have signs to suggest subarachnoid hemorrhage should have a noncontrast head CT. If subarachnoid blood is found, then cerebral angiography to detect vascular injury is recommended (17,18,28).

Complications of sinus disease such as intracranial and intraorbital infections can occur. These are emergent problems and are best evaluated by axial CT scans after contrast injections.

V. CT for Staging of Sinus Pathology

CT is the modality of choice, then, for evaluation of sinus disease. Recently, however, the value of CT in staging of sinus pathology has been explored. Particularly with regard to outcome, CT scanning preoperatively is indicative of disease severity and is related to outcome (30). Gliklich and Metson compared four proposed sinus CT staging systems with regard to their value in outcomes research. They emphasized that the statistical attributes of a staging system directly affect its usefulness in clinical trials, and concluded that a staging system based on anatomical disease site would be most beneficial with regard to outcomes research (31).

In another study by Friedman and Katsantonis, a four-stage system was proposed. *Stage I* disease includes single-focus disease radiographically, either unilaterally or bilaterally. *Stage II* is defined as discontiguous or patchy areas of disease radiographically with symptomatic response to medication. *Stage III* includes contiguous disease throughout the ethmoid labyrinth, with or without other major sinus opacity, with symptomatic response to medication. *Stage IV* disease includes contiguous hyperplastic disease involving all sinuses with minimal or no symptomatic response to medication. Stage I disease indicates primarily medical treatment while Stages II–IV indicate surgical treatment (32). These authors conclude that this four-stage system is most indicative of clinical course and eventual outcome.

It is clear that careful radiographic evaluation, particularly the use of CT for staging of sinus pathology, is a crucial component, if not the prime determinant, for staging and clinical outcome.

Acknowledgment

The author is currently a grant recipient of ISG Technologies Inc., Toronto, Ontario, Canada.

References

1. Moss A, Parsons V. Current Estimates from the National Health Interview Survey, United States—1985. Hyattsville, MD: National Center for Health Statistics, 1986.
2. Messerklinger W. Endoscopy of the Nose. Baltimore: Urban and Schwartzenberg, 1978.
3. Messerklinger W. Zur Endoskopietchnik des mittleren Nassenganges. Arch Otorhinolaryngol 1978; 221:297–305.
4. Wigand ME, Steiner W, Jaumann MP. Endonasal sinus surgery with endoscopic control: from radical operation to rehabilitation of the mucosa. Endoscopy 1978; 10: 255–260.
5. Stammberger H. Functional Sinus Surgery. Philadelphia: BC Decker, 1991:273–282.
6. Kennedy DW, Zinreich SJ. The functional endoscopic approach to inflammatory sinus disease: current perspectives and technique modifications. Am J Rhinol 1988; 2:89–93.
7. Zinreich S, Kennedy D, Rosenbaum A, Gayler B, Kumar A, Stammberger H. Paranasal sinuses: CT imaging requirements for endoscopic surgery. Radiology 1987; 163:769–775.
8. Shankar L, Evans K, Hawke M, Stammberger H. An Atlas of Imaging of the Paranasal Sinuses. Toronto: Imago Publishing, 1994:41–72.
9. Harnsberger R. Imaging for the sinus and nose. In: Head and Neck Imaging Handbook. St. Louis: Mosby Yearbook, 1990:387–419.
10. Hosemann W. Dissection of the lateral nasal wall in eight steps. In: Wigand ME,

ed. Endoscopic Surgery of the Paranasal Sinuses and Anterior Skull Base. New York: Thieme Medical Publishers, 1990:36–41.

11. Zinreich S. Paranasal sinus imaging. Otolaryngol Head Neck Surg 1990; 103:863–868.

12. Zinreich S. Imaging of inflammatory sinus disease. Otolaryngol Clin North Am 1993; 26:535–547.

13. Zinreich S, Abidin M, Kennedy D. Cross-sectional imaging of the nasal cavity and paranasal sinuses. Oper Techn Otolaryngol Head Neck Surg 1990; 1:93–99.

14. Zinreich S. Imaging of chronic sinusitis in adults: X-ray, computed tomography, and magnetic resonance imaging. J Allergy Clin Immunol 1992; 90:445–451.

15. Yousem D. Imaging of sinonasal inflammatory disease. Radiology 1993; 188:303–314.

16. Buus D, Tse D, Farris B. Ophthalmic complications of sinus surgery. Ophthalmology 1990; 97:612–619.

17. Hudgins P. Complications of endoscopic sinus surgery—the role of the radiologist in prevention. Radiol Clin North Am 1993; 31:21–31.

18. Hudgins P, Browning D, Gallups J. Endoscopic paranasal sinus surgery: radiographic evaluation of severe complications. AJNR 1992; 13:1161–1167.

19. Maniglia A. Fatal and major complications secondary to nasal and sinus surgery. Laryngoscope 1989; 99:276–283.

20. Maniglia A. Fatal and other major complications of endoscopic sinus surgery. Laryngoscope 1991; 101:349–354.

21. Laine F, Smoker W. The ostiomeatal unit and endoscopic surgery: anatomy, variations, and imaging findings in inflammatory diseases. AJR 1992; 159:849–857.

22. Mafee M. Preoperative imaging anatomy of the nasal-ethmoid complex for functional endoscopic sinus surgery. Radiol Clin North Am 1993; 31:1–20.

23. Bolger W, Butzin C, Parsons D. Paranasal sinus bony anatomic variations and mucosal abnormalities: CT analysis for endoscopic sinus surgery. Laryngoscope 1991; 101:56–64.

24. Yousem D, Kennedy D, Rosenberg S. Ostiomeatal complex risk factors for sinusitis: CT evaluation. J Otolaryngol 1991; 20:419–424.

25. Laine FJ, Kuta AJ. Imaging the sphenoid bone and basiocciput: pathologic considerations. Semin Ultra CT MRI 1993; 14:160–177.

26. Dessi P, Moulin G, Triglia JM, Zanaret M, Cannoni M. Difference in height of the right and left ethmoidal roofs: a possible risk factor for ethmoidal surgery. Prospective study of 150 CT scans. J Laryngol Otol 1994; 108:261–262.

27. Neuhaus RW. Orbital complications secondary to endoscopic sinus surgery. Ophthalmology 1990; 97:1512–1518.

28. Stankiewicz JA. Complications of endoscopic intranasal ethmoidectomy. Laryngoscope 1987; 97:1270–1273.

29. Stankiewicz JA. Complications in endoscopic intranasal ethmoidectomy: an update. Laryngoscope 1987; 99:686–670.

30. Kennedy DW. Prognostic factors, outcomes and staging in ethmoid sinus surgery. Laryngoscope 1992; 102:1–18.

31. Gliklich RE, Metson R. A comparison of sinus computed tomography (CT) staging systems for outcomes research. Am J Rhinol 1994; 8:291–297.
32. Friedman WH, Katsantonis GP. Staging systems for chronic sinus disease. ENT J 1994; 73:480–484.

13

Intranasal Corticosteroids

NIELS MYGIND

University of Aarhus
Aarhus, Denmark

ROBERT M. NACLERIO

University of Chicago
Chicago, Illinois

I. Introduction

The introduction, in 1973 (1), of local intranasal glucocorticosteroids or corticosteroids (CSs) without significant risk of adverse systemic effects revolutionized the treatment of allergic rhinitis, perennial nonallergic rhinitis, and nasal polyposis. Intranasal GCs are currently the most potent medication available for the treatment of these diseases. Intranasal preparations eliminate the systemic side effects and equal or exceed the efficacy of their systemic counterparts. Initially reserved as second-line agents, intranasal CSs may now be changing to first-line treatment in most cases (2).

This chapter combines a review of the literature and more than 20 years' clinical experience of topical steroid treatment for rhinitis.

II. Mechanisms of Action

After establishing the efficacy of modern CS sprays, a series of studies have elucidated the effect of CSs on the various components of the inflammatory reaction in airway mucosa. Studies of allergen challenges have helped define the pathophysiology of allergic rhinitis. An initial (early) response is followed by an inflammatory response (referred to as a late reaction). The effect of CSs on both phases will be discussed.

A. Early Response to Allergen Challenge

Symptoms

It was formerly believed that CSs inhibited the allergen-induced late response without effect on the early response (3). This was mainly based on studies using short-term pretreatment with oral CSs. However, there is now convincing evidence that CSs have some inhibitory effect on the symptoms of the early response, which becomes apparent after prolonged treatment with topical use of the drug (4–12) (Fig. 1). Similar results have been found in the lower respiratory tract (13). Thus, in addition to the anti-inflammatory activity of topical CSs, they possess a prophylactic potential that may be important for clinical application.

The protective effect of topical CSs differs from one study to another, probably because of differences in study design and intensity of challenge (4–12). The degree of protection may also vary with the specific symptom or parameter recorded (Table 1).

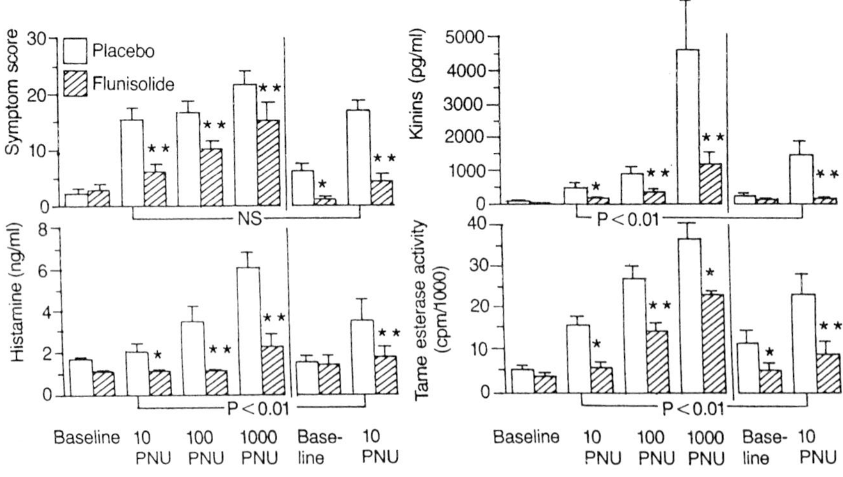

Figure 1 Levels of histamine, TAME esterase activity, and kinins and symptom scores 10 min after each challenge (mean ± SEM). The vertical line indicates 11-hr separation in time between challenges. (From Ref. 9.)

Table 1 Effect of Pretreatment with Budesonide (400 μg/day for 14 days) on Symptoms Following an Allergen Challenge

	Early-phase symptoms	Late-phase symptoms
Sneezing	72%	97%
Nose blowing	37%	76%
Nasal peak flow	17%	96%

Source: From Ref. 13.

Mast Cells

A series of studies using a 1-week pretreatment period with potent topical CSs in asymptomatic hay fever patients (seasonal allergic rhinitis) has shown a reduction of the early symptom response in association with a reduction in the generation of histamine and other inflammatory mediators (8,9,14–16). The reduced level of histamine in lavage fluid has been confirmed in other studies (10), and tryptase levels have also been reduced by topical steroids (11), although the effect was not statistically significant (12). Although topical CS treatment in one study (17) resulted in a 50% reduction of allergen-induced mediator release, it failed to induce any significant change in the number of mast cells in the mucous membrane. As CSs do not appear to stabilize mast cells in vitro, there is no obvious explanation for their inhibition of the early response.

Blood Vessels

Following dermal application, the CSs induce a pallor of the skin, which has been used to grade their anti-inflammatory potency. It was therefore reasonable to believe that a similar "vasoconstriction" might explain a part of the clinical efficacy of the drugs in rhinitis. However, treatment with budesonide in normal persons had no effect either on the capacitance vessels, as determined by measurement of nasal airway resistance (7,18), or on the resistance vessels, as determined by the xenon wash-out technique (19). Furthermore, there is no apparent CS-induced change in the responsiveness of the capacitance vessels to α- or β-adrenergic stimulation (18).

Another vascular characteristic that may play a role in the allergic response is the increase in vascular permeability. Not only cells, but also several active plasma components, such as kininogen, leak into the nasal mucosa during the allergic reaction (20,21). Daily topical CS treatment in rhinitis reduces the allergen-induced increased levels of both albumin (9,22) and bradykinin in nasal lavage fluid (23). This antiexudative effect of topical CSs reflects their anti-inflammatory action rather than a direct vascular effect (23).

B. Late Inflammatory Response to Allergen Challenge

Symptoms

The late response in the nose does not occur at a fixed point in time; the symptoms are weak and variable, and they do not follow a strict biphasic pattern (13). Nasal symptoms occurring 2–12 hr after allergen provocation can be almost completely eliminated by either systemic or topical pretreatment with CSs (8,9,13) (Table 1).

Kinetics and Activation of Inflammatory Cells

Exposure of the nasal mucosa to allergen increases the number of eosinophils, basophils, neutrophils, and lymphocytes (24–26). All these cells become activated, releasing a multitude of mediators and cytokines that potentially contribute to the inflammatory process and the rhinitis symptoms. Short-term pretreatment with oral CS (prednisone, 60 mg/day for 2 days) blocks the influx and activation of eosinophils, but the influx of neutrophils and mononuclear cells appears unaffected (27). Two-week treatment with topical CSs, on the other hand, blocks the influx of all inflammatory cells (24,28–31).

CSs inhibit the influx of basophils and mast cells of the MC_T (mast cell tryptase only) type to the surface epithelium (29,32–35) (Fig. 2) and the influx of eosinophils to the entire mucous membrane and the activation of the eosinophils (31–34) both following allergen challenge (Fig. 3) and during allergen exposure in the pollen season (Fig. 4).

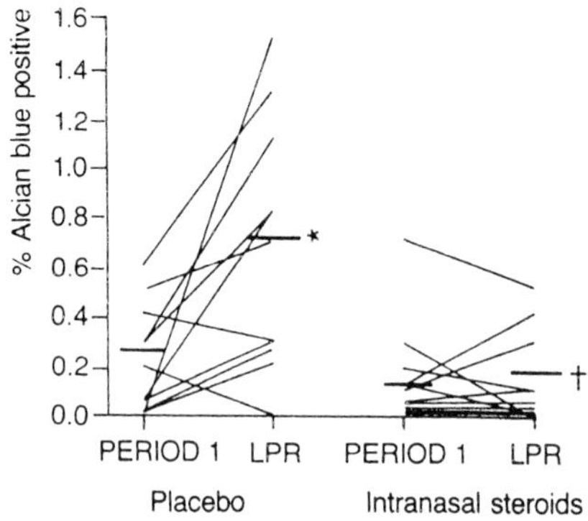

Figure 2 Influx of mast cells and basophils (Alcian-blue-positive cells) after nasal allergen challenge in allergic subjects. The late-phase response (LPR) is 3–11 hr after allergen challenge. Placebo versus intranasal steroid LPR, $p < 0.01$. (From Ref. 24.)

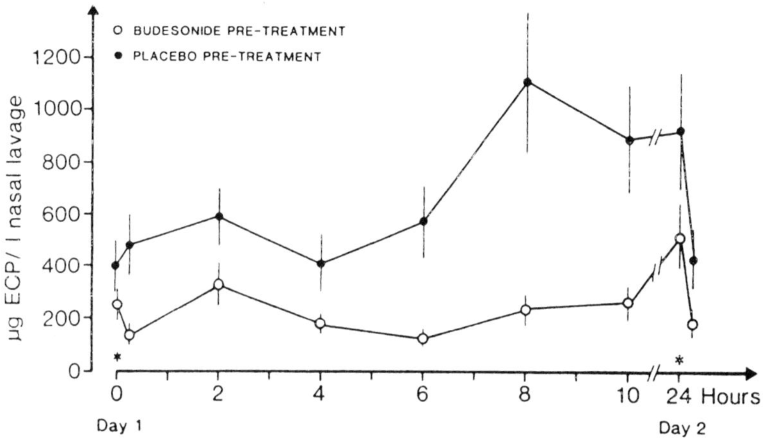

Figure 3 Nasal lavage eosinophil cationic proteins (ECP) (mean ± SEM) following allergen provocation and pretreatment with budesonide (400 μg/day for 14 days). *Nasal allergen provocation. (From Ref. 37.)

Nasal Reactivity

The inflammatory response following allergen exposure changes reactivity to specific (allergen) and nonspecific (e.g., histamine) stimulation. Short-term oral, as well as topical, CSs block the allergen-induced increase in reactivity to specific and nonspecific stimuli (13,39). This reduction occurs even when the CS is given after the allergen challenge (40). A possible explanation for this reduction in the increase to antigen is a reduction of basophils on the surface of the nasal mucosa, cells that can be activated following antigen exposure. Since topical CSs are equally successful in blocking the increase in reactivity to a nonspecific stimulus (41), other explanations, such as an effect on the sensory nerves and/or the epithelial barrier, might also be valid.

One of the major beneficial effects of CSs in asthma is a reduction of bronchial hyperreactivity (42). In the nose, topical CS treatment usually reduces the increase in responsiveness to histamine and methacholine (15,38,43–46). The clinical significance of this reduction is not clear.

C. Langerhans Cells

Holm and co-workers (47) identified antigen-presenting dendritic cells, having the characteristics of Langerhans cells, in the human nasal epithelium and lamina propria and showed that their number increased following allergen exposure. Treatment with a topical CSs markedly reduce their number in perennial rhinitis

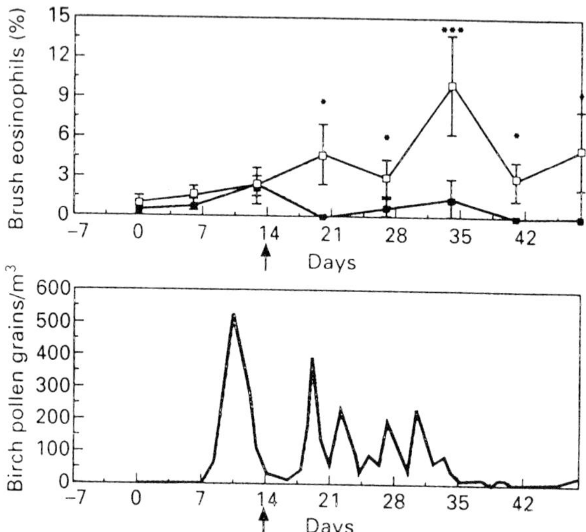

Figure 4 Proportion of eosinophils harvested from the nasal mucosa prior to and during the pollen season. (Open squares) Mean ± SEM for placebo group. (Filled squares) Values obtained during budesonide treatment. The arrow indicates start of treatment. *$p < 0.04$; ***$p < 0.001$, for comparison between placebo and active. (From Ref. 38.)

(47) (Fig. 5). This interesting finding concurs with experience from CS treatment of the skin, but its exact meaning for rhinitis symptomatology remains to be established. Godthelp and co-workers (48) have advanced the hypothesis that the Langerhans cells, by their possession of high-affinity receptors for IgE, are responsible for the stimulation of T cells and their cytokine production, and that topical steroids inhibit this stimulation, with its subsequent inflammation and IgE synthesis, by their effect on the Langerhans cells.

D. Lymphocytes and Cytokines

Evidence has accrued that T cells and their humoral products, cytokines, play important roles in the inflammatory reaction in both asthma (49) and rhinitis (48). As T-cell kinetics, activation, and cytokine production are highly sensitive to CSs (49), it seems likely that an important part of the clinical benefit from this type of treatment is due to a downregulation of T-cell function. At present, there are only a few publications on the effect of CSs on lymphocytes and cytokines in the nasal airways. In a study by Rak and co-workers (50) of nasal allergen challenge, pretreatment with topical CSs significantly reduced the number of epi-

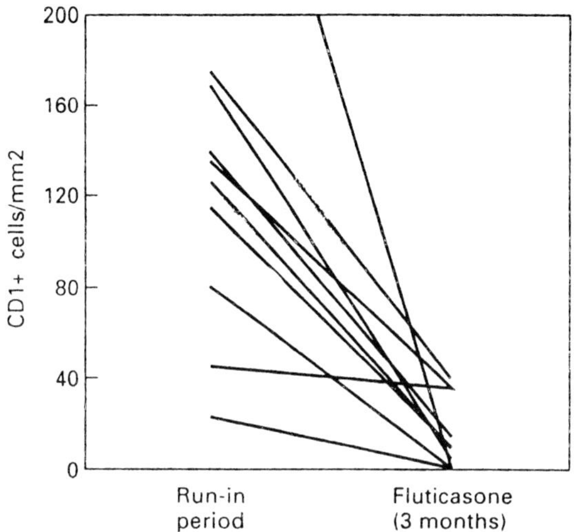

Figure 5 The number of Langerhans cells (CD1+ cells) in the nasal epithelium of patients with perennial allergic rhinitis before and during fluticasone therapy. (From Ref. 47.)

thelial CD3+ (total T cells), CD4+ (T-helper cells), CD8+ (T-effector cells), CD25+ cells (activated T cells), and IL-4-producing cells (42,51) (Fig. 6). Bradding and co-workers (52) also found a CS reduction of allergen induced increased number of IL-4-containing cells. Godthelp and co-workers (48) found a reduction of T-cell-produced cytokines but not of the number of cells. In clinical disease, the numbers of subepithelial CD3+, CD4+, and CD8+ cells were reduced in nasal polyps treated with topical CS (53).

However, other cells, such as epithelial cells, also produce cytokines, and recent in vitro studies have indicated that the expression of GM-CSF, IL-6, and IL-8 in airway epithelial cells is reduced by CSs (54,55). It seems likely, though not yet proven, that CS treatment may also downregulate the expression of adhesion molecules, such as ICAM-1, on nasal epithelial cells (53).

E. Th2 Cell Cytokines, IgE Isotype Switching

There is increasing evidence that the cytokine profile in the microenvironment of naïve T-helper cells (Th0 cells) is important for determining their transformation into Th1 or Th2 cells (56,57). Pawankar and co-workers (58) have recently shown a marked upregulation of the Th2 cytokine, IL-13, in nasal epithelial cells following allergen challenge. As an in vitro study of nasal epithelial cells has

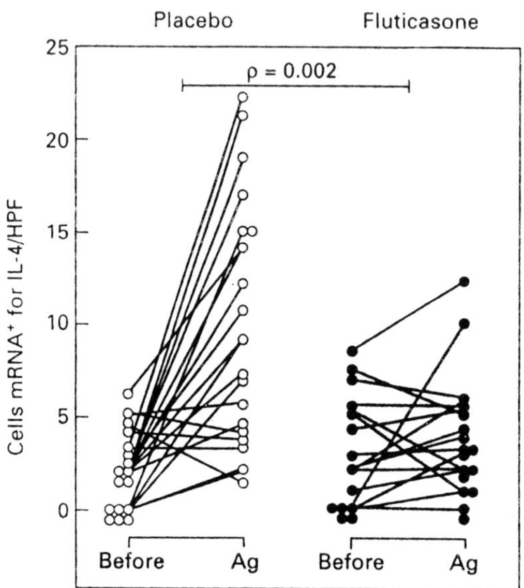

Figure 6 Effect of fluticasone on the number of cells in the nasal mucosa expressing mRNA for IL-4. Data are shown from baseline (before) and at 24 hours after allergen challenge (Ag) following 6-week treatment with fluticasone (closed circles) or placebo (open circles). (From Ref. 177.)

shown CS-induced inhibition of cytokine gene expression and release (59), it is tempting to speculate that CSs, in particular when applied topically, may inhibit this upregulation of the allergy-promoting cytokine, IL-3, and as a consequence inhibit Th2 cell formation, IgE isotype switching of B cells, and the synthesis of IgE antibody. In favor of this hypothesis Naclerio and co-workers (60) in two studies found that intranasal CS treatment during the pollen season inhibits the allergen-induced increase of specific IgE antibody in plasma. Furthermore, Karlsson et al. (61), using a sensitive reverse-transcriptase polymerase chain reaction for the demonstration of IL-4 in nasal tissues, have recently shown an upregulation of this allergy-associated cytokine during allergen challenge and exposure, and an inhibitory effect of topical CSs.

   In summary, CSs have multiple effects on the inflammatory effects associated with allergic rhinitis. This multiplicity of events probably explains their tremendous clinical utility.

III. Clinical Usage of Corticosteroids

Hydrocortisone is the parent molecule from which natural and synthetic CSs are derived (Figs. 7 and 8). The structure-activity relationships of the CS molecule have been intensively investigated. The lipophilic nature of CSs permits rapid absorption across mucosal surfaces. Systemically absorbed CSs bind to plasma proteins and undergo metabolism in the liver before being excreted in the urine. Their action on individual cells begins when the free CS molecule diffuses across the cell membrane and binds to steroid receptors within the cytoplasm of the cell. The complex interacts with the nucleus to eventually form messenger RNA transcripts. The posttranscriptional proteins then mediate drug effects. The need for transcription and translation accounts for the time delay between administration and clinical activity.

The CS molecules that are widely used today for intranasal treatment are beclomethasone dipropionate, flunisolide, budesonide, fluticasone propionate, and triamcinolone acetonide (62–65).

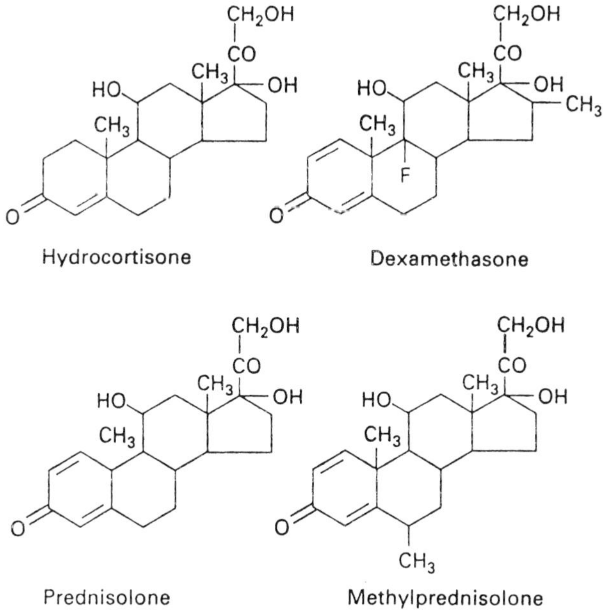

Figure 7 Chemical structures of some important corticosteroids for systemic use.

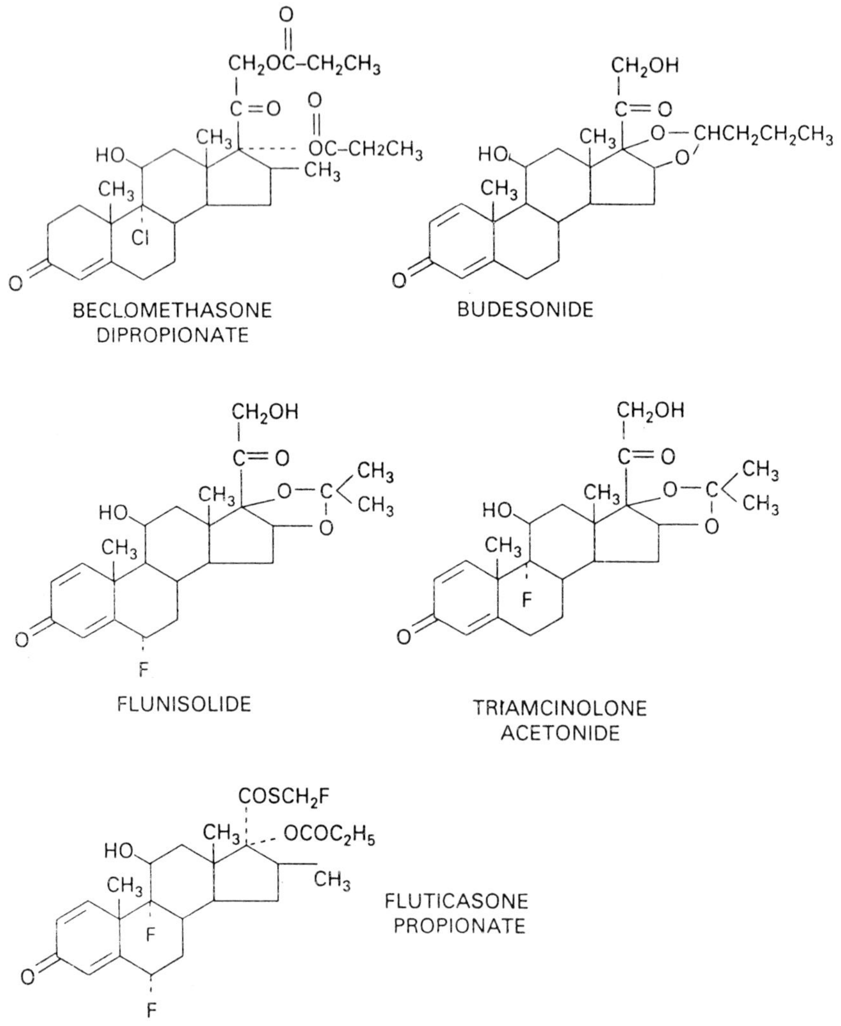

Figure 8 Chemical structures of some important corticosteroids for topical application. They are ester derivatives of hydrocortisone. The ester side chains are readily cleaved in the liver following absorption and this dramatically reduces systemic effects.

A. Drugs

Dexamethasone

This drug has been used as a nasal spray for many years, and remains on the market in some countries. However, it was shown as early as 1967, by Norman et al. (66), that the recommended therapeutic dosage reduces HPA responsiveness. This results from the lack of first-pass metabolism of the drug in the liver and from its long plasma half-life.

Betamethasone Sodium Phosphate

This drug, which is available in some countries in drop form, also has a small systemic effect when used at the recommended dose. Like dexamethasone it should be replaced by one of the molecules described below. It is claimed to have a beneficial effect on olfaction when used as drops in the head-hanging position.

Betamethasone Valerate

In 1968, Czarny and Brostoff (67) reported promising results with this molecule as a nasal spray. Although it seems to have properties similar to those of beclomethasone dipropionate, it has not been marketed for nasal use except in the United Kingdom.

Beclomethasone Dipropionate (Beclomethasone)

Beclomethasone, which is slightly more potent than betamethasone valerate, has been studied extensively since the first report in 1973 (1). It was marketed in the United Kingdom in 1974 and is now available in more than 100 countries. It is the CS molecule with which we have the longest and most extensive experience in the airways, and it serves as the reference drug for the study of new CSs.

Flunisolide

The first report on intranasal use of this CS appeared in 1976 (68). Like other CS molecules in this group, flunisolide is poorly water-soluble, and it is therefore dissolved in a mixture of polyethylene glycol and propylene glycol; it is delivered as a solution from a metered-dose pump spray. This preparation has been on the market since 1978 and is available in many countries.

Budesonide

Budesonide, a nonhalogenated molecule, is more completely inactivated in the liver than beclomethasone. Whereas beclomethasone has a plasma elimination time of about 15 hr, flunisolide and budesonide have a plasma half-life of about 2 hr. Budesonide was first studied in 1980 (69) and it is now on the market in most countries.

Fluticasone Propionate (Fluticasone)

Fluticasone is a more recently synthesized and extensively tested molecule claimed to have negligible oral bioavailability (70–72). It has been launched in an increasing number of countries.

Triamcinolone Acetonide (Triamcinolone)

Triamcinolone is a well-known CS molecule widely used in dermatology. It has been launched as a pressurized nasal aerosol in the United States and Canada (73), and recently also as an aqueous spray.

Fluocortin Butylester

This molecule is a weak CS with negligible systemic activity. It is delivered as a powder from a special device (74). It is on the market in a few countries.

B. Drug Comparisons

Controlled studies have indicated that flunisolide 200 µg (75,76) has the same antirhinitis effect as the reference molecule beclomethasone 400 µg, indicating a higher potency for flunisolide.

Three studies showed an equal antirhinitis effect of fluticasone 200 µg o.d. and beclomethasone 168 µg b.d. (77,78) and 200 µg b.d. (79), and two other large multicenter studies showed a better effect of fluticasone 200 µg o.d. than of beclomethasone 168 µg b.d. (80) and of fluticasone 200 µg b.d. than of beclomethasone 200 µg b.d. (81). Two studies showed equal efficacy of fluticasone 100 µg o.d. and b.d. and of beclomethasone 200 µg b.d. (82).

Nine open studies (63,83,84) and two double-blind studies (85–87) have shown a higher antirhinitis effect for budesonide 400 µg than for beclomethasone 400 µg, particularly for nasal blockage (Fig. 9). Thus, the two molecules do not seem to be equipotent on a microgram basis. As dose-response curves for the two drugs are not available for comparison, it is not possible to say whether budesonide and beclomethasone differ not only in potency but also in efficacy.

An open comparison of budesonide as a powder (Rhinocort Turbuhaler), 200 µg or 400 µg o.d. (25% retained in the inhaler), and fluticasone aqueous nasal spray (Flixonase), 200 µg o.d., did not reveal any statistically significant differences with regard to efficacy or short-term safety (88).

Triamcinolone is superior to placebo and seems equally effective as beclomethasone (60,89,90).

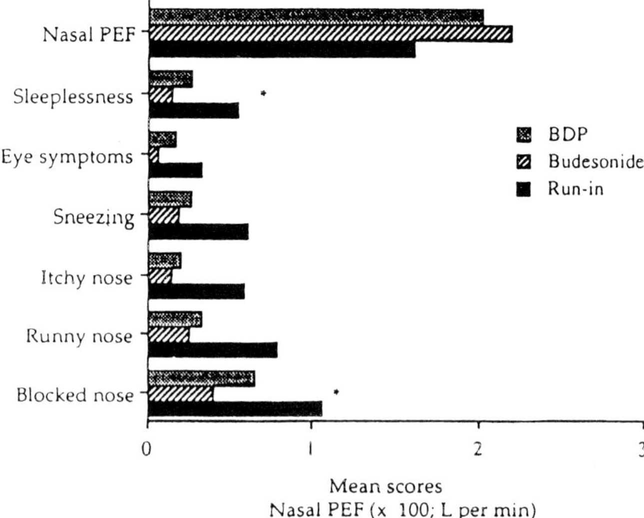

Figure 9 Effect of budesonide and beclomethasone dipropionate treatment on morning symptom scores, sleeplessness score, and nasal peak flow values in patients with perennial rhinitis. *$p < 0.05$ for drug comparisons. Nasal PEF reached a significant value only in the evening. (From Ref. 87.)

With regard to the risk of local side effects, there is no reason to believe that there are significant differences between the aforementioned CS molecules. With respect to systemic CS effects, it has been shown that fluticasone has less systemic activity than beclomethasone when given in equipotent doses (70,91). Nonetheless the more than 20-year experience with beclomethasone has not demonstrated any significant systemic side effects.

In summary, there appear to be only minor differences between beclomethasone, flunisolide, budesonide, fluticasone, and triamcinolone with regard to efficacy and safety.

C. Topical Versus Systemic Mode of Action

There is no doubt that the modern CS sprays exert their antirhinitis effect by a local, not systemic, mode of action. Convincing clinical proof comes from the marked effect on nasal symptoms in hay fever (seasonal allergic rhinitis), together with the absence or negligible effect on eye symptoms (Fig. 10). Definite proof of topical activity has been provided for flunisolide and budesonide, which were given intranasally and orally in double-blind trials, with only nasal application having an antirhinitis effect (92,93) (Fig. 11).

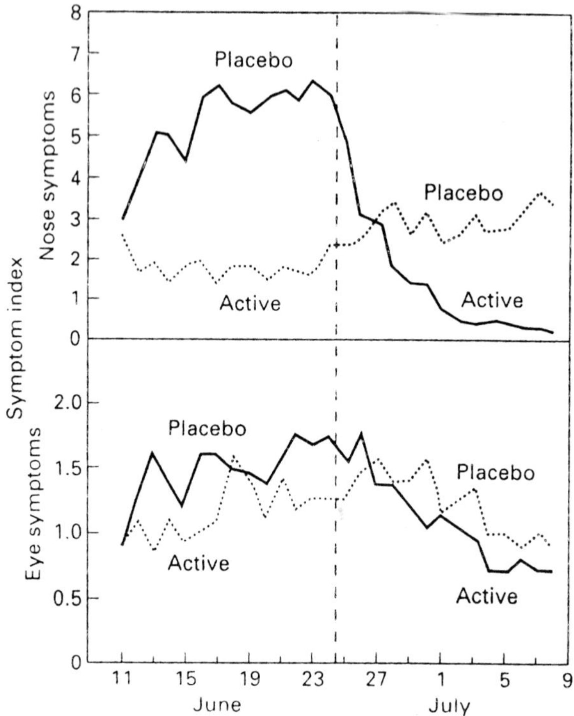

Figure 10 The marked effect of intranasal corticosteroid (beclomethasone) on nasal symptoms as compared to eye symptoms is good indirect evidence for a local mode of action. (From Ref. 1.)

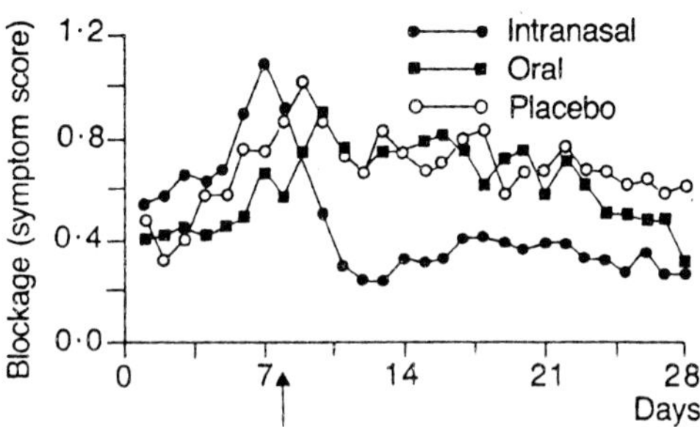

Figure 11 While intranasal budesonide 400 µg/day has a marked antirhinitis effect, a similar dose given orally has no effect, showing that a local application is essential. (From Ref. 93.)

It was previously believed that the difference between topical and systemic activity was due to a lack of absorption from the nose, but it is now evident that these molecules are readily absorbed from the mucous membrane. The lack of systemic effect is due rather to the rapid hepatic metabolism and short plasma half-life.

D. Delivery Systems

The poor water solubility of topical CS molecules led to their introduction as CFC- or Freon-propelled pressurized aerosols. Although such sprays were easy to use, the high linear velocity of the aerosol close to the nozzle resulted in a poor drug distribution in the nasal cavity (94–96). The drug simply hits the mucous membrane ''like a bullet from a gun.'' Theoretically, it is less than ideal that the bulk of such potent drugs should be deposited in a small area at the front of the nose. In particular, the previously used U.S. type of beclomethasone spray with a 3-mm nozzle resulted in major drug deposition in the skin-covered vestibule. As local side effects from CSs are well known from dermatology, it is astonishing that they have not occurred in the nostril.

Flunisolide is dissolved in polyethylene glycol and propylene glycol, and can therefore be delivered from a metered-dose pump spray, but this solution causes some immediate stinging. Beclomethasone, budesonide, and fluticasone are available as aqueous suspensions, also delivered from pump sprays. This type of delivery system gives a better intranasal distribution than a pressurized aerosol (94–96). However, the preservative (benzalkonium chloride not in budesonide spray) is known to inhibit ciliary activity (97,98). It has been questioned whether this in vitro finding has any significance for continuous treatment in vivo. Benzalkonium chloride, in topical adrenergic agents, contributes to the development of the symptoms of rhinitis medicamentosa (99) indicating that continuous use of this preservative might contribute to morbidity. The solvent used for flunisolide causes even greater inhibition of ciliary beat frequency (100).

CSs delivered from pressurized aerosols and aqueous pump sprays seem to produce an equivalent degree of symptom reduction (101,102).

Newman et al. (96) have shown that only a part of the drug delivered to the nose actually reaches the ciliated mucous membrane. This portion is about 50% for aqueous pump sprays and may be as little as 20% for pressurized aerosols. The 80% of the drug from a pressurized aerosol deposited in the nonciliated anterior part of the nose may be lost, but it is also possible that some of the drug is subsequently carried to the ciliated epithelium, thus serving as a depot. Another intranasal medication, ipratropium bromide, has a longer-lasting effect when given from a pressurized aerosol as compared with an aqueous pump spray (103).

In recent years a pure powder formulation of budesonide, delivered from a multidose device, has become available (104,105). It is equally effective as the pressurized aerosol (104) and causes little immediate irritation. This formulation has the advantage of not containing Freon, preservatives, lubricants, or carrier powder. A relatively large proportion of the drug is retained in the nozzle of the device (mean 26%) and children seem to have difficulty in creating sufficient inspiratory flow to inhale enough powder for therapeutic efficacy (107). A small amount (mean 4.7%) passes through the nasal cavity and reaches the lower airways (106), which might be clinically beneficial in rhinitis patients with concurrent bronchial hyperreactivity and mild asthma.

Little information is available on the bioavailability and efficacy of single doses delivered by aerosols, pump sprays, and powder devices or how these delivery systems relate to inspiratory flow rate, degree of nasal blockage, and quantity of intranasal secretion (106,108). Despite this lack of knowledge they are highly effective clinically in controlling rhinitis symptoms. Possibly, new delivery systems, providing a more efficient deposition in the olfactory region and the osto-meatal complex, can improve the effect of topical CSs on anosmia and sinusitis symptoms.

E. Dosage

In clinical practice an adult dose of 200–400 µg/day is given, with half the dose in children (109). In recent years, asthma research has shown that the previously used standard dose (400 µg/day) is insufficient in severe cases, and a clear dose-response relationship has been demonstrated. Consequently, high-dose therapy is now widely used in the lower airways. However, in rhinitis, the results are less clear from the few dose-response studies that have been performed. A study of seasonal allergic rhinitis showed insignificant differences in symptomatic relief when fluticasone 50 µg was compared with 800 µg/day, although only the high dose increased nasal airflow (32). In children with hay fever there was no difference between fluticasone 100 µg and 200 µg daily (110). In two studies of patients with severe hay fever fluticasone 200 µg b.d. was significantly more effective than 200 µg o.d. (111,112). In perennial rhinitis, beclomethasone 800 µg was significantly better than 200 µg, but only for one effect indicator (113). In another study of perennial rhinitis, there was a tendency for a better effect from budesonide 800 µg than from 400 µg (114), and a study of fluticasone showed equal efficacy of 200 µg o.d. and b.d. (79). In nasal polyposis budesonide powder at doses of 400 and 800 µg/day was equally effective (115), but 200 µg was less effective than 400 µg in hay fever (104).

In conclusion, the dose-response curve for topical CSs is less well defined and probably flatter in rhinitis than in asthma. Therefore, high-dose therapy cannot in general be recommended for rhinitis, but a higher-than-normal dose may be tried for a shorter period in patients with severe symptoms and insufficient response to an ordinary dose.

F. Application Frequency

It is unclear why, on introduction, beclomethasone was prescribed on a four times daily regimen. Over the succeeding years this frequency was reduced to twice daily and most recently a number of controlled studies have convincingly shown that once-daily application is sufficient in the majority of patients (72,78,79, 82,116–118). Most of these studies are undertaken with fluticasone, but there does not seem to be any difference between CS molecules with regard to the applicability of a once-daily regimen.

It is possible, however, that some patients with severe symptoms need not only a higher dose but also twice-daily administration during periods with massive allergen exposure and severe symptoms (111,112).

G. Patient Instruction

Careful patient instruction is important for therapeutic success. Patients must be taught the correct usage of the spray, which may vary between the different devices.

To avoid trauma, the nozzle of a pressurized aerosol should be positioned in the sagittal plane and not be pointed toward the septal wall. Intranasal drug distribution will be improved by giving one puff toward the upper and one toward the lower part of the nose. The high linear velocity of the aerosol renders coordinated actuation and inhalation of little importance. When a pump spray is used, it is necessary to coordinate the actuation with a short sniff to obtain good intranasal distribution. With a powder device coordination is not required but a short inhalation is necessary for delivery and distribution of the drug.

Obviously the nasal airway should be as open and clear as possible prior to instillation of medication. The patient should, if appropriate, start by blowing the nose. In chronic nasal obstruction, a short course of systemic CS, or a topical decongestant, may be helpful to improve patency and instillation of topical medication (119). Patients should be told that immediate relief cannot be expected from a CS spray in contrast to the use of a vasoconstrictor. In seasonal allergic rhinitis, it will take some days before the full beneficial results of topical CSs can be expected. In chronic rhinitis it may take some weeks before the effectiveness of the spray can be evaluated.

It is also important that the spray be used regularly and not on an ad hoc basis. Once the maximal benefit is achieved, the dosage can in some patients be tapered down to 200 or even 100 µg/day. To determine whether continued therapy is required patients can be asked to discontinue the spray for short periods during a year. If the disease is still active, symptoms will recur, but in some patients it can take several weeks for this to manifest due to the prolonged action of the CS. This makes many patients doubt whether there is a cause-and-effect relationship between spraying and improvement in their disease.

H. Efficacy

Modern topical CSs are highly effective in the treatment of seasonal and perennial allergic rhinitis, perennial nonallergic rhinitis, and nasal polyposis, in both adults and children. With only one exception, all 95 placebo-controlled studies published have shown a significantly better effect with intranasal CS than from placebo: an impressive record, which is not matched by many other therapies in medicine.

I. Comparison with Other Treatments

A modern CS spray is definitely more effective in allergic rhinitis than sodium cromoglycate (120). In comparison with systemic and topical antihistamines, most (121–132), but not all (133–137), double-blind studies in allergic rhinitis show the CS spray to be more effective, especially for nasal blockage (Fig. 12).

J. Combined Therapy

A CS spray can further reduce nasal symptoms when it is combined with an antihistamine (138). Conversely, studies have failed to show increased efficacy when an antihistamine is given to patients on topical steroids (126,129,139) and

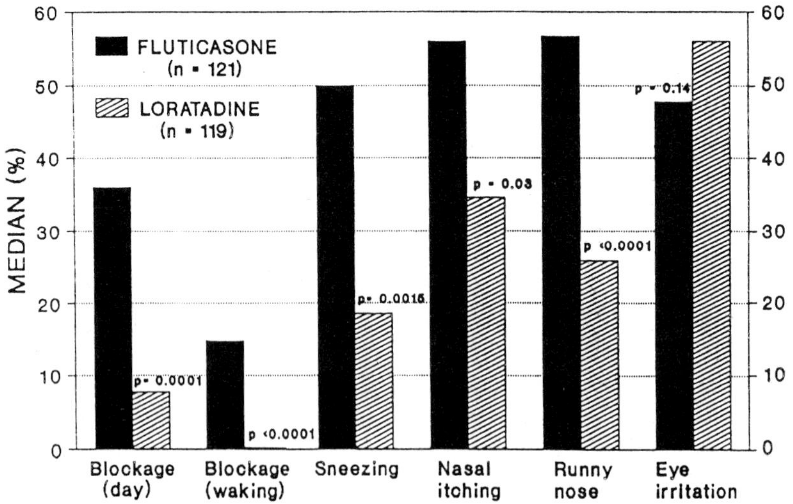

Figure 12 Median percentage of symptom-free days. Fluticasone has significantly higher percentages of symptom-free days than loratadine for all nasal symptoms scored. No difference was found for eye symptoms. (From Ref. 131.)

consequently the addition of an antihistamine to a current treatment with intranasal CSs will add to the cost without giving added benefit.

It is generally believed, but not proven, that systemic CSs can add to the efficacy of topical treatment in severe disease. At least, a short course of systemic CSs may improve the responsiveness to topical treatment by opening up a blocked nasal airway.

K. Seasonal Allergic Rhinitis

More than 50 studies have shown that topical CSs are highly effective in hay fever, with therapeutic results ranging from good to excellent in 70–90% of the patients (1,68,140,141). With this high degree of efficacy and the limited length of time requiring therapy in seasonal allergic rhinitis, one should have no hesitation in using this treatment modality as the first-line, when anything other than occasional antihistamines is contemplated (2).

In highly sensitive patients, on a recommended dose of nasal CS, there can be breakthrough of symptoms when the pollen count is high. A short course of systemic CS is often useful, although its additional benefit has not been quantified. It is possible that increasing the dosage of topical steroids may be equally sufficient. It is also important to inform patients that concomitant use of noncorticosteroid eyedrops may be required. Interestingly, a nasal CS spray can have a beneficial effect on cough, and also on bronchial reactivity and asthma symptoms (119,142–146).

L. Perennial Rhinitis

It is more difficult to treat perennial rhinitis than simple hay fever. Tarlo et al. (147) found that only 54% of patients with perennial allergic and nonallergic rhinitis achieved acceptable symptomatic improvement from a CS spray, but after administration of short-term oral prednisone, 73% of patients obtained moderate or marked symptomatic improvement from topical treatment. In severe cases, it is thus advisable to make a therapeutic trial with short-term systemic CSs, when the effect of a nasal CS is insufficient.

In patients suffering from perennial nonallergic rhinitis, CSs also offer an effective form of control of nasal symptoms in most, but not all, cases (69,147–150). The presence of eosinophils in a nasal smear before treatment suggests a degree of CS responsiveness in terms of symptomatic relief (69,151,152). However, the absence of these cells does not preclude a therapeutic trial as the methodology to detect eosinophils in nasal smears is poorly standardized (153).

M. Nasal Polyps

The precise etiology of nasal polyps is unclear. Eosinophils are commonly found in polyps, but the association with allergy appears to be coincidental (154,155).

Topical CS treatment reduces nasal symptoms, polyp size (115,156–159) (Figs. 13 and 14), and the number of recurrences after polypectomy, especially in patients who have previously been subjected to frequent polypectomies (159–162) (Fig. 15). Consequently, the use of CSs both before and following surgical removal of the polyps should be encouraged. Symptoms may be exacerbated by viral and bacterial upper respiratory tract infection. A short-term course of systemic steroids may help combat obstruction and improve intranasal spray distribution, and it does not increase the severity of the infection. Loss of the sense of smell can be an annoying symptom for many patients with nasal polyposis, and although this may improve following surgery and the use of systemic CSs, the long-term results with topical treatment are often disappointing.

Management of patients with severe polyposis is still unsatisfactory but it can be improved by the combination of long-term topical CSs, short-term systemic CSs, and surgery (159).

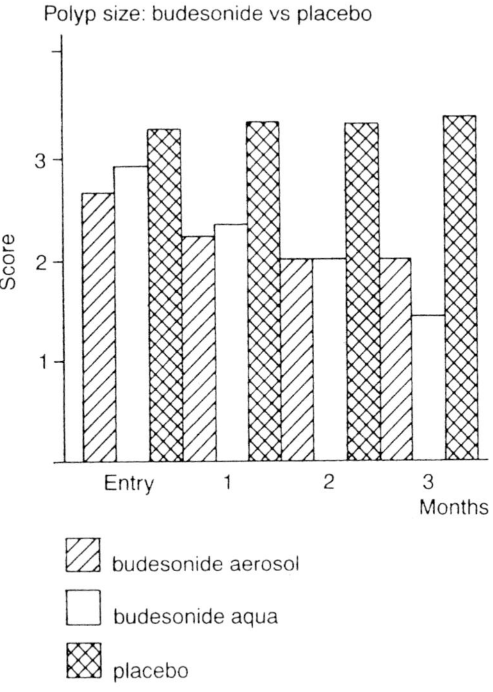

Figure 13 Mean polyp score in 86 patients before and after 3 months of treatment with budesonide aerosol 400 µg/day, budesonide aqua 400 µg/day, or placebo. (From Ref. 102.)

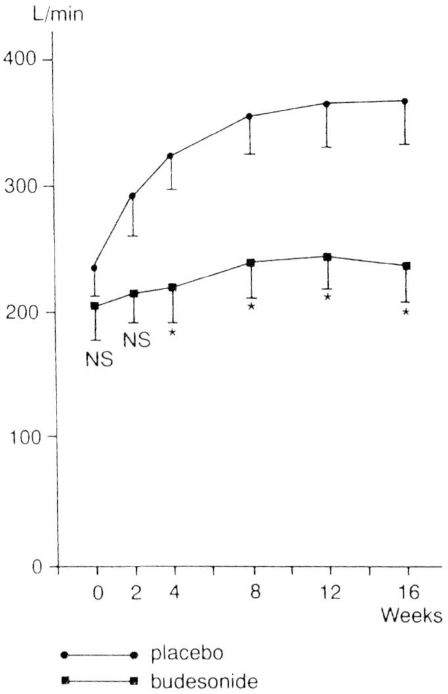

Figure 14 Effect of nasal steroid on nasal peak flow in patients with nasal polyposis (mean and SEM; $*p < 0.05$). (From Ref. 157.)

N. Infectious Rhinitis

The effect of topical CSs alone is marginal in infectious rhinitis (163) and sinus-itis (164), while there is a report on a beneficial effect of a CS preparation containing neomycyin on mucopurulent discharge in chronic rhinosinusitis (165). At present, such preparations have no place in clinical practice. CSs are highly effective in eosinophil-dominated inflammation and allergy but not in neutrophil-dominated inflammation and infection.

O. Treatment of Children

The principles of treatment of allergic rhinitis in children are the same as those in the adult, though the emphasis may differ somewhat. Prophylactic measures of allergen avoidance assume a greater importance in children than in adults. In preschool children it may be difficult to administer topical medication due to lack of cooperation, and oral antihistamines are then the primary agents. However, in

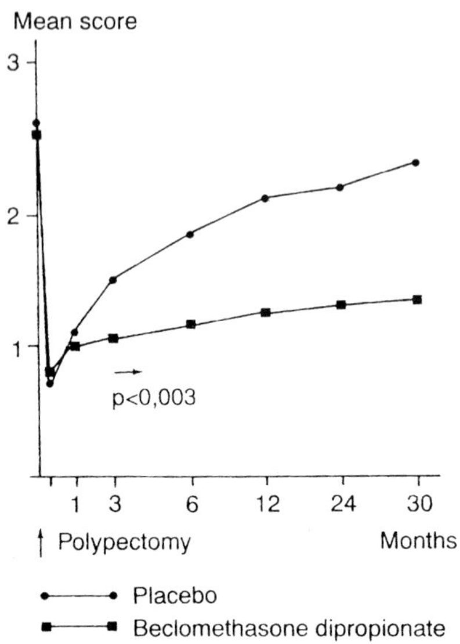

Figure 15   Mean nasal symptom scores before and after polypectomy in 20 patients receiving long-term therapy with beclomethasone dipropionate and in 20 untreated patients. (From Ref. 162.)

a multicenter study it was possible to treat even 4-year-old children with an aqueous spray (166).

Some physicians are reluctant to prescribe topical nasal CSs in children because of concerns about the long-term systemic and local adverse effects of these drugs. However, after more than 20 years' experience with topical nasal CSs there have been virtually no adverse reports and these agents may, therefore, be used at the prescribed dosage (generally half of the adult dose preferably given once daily in the morning), particularly where nasal obstruction is the most pronounced symptom (2) (Table 2). However, the clinician should consider all

Table 2   Safe Use of Intranasal Corticosteroids for Perennial Rhinitis in Children

Allergen avoidance carried out
Antihistamine (and cromoglycate) tried and found inadequate
Daily symptoms of significance for the child
The daily dose as low as possible (maximum 200 μg/day)
Medication given once in the morning
Spraying supervised by an adult
Regular checks

the possible differential diagnoses that may result in long-term nasal symptoms, undertaking a careful history and examination and other investigations as appropriate prior to starting medication.

P. Treatment in Pregnancy

Animal studies have suggested that CSs may have adverse effects on the developing fetus particularly with respect to cleft palate development. The association between systemic CSs and this developmental abnormality in humans is less definite and a large body of clinical data during the past 30 years has not confirmed the concerns generated by the animal studies (167). Though this controversy persists about systemic CSs, topical use of nasal CSs, particularly after the first trimester, is not contraindicated as it has not been associated with any teratogenic or adverse effects. However, as there are no adequate and well-controlled studies in pregnant women, the treatment should be used only if the expected benefit justifies the potential risk to the fetus.

Q. Side Effects

Discomfort and Irritation

When a topical CS is first instilled into a hyperreactive nose it can result in some sneezing. Patients should be encouraged to continue spraying, as this symptom usually disappears after some days (44). It is more a symptom of the disease than a true side effect. This does not apply to the immediate stinging experienced with flunisolide.

Dryness, Crusting, Epistaxis, and Septal Perforation

A sensation of dryness in the nostril, associated with slight blood staining and crusts, is frequently encountered, but it does not seem to worsen during long-term treatment. Rarely, treatment has to be temporarily stopped because of epistaxis. Usually, patients can continue therapy, if they change from a pressurized aerosol to an aqueous spray or a powder, reduce the dosage, medicate only once daily (78,118), and use a neutral ointment, e.g., petroleum jelly, on the nasal septum on a regular basis.

There are case reports of septal perforation after intranasal CS therapy (168). It is difficult to exclude other causes of the perforation such as direct mechanical trauma, but it seems to be a genuine adverse effect from intranasal CSs, probably the pressurized aerosols in particular. However, the risk appears to be small, as these sprays have now been in use since 1974, accumulating many million patient-years. It is advisable to do rhinoscopy routinely before starting long-term treatment of perennial rhinitis, and in children, to repeat the examination at regular intervals. Also, tell the patient to return for examination if frequent bleeding or crusting develops.

Risk of Atrophic Rhinitis

When CS sprays were first introduced, there was considerable concern about the risk of mucosal atrophy, based on the experience with CS treatment of the skin. However, extensive long-term clinical experience and a number of biopsy studies (169–171) have not indicated that such a risk exists in the nose (or in the bronchi treated with orally inhaled CSs).

There are two possible explanations of the striking difference between skin and airway mucosa with regard to the risk of atrophy. The first is that the CS molecule applied on the skin as an ointment or cream remains in situ for more than 24 hr, whereas it is removed by mucociliary clearance within a few hours from the airway mucosa. The second is that collagen fibers in the airways seem to be more resistant than those in the skin to the catabolic effect of CSs (172). It is in favor of this statement that Cushing's disease and long-term oral CS treatment result in skin atrophy, but do not adversely affect the airways.

Risk of Infectious Rhinosinusitis

There is no evidence that topical CS treatment can increase the frequency or the severity of viral or bacterial infections in the nose or paranasal sinuses, and CS-induced nasal candidiasis has apparently not been described.

Risk of Systemic Side Effects

Long-term intranasal treatment of adults with 200–400 µg/day of beclomethasone, flunisolide, budesonide, and fluticasone has shown that the risk of systemic CS adverse effects is small.

There is a single case report of posterior subcapsular cataract after intranasal CS use (173), but it may be coincidental and not causal (174). A cross-sectional study with slit-lamp examination of 95 children who had inhaled CSs in an average dosage of 750 µg/day for 5 years failed to show any cases of posterior subcapsular cataract (174).

Recent data indicate that children receiving an adult dose of budesonide (200 µg twice daily) show growth inhibition (175), whereas this is not the case when 200 µg is given once daily in the morning. Although it is too early to judge the clinical significance of these short-term results, obtained with a highly sensitive method (kneemometry), it seems advisable in children to use the lowest dose that can control the symptoms (maximum 200 µg/day), and to give the entire dose in the morning.

There are no reports of the development of osteoporosis in postmenopausal women, but on the other hand, there are no data that definitely can exclude a contributing effect of long-term nasal use of topical CSs.

Even though clinical experience has convincingly shown the risk of systemic adverse effects to be negligible, an ordinary dosage of an intranasal steroid is associated with a downregulation of local as well as systemic glucocorticoid receptors (176).

IV. Conclusions

The introduction of nasal CSs more than 20 years ago has been the most important therapeutic progress in rhinitis management. Our knowledge of the mode of action of CSs is still incomplete although a series of intranasal studies have shown multiple effects on the immune inflammatory reaction. Nasal CSs are a highly effective therapeutic modality for long-term therapy of allergic rhinitis, perennial nonallergic rhinitis, and nasal polyposis. Experience since 1973 has shown that the side effects from this type of treatment are negligible and far less serious than those occurring in the skin following long-term use of CS ointment. Intranasal CSs can therefore be considered as first-line treatment for allergic rhinitis, nonallergic rhinitis, and nasal polyposis. The major disadvantage of this type of treatment is the slow onset of action and the lack of effect on itchy eyes. While the second generation H_1 antihistamines are the drugs of choice in patients having occasional symptoms, intranasal CSs are, in our opinion, preferable in patients having daily rhinitis symptoms.

References

1. Mygind N. Local effect of intranasal beclomethasone dipropionate aerosol in hay fever. Br Med J 1973; 4:464–466.
2. Lund VJ. International consensus report on the diagnosis and management of rhinitis. Allergy 1994; 49(Suppl 19):1–34.
3. Pepys J, Hutchroft BJ. Bronchial provocation tests in etiologic diagnosis and analysis of asthma. Am Rev Respir Dis 1975; 112:928–959.
4. Vilsviik JS, Jenssen AO, Walstad R. The effect of beclomethasone dipropionate aerosol on allergen induced nasal stenosis. Clin Allergy 1975; 5:291–294.
5. Okuda M, Senba O. Effect of beclomethasone dipropionate nasal spray on subjective and objective findings in perennial rhinitis. Clin Otolaryngol 1980; 53:15–21.
6. Horak F, Matthew H. The protective action of fluocortin butylester (FCB) in the nasal antigen provocation test: a controlled double-blind crossover study. Ann Allergy 1982; 48:305.
7. Pipkorn U. Budesonide and nasal allergen challenge testing in man. Allergy 1982; 37:129–134.

8. Pipkorn U, Proud D, Schleimer RP, et al. Effects of short term systemic glucocorticoid treatment on human nasal mediator release after antigen challenge. J Clin Invest 1987; 80:957–961.

9. Pipkorn U, Proud D, Lichtenstein LM, Kagey-Sobotka A, Norman PS, Naclerio RM. Inhibition of mediator release in allergic rhinitis by pretreatment with topical glucocorticosteroids. N Engl J Med 1987; 316:1506–1510.

10. Scadding GK, Darby YC, Austin CE. Effect of short-term treatment with fluticasone propionate nasal spray on the response to nasal allergen challenge. Br J Clin Pharmacol 1994; 38:447–451.

11. Konno A, Yamakoshi T, Terada N, Fujita Y. Mode of action of a topical steroid on immediate phase reaction after antigen challenge and nonspecific hyperreactivity in nasal allergy. Int Arch Allergy Immunol 1994; 193:79–87.

12. de Graaf-in 't Veld C, Garrels IM, Jansen APH, et al. Effect of intranasal fluticasone on the immediate and late allergic reaction and nasal hyperreactivity in patients with a house dust mite allergy. Clin Exp Allergy 1995; 25:966–973.

13. Grønborg H, Bisgaard H, Rømeling F, Lindqvist N, Mygind N. Nasal symptom response to allergen provocation: effect of the glucocorticoid budesonide. Allergy 1993; 48:87–93.

14. Dahl R, Johansson S-Å. Importance of duration of treatment with inhaled budesonide on the immediate and late bronchial reaction. Eur J Respir Dis 1982; 63(Suppl 122):167–175.

15. Pipkorn U. Budesonide and nasal histamine challenge. Allergy 1982; 37: 359–363.

16. Pipkorn U. Effect of topical glucocorticoid treatment on nasal mucosal mast cells in allergic rhinitis. Allergy 1983; 38:125–129.

17. Pipkorn U, Andersson P. Budesonide and nasal mucosal histamine content and anti-IgE induced histamine release. Allergy 1982; 37:591–595.

18. Lindqvist N, Holmberg K, Pipkorn U. Intranasally administered budesonide, a glucocorticoid, does not exert its clinical effect through vasoconstriction. Clin Otolaryngol 1989; 14:519–523.

19. Bende M, Lindqvist N, Pipkorn U. The effect of a topical steroid, budesonide, on nasal mucosal blood flow as measured with ^{133}Xe wash-out technique. Allergy 1983; 38:461–464.

20. Baumgarten CR, Togias A, Naclerio RM, Norman PS, Lichtenstein LM, Proud D. Kininogens are generated following nasal challenge with allergen in aller-jygen individuals but not in non-allergic individuals. J Clin Invest 1985; 76:191–197.

21. Proud D, Togias A, Naclerio RM, Crush S, Norman PS, Lichtenstein LM. Kinins are generated in-vivo following nasal airway challenge of allergic individuals with allergen. J Clin Invest 1983; 72:1678–1685.

22. Sørensen H, Mygind N, Pedersen CB, Prytz S. Long term treatment of nasal polyps with beclomethasone dipropionate aerosol III. Acta Otolaryngol (Stockh) 1976; 82: 260–262.

23. Svensson C, Klementsson H, Andersson M, Pipkorn U, Alkner U, Persson CGA. Glucocorticoid-induced attenuation of mucosal exudation of fibrinogen and bradykinins in seasonal allergic rhinitis. Allergy 1994; 49:177–183.

24. Bascom R, Wachs M, Naclerio RM, Pipkorn U, Galli S, Lichtenstein LM. Basophil

influx occurs after nasal antigen challenge: effects of topical corticosteroid pretreatment. J Allergy Clin Immunol 1988; 81:580–589.

25. Naclerio RM. Inflammation in allergic rhinitis. Res Clin Forums 1992; 14(3):49–55.

26. Okuda M, Othsuka H, Sakaguchi K, Ohnishi M, Okubo K. Effect of anti-allergic treatment on nasal surface basophilic metachromatic cells in allergic rhinitis. Allergy Proc 1989; 10:23–26.

27. Bascom R, Pipkorn U, Lichtenstein LM, Naclerio RM. The influx of inflammatory cells into nasal washings during the late response to antigen challenge. Effect of systemic corticosteroids. Am Rev Respir Dis 1988; 138:406–412.

28. Andersson M, Andersson P, Venge P, Pipkorn U. Eosinophils and eosinophil cationic protein (ECP) in nasal lavages during allergen-induced hyperresponsiveness. Effect of topical glucocorticosteroid treatment. Allergy 1989; 44:342–348.

29. Gomez E, Clague J, Gatland D, Davies R. Effect of topical corticosteroids on seasonally induced increase in nasal mast cells. Br Med J 1988; 246:1572–1573.

30. Otsuka H, Denburg JA, Befus AD, et al. Effect of beclomethasone dipropionate on nasal metachromatic cell sub-population. Clin Allergy 1986; 16:589–595.

31. Pipkorn U, Enerbäck L. Nasal mucosal mast cells and histamine in hay fever: effect of topical glucocorticoid treatment. Int Arch Allergy Appl Immunol 1987; 84:123–128.

32. Meltzer EO, Orgel HA, Bronshy EA, et al. A dose-ranging study of fluticasone propionate aqueous nasal spray for seasonal allergic rhinitis assessed by symptoms, rhinomanometry, and nasal cytology. J Allergy Clin Immunol 1990; 86:221–230.

33. Meltzer EO, Orgel HA, Rogenes PR, Field EA. Nasal cytology in patients with allergic rhinitis: effects of intranasal fluticasone propionate. J Allergy Clin Immunol 1994; 94:708–715.

34. Bradding P, Feather IH, Wilson S, Holgate ST, Howarth PH. Cytokine immunoreactivity in seasonal rhinitis: regulation by a topical corticosteroid. Am J Respir Crit Care Med 1995; 151:1900–1906.

35. Juliusson S, Aldenborg F, Enerbäck L. Protease content of mast cells of nasal mucosa: effects of natural allergen exposure and of local corticosteroid treatment. Allergy 1995; 50:15–22.

36. Bascom R, Wachs M, Naclerio RM, Pipkorn U, Galli S, Lichtenstein LM. Basophil influx occurs after nasal antigen challenge: effects of topical corticosteroid pretreatment. J Allergy Clin Immunol 1988; 81:580–589.

37. Bisgaard H, Grønborg H, Mygind N, Dahl R, Venge P. Allergen-induced increase of eosinophil cationic protein in nasal lavage fluid: effect of the glucocorticoid budesonide. J Allergy Clin Immunol 1990; 85:891–895.

38. Klementsson H, Svensson C, Andersson M, Venge P, Pipkorn U, Persson CG. Eosinophils, secretory responsiveness and glucocorticoid-induced effects on the nasal mucosa during a weak pollen season. Clin Exp Allergy 1991; 21:705–710.

39. Andersson M, Andersson P, Pipkorn U. Allergen-induced specific and non-specific nasal hyperreactivity. Reciprocal relationship and inhibition by topical glucocorticosteroids. Acta Oto-laryngol (Stockh) 1989; 107:270–277.

40. Andersson M, Andersson P, Pipkorn U. Topical glucocorticosteroids and allergen-

induced increase in nasal reactivity. Relationship between treatment time and inhibitory effect. J Allergy Clin Immunol 1988; 82:1019–1026.

41. Baroody F, Lichtenstein LM, Kagey-Sobotka A, Proud D, Naclerio RM. Topical steroids inhibit antigen-induced nasal hyperreactivity to histamine. J Allergy Clin Immunol 1989; 82:163 (abstract).

42. Ryan G, Latimer KM, Juniper EF, Roberts RS, Hargreave FE. Effect of beclomethasone dipropionate on bronchial responsiveness to histamine in controlled nonsteroid-dependent asthma. J Allergy Clin Immunol 1985; 75:25–30.

43. Malm L, Wihl J-Å, Lamm CJ, Lindqvist N. Reduction of methacholine induced nasal secretions by the treatment with a new topical steroid in perennial non-allergic rhinitis. Allergy 1982; 36:209–214.

44. Toft A, Wihl J-Å, Toxman J, Mygind N. Double-blind comparison between beclomethasone dipropionate as aerosol and as powder in patients with nasal polyposis. Clin Allergy 1982; 12:391–401.

45. van Wijk RG. Nasal hyperresponsiveness to histamine, methacholine and phentolamine in allergic rhinitis patients and controls. Clin Allergy 1987; 17:563–570.

46. Birchall MA, Henderson JC, Studham JM, Phillips I, Pride NB, Fuller RW. The effect of topical fluticasone propionate on intranasal histamine challenge in subjects with perennial allergic rhinitis. Clin Otolaryngol 1995; 20:204–210.

47. Holm AF, Fokkens WJ, Godthelp T, Mulder PGH, Vroom TM, Rijntjes E. Effect of 3 months' nasal steroid therapy on nasal T cells and Langerhans cells in patients suffering from allergic rhinitis. Allergy 1995; 50:204–209.

48. Godthelp T, Holm AF, Blom H, Klein-Jan A, Rijntes E, Fokkens WJ. The effect of fluticasone propionate aqueous nasal spray on nasal mucosal inflammation in perennial allergic rhinitis. Allergy 1995; 50(Suppl 23):21–24.

49. Kay AB. Asthma and inflammation. J Allergy Clin Immunol 1991; 87:893–910.

50. Rak S, Jacobson MR, Sudderick RM, Masuyama K, Kay AB, Hamid Q, Löwhagen O, Durham SR. Influence of prolonged treatment with topical corticosteroid (fluticasone propionate) on early and late phase nasal responses and cellular infiltration in the nasal mucosa after allergen challenge. Clin Exp Allergy 1994; 24:930–939.

51. Masuyama K, Rak S, Jacobson MR, Löwhagen O, Hamid Q, Durham SR. Rhinitis at the cellular level. Eur Respir Rev 1994; 4:252–255.

52. Bradding P, Feather IH, Wilson S, Holgate ST, Howarth PH. Cytokine immunoreactivity in seasonal rhinitis: regulation by a topical corticosteroid. Am J Respir Crit Care Med 1995; 151:1900–1906.

53. Kanai N, Denburg JA, Evans S, Conway M, Jordana M, Dolovich J. Nasal polyp inflammation. Effect of topical nasal steroid. Am J Respir Crit Care Med 1994; 150:1094–1100.

54. Cox G, Ohtoshi T, Vancheri C, Denburg J, Dolovich J, Gauldie J, Jordana M. Promotion of eosinophil survival by human bronchial epithelial cells and its modulation by steroids. Am J Respir Cell Mol Biol 1991; 4:525–531.

55. Mattoli S, Vittori E, Marini M. Corticosteroids downregulate the increased expression off GM-CSF, IL6 and IL8 in bronchial epithelium of asthmatic patients (abstract). J Allergy Clin Immunol 1992; 89:164.

56. Scott P. IL-12: initiation cytokine for cell-mediated immunity. Science 1993; 260:496–497.

57. Holt P. Immune tolerance and protection against allergic sensitization. Allergy 1995; 50(Suppl 25):34–36.

58. Pawankar RU, Okuda M, Hasegawa S, et al. Interleukin-13 expression in the nasal mucosa of perennial allergic rhinitis. Am J Respir Crit Care Med 1995; 152:2059–2067.

59. Mullol J, Xaubet A, Gaya A, et al. Cytokine gene expression and release from epithelial cells. A comparison study between healthy nasal mucosa and nasal polyps. Clin Exp Allergy 1995; 25:607–615.

60. Naclerio RM, Adkinson NF Jr, Creticos PS, Baroody FM, Hamilton RG, Norman PS. Intranasal steroids inhibit seasonal increases in ragweed-specific immunoglobulin E antibodies. J Allergy Clin Immunol 1993; 92:517–521.

61. Karlsson MG, Davidsson A, Viale G, Graziani D, Hellquist HB. Nasal messenger RNA expression of interleukins 2, 4 and 5 in patients with allergic rhinitis. Diagn Mol Pathol 1995; 4:85–92.

62. Brogden RN, Heel RC, Speight TM, Avery GS. Beclomethasone dipropionate. A reappraisal of its pharmacodynamic properties and therapeutic efficacy after a decade of use in asthma and rhinitis. Drugs 1984; 28:99–126.

63. Clissold SP. Rhinitis. In: Barnes PJ, Mygind N, eds. Budesonide: Clinical Experience in Asthma and Rhinitis. Manchester: ADIS Press, 1988:51–64.

64. Pakes GE, Brogden RN, Heel RD, Speight TM, Avery GS. Flunisolide: a review of its pharmacological properties and therapeutic efficacy in rhinitis. Drugs 1980; 19:397–411.

65. Siegel SC. Topical intranasal corticosteroid therapy in rhinitis. J Allergy Clin Immunol 1988; 81:984–991.

66. Norman PS, Winkenwerder WL, Agbayani BF, Migeon CJ. Adrenal function during the use of dexamethasone aerosols in the treatment of ragweed hay fever. J Allergy Clin Immunol 1967; 40:57–61.

67. Czarny D, Brostoff J. Effect of intranasal betamethasone-17-valerate on perennial rhinitis and adrenal function. Lancet 1968; 2:188–190.

68. Turkeltaub PC, Norman PS, Crepea S. Treatment of ragweed hay fever with an intranasal spray containing flunisolide: a new synthetic corticosteroid. J Allergy Clin Immunol 1976; 58:597–606.

69. Balle VH, Pedersen U, Engby B. Allergic perennial and nonallergic vasomotor rhinitis treated with budesonide nasal spray. Rhinology 1980; 18:135–142.

70. Harding SM. The human pharmacology of fluticasone propionate. Respir Med 1990; 84(Suppl A):25–29.

71. Scadding GK, Lund VJ, Holmstrand M, Darby YC. Clinical and physiological effects of fluticasone propionate aqueous nasal spray in the treatment of perennial rhinitis. Rhinology 1991; (Suppl 11):37–43.

72. Dolovich J, Wong AG, Chodirker WB, Drouin MA, Hargreave FE, Hebert J, Knight A, Small P, Yang WH. Multicenter trial of fluticasone propionate aqueous nasal spray in ragweed allergic rhinitis. Ann Allergy 1994; 72:147–153.

73. Findley S, Huber F, Garcia J, Huang L. Efficacy of once-a-day intranasal administration of triamcinolone acetonide in patients with seasonal allergic rhinitis. Ann Allergy 1992; 68:228–232.

74. Orgel HA, Meltzer EO, Bierman CW, et al. Intranasal fluocortin butyl in patients

with perennial rhinitis: a 12-month efficacy and safety study including nasal biopsy. J Allergy Clin Immunol 1991; 88:257–264.

75.   Sahay JN, Chatterjee SS, Engler C. A comparative trial of flunisolide and beclomethasone dipropionate in the treatment of perennial allergic rhinitis. Clin Allergy 1980; 10:65–70.

76.   Welsh PW, Stricker WE, Chu CP, et al. Efficacy of beclomethasone nasal solution, flunisolide and cromolyn in relieving symptoms of ragweed allergy. Mayo Clin Proc 1987; 62:125–134.

77.   Radner PH, Paull BR, Findlay SR, Hampel F, Martin B, Krai KM, Rogenes PR. Fluticasone propionate given once daily is as effective for seasonal allergic rhinitis as beclomethasone dipropionate given twice daily. J Allergy Clin Immunol 1992; 90:285–291.

78.   van As A, Bronsky EA, Dockhorn RJ, Grossman J, Lumry W, Meltzer EO, Seltzer JM, Rogenes PR. Once daily fluticasone propionate is as effective in perennial rhinitis as twice daily beclomethasone dipropionate. J Allergy Clin Immunol 1993; 91:1146–1154.

79.   Scadding GK, Lund VJ, Jacques LA, Richards DH. A placebo-controlled study of fluticasone propionate aqueous nasal spray and beclomethasone dipropionate in perennial rhinitis: efficacy in allergic and non-allergic perennial rhinitis. Clin Exp Allergy 1995; 25:737–743.

80.   LaForce CF, Dockhorn RJ, Findlay SR, Meltzer EO, Nathan RA, Stricker W, Weakley S, Field FA, Rogenes PR. Fluticasone propionate: an effective alternative treatment for seasonal allergic rhinitis in adults and adolescents. J Fam Pract 1994; 38:145–152.

81.   Haye R, Gomez EG. A multicenter study to assess long-term use of fluticasone propionate aqueous nasal spray in comparison with beclomethasone dipropionate aqueous nasal spray in the treatment of perennial rhinitis. Rhinology 1993; 31:169–174.

82.   Davies DH, Milton CM. Fluticasone propionate aqueous nasal spray: a well-tolerated and effective treatment for children with perennial rhinitis. Pediatr Allergy Immunol 1996; 7:35–43.

83.   al Mohaimeid H. A parallel-group comparison of budesonide and beclomethasone dipropionate for the treatment of perennial allergic rhinitis in adults. J Intern Med Res 1993; 21:67–73.

84.   Adamapoulus G, Manolopoulus L, Giotakis I. A comparison of the efficacy and patient acceptability of budesonide and beclomethasone dipropionate aqueous nasal spray in patients with perennial rhinitis. Clin Otolaryngol 1995; 20:340–344.

85.   Vanzieleghem MA, Juniper EF. A comparison of budesonide and beclomethasone dipropionate nasal aerosols in ragweed-induced rhinitis. J Allergy Clin Immunol 1987; 79:887–892.

86.   McArthur JG. A comparison of budesonide and beclomethasone dipropionate sprays in the treatment of seasonal allergic rhinitis. Clin Otolaryngol 1994; 19:537–542.

87.   Basran GS, McGivern DV, Hanley S, Davies D. The efficacy of budesonide and beclomethasone dipropionate delivered via a pressurized metered dose inhaler, in

the treatment of perennial rhinitis: a randomized, double-blind, crossover study. Am J Rhinol 1995; 9:285–290.

88. Andersson M, Berglund R, Greiff L, et al. A comparison of budesonide nasal dry powder with fluticasone propionate aqueous nasal spray in patients with perennial allergic rhinitis. Rhinology 1995; 33:19–22.

89. Storms W, Bronsky E, Findley S, Pearlman D, Rosenberg S, Shapiro GG, et al. Once daily triamcinolone acetonide nasal spray is effective for the treatment of perennial allergic rhinitis. Ann Allergy 1991; 66:329–334.

90. Welch MJ, Bronsky EA, Grossman J, Shapiro GG, Tinkelman DG, Garcia JD, Gillen MS. Clinical evaluation of triamcinolone acetonide nasal aerosol in children with perennial allergic rhinitis. Ann Allergy 1991; 67:493–498.

91. van As A, Bronsky E, Grossman J, Meltzer EO, Ratner P, Reed C. Dose tolerance study of fluticasone propionate aqueous nasal spray in patients with seasonal allergic rhinitis. Ann Allergy 1991; 67:156–162.

92. Kwaselow A, MacLean J, Busse W, et al. A comparison of intranasal and oral flunisolide in the therapy of allergic rhinitis. J Allergy Clin Immunol 1985; 40: 363–367.

93. Lindqvist N, Andersson M, Bende M, Loeth S, Pipkorn U. The clinical efficacy of budesonide in hay fever treatment is dependent on topical nasal application. Clin Exp Allergy 1989; 19:71–76.

94. Hallworth GW, Padfield JM. A comparison of regional deposition in a model nose of a drug discharged from metered aerosol and metered-pump nasal delivery system. J Allergy Clin Immunol 1986; 77:348–353.

95. Mygind N, Vesterhauge S. Aerosol distribution in the nose. Rhinology 1978; 16: 79–88.

96. Newman SP, Moren F, Clarke SW. Deposition pattern from a nasal pump spray. Rhinology 1987; 25:77–82.

97. Batts AH, Marriott C, Martin GP, Bond SW. The effect of some preservatives used in nasal preparations on mucociliary clearance. J Pharm Pharmacol 1989; 41:156–159.

98. Berg ØH, Lie K, Steinvåg SK. The effect of decongestive nosedrops on human respiratory mucosa in vitro. Laryngoscope 1994; 104:1153–1158.

99. Graf P. Long-term use of oxy- and xylometazoline nasal sprays induces rebound swelling, tolerance and nasal hyperreactivity. Rhinology 1996; 34:9–13.

100. Stafanger G. In vitro effect of beclomethasone dipropionate and flunisolide on mobility of human nasal cilia. Allergy 1987; 42:507–511.

101. Orgel HA, Meltzer EO, Kemp JP, Welch MJ. Clinical, rhinomanometric, and cytological evaluation of seasonal allergic rhinitis treated with beclomethasone dipropionate as aqueous nasal spray or pressurized aerosol. J Allergy Clin Immunol 1986; 77:858–864.

102. Johansen LV, Illum P, Kristensen S, Winther L, Petersen SV, Synnerstad B. The effect of budesonide in the treatment of small and medium-sized nasal polyps. Clin Otolaryngol 1993; 18:524–527.

103. Borum S, Becker B, Mygind N, Borum P. Comparison between the effect of ipratropium bromide as a pressurized aerosol and as an aqueous pump spray on methacholine-induced rhinorrhea. Clin Otolaryngol 1997; 22:132–134.

104. Pedersen B, Larsen BB, Dahl R, Lindqvist N, Mygind N. Powder administration of pure budesonide for the treatment of seasonal allergic rhinitis. Allergy 1991; 46: 582–587.

105. Pedersen B, Larsen BB, Dahl R, Hedsby L, Mygind N. Budesonide powder administration for the treatment of grass-pollen-induced allergic rhinitis. Allergy 1994; 49:855–860.

106. Thorsson L, Newman SP, Weiz A, Trofast E, Móren F. Nasal distribution of budesonide inhaled via a powder inhaler. Rhinology 1993; 31:7–10.

107. Agertoft L, Wolthers OD, Fuglsang G, Pedersen S. Nasal powder administration for seasonal rhinitis in children and adolescents. Pediatr Allergy Immunol 1993; 4:152–156.

108. Larsen C, Jørgensen MN, Tommerup B, Mygind N, Dagrosa EE, Grigoleit H-G, Malerczyk V. Influence of experimental rhinitis on the gonadotropin response to intranasal administration of buserelin. Eur J Clin Pharmacol 1987; 33:155–159.

109. Grossman J, Banov C, Bronsky EA, et al. Fluticasone propionate aqueous nasal spray is safe and effective for children with seasonal allergic rhinitis. Pediatrics 1993; 92:594–599.

110. Boner A, Sette L, Martinati L, Sharma RK, Richards DH. The efficacy and tolerability of fluticasone propionate aqueous nasal spray in children with seasonal allergic rhinitis. Allergy 1995; 50:498–505.

111. Pedersen B, Dahl R, Richards DH, et al. Fluticasone propionate aqueous nasal spray controls symptoms of most patients with seasonal allergic rhinitis. Allergy 1995; 50:794–799.

112. Dolovich J, O'Connor M, Stepner N, Smith A, Sharma RK. Double-blind comparison of intranasal fluticasone propionate, 200 µg, once daily with 200 µg twice daily in the treatment of patients with severe seasonal allergic rhinitis to ragweed. Ann Allergy 1994; 72:435–440.

113. Malm L, Wihl J-Å. Intranasal beclomethasone dipropionate in vasomotor rhinitis. Acta Allerg (Kbh) 1976; 31:245–250.

114. Wight RG, Jones AS, Beckingham E, Andersson B, Ek L. A double-blind comparison of intranasal budesonide 400 µg and 800 µg in perennial rhinitis. Clin Otolaryngol 1992; 17:354–358.

115. Lildholdt T, Rundcrantz H, Lindqvist N. Effect of topical corticosteroid powder for nasal polyps: a double-blind, placebo-controlled study of budesonide. Clin Otolaryngol 1995; 20:26–30.

116. Munch E, Gomez G, Mygind N, et al. An open comparison of dosage frequency of beclomethasone dipropionate in seasonal allergic rhinitis. Clin Allergy 1981; 11: 303–309.

117. Nathan RA, Bronsky EA, Fireman P, et al. Once daily fluticasone propionate aqueous nasal spray is an effective treatment for seasonal allergic rhinitis. Ann Allergy 1991; 67:332–338.

118. Banov CH, Woehler TR, LaForce CF, et al. Once daily intranasal flutocasone propionate is effective for perennial allergic rhinitis. Ann Allergy 1994; 73:240–246.

119. Cockcroft DW, MacCormack DW, Newhouse MT, Hargreave FE. Beclomethasone dipropionate in allergic rhinitis. Can Med Assoc J 1976; 115:523–526.

120. Bousquet J, Chanal I, Alquié MC, et al. Prevention of pollen rhinitis. Comparison

of fluticasone propionate aqueous nasal spray versus disodium cromoglycate nasal spray. Allergy 1993; 48:327–333.

121. Beswick KB, Kenyon GS, Cherry JR. A comparative study of beclomethasone dipropionate aqueous nasal spray with terfenadine tablets in season allergic rhinitis. Curr Med Res Opin 1985; 9:560–567.

122. Bunnag C, Jareoncharsri P, Wong ECK. A double-blind comparison of nasal budesonide and oral astemizole for the treatment of perennial rhinitis. Allergy 1992; 47:313–317.

123. Charpin D, Vervloet D. Treating seasonal rhinitis: antihistamines or intranasal corticosteroids? Eur Respir Rev 1994; 4:256–259.

124. Frølund L. Efficacy of an oral antihistamine, loratadine, as compared with a nasal steroid spray, beclomethasone dipropionate, in seasonal allergic rhinitis. Clin Otolaryngol 1992; 16:527–531.

125. Harding SM, Heath S. Intranasal steroid aerosol in perennial rhinitis: comparison with an antihistamine compound. Clin Allergy 1976; 6:369–372.

126. Juniper EF, Kline PA, Hargreave FE, Dolovich J. Comparison of beclomethasone dipropionate aqueous spray, astemizole, and the combination in the prophylactic treatment of ragweed-induced rhinoconjunctivitis. J Allergy Clin Immunol 1989; 83:627–633.

127. Munch E, Søborg M, Nørreslet TT, Mygind N. A comparative study of dexchlorpheniramine maleate sustained tablets and budesonide nasal spray in seasonal allergic rhinitis. Allergy 1983; 38:517–524.

128. Salomonsson P, Gottberg L, Heilborn H, Norrlind K, Pegelow KO. Efficacy of an oral antihistamine, astemizole, as compared to a nasal steroid spray in hay fever. Allergy 1988; 43:214–218.

129. Simpson RJ. Budesonide and terfenadine, separately and in combination, in the treatment of hay fever. Ann Allergy 1994; 73:497–502.

130. Darnell A, Pecoud A, Richards DH. A double-blind comparison of fluticasone propionate aqueous spray, terfenadine tablets and placebo in the treatment of patients with seasonal allergic rhinitis to grass pollen. Clin Exp Allergy 1994; 24:1144–1150.

131. Jordana G, Dolovich J, Briscoe MP, et al. Intranasal fluticasone propionate versus loratadine in the treatment of adolescent patients with seasonal allergic rhinitis. J Allergy Clin Immunol 1996; 97:588–595.

132. van Bavel J, Findlay SR, Hampel F, et al. Intranasal fluticosone propionate is more effective than terfenadine tablets for seasonal allergic rhinitis. Arch Intern Med 1994; 154:2699–2704.

133. Davies RJ, Lund VJ, Harten-Ash VJ. The effect of intranasal azelastine and beclomethasone on the symptoms and signs of nasal allergy in patients with perennial allergic rhinitis. Rhinology 1993; 31:159–164.

134. Dorow P, Aurich R, Petzold U. Efficacy and tolerability of azelastine nasal spray in patients with allergic rhinitis compared to placebo and budesonide. Drug Res 1993; 43:909–912.

135. Gastpar H, Aurich R, Petzold U, et al. Intranasal treatment of perennial allergic rhinitis. Comparison of azelastine nasal spray and budesonide nasal aerosol. Arzneimittelforschung 1993; 43:475–479.

136. Negrini AC, Troise C, Voltolini S, Horak F, Bachert C, Janssens M. Oral antihistamine/decongestant treatment compared with intranasal corticosteroids in seasonal allergic rhinitis. Clin Exp Allergy 1995; 25:60–65.

137. Wood SFG. Oral antihistamine and nasal steroid in hay fever. Clin Allergy 1986; 16:195–201.

138. Wihl J-Å, Petersen BN, Petersen LN, Gundersen G, Bresson G, Mygind N. Effect of the nonsedative H_1-receptor antagonist asthemizole in perennial allergic and non-allergic rhinitis. J Allergy Clin Immunol 1985; 75:720–727.

139. Benincasa C, Lloyd RS. Evaluation of fluticasone propionate aqueous nasal spray taken alone and in combination with cetirizine in the prophylactic treatment of seasonal allergic rhinitis. Drug Invest 1994; 8:225–233.

140. Pipkorn U, Rundcrantz H, Lindqvist N. Budesonide—a new nasal steroid. Rhinology 1980; 18:171–175.

141. Siegel SC, Katz R, Rachelefsky GS, et al. Multicenter study of beclomethasone dipropionate in adults with seasonal allergic rhinitis. J Allergy Clin Immunol 1982; 69:345–353.

142. Henriksen J, Wenzel A. Effect of an intranasally administered corticosteroid (budesonide) on nasal obstruction, mouth breathing, and asthma. Am Rev Respir Dis 1984; 130:1014–1018.

143. Reed CE, Marcoux JP, Welsh PW. Effects of topical nasal treatment on asthma. J Allergy Clin Immunol 1988; 81:1042–1047.

144. Aubier M, Levy J, Clerici C, Neukirch F, Herman D. Different effects of nasal and bronchial glucocorticosteroid administration on bronchial hyperresponsiveness in patients with allergic rhinitis. Am Rev Respir Dis 1992; 146:122–126.

145. Corren J, Adinoff AD, Buchmeier AD, Irvin CG. Nasal beclomethasone prevents the seasonal increase in bronchial responsiveness in patients with allergic rhinitis and asthma. J Allergy Clin Immunol 1992; 90:250–256.

146. Wood RA, Egglestone PA. The effects of intranasal steroids on nasal and bronchial responses to cat exposure. Am J Respir Crit Care Med 1995; 151:315–320.

147. Tarlo SM, Cockroft DW, Dolovich J, Hargreave FE. Beclomethasone dipropionate aerosol in perennial rhinitis. J Allergy Clin Immunol 1977; 59:232–236.

148. Hansen I, Mygind N. Local effect of intranasal beclomethasone dipropionate aerosol in perennial rhinitis. Acta Allerg (Kbh) 1974; 29:281–287.

149. Lindqvist N, Balle V, Karma P, et al. Long term safety and efficacy of budesonide nasal aerosol in perennial rhinitis—a 12 month multicenter study. Allergy 1986; 41:179–186.

150. Löfkvist T, Svensson G. Treatment of vasomotor rhinitis with beclomethasone dipropionate. Acta Allerg (Kbh) 1976; 31:227–238.

151. Feiss G, Welch M, Meltzer E, Alderfer V, Smith J. The predictive value of nasal eosinophilia for therapeutic response intranasal corticosteroid treatment in perennial allergic rhinitis. J Allergy Clin Immunol 1992; 89:209 (abstract).

152. Small P, Black M, Frenkiel S. Effect of treatment with beclomethasone dipropionate in subpopulations of perennial rhinitis patients. J Allergy Clin Immunol 1982; 70:78–82.

153. Whelan CFA. Problems in the examination of nasal smears in allergic rhinitis. J Laryngol Otol 1980; 84:399–405.

154. Chaplin I, Haynes JT, Spahn I. Are nasal polyps an allergic phenomenon? Ann Allergy 1971; 29:63–64.

155. Delaney JC. Aspirin idiosyncrasy in patients admitted for nasal polypectomy. Clin Otolaryngol 1976; 1:27–30.

156. Deuschl H, Drettner B. Nasal polyps treated with beclomethasone nasal aerosol. Rhinology 1977; 15:17–23.

157. Holopainen E, Grahne B, Malmberg H, Makinen J, Lindqvist N. Budesonide in the treatment of nasal polyposis. Eur J Respir Dis 1982; 63(Suppl 122):221–228.

158. Mygind N, Pedersen CB, Prytz S, Sørensen H. Treatment of nasal polyps with intranasal beclomethasone dipropionate aerosol. Clin Allergy 1975; 5:159–164.

159. Lildholdt T, Mygind N. Corticosteroids: locally and systemically. In: Mygind N, Lildholdt T, eds. Nasal Polyposis: An Inflammatory Disease and Its Treatment. Copenhagen: Munksgaard 1997;160–169.

160. Drettner B, Ebbesen A, Nilsson M. Prophylactic treatment with flunisolide after polypectomy. Rhinology 1982; 20:149–158.

161. Holopainen E, Grahne B, Malmberg H, Mäkinen J, Lindqvist N. Budesonide in the treatment of nasal polyposis. Eur J Respir Dis 1982; 63(Suppl 122):221–228.

162. Karlsson G, Rundcrantz H. A randomized trial of intranasal beclomethasone dipropionate after polypectomy. Rhinology 1982; 20:144–148.

163. Farr BM, Gwaltney JM Jr, Hendley JO, Hayden FG, Naclerio RM, McBride T, Doyle WJ, Sorrentino JV, Proud D. A randomized controlled trial of glucocorticoid prophylaxis against experimental rhinovirus infection. J Infect Dis 1990; 162: 1173–1177.

164. Meltzer EO, Busse WW, Druce HM, Metzger WJ, Mitchell DO, Selner J, Shapiro GG, van Bavel JH. Assessment of flunisolide nasal spray versus placebo as an adjunct to antibiotic treatment of sinusitis. J Allergy Clin Immunol 1992; 89:301 (abstract).

165. Sykes DA, Wilson R, Chan KL, Mackay IS. Relative importance of antibiotic and improved clearance in topical treatment of chronic mucopurulent rhinosinusitis. Lancet 1986; 2:359–360.

166. Boner AL, Sette L. Rhinitis in children: efficacy and safety of a new intranasal corticosteroid. Eur Respir Rev 1994; 20:271–273.

167. Schatz M, Zeiger RS, eds. Asthma and Allergy in Pregnancy and Early Infancy. New York: Marcel Dekker, 1993:1–636.

168. Soderberg-Warner ML. Nasal septal perforation associated with topical corticosteroid therapy. J Pediatr 1984; 105:840–841.

169. Mygind N, Sørensen H, Pedersen CG. The nasal mucosa during long-term treatment with beclomethasone dipropionate aerosol. A light- and scanning electron microscopic study of nasal polyps. Acta Otolaryngol (Stockh) 1978; 85:437–443.

170. Brown HM, Storey G, Jackson FA. Beclomethasone dipropionate aerosol in treatment of perennial and seasonal rhinitis: a review of five years' experience. Br J Clin Pharmacol 1977; 4(Suppl 3):283–286.

171. Pipkorn U, Pukander J, Suonpaa J, Makinen J, Lindqvist N. Long-term safety of budesonide nasal aerosol—a 5½ year follow-up study. Clin Allergy 1988; 18:253–259.

172. Sarnstrand B, Jeppsson Å, Malmstrom A, Brattsand R. Effect of glucocorticoste-

roids on hyaluronic acid synthesis in vitro in human fibroblast-like cells from lung and skin. In: Hogg JC, Ellul-Micalef R, Brattsand R, eds. Glucocorticosteroids, Inflammation and Bronchial Hyperreactivity. Amsterdam: Excerpta Medica, 1985: 157–166.

173. Frauenfelder FT, Myer SM. Posterior subcapsular cataracts associated with nasal or inhalation corticosteroids. Am J Ophthalmol 1990; 109:489–490.

174. Simons FE, Persaud MP, Gillespie CA, Cheang M, Shuckett EP. Absence of posterior cataracts in young patients treated with inhaled glucocorticoids. Lancet 1993; 342:776–778.

175. Wolthers OD, Pedersen S. Kneemometry assessment of systemic activity of once daily intranasal dry-powder budesonide in children. Allergy 1994; 49:96–99.

176. Knutsson U, Stjärna P, Marcus C, Carlstedt-Duke J, Carlström K, Brönnegard M. Effects of intranasal glucocorticoids on endogenous glucocorticoid peripheral and central function. J Endocrinol 1995; 144:301–310.

177. Masuyama K, Jacobson MR, Rak S, et al. Topical glucocorticoid (fluticasone propionate) inhibits cells expressing cytokine mRNA for interleukin-4 in the nasal mucosa in allergen-induced rhinitis. Immunology 1994; 82:192–199.

14

Systemic Corticosteroids

**NIELS MYGIND and
RONALD DAHL**

University of Aarhus
Aarhus, Denmark

ROBERT M. NACLERIO

University of Chicago
Chicago, Illinois

I. Rationale

Since the introduction of topical corticosteroids for nasal use, the role of systemic steroids in the treatment of nasal disorders has greatly declined. Their current indications in the management of allergic rhinitis are not well defined. Theoretically a systemic administration of corticosteroids can have some advantages over topical treatment because: 1) the drug reaches all parts of the nasal cavity, including the olfactory airway and the middle meatus, where polyps form, 2) it reaches the mucous membrane of the paranasal sinuses, 3) it can be effective in a completely blocked nose or nostril, and 4) it has a direct effect on bone marrow and circulating precursor cells.

For these reasons, it is relevant to investigate the potential use of systemic steroids for rhinitis. While there are now over 100 published placebo-controlled trials of topical steroids (see Chapter 13), we have only been able to find three such studies of systemic steroids (1–3). Thus, the investigation of this therapy for rhinitis is remarkably insufficient, probably because of lack of interest and of support from the pharmaceutical industry, as well as the recognized long-term complications associated with the use of these agents. The long-term side effects must always be considered when describing their role in therapy. Since allergic rhinitis is a disease that spans decades, the yearly use of systemic steroids may cause problems such as osteoporosis and cataracts in the elderly.

II. Principles of Therapy

As the short-term risks of adverse effects from systemic corticosteroids depend largely on the duration of treatment, we believe that only short-term therapy (about 2 weeks) is justified for a benign disease such as rhinitis. Short-term systemic steroids for rhinitis can be both safe and useful, when the rules, given in Table 1, are followed.

III. Drug Administration and Dosage

Steroids can be given orally (prednisolone, 5–30 mg/day) or as a depot injection (methylprednisolone 80 mg or betamethasone 14 mg, corresponding to 100 mg of prednisolone).

The continuous release of corticosteroid from a depot injection will suppress the hypothalamopituitary-adrenal (HPA) axis more than a single oral dose given in the morning (4–6). However, this has little clinical consequence when drug release is confined to a few weeks. Although a single depot injection of 80 mg methylprednisolone reduces plasma cortisol for at least 1 week (7), but not for 3 weeks (8), it does not suppress the responsiveness of the HPA axis (7). It may be an advantage of a depot injection that the total dose of corticosteroid, necessary to suppress rhinitis symptoms seems to be smaller than when it is given as oral medication once daily for 2–3 weeks (8).

Our knowledge about the optimal dose of systemic steroid to be used for rhinitis is insufficient. There is only one published dose-response study, showing a significantly better effect of 24 mg methylprednisolone orally than of 6 and 12 mg on hay fever symptoms (3).

Table 1 Principles for Safe Use of Systemic Steroids for Rhinitis

---

Only short-term therapy (2 weeks)
Not used more frequently than every 3rd month
Not used instead of other treatments, but in addition to intranasal steroid
Not given to children, pregnant women, or patients with known contraindications

---

IV. Seasonal Allergic Rhinitis

The effect of a depot injection of corticosteroid in hay fever has been studied in a number of uncontrolled trials (9–16), while we have found only three placebo-controlled studies (1–3) and two controlled drug-comparative studies (7,8).

In 1960, Brown and co-workers (1) compared placebo with methylprednisolone, 240 mg, given as three weekly injections. Not surprisingly, the authors' overall impression was that this high-dose therapy, not used today, resulted in "a marked relief of symptoms."

In two consecutive placebo-controlled hay fever studies, Borum and co-workers (2) found a significant effect of a single depot injection of methylprednisolone (80 mg) on rhinoconjunctivitis symptoms. However, the degree of effect varied with the symptoms. The effect on sneezing and nose blowings was weak, and that on eye itching was moderate, but nasal blockage was markedly reduced (Fig. 1), and for a longer period than the duration of the reduction of plasma cortisol (8), suggesting that some vicious circle had been broken.

In the two studies of Borum and co-workers (2), the efficacy of a depot injection given at the beginning of the pollen season was compared to that of an injection given at the peak of the pollen season. The early injection gave a larger total reduction of symptoms than the injection at the peak of the season.

The only published placebo-controlled trial of oral steroids was undertaken in 31 patients with ragweed hay fever, who received either placebo or methylprednisolone, 6, 12, or 24 mg/day (3). There was a dose-related reduction in rhinitis symptoms, but not all symptoms responded equally well. Itching and sneezing were not effectively suppressed by low-dose systemic treatment, and even 24 mg of methylprednisolone did not have a statistically significant effect on nasal itching.

Another hay fever study compared a depot injection of betamethasone (14 mg, corresponding to about 100 mg prednisolone) with oral prednisolone (7.5 mg/day for 3 weeks, giving a total dose of 157.5 mg) (8). The two treatment regimens showed equal efficacy, but only the oral medication had a demonstrable effect on plasma cortisol level at the end of the treatment period.

Pichler and co-workers (7) compared the effect of 80 mg methylprednisolone as a depot injection with budesonide nasal spray (400 μg/day) in 31 hay fever patients. A comparison of the two treatment groups in relation to the pollen count yielded statistically significant less nasal itching ($p = 0.001$), sneezing ($p = 0.02$), and "runny nose" ($p = 0.01$) in the budesonide group, while there was no difference between the two groups with regard to nasal blockage.

When other treatments are inadequate in highly sensitive patients during periods of high pollen counts, it is often routine to add systemic corticosteroids. However, this therapy does not seem to be very effective on itching, sneez-

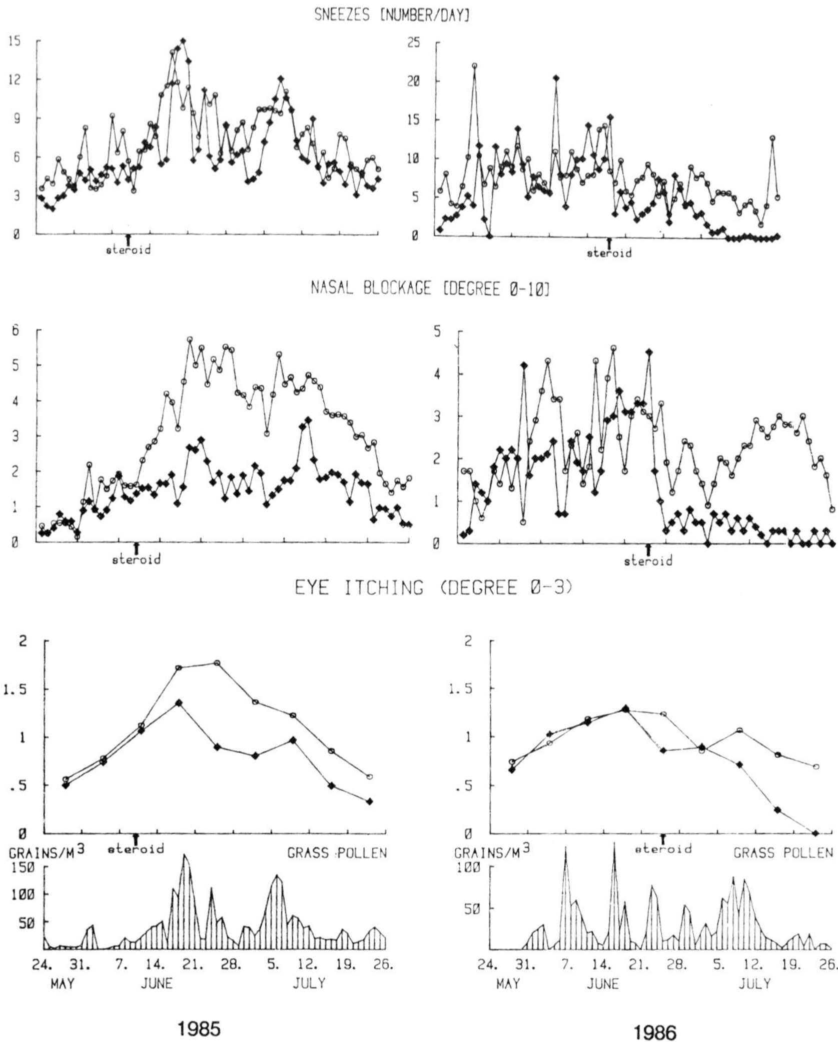

Figure 1   A depot-steroid injection of 80 mg methylprednisolone has a weak effect on sneezing in hay fever (top). However, the use of rescue medication (chlorpheniramine tablets) was higher in the placebo group than in the active group in the 1985 trial ($p <$ 0.001). The effect on nasal blockage is marked and long-lasting (middle). The effect on eye itching is moderate (bottom). The use of conjunctivitis rescue medication (antihistamine eye drops) was higher in the placebo group than in the active group in the 1985 trial ($p <$ 0.001). (From Ref. 2.)

ing, and rhinorrhea, and an additive effect has not been proven in controlled trials.

In seasonal allergic rhinitis, oral medication has, in principle, the advantage over a depot injection that the treatment can follow the pollen count, and in this way, unnecessary medication, e.g., during rainy periods, can be avoided. The patients can be supplied with prednisolone tablets and be instructed to take 5–20 mg in the morning during troublesome periods. However, there are no data to demonstrate the efficacy of this type of periodic steroid medication.

V. Perennial Rhinitis

Perennial rhinitis is associated with chronic inflammation and nasal blockage, which often is more severe than in seasonal allergic rhinitis. It is therefore remarkable that there is no published placebo-controlled study of the effect of systemic steroids in this disease.

Tarlo and co-workers (17) undertook an open study of the effect of a short course of oral prednisone in patients with perennial rhinitis, who were treated with nasal beclomethasone dipropionate. Only 54% of these patients achieved acceptable symptomatic improvement from the nasal steroid spray alone, but after administration of prednisone, 73% of the patients obtained moderate or marked symptomatic improvement from the topical treatment. These results suggest that a short course of systemic steroids can be helpful in patients with severe perennial rhinitis to open up a blocked nose before topical therapy. It may also be indicated when there is a temporary failure of intranasal treatment, for example after a common cold.

VI. Nasal Polyposis

Three studies describe the effect of systemic steroids in nasal polyposis. Lildholdt and co-workers (18), in their first study, randomized 53 patients to either surgical removal of visible polyps with a snare or a depot injection of steroid (betamethasone 14 mg). Both regimens caused substantial and equal increase in nasal expiratory peak flow. The improvement was maintained during a 1-year observation period (Fig. 2), in which the patients were treated with topical steroids. The sense of smell improved significantly in the systemic steroid group at 2 weeks but was not maintained 2–12 months into topical therapy.

In a second study of 124 patients, Lildholdt and co-workers (19) randomized 33 patients, who failed to respond to the initial treatment with topical steroid, to treatment with a depot injection of 14 mg betamethasone or polypectomy with a snare. After 1 year of continuous topical therapy there was no difference between the two groups with regard to any effect parameter (Fig. 3). The authors

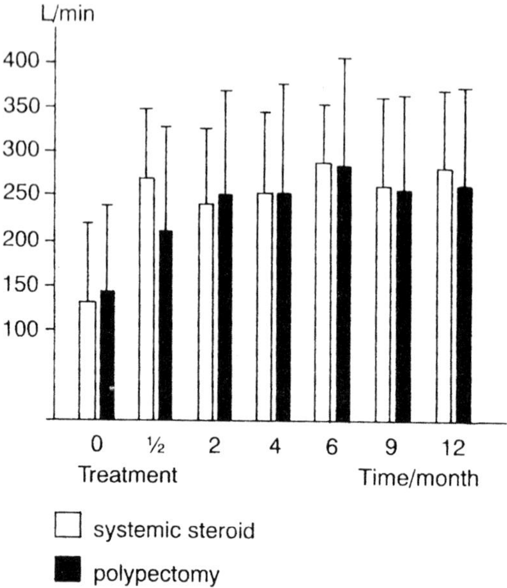

Figure 2 Mean nasal peak flow (± SD) in 53 patients treated with beclomethasone dipropionate following an initial depot injection of corticosteroid (betamethasone 14 mg) (white bars) or polypectomy with a snare (black bars). (From Ref. 18.)

found that only 15% of all patients did not respond satisfactorily to the treatment given and needed surgery. They conclude that ''the primary treatment of nasal polyps should be systemic and local steroids.''

Van Camp and Clement (20) gave 25 patients with massive nasal polyposis a large dosage of oral prednisolone (60 mg/day for 4 days and then tapered off by 5 mg daily, giving a total dose of 570 mg). There was a considerable reduction in the frequency of all symptoms, in particular nasal obstruction, and the sense of smell improved. Nasal polyps became invisible at rhinoscopy in 10 of 25 patients. Half of the patients (13 of 25) showed improvement judged by a computed-tomography scan of the sinuses. Although these 13 patients, called responders, continued on topical steroids, ''there was a strong tendency of recurrence . . . which made surgical intervention inevitable.'' The authors conclude that ''systemic steroid treatment should be reserved for those cases that require surgery.'' They emphasize that surgery can be considerably facilitated by preoperative systemic steroid therapy.

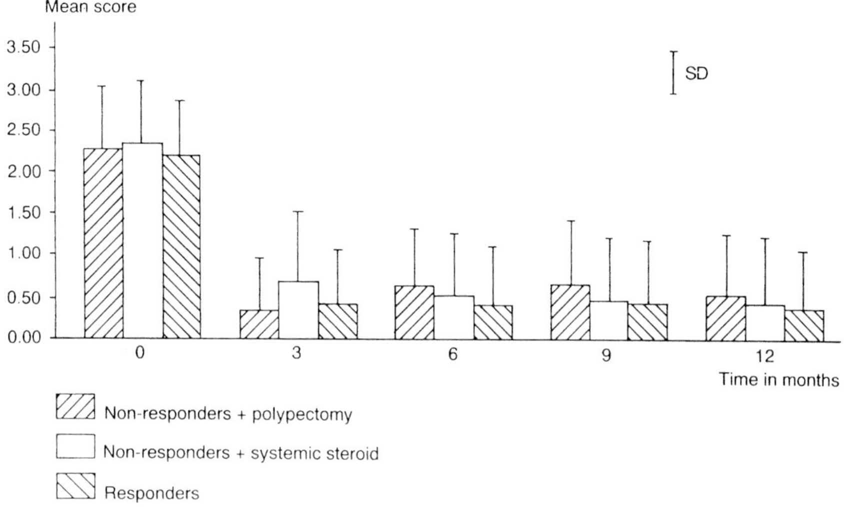

Figure 3 Scores for nasal blockage (mean ± SD) in 119 patients treated with topical corticosteroid (budesonide powder 400 or 800 µg/day) for 12 months. Initially all patients were treated with budesonide for 1 month. "Responders" (85 of 119) continued on topical therapy only, while "nonresponders" (34 of 119) also received either systemic steroid (betamethasone 14 mg as a depot injection) or polypectomy. (From Ref. 19.)

Although systemic steroid treatment of nasal polyposis has not been studied in placebo-controlled trials, there is little doubt that it is highly effective. Rhinitis symptoms and polyp size are reduced, and, in contrast to topical steroids, there is a good effect on the sense of smell and an effect on the paranasal sinuses. A short course of systemic steroids is equally effective to polypectomy with a snare (18), and preoperative use of systemic steroids will facilitate surgery.

Only a single course of systemic steroids has been given in published studies. However, we believe that some patients with severe, recurrent polyposis may benefit from repeated use of short-term systemic steroids, but there are, at present, no analysis of the pro's and con's of this type of management. If, for example, a depot injection (methylprednisolone 80 mg or betamethasone 14 mg) is given no more frequently than every 3 months, it will correspond to continuous treatment with 1–2 mg prednisolone a day. Adverse effects from this therapy may, in some patients with severe disease and abolished olfaction, be outweighed by increased quality of life.

VII. Contraindications and Side Effects

Contraindications to systemic steroid treatment are glaucoma, herpes keratitis, diabetes mellitus, psychic instability, advanced osteoporosis, severe hypertension, tuberculosis, or other chronic infection. We do not find it correct to use systemic steroids for rhinitis in children and during pregnancy.

The side effects from a 2-week treatment are few and mild. Depot injections can, in rare cases, cause a depression over the injection site. Some authors recommend depot injections into swollen nasal turbinates and polyps, but this must be discouraged as blindness has been reported.

VIII. Conclusions

The role of systemic steroids in the treatment of allergic rhinitis is not well defined. In most cases topical treatment provides sufficient relief. In theory, treatment with the nasal steroids may be improved in severe cases by short courses of systemic steroids, which can reach all parts of the nasal cavity and paranasal sinuses. When the duration of the treatment period is limited to about 2 weeks, and when the relevant contraindications are considered, systemic steroids can be safe without risk of short-term serious adverse effects. Three placebo-controlled studies have shown such therapy to have a significant effect on nasal blockage, but the effect on itching, sneezing, and rhinorrhea is weak. In severe cases of seasonal allergic rhinitis, short-term systemic steroids are often added to other types of treatment, but there is no proof of added efficacy. In perennial rhinitis, a short course of systemic steroids can probably increase the response rate to topical steroids. In nasal polyposis, the treatment can reduce rhinitis symptoms, improve the sense of smell, facilitate nasal surgery, prevent the recurrence of polyps after polypectomy, and can be used as a substitute for simple polypectomy. Used in this way, short-term systemic steroids may be an effective and safe additive to a basic treatment with topical treatment. However, there is a striking shortage of placebo-controlled studies of systemic steroids for rhinitis and polyposis, and further studies of dose-response relationship, effect profile, and mode of administration (tablets versus depot injections) are needed.

References

1. Brown EB, Seideman T, Siegelaub BA, Popovitz FACA. Depo-methylprednisolone in the treatment of ragweed hay fever. Ann Allergy 1960; 18:1321–1330.
2. Borum P, Grønborg H, Mygind N. Seasonal allergic rhinitis and depot injection of a corticosteroid. Allergy 1987; 42:26–32.

3. Brooks CD, Karl KJ, Francom SF. Oral methylprednisolone acetate (Medrol tablets) for seasonal rhinitis. J Clin Pharmacol 1993; 33:816–822.

4. Hedner P, Persson G. Suppression of hypothalamo-pituitary-adrenal axis after a single intrammuscular injection of methylprednisolone acetate. Ann Allergy 1981; 47: 176–179.

5. Ganderton MA, James VHT. Clinical and endocrine side-effects of methylprednisolone acetate as used in hay fever. Br Med J 1970; 1:267–269.

6. Helfer EL, Rose LI. Corticosteroids and adrenal suppression characterizing and avoiding the problem. Drug 1989; 38:838–845.

7. Pichler WJ, Klint T, Blaser M, Graf W, Sauter S, Weiss S, Witschi K. Clinical comparison of systemic methylprednisolone acetate versus topical budesonide in patients with seasonal allergic rhinitis. Allergy 1988; 43:87–92.

8. Laursen LC, Faurschou P, Pals H, Svendsen UG, Weeke B. Intramuscular betamethasone dipropionate vs. oral prednisolone in hay fever. Allergy 1987; 42:168–172.

9. Brown EB, Siegelaub BA. Treatment of ragweed hay fever with methylprednisolone. J Allergy 1958; 29:227–232.

10. Arbeiter H, Knapp RD. Allergic rhinitis and bronchial asthma treatment with parenteral methylprednisolone acetate. Ann Allergy 1961; 19:633–635.

11. Marshall BY. Short-term parenteral corticosteroid therapy for hay-fever and allergic rhinitis. Practitioner 1965; 194:676–679.

12. Lewin RA. Methylprednisolone acetate in the treatment of hay fever. Br J Clin Pract 1968; 22:173–175.

13. Ganderton MA, Brostoff J, Frankland AW. Comparison of preseasonal and coseasonal Allpyral with Depo-Medrone in summer hay-fever. Br Med J 1969; 1:357–358.

14. Kronholm A. Injectable depot corticosteroid therapy in hay fever. J Intern Med Res 1979; 7:314–317.

15. Ohlander B, Hansson R, Karlsson K-E. A comparison of three injectable corticosteroids for the treatment of patients with seasonal hay fever. J Intern Med Res 1980; 8:63–69.

16. Walander A. Treatment of allergic rhinitis with a long-acting steroid preparation. Clin Trials J 1986; 5:907–909.

17. Tarlo SM, Cockroft DW, Dolovich J, Hargreave FE. Beclomethasone dipropionate aerosol in perennial rhinitis. J Allergy Clin Immunol 1977; 59:232–236.

18. Lildholdt T, Fogstrup J, Gammelgaard N, Kortholm B, Ulsøe C. Surgical versus medical treatment of nasal polyps. Acta Otolaryngol (Stockh) 1988; 105:140–143.

19. Lildholdt T, Rundcrantz H, Bende M, Larsen K. Glucocorticoid treatment for nasal polyps. A study of budesonide powder and depot-steroid injection. Arch Otolaryngol Head Neck Surg 1997; 123:595–600.

20. van Camp P, Clement PAR. Results of oral steroid treatment in nasal polyposis. Rhinology 1994; 32:5–9.

15

Antihistamines

F. ESTELLE R. SIMONS

University of Manitoba
Winnipeg, Manitoba, Canada

I. Introduction

Antihistamines (H_1-receptor antagonists) are the most commonly used medications in the world for allergic rhinitis treatment (Fig. 1). They are usually the medications to which people suffering from rhinitis turn first for relief. In many countries, they are available without a physician's prescription.

We will review the rationale for use of H_1-receptor antagonists in this disorder, their mechanisms of action, clinical pharmacology, efficacy in allergic rhinitis and other respiratory tract disorders, and potential adverse effects (1).

II. Rationale for Use of H_1-Receptor Antagonists in Allergic Rhinitis

Allergic rhinitis is characterized by mucosal inflammation, evidenced by accumulation of mast cells, basophils, and eosinophils; endothelial and epithelial cell activation; expansion of dendritic antigen-presenting cells; and, in chronic disease, T-lymphocyte accumulation and activation (2). Release of chemical mediators from activated mast cells, basophils, and eosinophils causes the end-organ effects of nasal itch, sneeze, rhinorrhea, and obstruction.

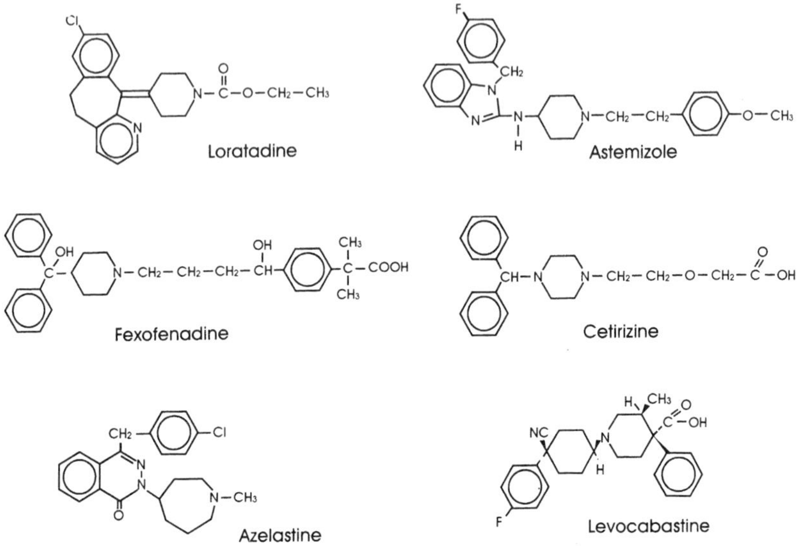

Figure 1   Chemical structures of selected H_1-receptor antagonists.

Histamine is the major granule constituent of tissue mast cells and circulating basophils and is, quantitatively, the major mediator generated on immunological activation of these cells. Histamine concentrations in nasal secretions are not a reliable marker of the inflammatory process in the nasal mucosa, as they are not increased in all subjects with allergic rhinitis. This may be due to rapid degradation of histamine by histaminase or rapid uptake of histamine at the H_1 receptors in the nasal mucosa; also, histamine may be generated locally by bacteria, thus further confounding the issue.

In allergic rhinitis, histamine plays an important role in the early-phase response to allergen (3). Acting at the H_1 receptor, it causes sneezing and itching via sensory nerve stimulation and leads to rhinorrhea and congestion via vasodilation, increased vascular permeability, extravasation of protein, and reflex stimulation of glandular secretions. It may also contribute to the late-phase response, specifically to recruitment, adherence, and activation of eosinophils and other inflammatory cells, generation of leukotrienes, and induction of interleukin secretion by endothelial cells. It upregulates the expression and mobilization of the cell adhesion molecule P-selectin in the vascular endothelium, and may indirectly upregulate the epithelial expression of intercellular adhesion molecule 1 (ICAM-1).

Histamine H_1 receptors are found primarily on the vascular endothelium of the postcapillary venules in the nasal mucosa, and are increased in number in the nasal mucosa of subjects with allergic rhinitis symptoms (4) (Fig. 2). When these subjects are asymptomatic, nasal allergen challenge in the laboratory is followed by an increase in histamine responsiveness, which elicits sneezing, itching, and rhinorrhea within minutes of insufflation. This phenomenon also occurs, although somewhat less consistently, during natural seasonal exposure to allergens. Pretreatment with H_1-receptor antagonists inhibits nasal symptoms after histamine or allergen challenge.

The histamine H_1 receptor was characterized historically using a pharmacologic approach. It is now being studied using a molecular genetic approach. The gene for the H_1 receptor has been cloned in human leucocytes and has been expressed in heterologous cell lines. It maps to the short arm of chromosome 3. The H_1 receptor has the typical characteristics of G-protein-coupled receptors, with seven transmembrane domains connected by alternating extracellular loops (5).

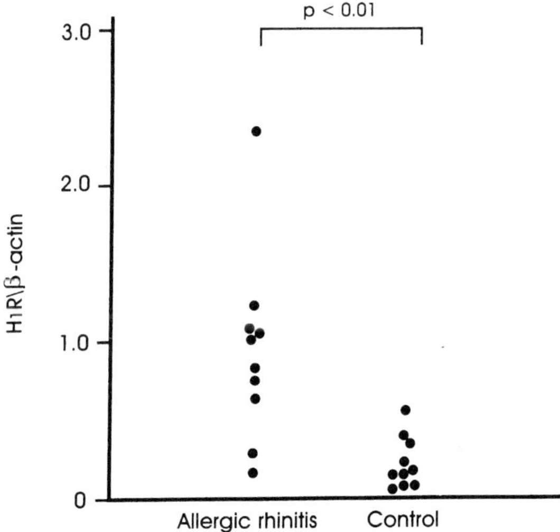

Figure 2 H_1-receptor mRNA expression was studied in 10 subjects with allergic rhinitis and in 10 healthy subjects. RNA was extracted from scrapings of inferior turbinate mucosa. RNA pellets were treated with DNase. The histamine$_1$-receptor and beta-actin mRNA were amplified for 35 cycles by reverse transcription polymerase chain reactions (PCR). The PRC products were hybridized with internal probes and band intensities were quantitated by a densitometer. The mean H_1-receptor/β-actin ratio was 0.88 ± 0.62 in allergic rhinitis and 0.29 ± 0.17 in normal subjects ($p < 0.01$). Expression of H_1-receptor mRNA is increased in the nasal mucosa of subjects with allergic rhinitis. (From Ref. 4.)

III. Mechanisms of Action

A. H_1 Blockade

Histamine H_1-receptor antagonists are highly selective for H_1 receptors and have little effect at H_2 or H_3 receptors. Although old, relatively non-selective H_1-receptor antagonists may also activate muscarinic, cholinergic, 5-hydroxytryptamine (serotonin) or alpha-adrenergic receptors, few of the new selective H_1 antagonists have any of these properties. The precise structural requirements for selectivity and affinity for H_1 receptors are being elucidated (6).

At low concentrations, H_1-receptor antagonists are competitive antagonists of histamine (7). They bind to H_1 receptors, but do not activate them, thus preventing histamine binding and activity. At higher concentrations, some new H_1-receptor antagonists such as astemizole, ebastine, and loratadine also exhibit non-competitive inhibition. The binding of most H_1 antagonists is readily reversible, but some do not dissociate as readily from H_1 receptors as others.

During the immediate hypersensitivity reaction, histamine concentrations may reach $10^{-6}-10^{-3}$ M. The concentration of an H_1-receptor antagonist in tissue varies with its physicochemical properties, pharmacokinetic activity, and dose; however, peak concentrations seldom exceed 10^{-6} M. For H_1-receptor antagonists such as astemizole, ebastine, and loratadine, tissue concentrations of active H_1-antagonist metabolites may be more relevant than those of the parent compound (1).

B. Antiallergic Effects

H_1-receptor antagonists decrease release of chemical mediators of inflammation from mast cells and basophils. These antiallergic effects generally occur only at high concentrations of H_1-antagonists. They are unrelated to histamine H_1-blockade; rather, they are non-specific biochemical effects that occur when H_1-antagonists form an ionic association with cell membranes, prevent calcium binding, and inhibit calmodulin and other membrane-associated enzymes (8).

When nasal allergen challenge is performed after several days of treatment with terfenadine, cetirizine, or loratadine by mouth, or azatadine, azelastine, or levocabastine intranasally, sneezing and other symptoms of allergic rhinitis are reduced, microvascular leakage is reduced, and chemical mediators of inflammation such as histamine, prostaglandin D2, and leukotriene C4 are released in smaller amounts. Inhibition of the response to allergen challenge is often partial, with significant decrease in release of one mediator, but not others (9) (Fig. 3).

The relative importance of the antiallergic effects of H_1-receptor antagonists in contributing to their overall clinical efficacy is not known. H_1-receptor antagonists with antiallergic effects are not convincingly more effective than those without them. Although there are comparative studies of the *clinical* effi-

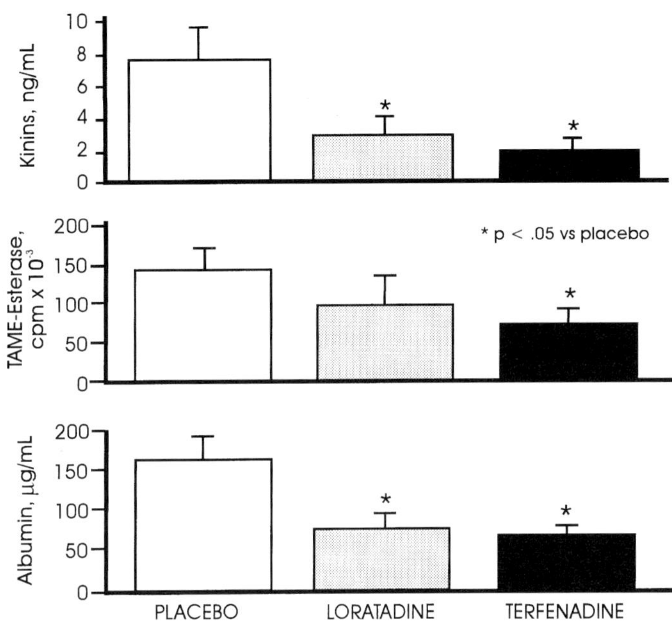

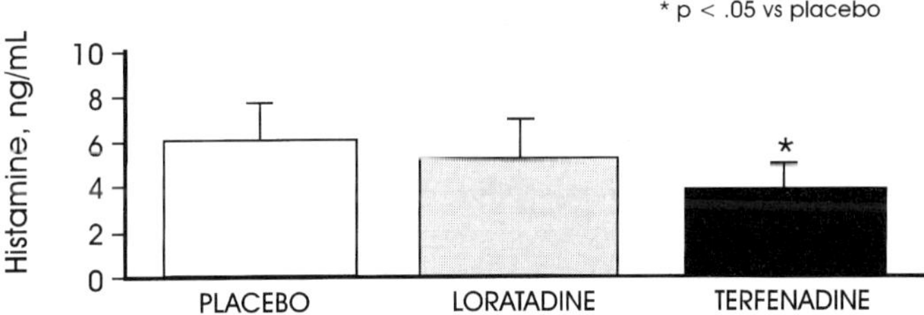

Figure 3 In a double-blind, placebo-controlled, crossover study, 14 asymptomatic allergic subjects were treated with either placebo, loratadine 10 mg od, or terfenadine 60 mg bid for 1 week. Nasal allergen challenge with lavages and quantitation of mediator levels were performed. Cells were counted in lavage fluid 24 hr postchallenge. Methacholine challenges were also performed at 24 hr. Compared to placebo, both loratadine and terfenadine significantly decreased allergen-induced sneezing and secretions (not shown) and decreased (a) kinins, TAME-esterase activity, and albumin, and (b) histamine in lavage fluid. There was no effect on levels of tryptase, PGD_2, or LTC_4 in lavage fluid, or on eosinophil influx. Loratadine and terfenadine partially inhibited the early nasal response to allergen challenge, in addition to decreasing sneezing and secretions. (From Ref. 9.)

cacy of H_1-receptor antagonists with cromolyn, nedocromil, and glucocorticoids in subjects with rhinitis, there are few direct comparisons of the *antiallergic* effects of H_1-receptor antagonists with those of these other classes of medications in allergic disorders.

IV. Clinical Pharmacology

A. Pharmacokinetics

The pharmacokinetics of some of the first-generation and most of the second-generation H_1-receptor antagonists have been investigated in healthy subjects, in subjects with allergic rhinitis, and in special populations such as persons with hepatic or renal dysfunction, the elderly, and children. H_1-receptor antagonists are well absorbed after oral administration, with time from oral intake to peak plasma concentration often being less than 1 hr (1,10–17) (Table 1). Protein binding ranges from 78 to 99%.

Most H_1-receptor antagonists are metabolized by the hepatic microsomal mixed-function oxygenase system. Plasma concentrations are relatively low after single oral doses, which indicates considerable first-pass extraction by the liver. Terminal elimination half-life values are variable, ranging from about 2 hr for acrivastine to about 24 hr for older H_1-receptor antagonists such as chlorpheniramine and hydroxyzine, and for newer ones such as astemizole and azelastine. The terminal elimination half-life values of H_1-receptor antagonist active metabolites such as desmethylastemizole, descarboethoxyloratadine, desmethylastemizole, and desmethylazelastine differ from those of their respective parent compounds. Half-life values of H_1-receptor antagonists which undergo hepatic metabolism are shorter in children and prolonged in the elderly, in subjects with hepatic dysfunction, and in those receiving hepatic microsomal oxygenase inhibitors such as macrolide antibiotics or imidazole antifungals.

Some H_1-receptor antagonists such as cetirizine, acrivastine, and levocabastine are eliminated largely unchanged in the urine; fexofenadine is eliminated largely unchanged in the urine and feces. The terminal elimination half-life values for acrivastine, cetirizine, and levocabastine may be prolonged in subjects with renal insufficiency.

B. Pharmacodynamics

Suppression of the wheal-and-flare reaction in the skin induced by histamine or antigens provides a useful biological assay of H_1-receptor antagonists at peripheral H_1-receptors (1,10–17). This assay has been well standardized and digitized for use in clinical research. H_1-receptor antagonists decrease the size of the wheal by decreasing vascular permeability and leakage of plasma protein, and decrease the size of the flare by reducing indirect vasodilation caused by stimulation of the

Table 1 Pharmacokinetics of Representative H_1-Receptor Antagonists

H_1-receptor antagonist[a] (metabolite)	t_{max}[c] (hr)	$t_{1/2}$[d] (hr)	Duration of action (hr)[e]
Old, first-generation			
Chlorpheniramine	2.8 ± 0.8	27.9 ± 8.7	1–24
New, second-generation			
Acrivastine	1.4 ± 0.4	1.7 ± 0.2	1–6
	0.85–1.4	1.4–2.1	
Astemizole (desmethylastemizole)	0.5 ± 0.2 to 0.7 ± 0.3	1.1 days 9.5 days	1–24
Azelastine (demethylazelastine)	5.3 ± 1.6 (20.5)	22 ± 4 (54 ± 15)	1–12
Cetirizine	1.0 ± 0.5	7.4 ± 1.6	1–24
Ebastine[b] (carebastine)	(3.6 ± 1.0)	(10.3 ± 2.6)	1–24
Fexofenadine	1–3	14.4	1–24
Levocabastine	2	33	0.5–12
Loratadine (descarboethoxyloratadine)	1.0 ± 0.3 (1.5 ± 0.7)	11.0 ± 9.4 (17.3 ± 6.9)	1–24
Mizolastine[b]	1	8.9 ± 2.5	1–24

[a]Results are mean $\pm$ standard deviation, in healthy young adults.
[b]Not approved for use in the United States at time of publication.
[c]Time from oral intake to peak plasma concentration.
[d]Plasma terminal elimination half-life.
[e]Assessed using the wheal-and-flare reaction in human skin.

histamine-induced axon reflex. All H_1-receptor antagonists inhibit this reaction in the skin to some extent, but the magnitude of the effect, the time to peak effect, and the duration of the effect are medication- and dose-related. Inhibition correlates with onset of relief of symptoms of allergic rhinitis. It usually begins within 1 hr and is greatest 5–7 hr after a dose, several hours after maximal plasma concentration is reached. There is therefore a pharmacodynamic as well as a pharmacological rationale for giving an H_1-receptor antagonist *before* an anticipated allergic reaction, if possible, to achieve greatest efficacy. The delay in response is probably not due to delay of the medication in reaching the skin, as skin concentrations are as high as or higher than plasma concentrations throughout the dosing interval.

The duration of action of a single dose of an H_1-receptor antagonist is more prolonged than might be expected in view of the terminal elimination half-life. For many of the medications, it is approximately 24 hr, and once-a-day dosing is possible (18) (Fig. 4; Table 2). After a 7-day course of H_1-receptor antagonists

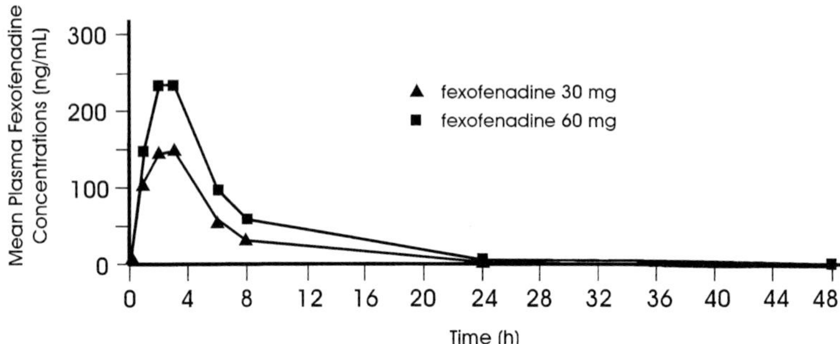

a

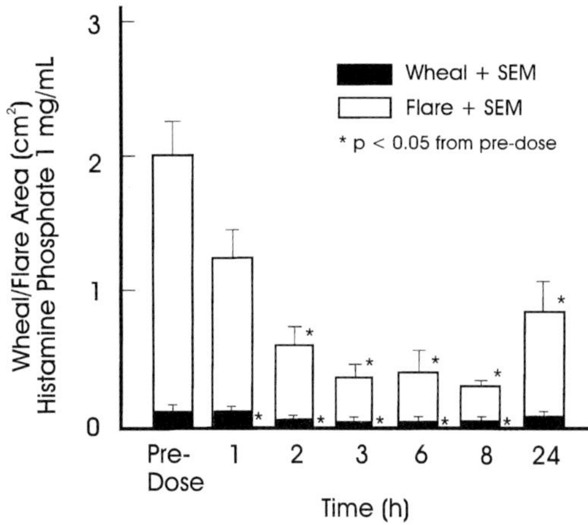

b

Figure 4 In a double-blind, crossover study, 15 children received fexofenadine 30 mg or 60 mg on two separate study days, at least 1 week apart. Plasma fexofenadine concentrations were measured and suppression of the histamine-induced wheal-and-flare reaction was monitored before each dose and from 1 to 24 hr after the dose. (a) The terminal elimination half-life was 18 hr. (b) Prompt, sustained wheal-and-flare suppression was noted after fexofenadine 30 mg (shown) and 60 mg (not shown). (From Ref. 18.)

Table 2 Formulations and Dosages of Representative H_1-Receptor Antagonists

	Formulation	Recommended dose
Old, first-generation		
Chlorpheniramine maleate (Chlortrimeton)	Tablets 4 mg, 8 mg[b], 12 mg[b] Syrup 2.5 mg/5 ml Parenteral solution 10 mg/ml	Adult: 8–12 mg bid[b] Pediatric[c]: 0.35 mg/kg/ 24 hr
New, second-generation		
Acrivastine (Semprex)	Tablets 8 mg (with pseudoephedrine 60 mg)	Adult: 8 mg tid
Astemizole (Hismanal)	Tablets 10 mg Suspension 10 mg/5 ml[a]	Adult: 10 mg od Pediatric[a]: 0.2 mg/kg/ 24 hr
Azelastine (Astelin)	Nasal solution 0.1% (0.137 mg/spray) Tablets 2 mg[a]	Intranasal: 2 sprays in each nostril od or bid; adult: 2–4 mg bid[a]
Cetirizine (Reactine)	Tablets 10 mg	Adult: 5–10 mg od
Ebastine[a] (Ebastel)	Tablets 10 mg[a]	Adult: 10 mg od[a]
Fexofenadine (Allegra)	Tablets 60 mg, 120 mg[a]	Adult: 60 mg bid *or* 120 mg od[a]
Levocabastine (Livostin)	Microsuspension: ophthalmic 50 µg/ml (15 µg/ drop); nasal[a] 50 µg/ml (50 µg/spray)	Ophthalmic: adults and children (12–65 yr): 1 drop in each eye bid (may be increased to tid or qid) Intranasal: 2 sprays in each nostril bid–qid[a]
Loratadine (Claritin)	Tablets 10 mg Syrup 1 mg/ml	Adult: 10 mg od Pediatric: (2–12 yr): 5 mg/day (>12 yr and >30 kg): 10 mg/day
Mizolastine[a] (Mizollen)	Tablets 10 mg[a]	Adult: 10 mg od[a]

od, once daily; bid, twice daily; tid, three times daily; qid, four times daily.
[a] Not approved for use in the United States at time of publication.
[b] Timed-release.
[c] For subjects $\leq$40 kg.

such as cetirizine, fexofenadine, or loratadine, histamine blockade persists for a few days after the medication is stopped; for astemizole, the blockade may persist for 4–6 weeks.

Long-term administration of H_1-receptor antagonists does not lead to autoinduction of hepatic metabolism or an increased rate of elimination. In studies lasting 4–12 weeks, during which compliance was closely monitored, peripheral H_1-receptor blockade in the skin and efficacy in allergic rhinitis did not decrease significantly (1).

The diversity in the clinical pharmacology of H_1-receptor antagonists is an advantage, as it enables physicians to make a rational choice of medications for use in various clinical circumstances.

V. Clinical Efficacy

A. H_1-Receptor Antagonists Used for Allergic Rhinitis Treatment

The efficacy of H_1-receptor antagonists in seasonal or perennial allergic rhinitis has been well documented in prospective, randomized, double-blind, placebo-controlled clinical trials in large numbers of subjects (10–17). These studies have contributed significantly to improved understanding of the pathophysiology of allergic rhinitis, as well as to knowledge about individual H_1-receptor antagonists.

In the clinical investigation of H_1-receptor antagonists, as in the investigation of efficacy and safety of other classes of medication used for allergic rhinitis treatment, standards have improved greatly during the past decade. In seasonal allergic rhinitis studies, pollen counts are monitored throughout and subjects in the active treatment and placebo groups are matched for sensitivity to the allergens likely to be encountered during the study. In perennial rhinitis studies, although subjects' sensitivity to allergen is always documented, allergen exposure has not, to date, generally been quantitated.

The design of many seasonal and perennial rhinitis studies incorporates a pre-H_1-receptor anatagonist treatment run-in period, during which baseline symptoms are recorded and subjects qualify for the study by demonstrating a minimal baseline pretreatment level of nasal symptoms: itch, sneezing, and rhinorrhea, and ancillary symptoms: itchy, watery eyes, itchy throat or ears, and cough. In some studies, subjects responding to placebo during this run-in period are eliminated from the study population. In many clinical trials the symptom of obstruction is scored separately from other rhinitis symptoms; subjects with anatomical problems contributing to nasal obstruction are excluded from participation. Increasingly, in addition to assessment of rhinitis symptoms, per se, studies are designed to include assessment of the impact of rhinitis on quality of life, that is, how the disorder affects daily functioning (19).

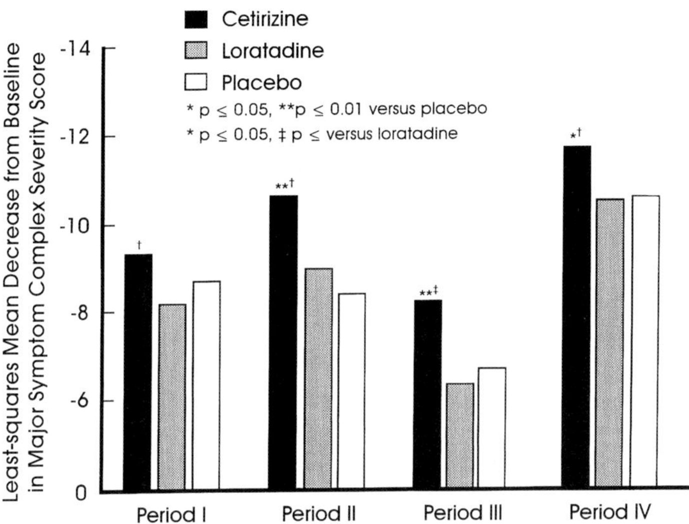

Figure 5 In a double-blind, parallel-group, 2-day study conducted in outdoor parks, 279 subjects during the spring allergy season, cetirizine 10 mg, loratadine 10 mg, or placebo was administered at 10:00 A.M. on both days. Symptom scores were obtained hourly from 11:00 A.M. to 4:00 P.M. in the park (period I); at 6:00, 8:00, and 10:00 P.M. at home (period II); the next day in the park hourly from 8:00 to 10:00 A.M. (period III); and from 11:00 A.M. to 4:00 P.M. at home (period IV). Cetirizine produced significantly greater mean reductions than loratadine or placebo in major symptom complex severity scores at all time periods ($p \leq 0.05$), except period I for placebo. The study medications were well tolerated. The incidence of somnolence was 13% with cetirizine versus 2% with placebo ($p < 0.05$), versus 5% with loratadine. Headache occurred more frequently with loratadine (23%) than with cetirizine (11%) ($p = 0.03$). (From Ref. 20.) MSC = major symptom complex. In "real life," beyond clinical trials, H_1-antagonists seem to have similar effectiveness.

The duration of seasonal allergic rhinitis studies is usually 1–2 weeks, starting at the beginning of the pollen season. "Day in the park" studies of about 48-hr duration (20) (Fig. 5) and even shorter studies incorporating allergen challenge in a room or chamber (21) also provide useful information, especially about onset of action. The duration of perennial allergic rhinitis studies is usually 4–8 weeks. In most studies, the H_1-receptor antagonist is administered on a regular daily or twice-daily basis. Although H_1-receptor antagonists are commonly used on an "as-needed" basis for prevention or relief of symptoms in rhinitis, there are few formal studies of this clinical application.

In the hundreds of trials of H_1-receptor antagonists that have been conducted in rhinitis, although there are minor differences in outcome attributable to study design (number of subjects enrolled, criteria for study entry, and pollen counts or other local environmental factors), a general efficacy profile for these medications emerges. They modify the subjective symptoms of nasal itch, sneeze, and rhinorrhea to a greater extent than placebo does, but are not much more effective than placebo in relieving nasal obstruction. In subjects with concomitant allergic conjunctivitis, itching, watering, and redness of the eyes are also very effectively treated using H_1-receptor antagonists. Overall, about 50–60% reduction in symptoms, compared to 30–40% reduction produced by placebo, can be documented (10–17). In seasonal allergic rhinitis, results are best if the medications are started early in the pollen season.

The efficacy profiles of newer, relatively nonsedating H_1-receptor antagonists such as cetirizine, ebastine, fexofenadine, loratadine, and mizolastine are similar to the profiles of potentially sedating medications such as chlorpheniramine (1,10–17). Furthermore, the efficacy profiles of orally administered medications are similar to those of intranasal agents such as azelastine or levocabastine (22). Although the intranasal agents have a slightly more rapid onset of action and are quite effective in relieving pruritus, sneezing, and rhinorrhea, like H_1-receptor antagonists administered orally, they are not highly effective in relieving nasal blockage.

There are few published dose-response studies of H_1-receptor antagonists in allergic rhinitis. Although a dose-response effect may be noted for some symptoms, doubling the manufacturers' recommended dose does not usually result in a significant increase in overall symptom relief. While nonresponders to one H_1-receptor antagonist may respond to another, in general, subjects with allergic rhinitis who do not respond to an H_1-receptor antagonist should be considered strong candidates for intranasal glucocorticoid treatment.

Although manufacturers can always find one or more studies to support claims for superiority of ''their'' particular H_1-receptor antagonist, when all published studies are reviewed, overall, no H_1-receptor antagonist, old or new, oral or intranasal, emerges with a clinically important superior efficacy profile (1,22). Selection of an H_1-receptor antagonist for allergic rhinitis treatment is thus based on considerations such as safety profile, cost (23), and individual preference.

B. H_1-Receptor Antagonists and Other Medications Used for Allergic Rhinitis Treatment

To provide increased relief of nasal blockage, H_1 antagonists are marketed in fixed-dose combinations with decongestants such as pseudoephedrine (22,24) (Fig. 6).

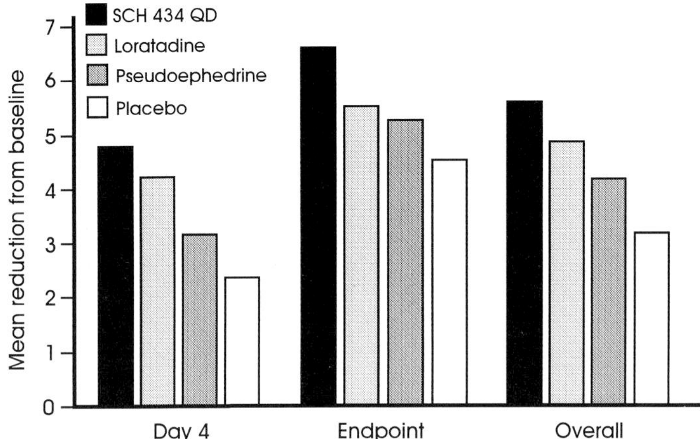

Figure 6 In a double-blind, placebo-controlled study, 874 subjects with moderate-severe seasonal allergic rhinitis were treated for 2 weeks with loratadine 10 mg/pseudoephedrine 240 mg (extended-release) or loratadine 10 mg or pseudoephedrine 120 mg every 12 hr or placebo. The combination was more effective than either of the components alone or than placebo in the treatment of seasonal allergic rhinitis; specifically, it was superior to pseudoephedrine in reducing nonnasal symptoms at all time points ($p < 0.01$) and superior to loratadine in relieving nasal stuffiness at end-point ($p < 0.01$). (From Ref. 24.)

H_1-receptor antagonists, whether administered orally or applied to the nasal mucosa or conjunctivae, provide comparable or slightly greater relief of allergic rhinoconjunctivitis to that provided by intranasal sodium cromoglycate in a 4% solution administered four times daily (25). Intranasal H_1-receptor antagonists also have similar efficacy to nedocromil.

H_1-receptor antagonists are less effective than intranasal glucocorticoids for relief of nasal symptoms in allergic rhinitis. In a few studies in which representative medications from these two classes have been compared, subjects treated with an H_1-receptor antagonist alone or with an H_1-receptor antagonist in combination with an intranasal glucocorticoid have had superior relief of ocular symptoms, compared with subjects treated with the intranasal glucocorticoid alone (26).

H_1-receptor antagonists administered simultaneously with H_2-receptor antagonists intranasally or by mouth are significantly more effective in decreasing nasal airflow resistance induced by intranasal histamine provocation than either the H_1 or the H_2 antagonists are alone, but the added effectiveness is small and has not been found in all studies (27). Intranasal pretreatment with an H_2-receptor antagonist alone decreases rhinorrhea but not sneezing, in contrast to pretreatment with the H_1-receptor antagonist alone, which decreases both rhinorrhea and sneezing.

C. H_1-Receptor Antagonists in Other Respiratory Tract Disorders

Upper Respiratory Tract Infections

H_1-receptor antagonists are widely used for treatment of viral upper respiratory tract infections, although until recently there has been little scientific rationale for this practice (28). Histamine concentrations are increased in urine, but not nasal secretions in subjects with symptomatic rhinovirus-induced colds, in contrast to the increased levels of kinins, TAME-esterase activity, and albumin found in secretions.

Asthma

Historically, there have been concerns about using H_1-receptor antagonists in subjects with rhinitis who also have concomitant asthma, because of the possibility of increased drying of secretions and of bronchoconstriction. These concerns are no longer valid. During the past two decades, H_1-receptor antagonists have been thoroughly investigated in asthma.

Pretreatment with an H_1-receptor antagonist provides some protection against bronchospasm induced by histamine, exercise, hyperventilation of cold, dry air, hypertonic or hypotonic saline, distilled water, adenosine $5'$-monophosphate, or allergen, especially the early allergic response. The amount of protection varies with the H_1 antagonist, the dose, and the stimulus used for bronchoconstriction (29) (Fig. 7).

H_1-receptor antagonists also relieve mild persistent asthma symptoms. This effect may be due, at least in part, to improvement in concomitant allergic rhinitis, as in usual doses, the direct bronchodilator effect of H_1-antagonists is minimal. H_1-antagonists are not effective in severe persistent asthma.

Otitis Media

Acute otitis media and otitis media with effusion have high spontaneous remission rates. H_1-receptor antagonists, often in combination with α-adrenergic decongestants, are frequently prescribed for children with otitis media, but there are no placebo-controlled, double-blind studies incorporating repeated objective assessment of tympanic membrane compliance to support a beneficial effect of H_1-receptor antagonists on eustachian tube function in these disorders. Despite several negative studies of the efficacy of H_1-receptor antagonists in otitis media (30), it is of interest that histamine concentrations are elevated in the middle ear

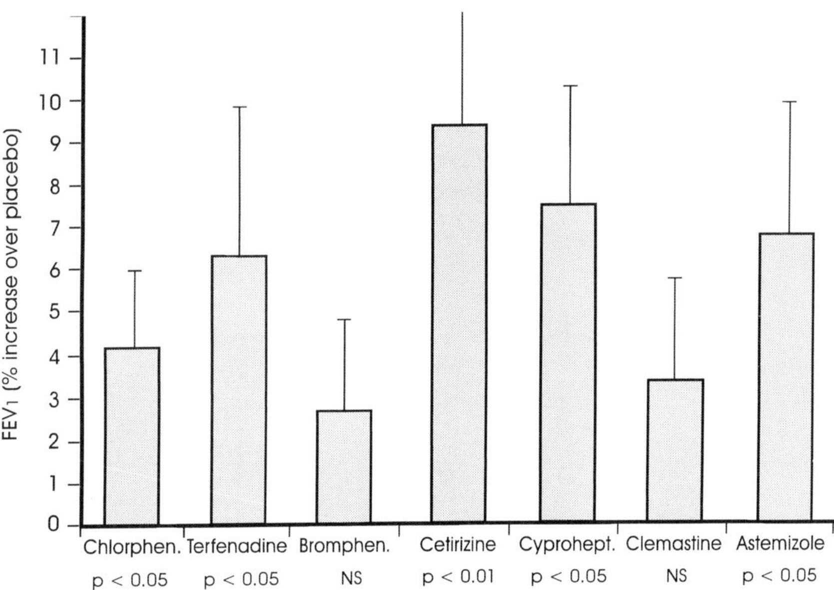

Figure 7 In a single-blind, placebo-controlled study, 20 volunteers with stable asthma received chlorpheniramine (4 mg), terfenadine (60 mg), brompheniramine (4 mg), cetirizine (10 mg), cyproheptadine (4 mg), clemastine (1 mg), or astemizole (10 mg). Subjects had FEV_1 measurements, bronchial challenge with histamine phosphate in doubling concentrations of 0.03–32 mg/ml, and epicutaneous tests with doubling concentrations of histamine phosphate from 2 to 32 mg/ml. All H_1-antagonists had some bronchodilator effect (shown). The mean increase in FEV_1 ranged from 2.58% after brompheniramine to 9.28% after cetirizine. All H_1-receptor antagonists displaced the histamine concentration-response curve to the right, but only cetirizine and terfenadine had a significant effect. There was good correlation between the protective effect of the H_1 antagonists in the skin and in the airways ($r = 0.85$, $p < 0.01$).(From Ref. 29.)

effusions in otitis media and that the eustachian tube response to intranasal histamine and other chemical mediators of inflammation is increased in subjects with allergic rhinitis compared to healthy subjects.

Other

Allergic rhinitis and chronic sinusitis often coexist. Although H_1-receptor antagonists may be useful as adjunctive medications for the treatment of rhinorrhea and other nasal symptoms in this situation, they are not recommended as primary medications for the treatment of sinusitis. There is also no rationale for using H_1-receptor antagonists in the treatment of nasal polyposis.

VI. Potential Adverse Effects of H_1-Receptor Antagonists

A. Central Nervous System Adverse Effects

Old H_1-Receptor Antagonists

Some H_1-receptor antagonists were discovered during programmed searches for antipsychotic medications. In recommended doses, old H_1-receptor antagonists such as triprolidine, diphenhydramine, and chlorpheniramine may have adverse effects on the central nervous system. While nearly all studies have focused on subjective somnolence and objective impaired performance, many other adverse neurological effects may occur (31) (Table 3). Even chlorpheniramine, not usually considered to be a highly sedating first-generation H_1-receptor antagonist, has been reported to cause CNS impairment in over 40% of users (32,33).

Gastrointestinal upset, appetite stimulation, or anticholinergic effects such as dry mouth, blurred vision, urinary retention, or impotence may also be noted. Rarely, jaundice and cytopenias have been reported. An overdose may result in coma, or in paradoxical stimulatory central nervous system effects such as seizures, dyskinesia, or dystonia, or neuropsychiatric effects such as hallucinations or psychosis. Tachycardia, prolongation of the QTc interval, heart block, and arrhythmias have been reported.

Old H_1-receptor antagonists are still used because they are effective and relatively inexpensive, especially if generic formulations are used (23). Some physicians recommend giving these medications at bedtime only, because somnolence and impaired performance are of no concern during the night, and peripheral H_1-blockade may be present the next morning. Indeed, the older H_1-antagonists, diphenhydramine, doxylamine, and pyrilamine, are widely used as nonprescription sleeping aids. Other physicians advocate regular daytime use, anticipating that the subjects will become tolerant of the central nervous system adverse effects but not of the peripheral H_1 blockade; however, development of tolerance to the sedative effect of H_1-receptor antagonists has not occurred consistently in double-blind studies of the phenomenon (32).

Physicians should be cautious about recommending old H_1-receptor antagonists, bearing in mind that pilots are not allowed to use these medications, and that in many jurisdictions, motorists involved in an accident and found to be driving under the influence of one of these medications can be fined or jailed or have their licenses revoked. It is unknown how many students have failed examinations or how many employees have made errors in their work after ingesting an older H_1-receptor antagonist. The warning that appears on the package

Table 3 Adverse Neurological Effects of Old First-Generation Antihistamines

Stimultory	
Dyskinesia	Irritability
Dystonia	Headaches
Seizures	Muscle twitching
Euphoria	Nervousness
Hyperreflexia	Tremor
Insomnia	
Neuropsychiatric	
Anxiety	Hysteria
Catatonia	Impaired mental efficiency
Confusion	Impaired judgment
Delusion	Psychosis
Depression	Hallucinations
Peripheral	
Areflexia	Paralysis
Blurred vision	Paresthesias
Dilated pupils	Toxic neuritis
Depressive	
Ataxia	Lassitude
Coma	Narcolepsy
Delirium	Sedation
Dizziness	Somnolence
Drowsiness	Weakness
Fatigue	

inserts for these medications, to avoid use if driving a vehicle or operating heavy machinery, is outdated in this high-technology era.

New H_1-Receptor Antagonists

Compared to the old H_1-receptor antagonists, the new medications, cetirizine, fexofenadine, loratadine, and mizolastine have relatively fewer adverse central nervous system effects such as somnolence or impaired performance (10–17,34) (Fig. 8), as documented in over 70 objective studies using electroencephalographic monitoring, sleep latency investigations, and standardized performance tests, including clerical tasks, school learning, simulated or actual driving, and simulated aircraft piloting. Most studies have been performed in healthy subjects. The improved margin of safety with regard to central nervous system adverse effects provided by the newer medications may be especially important in sub-

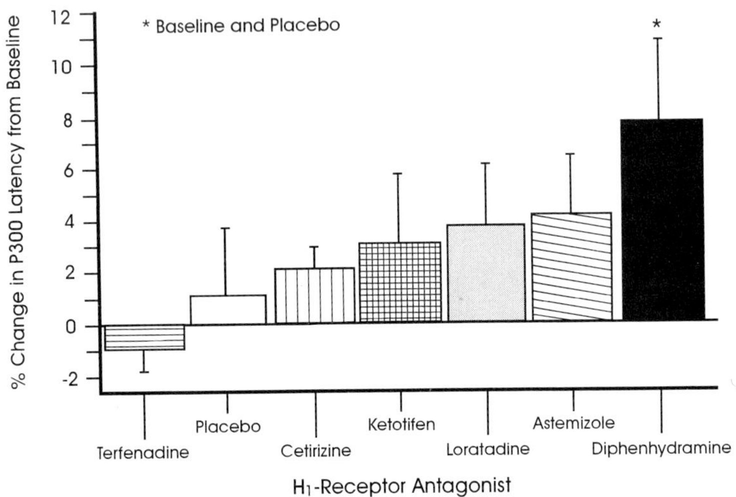

Figure 8 In a double-blind, placebo-controlled, crossover study, 15 healthy men received six different H_1-receptor antagonists. In rank order from least to greatest effect on the P300 latency, the medications were: terfenadine 60 mg, placebo, cetirizine 10 mg, ketotifen 2 mg, loratadine 10 mg, astemizole 10 mg, and diphenhydramine 50 mg. Only diphenhydramine increased the P300 latency significantly compared to baseline and placebo. *The increase in subjective somnolence was significantly greater than placebo after cetirizine, ketotifen, and diphenhydramine.* All H_1-receptor antagonists produced peripheral H_1-blockade. (From Ref. 34.)

jects with allergic rhinitis (35), which may itself affect the duration and quality of nocturnal sleep, with resulting impairment of performance the following day.

No new H_1-receptor antagonist is entirely free from these adverse effects under all circumstances. Among new H_1-receptor antagonists, some are more central-nervous-system-impairing than others. The new H_1-receptor antagonists acrivastine (10), azelastine (15), and levocabastine (11), although not as well studied from the point of view of central nervous system safety, do seem to cause somnolence when administered by mouth; acrivastine is sold only in combination with a decongestant that has central-nervous-system-stimulating effects. When administered intranasally, azelastine and levocabastine do not seem to increase somnolence. The central nervous system effects of cetirizine have been well studied, and while it selsom causes significant impairment of performance, it seems more likely to cause subjective somnolence than placebo (16,20,34).

If the manufacturers' recommended doses of new H_1-receptor antagonists are exceeded, central nervous system function may become impaired. When these medications are administered concomitantly with alcohol, diazepam, or related substances, they do not increase the somnolence and the impaired performance produced by these CNS-active chemicals alone (32,33). The decongestant component of second-generation H_1-antagonist/decongestant formulations may cause insomnia and other central nervous system stimulatory symptoms.

B. Cardiovascular Adverse Effects

Although old H_1-receptor antagonists are not entirely free from these effects, recent attention has focused on the rare and usually preventable cardiovascular adverse effects produced by astemizole and terfenadine (36) (Fig. 9). These H_1-receptor antagonists may prolong the QTc interval and cause cardiac dysrhythmias after overdose or under other specific conditions such as: pre-existing cardiovascular disorders including congenital or acquired prolonged QT syndrome or bradycardia; metabolic problems such as hypokalemia or hypocalcemia; hepatic dysfunction; or concomitant use of hepatic mixed-function oxygenase inhibitors such as macrolide antibiotics (erythromycin, clarithromycin) or imidazole antifungals (ketaconazole, itraconazole) (32,37). Not all individuals at risk actually develop dysrhythmias. Important warning symptoms include syncope at rest or with exercise, loss of consciousness, and palpitations.

The mechanism involves excessive delay in repolarization that induces early after-depolarizations and delayed repolarization, and produces marked QTc prolongation, bizarre T-wave changes, and a variety of dysrhythmias, including polymorphic ventricular tachycardia or torsades de pointes (37). Central nervous system adverse effects such as somnolence are caused by a completely different mechanism, and their presence or absence does not have any predictive value for cardiovascular system adverse effects.

Use of astemizole or terfenadine has declined worldwide in recent years, and terfenadine has recently been withdrawn from the market in some countries. Newer H_1-antagonists can now be screened with regard to their proclivity to cause cardiovascular effects in humans before clinical trials are conducted; patch clamp studies using isolated human ventricular myocytes, or cloned human ion channels are used for this purpose.

C. Other Potential Adverse Effects

Astemizole and ketotifen, like the old H_1-receptor antagonist cyproheptadine, may stimulate the appetite and lead to inappropriate weight gain. Azelastine may cause a transient bitter or metallic taste when administered orally or even intranasally. Azelastine or levocabastine administered intranasally may cause mucosal irritation, but they have not been reported to induce sensitization during short-term topical treatment, in contrast to the sensitization induced by topical application

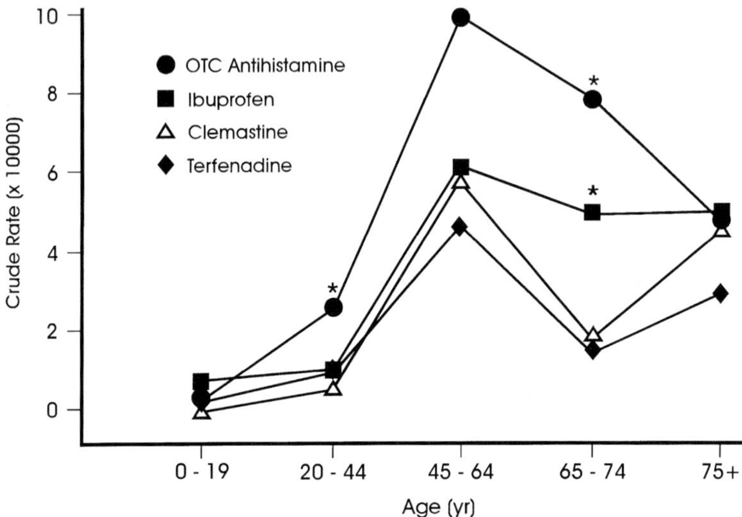

Figure 9 The investigators tested the hypothesis that terfenadine exposure increased the risk of arrhythmias, using an observational historical cohort study design and a medication exposure period of 30 days in people receiving terfenadine ($n = 181,672$), over-the-counter (OTC), nonprescription antihistamines ($n = 150,689$), ibuprofen ($n = 181,672$) (* = P < 0.01), and clemastine ($n = 83,156$). Ibuprofen was studied as a "control" because it is free from cardiovascular effects. The incidence of ventricular arrhythmias and cardiac arrest was higher in the OTC antihistamine group than in the terfenadine, ibuprofen, and clemastine groups. Crude rates per 10,000 prescription exposures of developing a life-threatening ventricular arrhythmia are represented for the four medication cohorts over the age categories assessed in the study. Interaction ($\uparrow$ = increased relative risk) between terfenadine and ketoconazole was identified ($n = 648$, relative risk = 26.08, $p < 0.001$). There was a trend toward interaction between terfenadine and erythromycin ($n = 41,308$, relative risk = 1.36, p = NS) (not shown). (From Ref. 36.)

of H_1-receptor antagonists to the skin. There is no evidence that any H_1-receptor antagonist currently approved for use has a carcinogenic or tumor-promoting effect in humans.

D. Safety Issues in Special Populations

Pregnancy and Lactation

H_1-receptor antagonists cross the placenta. Some old H_1 antagonists are teratogenic in animals, and have been suspected, although never proven, of causing fetal anomalies in humans. There is no evidence that new H_1-receptor antagonists cause fetal anomalies in humans. Some of the new ones, including cetirizine and loratadine, are classified as FDA Pregnancy Category B, indicating no evidence of risk in humans. Other new H_1-anatagonists are classified as FDA Pregnancy Category C and should be used during pregnancy only if the expected benefits to the mother exceed the unknown risks to the fetus (38).

H_1-receptor antagonists are excreted in breast milk and the old ones can cause drowsiness or irritability in infants when transmitted via this route.

Children

Although the new H_1-receptor antagonists have been studied in children with seasonal or perennial allergic rhinitis (38), some of these medications are not yet approved for use in children under age 12 years and are not yet available in liquid formulations.

Athletes

Old H_1-receptor antagonists that may potentially affect performance should not be recommended for competitive athletes. Labels of prescription and nonprescription H_1-receptor antagonists alike should be scrutinized with particular care by this group of individuals, as in addition to the H_1-receptor antagonists, these products may contain "banned" substances such as pseudoephedrine or phenylpropanolamine.

Rhinitis in the Workplace

Occupational rhinitis, defined as episodic work-related occurrence of sneezing, rhinorrhea, and nasal obstruction, triggered by dust fumes or vapors in the workplace is common. Old H_1-receptor antagonists are contraindicated in this population because of their potential not only for impairing job performance, but also for placing workers at risk of injury to themselves or others while on the job. Other employees, such as sleep-deprived shift workers and workers who have to perform boring, repetitive tasks, may be at increased risk for somnolence and similar problems after ingesting an old H_1-receptor antagonist (39).

Elderly

There are few specific studies of H_1-receptor antagonists in elderly subjects. The limited numbers of safety studies that have been performed suggest that the elderly may be at increased risk for adverse central nervous system effects from old H_1 antagonists, a special concern in view of the widespread use of these medications as sedatives in nursing homes and similar facilities. The elderly may also be at increased risk for adverse cardiovascular effects from astemizole and terfenadine (40).

VII. Conclusions

Histamine is, quantitatively, the most important chemical mediator of inflammation in allergic rhinitis. Its role in the pathophysiology of this disorder is well studied and well established. The diverse clinical pharmacology of H_1-receptor antagonists contrasts markedly with their rather similar efficacy profiles. H_1-receptor antagonists effectively prevent and relieve occasional or chronic allergic rhinitis symptoms of sneezing, itching, and rhinorrhea, but not of nasal blockage. They improve the quality of life for many people suffering from mild or moderate allergic rhinitis. Even in those with severe disease, addition of an H_1-receptor antagonist to the intranasal glucocorticoid treatment regimen may enhance relief of and systemic symptoms. The new H_1-receptor antagonists should supplant the old ones in the treatment of allergic rhinitis because of their more favorable benefit/risk ratios. Impaired central nervous system function after ingestion of the old H_1-receptor antagonists is more common than generally realized. In view of this, in addition to efficacy, safety issues, rather than cost, should be the determining factor when recommending an H_1-receptor antagonist for use in allergic rhinitis treatment.

References

1.   Simons FER, Simons KJ. The pharmacology and use of H_1-receptor antagonist drugs. N Engl J Med 1994; 330:1663–1670.
2.   Naclerio RM. Allergic rhinitis. N Engl J Med 1991; 325:860–869.
3.   Howarth P. H_1-receptor antagonists in rhinoconjunctivitis. In: Simons FER, ed. Histamine and H_1-Receptor Antagonists in Allergic Disease. New York: Marcel Dekker, 1996:215–249.
4.   Iriyoshi N, Takeuchi K, Yuta A, Ukai K, Sakakura Y. Increased expression of histamine H_1 receptor mRNA in allergic rhinitis. Clin Exp Allergy 1996; 26:379–385.
5.   Chowdhury BA, Kaliner MA. Molecular cloning and characterization of the human histamine H_1 receptor gene. ACI News 1995; 7:24–28.
6.   Zhang MQ, ter Laak AM, Timmerman H. Structure-activity relationships within a series of analogues of the histamine H_1-antagonist terfenadine. Eur J Med Chem 1993; 28:165–173.
7.   Casy AF. Antagonists of H_1 receptors of histamine: recent developments. In: Uvnäs B, ed. Histamine and Histamine Antagonists. Berlin: Springer-Verlag, 1991:549–572.
8.   Rimmer SJ, Church MK. The pharmacology and mechanisms of action of histamine H_1-antagonists. Clin Exp Allergy 1990; 20:3–17.
9.   Baroody FM, Lim MC, Proud D, Kagey-Sobotka A, Lichtenstein LM, Naclerio RM. Effects of loratadine and terfenadine on the induced nasal allergic reaction. Arch Otolaryngol Head Neck Surg 1996; 122:309–316.
10. Brogden RN, McTavish D. Acrivastine. A review of its pharmacological properties

and therapeutic efficacy in allergic rhinitis, urticaria and related disorders. Drugs 1991; 41:927–940.

11. Dechant KL, Goa KL. Levocabastine. A review of its pharmacological properties and therapeutic potential as a topical antihistamine in allergic rhinitis and conjunctivitis. Drugs 1991; 41:202–224.

12. Haria M, Fitton A, Peters DH. Loratadine. A reappraisal of its pharmacological properties and therapeutic use in allergic disorders. Drugs 1994; 48:617–637.

13. Janssens MM-L. Astemizole. A nonsedating antihistamine with fast and sustained activity. Clin Rev Allergy 1993; 11:35–63.

14. McTavish D, Goa KL, Ferrill M. Terfenadine: an updated review of its pharmacological properties and therapeutic efficacy. Drugs 1990; 39:552–574.

15. McTavish D, Sorkin EM. Azelastine: a review of its pharmacodynamic and pharmacokinetic properties, and therapeutic potential. Drugs 1989; 38:778–800.

16. Spencer CM, Faulds D, Peters DH. Cetirizine. A reappraisal of its pharmacological properties and therapeutic use in selected allergic disorders. Drugs 1993; 46:1055–1080.

17. Wiseman LR, Faulds D. Ebastine. A review of its pharmacological properties and clinical efficacy in the treatment of allergic disorders. Drugs 1996; 51:260–277.

18. Simons FER, Bergman JN, Watson WTA, Simons KJ. The clinical pharmacology of the new H_1-receptor antagonist fexofenadine in children. J Allergy Clin Immunol 1996; 98:1062–1064.

19. Harvey RP, Comer C, Sanders B, et al. Model for outcomes assessment of antihistamine use for seasonal allergic rhinitis. J Allergy Clin Immunol 1996; 97:1233–1241.

20. Meltzer EO, Weiler JM, Widlitz MD. Comparative outdoor study of the efficacy, onset and duration of action, and safety of cetirizine, loratadine, and placebo for seasonal allergic rhinitis. J Allergy Clin Immunol 1996; 97:617–626.

21. Day JH, Briscoe MP, Welsh A, Smith J, Mason J. Onset of action, efficacy and safety of a single dose of 60 mg and 120 mg fexofenadine HCl for ragweed allergy using controlled antigen exposure in an environmental exposure unit. J Allergy Clin Immunol 1996; 97:434.

22. Janssens MM-L, Howarth PH. The antihistamines of the nineties. Clin Rev Allergy 1993; 11:111–153.

23. Meltzer EO. An overview of current pharmacotherapy in perennial rhinitis. J Allergy Clin Immunol 1995; 95:1097–1110.

24. Bronsky E, Boggs P, Findlay S, et al. Comparative efficacy and safety of a once-daily loratadine-pseudoephedrine combination versus its components alone and placebo in the management of seasonal allergic rhinitis. J Allergy Clin Immunol 1995; 96:139–147.

25. Davies BH, Mullins J. Topical levocabastine is more effective than sodium cromoglycate for the prophylaxis and treatment of seasonal allergic conjunctivitis. Allergy 1993; 48:519–524.

26. Juniper EF, Kline PA, Hargreave FE, Dolovich J. Comparison of beclomethasone dipropionate aqueous nasal spray, astemizole, and the combination in the prophylactic treatment of ragweed pollen–induced rhinoconjunctivitis. J Allergy Clin Immunol 1989; 83:627–633.

27. Holmberg K, Pipkorn U, Bake B, Blychert L-O. Effects of topical treatment with

H$_1$ and H$_2$ antagonists on clinical symptoms and nasal vascular reactions in patients with allergic rhinitis. Allergy 1989; 44:281–287.

28. Smith MBH, Feldman W. Over-the-counter cold medications. A critical review of clinical trials between 1950 and 1991. JAMA 1993; 269:2258–2263.

29. Wood-Baker R, Holgate ST. The comparative actions and adverse effect profile of single doses of H$_1$-receptor antihistamines in the airways and skin of subjects with asthma. J Allergy Clin Immunol 1993; 91:1005–1014.

30. Cantekin EI, Mandel EM, Bluestone CD, et al. Lack of efficacy of a decongestant-antihistamine combination for otitis media with effusion ("secretory" otitis media) in children. N Engl J Med 1983; 308:297–301.

31. Meltzer EO. Comparative safety of H$_1$ antihistamines. Ann Allergy 1991; 67:625–633.

32. Simons FER. H$_1$-receptor antagonists. Comparative tolerability and safety. Drug Safety 1994; 10:350–380.

33. Hindmarch I, Bhatti JZ. Psychomotor effects of astemizole and chlorpheniramine, alone and in combination with alcohol. Int Clin Psychopharmacol 1987; 2:117–119.

34. Simons FER, Fraser TG, Reggin JD, Simons KJ. Comparison of the central nervous system effects produced by six H$_1$-receptor antagonists. Clin Exp Allergy 1996; 26:1092–1097.

35. Vuurman EFPM, van Veggel LMA, Uiterwijk MMC, Leutner D, O'Hanlon JF. Seasonal allergic rhinitis and antihistamine effects on children's learning. Ann Allergy 1993; 71:121–126.

36. Pratt CM, Hertz RP, Ellis BE, Crowell SP, Louv W, Moyé L. Risk of developing life-threatening ventricular arrhythmia associated with terfenadine in comparison with over-the-counter antihistamines, ibuprofen and clemastine. Am J Cardiol 1994; 73:346–352.

37. Woosley RL. Cardiac actions of antihistamines. Annu Rev Pharmacol Toxicol 1996; 36:233–252.

38. Simons FER. H$_1$-receptor antagonists in children. In: Simons FER, ed. Histamine and H$_1$-Receptor Antagonists in Allergic Disease. New York: Marcel Dekker, 1996:329–356.

39. Walsh JK, Muehlbach MJ, Schweitzer PK. Simulated assembly line performance following ingestion of cetirizine or hydroxyzine. Ann Allergy 1992; 69:195–200.

40. Tan R, Corren J. Optimum treatment of rhinitis in the elderly. Drugs Aging 1995; 7:168–175.

16

Nasal Airflow and Decongestants

RONALD ECCLES

Cardiff University
Cardiff, Wales, England

I. Introduction

Nasal congestion is related to engorgement of the nasal venous sinuses and these blood vessels can be decongested by treatment with topical and oral alpha-adrenergic agents. Nasal congestion is a very common and troublesome symptom associated with infective and allergic rhinitis. When nasal congestion occurs, it is often asymmetrical with one side of the nose almost obstructed while the other side may be quite open. Each side of the nose has a separate sensory and autonomic nerve supply and each side can react independently. To clarify the nature of nasal congestion and how nasal decongestants act this chapter will discuss the control of the nasal venous sinuses, the so-called "nasal cycle," and the factors that control nasal congestion.

Since the pharmacology of nasal decongestants is based on a sympathomimetic action, some description of the sympathetic nervous control of nasal blood flow and its effects on nasal airflow is required. The pharmacology of decongestant medications is discussed only in general terms to provide some understanding of their efficacy and limitations of use.

II. Control of Nasal Airflow

The nose acts as an air-conditioning system to warm, humidify, and filter the inspired air. To effectively mix and condition the airstream, the airflow must be turbulent (1). If the airflow was laminar, only the layer of air in contact with the nasal mucosa would be conditioned and the bulk of the airflow would not contact the nasal mucosa. Turbulent nasal airflow is generated by rapid changes in the direction and velocity of the inspired airstream. Suspended particulate matter is thrown onto the mucous blanket lining the nasal mucosa as the airstream changes direction and velocity as it passes from the narrow nasal valve region into the wider nasal cavity.

To act as an efficient air conditioner the nose must offer a considerable resistance to airflow, and nasal airway resistance is up to two-thirds of the total respiratory resistance (2). The major site of nasal resistance is situated at the narrowest point of the nasal airway, the nasal valve. The nasal valve is the area of the nose situated between the compliant nasal vestibule and the rigid bony cavum of the nose (3). The nasal valve is a dynamic valve, as nasal airway resistance is influenced by two compliant components: the lateral wall of the nasal vestibule, and the extensive venous sinuses or erectile tissue of the inferior turbinate and the nasal septum.

The compliant walls of the nasal vestibule are prone to collapse inward as inspiration generates a pressure difference across the walls of the nasal vestibule. The tendency for the walls of the nasal vestibule to collapse inward during inspiration is overcome by the splinting action of accessory respiratory muscles such as the alae nasi muscles, which attach to the alar cartilage (4). Contraction of the alae nasi muscles causes a dilation or flaring of the nostrils that stabilizes the walls of the nasal vestibule during the high nasal flow rates obtained with a maximal inspiratory effort and during exercise.

With normal quiet respiration the nasal airway resistance is mainly determined by the degree of engorgement of the venous sinuses in the nasal mucosa lining the tip of the inferior turbinate and the anterior end of the nasal septum. The nasal venous sinuses have some similarities with the erectile tissue of the male sexual apparatus as they have a great capacity for congestion, and filling of the venous sinuses can cause the tip of the inferior turbinate to swell forward by as much as 0.5 cm and cause complete obstruction of the nasal passage (5).

The mechanism controlling the filling of the venous sinuses is poorly understood. Throttle veins may control the emptying of the sinuses. Contraction of these veins would dam the venous drainage and cause congestion (6). The close apposition of arteries and veins in the bony canals of the nasal turbinates may be significant as dilation of the arterioles would increase the flow of blood into the sinuses and also compress the venous plexus, which drains the venous sinuses, and cause congestion (7,8). With a fixed outlet to the venous sinuses, the filling pressure determines the degree of congestion. Dilation of the arterioles in response to vasodilator inflammatory mediators may be a major factor determining the filling pressure of the venous sinuses and therefore the degree of congestion of the venous sinuses in rhinitis.

The venous sinuses are not simply passive vessels that dilate in response to changes in nasal blood flow. The venous sinuses have a wall of contractile smooth muscle with a dense adrenergic nerve supply from the sympathetic division of the autonomic nervous system (9). Electrical stimulation of the sympathetic nerves to the nose in animals causes a pronounced vasoconstriction, with shrinkage of the venous sinuses and a subsequent decrease in nasal airway resistance (10,11). Exercise causes nasal decongestion by an increase in sympathetic tone to the nasal blood vessels and a short period of exercise is often used as a means of decongesting the nose (1).

Under normal conditions there is a continuous sympathetic vasoconstrictor tone to the smooth muscle of the venous sinuses, and section or local anesthesia of the cervical sympathetic nerves that supply the nose causes relaxation of the vascular smooth muscle around the venous sinuses and nasal congestion (12–14). This observation indicates that the degree of congestion of the venous sinuses is determined by a balance between the filling pressure to the venous sinuses and the tension in the smooth muscle walls of the sinuses (15). The degree of congestion of the venous sinuses is therefore determined by two factors: nasal blood flow, which determines the filling pressure, and sympathetic tone, which determines the tone in the smooth muscle wall of the venous sinuses.

III. Nasal Cycle

The airflow through the nasal passages is normally asymmetrical with one nasal passage having the dominant airflow. This asymmetry of nasal airflow is not fixed, as the dominant airflow alternates from one nasal passage to the other over a period of several hours (16–20). The oscillations in nasal airflow are commonly referred to in the literature as the "nasal cycle," but Gilbert states that this term is confusing as there is little evidence for true cyclical changes in the majority of subjects who exhibit reciprocal changes in unilateral nasal airflow (21,22).

Because of the reciprocal changes in nasal airflow, one nasal passage usually has a higher airflow than the other. The airflow through the nasal passages is determined by the airway pressure changes during inspiration and expiration, and it is the negative or positive pressure at the level of the posterior nares that causes air to move through the nasal passages. Each nasal passage is exposed to the same pressure gradient and therefore it is the resistance of each nasal passage that determines the nasal airflow. The resistance is determined by the cross-sectional area of the nasal passage. Swelling of the venous sinuses narrows the nasal passage and therefore decreases the cross-sectional area and increases the resistance to airflow.

The reciprocal changes in nasal resistance are caused by changes in sympathetic nervous tone to the nasal venous sinuses, with the low-resistance side having the greatest sympathetic vasoconstrictor tone (13,14). Animal experiments indicate that reciprocal changes in nasal resistance are controlled from the respiratory areas of the brainstem with control of nasal resistance closely integrated with respiratory activity (23,24). A model illustrating the central control of the sympathetic tone to nasal venous sinuses is illustrated in Figure 1. The asymmetrical sympathetic tone is generated from two half-centers in the brainstem area with reciprocal connections across the brainstem (23).

The degree of unilateral nasal congestion is usually increased with inflammation of the nasal mucosa associated with nasal allergy and infection, and sub-

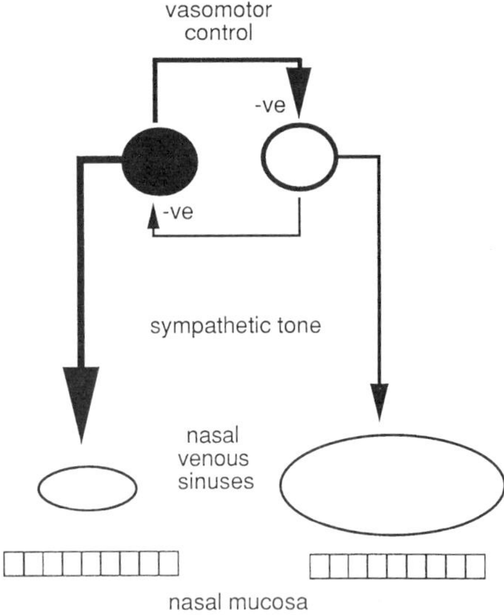

Figure 1 Model illustrating the sympathetic nervous control of nasal venous sinuses. Vasomotor control is proposed to reside in two half-centers in the brainstem. The half-centers have reciprocal connections, so that the dominance of activity oscillates over a period of hours, with only one center having dominance at any time. The sympathetic vasoconstrictor tone exerted by the right and left cervical sympathetic nerves, which supply the two halves of the nose, is normally asymmetrical. The asymmetrical sympathetic tone cause causes decongestion of the venous sinuses on one side of the nose and congestion on the other side. The spontaneous changes in nasal congestion over a period of hours are often called a ''nasal cycle.''

jects are often aware of periods of alternating unilateral nasal congestion when one nasal passage may be completely occluded (25,26). The amplitude of the spontaneous reciprocal changes in nasal resistance (nasal cycle) is increased during periods of upper respiratory tract infection, as illustrated in Figure 2.

The increase in the amplitude of the reciprocal changes in nasal airway resistance observed during upper respiratory tract infection may be explained on the basis of an increase in the filling pressure to the nasal venous sinuses rather than any difference in sympathetic nervous activity between the two conditions. The inflammation of the nasal mucosa in response to nasal infection is likely to cause vasodilation and an increase in the filling pressure to these veins.

The nasal venous sinuses have been shown to be sensitive to changes in venous pressure caused by changes in posture, as tilting head down causes an increase in nasal airway resistance (27,28). This postural response is exaggerated in subjects suffering from nasal inflammation due to allergic rhinitis, and tilting head downward often causes complete obstruction of one nasal passage in these patients (29).

The changes in nasal airway resistance observed when subjects are tilted head down support the hypothesis that nasal congestion is mainly caused by an increase in the filling pressure to the nasal venous sinuses as the major change in nasal airway resistance occurs on the high-resistance side of the nose with little or no change on the low-resistance side (28).

The change in posture associated with sleep is likely to cause an increase in nasal airway resistance due to the increase in venous pressure, but reciprocal changes in nasal airway resistance can also be induced by asymmetrical pressures to the body surface in dorsally recumbent or even in seated individuals (1). This reflex response to asymmetrical skin pressure is termed a ''corporonasal reflex'' and it helps to explain the alternation in nasal congestion as one turns from one side to the other in bed.

IV. Nasal Congestion

Nasal congestion is a common complaint that afflicts everyone, old and young, as we are all familiar with the blocked nose associated with the common cold. Nasal congestion is also commonly associated with allergic rhinitis and nasal irritation caused by air pollution. The mechanisms leading to nasal congestion associated with infection or allergy are similar, in that the end-result is nasal inflammation associated with an increased blood flow through the nasal mucosa. The increased mucosal blood flow causes an increase in the filling pressure to the venous sinuses and swelling of the nasal venous sinuses.

The nose is the most commonly infected organ of the body with over 200 viruses causing the common cold syndrome. The nasal inflammatory response

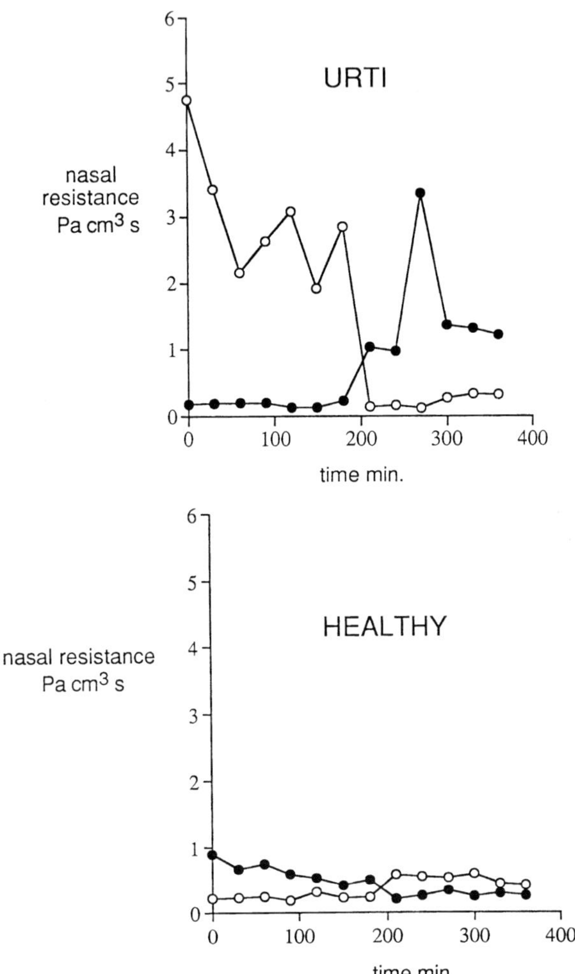

Figure 2 Spontaneous reciprocal changes in unilateral nasal airway resistance recorded in one subject while suffering from symptoms of acute upper respiratory tract infection (top) and 6–8 weeks later when healthy (bottom). Open symbols are left nasal airway resistance and closed symbols right nasal airway resistance. Each point represents the mean nasal airway resistance calculated from 12 breaths. (Redrawn from Ref. 93.)

caused by infection is poorly understood but may involve the peptide bradykinin and other inflammatory mediators such as prostaglandins and cytokines. Bradykinin is found in the nasal secretions of subjects with common cold, and nasal challenge with bradykinin causes nasal congestion, rhinorrhea and a sore throat (30,31). Bradykinin is a potent vasodilator substance and the vasodilation associated with bradykinin generation may cause an increase in nasal blood flow and congestion of the nasal venous sinuses.

As bradykinin is associated with infective rhinitis, histamine is mainly implicated with allergic rhinitis (32). Histamine can be detected from nasal washings in patients with allergic rhinitis and nasal challenge with histamine causes nasal congestion, itching, sneezing, and rhinorrhea. Like bradykinin, histamine is a potent vasodilator and thus causes an increase in nasal blood flow and nasal congestion.

Nasal irritation with air pollutants such as ozone, sulfur dioxide, and particulate matter causes irritation of trigeminal sensory nerves in the nose and release of the peptide substance P (33). Substance P is a potent vasodilator substance and the increase in nasal blood flow associated with substance P will lead to nasal congestion.

V. Assessment of Nasal Congestion

The degree of nasal congestion is usually assessed by symptom scores. Nasal airway resistance as determined by rhinomanometry, and more recently as nasal cross-sectional area, and nasal volume as determined by acoustic rhinometry, provide objective correlates. The principles of rhinomanometry and acoustic rhinometry have been described in detail elsewhere (4,34–36), and only the general principles associated with the assessment of nasal congestion will be discussed in this chapter.

The objective measures of nasal airway resistance and minimum nasal cross-sectional area are often used in clinical trials to assess the efficacy of nasal decongestants. However, these objective measures of the degree of nasal congestion may not always correlate to the subjective sensation of nasal congestion as felt by the patient (37–39). This is because the objective measures concentrate on the degree of congestion of venous sinuses in the narrowest part of the nose, i.e., the nasal valve region, whereas subjective scores as provided by the patient give an overall impression of nasal congestion.

The subjective score may be influenced by a general feeling of pressure and congestion due to pressure changes in the paranasal sinuses and middle ear and swelling of the nasal mucosa in the ethmoidal regions of the nose. The congestion in these areas of the upper airway is not measured by rhinomanometry and acoustic rhinometry although it is appreciated by the patient. In particular, swelling of the ethmoid region may cause a sensation of pressure and arterial throbbing as the mucosal surfaces come into contact. This may be perceived by the patient as nasal congestion but the nasal airway resistance may be in the normal range.

Nasal congestion is often asymmetrical with one nasal passage severely congested while the other passage has a low or normal resistance. In this case the total nasal resistance will be in the normal range but the patient will feel obstructed and uncomfortable and the subjective score for congestion will not be related to the total nasal resistance (39).

In general, the objective measures of the nose as provided by rhinomanometry and acoustic rhinometry are very useful for assessing the efficacy of topical nasal decongestants where the medication is applied directly to the nasal valve area, but they may not be so useful in assessing the efficacy of oral decongestants, which have a generalized decongestant action on the upper airway. Nasal volume measurements by acoustic rhinometry, in theory, should provide more information about generalized decongestion in the nose. However, in practice, acoustic rhinometry has major limitations when used to assess the congested nose, as the sound signal is greatly attenuated and prone to artifacts when transmitted through the narrowed airway (36).

VI. Sympathetic Neuroeffector Junction

The sympathetic nerves to the nasal mucosa form a dense plexus around the nasal venous sinuses and the nerves are also distributed to the arterioles (6). In the sympathetic adrenergic nerve terminal, norepinephrine is biosynthesized, stored in vesicles, and released by exocytosis as shown in Figure 3. Norepinephrine is released from the sympathetic nerve terminal on the arrival of an action potential and rapidly diffuses across the neuroeffector junction to bind to α_1- and α_2-adrenoceptors on the smooth muscle cells to initiate contraction of the smooth muscle (40). The effects of norepinephrine are terminated mainly by reuptake into the nerve ending (uptake 1), by diffusion from the junction, and by uptake into the smooth muscle cells (uptake 2). Neuronal uptake of norepinephrine can be blocked by antidepressants such as desmethylimipramine, which has been shown to potentiate the nasal vasoconstrictor effect of sympathetic nerve stimulation in animal experiments (41).

Neuropeptide Y has been identified as a potent vasoconstrictor neurotransmitter that is released with norepinephrine on stimulation of the nasal sympathetic nerves (42). The corelease of neuropeptide Y and norepinephrine helps to explain why it is difficult to block the sympathetic nasal vasoconstrictor response with alpha-receptor antagonists such as phenoxybenzamine and why depletion of nor-

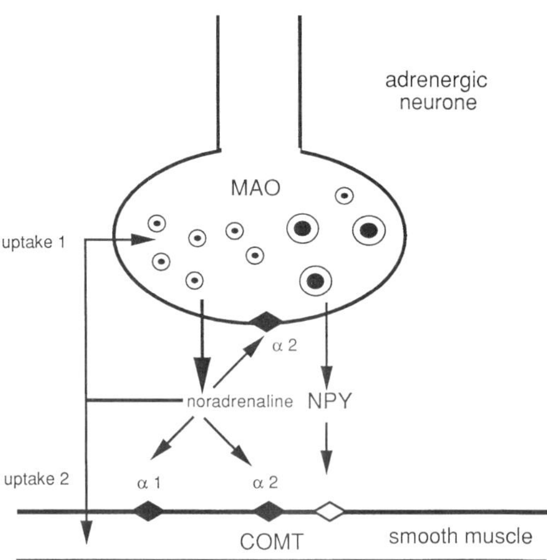

Figure 3 Diagram of sympathetic neuroeffector junction. Norepinephrine and neuropeptide Y (NPY) are released from vesicles in the nerve ending on arrival of the nerve action potential. Norepinephrine acts on α_1- and α_2-receptors on the vascular smooth muscle to cause vasoconstriction. Norepinephrine also acts on neuronal α_2-receptors, which inhibit and limit the release of norepinephrine in a negative feedback mechanism. The effects of norepinephrine are terminated by uptake into the nerve ending (uptake 1) and uptake into the smooth muscle cells (uptake 2). NPY is a cotransmitter with norepinephrine and causes a vasoconstrictor response.

epinephrine following treatment with reserpine does not abolish the nasal vasoconstrictor response (41,43).

Topical application of neuropeptide Y to the human nasal mucosa in healthy volunteers and patients with allergic rhinitis causes a pronounced vasoconstriction with a concomitant reduction in nasal airway resistance and plasma exudation (44). Neuropeptide Y is not used clinically as a nasal decongestant, but in the future, analogs of neuropeptide Y may prove useful as topical nasal decongestants.

The main factor determining the release of norepinephrine and neuropeptide Y from the sympathetic nerve endings in the nose is the frequency of nerve action potentials. However, the rate of release of norepinephrine and neuropeptide Y is also influenced by the concentration of norepinephrine in the neuroeffector junction. Norepinephrine acts on prejunctional α_2 receptors to inhibit its own release and the release of neuropeptide Y. This mechanism helps conserve neurotransmitter by inhibiting release when there is a high concentration of norepinephrine in the neuroeffector junction (45).

The pre- and postjunctional α-adrenoceptors have been shown to differ in their sensitivity to both agonists and antagonists and they are classified as α_1- and α_2-adrenoceptors (40). α_2-Adrenoceptors are found on the prejunctional nerve endings and regulate neurotransmitter release whereas both α_1- and α_2-adrenoceptors are found on nasal vascular smooth muscle cells (46,47).

There is some evidence that there may be a difference in the distribution of α_1- and α_2-receptors on nasal resistance vessels and venous sinuses, with α_2-receptors mediating constriction of nasal resistance vessels, and both α_1- and α_2-receptors mediating constriction of venous sinuses (48). This has led to the suggestion that nasal decongestants with α_1-receptor activity would act predominantly on nasal venous sinuses and would not constrict the resistance vessels that supply nutrients to the nasal mucosa (48).

The nasal blood vessels are extremely sensitive to circulating catecholamines such as epinephrine and norepinephrine, which are released from the adrenal medulla in response to fear and anxiety. Intravenous administration of epinephrine causes a pronounced vasoconstriction of nasal capacitance vessels and a reduction in nasal volume (49,50). The nasal blood vessels are up to five times more sensitive than the heart in responding to circulating epinephrine, and this great sensitivity of nasal blood vessels to circulating sympathomimetics means that nasal decongestion can be achieved by low doses of oral decongestants with little or no action on the rest of the cardiovascular system.

Circulating epinephrine and norepinephrine are degraded by the enzymes monoamine oxidase (MAO) and catechol-*O*-methyltransferase (COMT), but the metabolic transformation of these catecholamines is relatively slow compared to the degradation of acetylcholine via acetylcholine esterase. Both MAO and COMT are located intracellularly and therefore uptake of catecholamines into cells is necessary for metabolic degradation. Norepinephrine that is taken up into nerve endings is metabolized by MAO. COMT in the liver plays a major role in the metabolism of circulating catecholamines. MAO inhibitors are used for the treatment of depression as they increase the concentrations of norepinephrine dopamine and 5-hydroxytryptamine in the brain. No significant pharmacological action can be attributed to the inhibition of COMT.

Sympathomimetic nasal decongestants may act on the neuroeffector junction in three different ways: first, by direct action as they mimic the effects of norepinephrine by interacting with α_1- and α_2-receptors mediating constriction of venous sinuses; second, by indirect action by displacing neurotransmitters such as norepinephrine from the sympathetic nerve terminals; and third, by blocking the reuptake of norepinephrine into the nerve ending (uptake 1) and the smooth muscle (uptake 2). These actions will be discussed below for each of the nasal decongestant medications.

VII. Nasal Decongestant Medication

Nasal congestion is a common and troublesome symptom associated with upper respiratory tract infection, seasonal and perennial allergic rhinitis, and nonallergic rhinitis. Only six or seven sympathomimetics are commonly used as active ingredients; these can be broadly divided into oral and topical medications. Ephedrine, pseudoephedrine, and phenylpropanolamine are used as oral medications; phenylephrine is used in both oral and topical medications; oxymetazoline, xylometazoline, cocaine, and naphazoline are used as topical medications.

In general, topical medications are used for short courses of treatment especially for nasal congestion associated with upper respiratory tract infection, and the oral medications are used for longer courses of treatment for nasal congestion associated with sinusitis and nasal allergy. Topical nasal decongestants have a more rapid onset of action and a longer duration of action than oral decongestants (51). However, oral decongestants may be used to treat conditions such as sinusitis and otitis, where it is difficult to apply a topical decongestant to the swollen mucosa, and where congestion of the mucosa around the entrance to the sinus ostia and the eustachian tube contributes to the pathophysiology (52). The duration of action of some oral decongestants has been increased by the development of slow-release formulations.

The rationale for the use of topical nasal decongestants for only short courses of treatment is that prolonged use may cause nasal irritation and the development of rhinitis medicamentosa with rebound nasal congestion. However, there has been a recent trend to include topical sympathomimetics in nasal sprays containing medications for the treatment of nasal allergy where the period of treatment may be more than several weeks.

An effective nasal decongestant will act as a vasoconstrictor and there is always the possibility of side effects on the cardiovascular system. Information on the efficacy, pharmacokinetics, metabolism, and side effects of nasal decongestants is available in reference texts (53,54). In general, the topical sympathomimetics are less likely to affect the cardiovascular system than oral sympathomimetics as their vasoconstrictor action is localized to the blood vessels of the nasal mucosa. However, topical medications may be absorbed into the systemic circulation, especially if excess medication is swallowed, as may occur in children.

Care should be exercised when giving sympathomimetic medications to (1) patients with cardiovascular diseases such as hypertension and myocardial ischemia, because of the vasoconstrictor action of the medications; (2) patients with glaucoma, diabetes mellitus, and hyperthyroidism; (3) patients on medication with MAO inhibitors; and (4) the elderly, as there is a risk of precipitating urinary retention in patients with prostate enlargement.

When oral sympathomimetic decongestants are given to pregnant women, the medication will enter the fetus via the systemic circulation.

A. Ephedrine

Ephedrine is one of the oldest sympathomimetic medications. The alkaloid occurs naturally in the ephedra plant and it has been in use in Chinese medicine for over 5000 years as a tea infusion (Ma Huang). Ephedrine hydrochloride can be obtained from the plant source or prepared synthetically, and the levo-isomer is used clinically. Ephedrine is a sympathomimetic with both direct and indirect effects on adrenergic receptors. It acts indirectly by releasing neurotransmitter from sympathetic nerve endings and also has a direct action on α_1, α_2, β_1, and β_2 receptors. Ephedrine is rapidly absorbed after oral administration with a mean plasma half-life of around 6 hr. Ephedrine is metabolized in the liver, and both ephedrine and metabolites are excreted in the urine. Tolerance or tachyphylaxis occurs with prolonged use of ephedrine.

The usefulness of ephedrine as an oral decongestant is limited by its mild stimulant action on the central nervous system and insomnia is a common side effect. Ephedrine has been used as a bronchodilator for the treatment of reversible airway obstruction but its use has declined with the introduction of more selective β_2-agonists that produce less cardiac stimulation.

In addition to being widely used as an oral medication, ephedrine is used as a topical nasal decongestant in nasal drops containing ephedrine hydrochloride 0.5% and 1%. Some early clinical studies have demonstrated nasal decongestant efficacy of ephedrine, on nasal inhalation (55,56) and on oral administration (57), but there has been little interest in repeating this early work with more modern clinical methods as pseudoephedrine has in general superseded ephedrine as an oral nasal decongestant. Ephedrine nasal drops provide effective relief of nasal congestion for some hours, but with repeated use tolerance may develop, perhaps due to depletion of neurotransmitter in the nasal sympathetic nerve endings.

B. Pseudoephedrine

Pseudoephedrine like ephedrine is found as a natural constituent of the ephedra plant and it is a stereoisomer of ephedrine with similar, but less potent, pharmacological activity. It is widely used in oral nasal decongestant preparations especially in combination with analgesics and antihistamines.

Like ephedrine, pseudoephedrine has both direct and indirect sympathomimetic effects. It has direct effects on cardiac β-receptors and peripheral α_1-receptors and has a weak central nervous stimulant action.

Pseudoephedrine is readily and completely absorbed from the gastrointestinal tract and achieves peak plasma concentrations 1–3 hr after dosing. It is eliminated largely unchanged in the urine.

Although there are many publications investigating the efficacy of pseudoephedrine in combination with antihistamines and other medications, data on the tolerance and dose-response relationships of the nasal decongestant activity of pseudoephedrine are limited and incomplete (53,58,59).

Since pseudoephedrine has a short half-life, the blood concentrations may fluctuate excessively unless the dose is administered every 6 hr (60). This has led to the development of slow-release formulations of pseudoephedrine, which allow a longer dosing interval. However, there is little information as regards the bioequivalence of the slow-release formulations of pseudoephedrine compared to the standard pseudoephedrine formulations. Studies are necessary to determine the absorption characteristics of these products and whether differences in blood concentrations have clinical relevance (61).

C. Phenylpropanolamine

Phenylpropanolamine is used as an oral decongestant especially in combination with analgesics and antihistamines for the treatment of the common cold. It has both indirect and direct sympathomimetic activity as it causes the release of sympathetic neurotransmitter and has both α_1- and β_1-receptor-agonist activity.

Phenylpropanolamine is rapidly and completely absorbed from the gastrointestinal tract, and peak plasma concentrations are achieved 1–2 hr after dosing. The half-life is approximately 3–4 hr and the drug is largely excreted unchanged in the urine (60).

The nasal decongestant action of both oral and topically applied phenylpropanolamine has been demonstrated in clinical trials on patients with nasal obstruction and the common cold (56,62–64).

D. Phenylephrine

Phenylephrine is widely available as an oral decongestant in combination with antihistamines and analgesics, and is also available as nasal drops and nasal sprays for topical administration. Phenylephrine is a relatively selective α_1-receptor agonist but it also has weak α_2- and β-receptor activity, and some indirect action on sympathetic nerve endings.

After oral administration phenylephrine is readily absorbed but is subject to extensive presystemic metabolism, much of which occurs in the wall of the gut.

As a consequence of metabolism, systemic bioavailability is only around

Cocaine has a stimulant action on the central nervous system similar to that of amphetamine and its availability is closely regulated in most countries because of problems of drug abuse.

The sympathomimetic activity of cocaine is mainly due to blockade of neuronal uptake of norepinephrine (uptake 1) thus potentiating vasoconstrictor activity of endogenous norepinephrine at the neuroeffector junction. Cocaine also stabilizes nerve cell membranes and has a local anesthetic activity. The combined vasoconstrictor and local anesthetic actions of cocaine make it a useful topical medication to control bleeding and aid decongestion in the surgical operative field. However, cocaine is readily absorbed into the systemic circulation when applied to the nose, hence the prevalence of "cocaine sniffing" as a form of drug abuse. To reduce absorption of cocaine from the nose a topical vasoconstrictor such as oxymetazoline may be applied before application of cocaine (91). Norepinephrine and epinephrine should not be used as topical vasoconstrictors in conjunction with cocaine because cocaine greatly potentiates their actions on the cardiovascular system and the combination could cause hypertensive side effects (53).

XI. Effects of Nasal Decongestants on Airway Resistance

The asymmetry in unilateral nasal airway resistance has been previously reported by Williams and Eccles (26), who demonstrated that application of a topical sympathomimetic caused a marked decrease in nasal airway resistance on the congested side of the nose, yet no change in nasal resistance when applied to the low-resistance side of the nose. A similar observation was also made by Principato and Ozenberger (92), who reported that various topical nasal decongestants did not affect the nasal airway resistance when applied to the nasal passage in the low-resistance phase of the nasal cycle.

The asymmetrical effects of a topical nasal decongestant on unilateral nasal resistance in patients with nasal congestion associated with upper respiratory tract infection is illustrated in Figure 4, which clearly demonstrates that the major effect of the decongestant is restricted to the congested, or high-resistance, side of the nose. These findings indicate that the venous sinuses on the low-resistance side of the nose are already maximally constricted due to the presence of a high sympathetic vasoconstrictor tone and that application of an exogenous sympathomimetic does not cause any further vasoconstriction (26).

XII. Conclusions

Nasal congestion is a common and disturbing symptom associated with nasal infection and allergy. To understand the pathophysiology of nasal congestion we

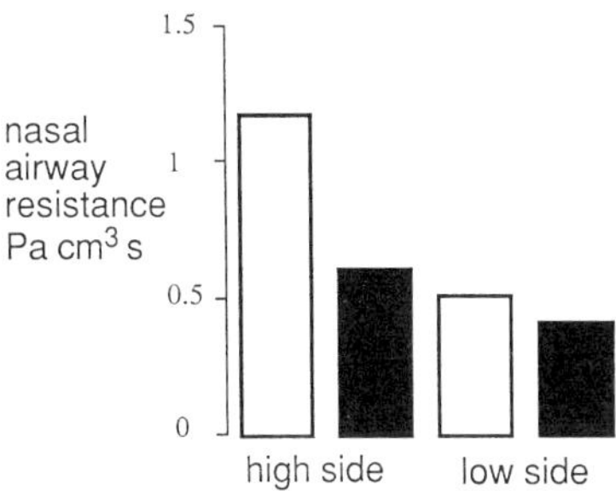

Figure 4 Asymmetrical effects of a topical nasal decongestant. Shown are the effects of a single dose of a topical nasal decongestant (0.1% xylometazoline) on unilateral nasal airway resistance (classed as high and low sides) in 35 patients with nasal congestion associated with the common cold. Shown are mean nasal resistance values before treatment (open bars) and after treatment (black bars). Note that the main action of the medication is to decongest the congested side of the nose with no significant decongestant action on the low-resistance side of the nose. (Redrawn from Ref. 26.)

must understand that we are dealing with two independent nasal passages, which have a separate autonomic innervation and which are subject to spontaneous changes in nasal resistance associated with the "nasal cycle." Nasal congestion is often unilateral and the effects of topical nasal decongestants are often asymmetrical. Topical nasal decongestants provide superior and more prolonged decongestion than the oral medications. However, prolonged therapy with topical nasal decongestants is prone to cause rebound congestion and rhinitis medicamentosa, and effective therapy with oral decongestants is limited by cardiovascular side effects. At best, nasal decongestants treat only one of the symptoms of rhinitis and this treatment is not aimed at the cause of the disease process. Menthol, which is widely marketed as a "decongestant," has no decongestant activity but does provide subjective relief. With the discovery of vasoconstictor peptide neurotransmitters in the nose, the time is ripe for development of a new generation of nasal decongestant medications that should aim to provide safe, effective, and prolonged decongestion without the nasal irritation, rebound, and cardiovascular side effects associated with the present generation of medications.

References

1. Cole P. Nasal airflow resistance. In: Mathew OP, Sant' Ambrogio GNY, eds. Respiratory Function of the Upper Airway. New York: Marcel Dekker, 1988:391–414.
2. Ferris BG, Mead J, Opie LH. Partitioning of respiratory flow resistance in man. J Appl Physiol 1964; 19:653–658.

3. Cole P. The nasal valve and current technology. Am J Rhinol 1996; 10:23–31.

4. Eccles R. Rhinomanometry and nasal challenge. In: Mackay IS, Bull TR, eds. Scott-Brown's Otolaryngology. London: Butterworths, 1987:40–53.

5. Haight JSJ, Cole P. Site and function of the nasal valve. Laryngoscope 1983; 93:49–55.

6. Cauna N. Blood and nerve supply of the nasal lining. In: Proctor DF, Andersen I, eds. The Nose: Upper Airways Physiology and the Atmospheric Environment. Amsterdam: Elsevier, 1982:45–69.

7. Wright JW. A consideration of the vascular mechanism of the nasal mucous membrane and its relations to certain pathological processes. Am J Med Sci 1995; 109:516–523.

8. Burnham HH. An anatomical investigation of blood vessels of the lateral nasal wall and their relation to turbinates and sinuses. J Laryngol Otol 1935; 50:569–593.

9. Dahlström A, Fuxe K. The adrenergic innervation of the nasal mucosa of certain mammals. Acta Otolaryngol (Stockh) 1964; 59:65–72.

10. Änggard A, Edwall L. The effects of sympathetic nerve stimulation on the tracer disappearance rate and local blood content in the nasal mucosa of the cat. Acta Otolaryngol (Stockh) 1974; 77:131–139.

11. Eccles R, Wilson H. The autonomic innervation of the nasal blood vessels of the cat. J Physiol 1974; 238:549–560.

12. Beickert P. Halbseitenrhythmus der vegetativen innervation. Arch Ohren-Nasen Kehlk-Heilk 1951; 157:404–411.

13. Stoksted P, Thomsen K. Changes in the nasal cycle under stellate ganglion blockade. Acta Otolaryngol (Stockh) 1953; (Suppl 109):176–181.

14. Eccles R. The domestic pig as an experimental animal for studies on the nasal cycle. Acta Otolaryngol (Stockh) 1978; 85:431–436.

15. Eccles R, Reilly M, Eccles KSJ. Changes in the amplitude of the nasal cycle associated with symptoms of acute upper respiratory tract infection. Acta Otolaryngol (Stockh) 1996; 116:77–81.

16. Sen H. Observations on the alternate erectility of the nasal mucous membrane. Lancet 1901; 1:564.

17. Heetderks DL. Observations on the reaction of normal nasal mucous membrane. Am J Med Sci 1927; 174:231–244.

18. Stoksted P. Rhinometric measurements for determination of the nasal cycle. Acta Otolaryngol (Stockh) 1953; (Suppl 109):159–175.

19. Hasegawa M, Kern EB. The human nasal cycle. Mayo Clin Proc 1977; 52:28–34.

20. Eccles R. The central rhythm of the nasal cycle. Acta Otolaryngol (Stockh) 1978; 86:464–468.

21. Gilbert AN, Rosenwasser AM. Biological rhythmicity of nasal airway patency—a re-examination of the nasal cycle. Acta Otolaryngol (Stockh) 1987; 104:180–186.

22. Gilbert AN. Reciprocity versus rhythmicity in spontaneous alternations of nasal airflow. Chronobiol Int 1989; 6:251–257.

23. Bamford OS, Eccles R. The central reciprocal control of nasal vasomotor oscillations. Pflügers Arch Eur J Physiol 1982; 394:139–143.

24. Eccles R. Sympathetic control of nasal erectile tissue. Eur J Respir Dis 1983; 64: 150–154.

25. Bende M, Barrow I, Heptonstall J, Higgins PG, Al-Nakib W, Tyrrell DAJ, Akerlund A. Changes in human nasal mucosa during experimental coronavirus common colds. Acta Otolaryngol (Stockh) 1989; 107:262–269.

26. Williams RG, Eccles R. Nasal airflow asymmetry and the effects of a topical nasal decongestant. Rhinology 1992; 30:277–282.

27. Rundcrantz H. Postural variations of nasal patency. Acta Otolaryngol (Stockh) 1969; 68:435–443.

28. Hasegawa M. Nasal cycle and postural variations in nasal resistance. Ann Otol Rhinol Laryngol 1982; 91:112–114.

29. Hasegawa M. Posture induced nasal obstruction in patients with allergic rhinitis. Clin Otolaryngol 1994; 19:135–137.

30. Proud D, Reynolds CJ, Lacapra S, Kagey-Sobotka A, Lichenstein LM, Naclerio RM. Nasal provocation with bradykinin induces symptoms of rhinitis and a sore throat. Am Rev Respir Dis 1988; 173:613–616.

31. Rajakulasingam K, Polosa R, Lau LCK, Church MK, Holgate ST, Howarth PH. Nasal effects of bradykinin and capsaicin: influence on plasma protein leakage and role of sensory neurons. J Appl Physiol 1992; 72:1418–1424.

32. Kaliner MA. Allergic rhinitis. In: Mygind N, Naclerio RM, eds. Allergic and Non-allergic Rhinitis. Clinical Aspects, Copenhagen: Munksgaard, 1993:153–158.

33. Eccles R. Rhinitis as a mechanism of respiratory defense. Eur Arch Oto-Rhino-Laryngol 1995; 252:S2–S7.

34. Eccles R. Other techniques for assessing nasal surgery. Facial Plast Surg 1990; 7: 260–265.

35. Cole P. The Respiratory Role of the Upper Airways. A Selective Clinical and Pathological Review. St Louis: Mosby-Year Book, 1993.

36. Tomkinson A, Eccles R. The identification of the potential limitations of acoustic rhinometery using computer-generated, 3-dimensional reconstructions of simple models. Am J Rhinol 1996; 10:77–82.

37. Jones AS, Willatt DJ, Durham LM. Nasal airflow: resistance and sensation. J Laryngol Otol 1989; 103:909–911.

38. Eccles R. Relationship between measured nasal airway resistance and the sensation of nasal airflow. Facial Plast Surg 1990; 7:278–282.

39. Sipila J, Suonpaa J, Silvoniemi P, Laippala P. Correlations between subjective sensation of nasal patency and rhinomanometry in both unilateral and total nasal assessment. J ORL 1995; 57:260–263.

40. Lefkowitz RJ, Hoffmab BB, Taylor P. Neurotransmission. The autonomic and somatic motor nervous systems. In: Hardman JG, Limbird LE, Molinoff PB, et al, eds. Goodman and Gilman's The Pharmacological Basis of Therapeutics. New York: McGraw-Hill, 1996:105–139.

41. Eccles R, MacLean AG. Relaxation of smooth muscle following contraction elicited by sympathetic nerve stimulation in vivo. Br J Pharmacol 1977; 61:551–558.

42. Lacroix JS, Stjarne P, Anggard A, Lundberg JM. Sympathetic vascular control of the pig nasal mucosa (III): co-release of noradrenaline and neuropeptide Y. Acta Physiol Scand 1989; 135:17–28.

43. Lacroix JS, Stjarne P, Anggard A, Lundberg JM. Sympathetic vascular control of the pig nasal mucosa (2): reserpine resistant, non adrenergic nervous responses in relation to neuropeptide Y and ATP. Acta Physiol Scand 1988; 133:183–197.

44. Baraniuk JN, Silver PB, Kaliner MA, Barnes PJ. Neuropeptide Y is a vasoconstrictor in human nasal mucosa. J Appl Physiol 1992; 73:1867–1872.

45. Lacroix JS. Adrenergic and non-adrenergic mechanisms in sympathetic vascular control of the nasal mucosa. Acta Physiol Scand 1989; 136(Suppl 581):1–63.

46. Ichimura K, Jackson RT. Evidence of alpha-2 adrenoceptors in the nasal blood vessels of the dog. Arch Otolaryngol 1984; 110:647–651.

47. Van Megen YJB, Klaassen ABM, Rodrigues de Miranda JF, Wentges RTR, Van Ginneken CAM. Demonstration of alpha 1 adrenoceptors in rat nasal mucosa. J Receptor Res 1989; 9:221–234.

48. Andersson KE, Bende M. Adrenoceptors in the control of human nasal mucosal blood flow. Ann Otol Rhinol Laryngol 1984; 93:179–182.

49. Malcolmson KG. The vasomotor activities of the nasal mucous membrane. J Laryngol Otol 1959; 37:73–98.

50. Eccles R, Eccles KSJ. Sympathetic innervation of the nasal mucosa of the pig. Res Vet Sci 1981; 30:349–352.

51. Connell JT, Linzmaye MI. Comparison of nasal airway patency changes after treatment with oxymetazoline and pseudoephedrine. Am J Rhinol 1987; 1:87–94.

52. Melen I, Andreasson L, Ivarsson A, Jannert M, Johansson CJ. Effects of phenylpropanolamine on ostial and nasal airway resistance in healthy-individuals. Acta Otolaryngol (Stockh) 1986; 102:99–105.

53. Dollery C. Therapeutic Drugs. Edinburgh: Churchill Livingstone, 1991.

54. Physicians Desk Reference. New Jersey: Medical Economics Data, 1995.

55. Butler DB, Ivy AC. Effects of nasal inhalers on erectile tissues of the nose. Arch Otolaryngol 1943; 38:309–317.

56. Dressler WE, Myers T, London SJ, Rankell AS, Poetsch CE. A system of rhinomanometry in the clinical evaluation of nasal decongestants. Ann Otol 1977; 86:310–317.

57. Thackray P. A double-blind, crossover controlled evaluation of a syrup for the night-time relief of the symptoms of the common cold, containing paracetamol, dextromethorphan hydrobromide, doxylamine succinate and ephedrine sulphate. J Intern Med Res 1978; 6:161–165.

58. Roth R, Canterkin E, Bluestone C, Welch R, Cho Y. Nasal decongestant activity of pseudoephedrine. Ann Otol 1977; 86:235–242.

59. Empey DW, Young GA, Letley E, John GC, Smith P, Macdonnell KA, Bagg LR, Hughes DTD. Dose response study of the nasal decongestant and cardiovascular effects of pseudoephedrine. Br J Clin Pharmacol 1980; 9:351–358.

60. Kanfer I, Dowse R, Vuma V. Pharmacokinetics of oral decongestants. Pharmacotherapy 1993; 6:S116–S128.

61. Hendeles L. Selecting a decongestant. Pharmacotherapy 1993; 13:130S–134S.

62. Bende M, Andersson KE, Johansson CJ, Sjogren C, Svensson G. Dose response relationship of a topical nasal decongestant: phenylpropanolamine. Acta Otolaryngol (Stockh) 1984; 98:543–547.

63. Gronborg H, Winther B, Brofeldt S, Borum P, Mygind N. Effects of oral norephedrine on common cold systems. Rhinology 1983; 21:3–12.
64. Darmansjah I, Akib HT, Setiawati A, Muchtar A, Rifki N. A dose-ranging study of phenylproanolamine on nasal air-flow. Int J Clin Pharmacol Ther Toxicol 1990; 28: 282–285.
65. Connell JT. Effectiveness of topical nasal decongestants. Ann Allergy 1969; 27: 541–546.
66. Hamilton LH. Effect of topical decongestants on nasal airway resistance. Curr Ther Res 1978; 24:261–268.
67. Covington TR, Pau AK. Oxymetazoline: a monograph. Am Pharm 1985; 25:21–26.
68. Bende M, Loth S. Vascular effects of topical oxymetazoline on human nasal mucosa. J Laryngol Otol 1986; 100:285–288.
69. Akerlund A, Klint T, Olen L, Rundcrantz H. Nasal decongestant effect of oxymetazoline in the common cold: an objective dose response study. J Laryngol Otol 1989; 103:743–746.
70. Osguthorpe JD, Shirley R. Neonatal respiratory distress from rhinitis medicamentosa. Laryngoscope 1987; 97:829–831.
71. Elwany SS, Stephanos WM. Rhinitis medicamentosa, an experimental histopathological and histochemical study. J ORL 1983; 45:187–193.
72. Graf P. Long-term use of oxy- and xylometazoline nasal sprays induces rebound swelling, tolerance, and nasal hyperreactivity. Rhinology 1996; 34:9–13.
73. Toohill RJ, Lehman RH, Grossman TW, Belson TP. Rhinitis medicamentosa. Laryngoscope 1981; 91:1614–1621.
74. Graf P, Juto JE. Decongestion effect and rebound swelling of the nasal mucosa during 4-week use of oxymetazoline. ORL 1996:157–160.
75. Graf P, Hallen H, Juto JE. Four-week use of oxymetazoline nasal spray (Nezeril®) once daily at night induces rebound swelling and nasal hyperreactivity. Acta Otolaryngol (Stockh) 1995; 115:71–75.
76. Stride RD. Nasal decongestant therapy. Br J Clin Pract 1967; 21:541–548.
77. Connell JT. Studies of rebound phenomena and oxymetazoline. J Clin Allergy 1988; 81:179.
78. Svensson C, Pipkorn U, Alkner U, Baumgarten CR, Persson CGA. Topical vasoconstrictor (oxymetazoline) does not affect histamine-induced mucosal exudation of plasma in human nasal airways. Clin Exp Allergy 1992; 22:411–416.
79. Eccles R. Plasma exudation in rhinitis. Clin Exp Allergy 1992; 22:319–320.
80. Graf P, Juto JE. Histamine sensitivity in the nasal mucosa during four-week use of oxymetazoline. Rhinology 1994; 32:123–126.
81. Graf P. Rhinitis medicamentosa: aspects on pathophysiology and treatment. Clin Exp Allergy 1997; 52:S30–S36.
82. Eccles R. Menthol and related cooling compounds. J Pharm Pharmacol 1994; 46: 618–630.
83. Schafer K, Braun HA, Isenberg C. Effect of menthol on cold receptor activity. J Gen Physiol 1986; 88:757–776.
84. Fox N. Effect of camphor, eucalyptol, and menthol on the vascular state of the mucous membrane. Arch Otolaryngol 1927; 6:112–122.

85. Burrow A, Eccles R, Jones AS. The effects of camphor, eucalyptus and menthol vapour on nasal resistance to airflow and nasal sensation. Acta Otolaryngol (Stockh) 1983; 96:157–161.
86. Eccles R, Jawad MS, Morris S. The effects of oral administration of menthol on nasal resistance to airflow and nasal sensation of airflow in subjects suffering from nasal congestion associated with the common cold. J Pharm Pharmacol 1990; 42: 652–654.
87. Sant'ambrogio FB, Anderson JW, Sant'ambrogio G. Menthol in the upper airway depresses ventilation in newborn dogs. Respir Physiol 1992; 89:299–307.
88. De Cort SC, Rowe JS, Eccles R. Cardiorespiratory effects of inhalation of L-menthol in healthy humans. J Physiol (Lond) 1993; 473:54P.
89. Orani GP, Anderson JW, Sant'Ambrogio FB. Upper airway cooling and menthol reduces ventilation in the guinea pig. J Appl Physiol 1991; 70:2080–2086.
90. Wynne JW. Obstruction of the nose and breathing during sleep. Chest 1982; 82: 657–658.
91. Malm L, Anggard A. Vasoconstrictors. In: Mygind N, Naclerio RM, eds. Allergic and Non-allergic Rhinitis: Clinical Aspects. Copenhagen: Munksgaard, 1993:95–100.
92. Principato, J. Ozenberger, J. Cyclical changes in nasal resistance. Arch Otolaryngol 1990; 91:71–77.
93. Eccles R, Reilly M, Eccles KSJ. Changes in the amplitude of the nasal cycle associated with symptoms of acute upper respiratory tract infection. Acta Otolaryngol (Stockh) 1996; 116:77–81.

17

Anticholinergic Medication

NIELS MYGIND

University of Aarhus
Aarhus, Denmark

FUAD M. BAROODY
and ROBERT M. NACLERIO

University of Chicago
Chicago, Illinois

PETER BORUM

Roskilde Hospital
Roskilde, Denmark

I. Introduction

Everyone has had watery rhinorrhea and has realized that it is a nuisance constantly to be aware of excess fluid in the nose, which distracts one's attention from work and social activities. Other people find it unsavoury and believe that it is potentially infectious.

When rhinorrhea is associated with sneezing, it is often caused by an allergic disease, and the patients can be offered efficient treatment with intranasal steroids or second-generation H_1 antihistamines. This modern therapy, however, often fails when rhinorrhea is the only, or the predominant, symptom (1).

As the seromucous glands in the nose have an abundant parasympathetic innervation (2,3), it is logical to test anticholinergic medication in patients suffering from watery rhinorrhea. Topical administration is necessary as systemic anticholinergic effects, such as mouth dryness, are unpleasant. In this chapter we shall review the studies of topical anticholinergic medication, in particular ipratropium bromide, which is now increasingly used for the treatment of watery rhinorrhea.

Excess nasal fluid or discharge can theoretically be derived from a number of sources: 1) anterior serous glands in the nose (a few hundred) (4), 2) small seromucous glands in the nose (about 90,000) (5), 3) seromucous glands in the paranasal sinuses (a few hundred) (5), 4) goblet cells in the nose and in the paranasal sinuses ($6000-11,000/mm^2$) (5), 5) plasma exudation (6), 6) tears, and (7) condensed water in the expiratory air. As intranasal anticholinergic medication can counteract only the first two sources, the efficacy of such treatment can give us pathophysiologically relevant information, as it is an indicator of the relative contribution of nasal glandular secretion to the volume of nasal fluids produced under different conditions.

II. Drugs and Drug Administration

The best-studied and clinically most widely used anticholinergic drug is ipratropium bromide (IB). Being a quaternary derivative of isopropyl noratropine it has a low lipid solubility and thus does not readily pass the blood-brain barrier and, therefore, it has fewer CNS effects than atropine (7–9). It is also claimed that IB is poorly absorbed from the airway mucosa (7–9), but we have little knowledge about the pharmacokinetics of intranasally administered IB.

IB was first delivered as an aerosol from a pressurized canister (commercially available in Europe and Canada), but recently an aqueous solution in a pump spray has been marketed in the United States. The recommended dosage of the pressurized aerosol is two puffs of 20 µg into each nostril four times daily (total daily dose 320 µg). The aqueous solution is available in two concentrations, 0.03% and 0.06%. The recommended dosage in perennial rhinitis is two puffs of 0.03% into each nostril two to three times daily (total daily dose 168–252 µg). In the common cold the recommended dosage is two puffs of 0.06% per nostril three to four times daily (total daily dose 504–672 µg). It is possible that the pressurized aerosol and the aqueous pump spray vary with regard to equipotent doses, duration of action, and occurrence of local side effects, as discussed below.

Atropine sulfate has been used in a few single-dose studies (10–14), and the antirhinorrhea effect seems comparable to that obtained with IB. However, we are not aware of any study that directly compares IB with atropine or with its quaternary derivative, atropine methonitrate.

III. Nasal Challenge Testing

A nasal challenge test can serve as an easy and fairly reliable experimental model for nasal disease. It can be used to characterize the response to nasal application of different immunological, chemical, and physical stimuli, and to study the pharmacological effects of various drugs. The ability of anticholinergic medication to inhibit the secretory response to methacholine, histamine, allergen, and cold air challenges, as described below, provides a rationale for treating the clinical disease.

A. Methacholine

Methacholine, a synthetic acethylcholine analog, stimulates muscarinic cholinoceptors, which are of the M1 and M3 subtypes in the nasal glands, with the M3 receptors predominating (15,16). Intranasal challenge with methacholine induces measurable rhinorrhea without sneezing or significant changes in nasal airway resistance (17,18).

Borum (19), measuring the volume of secretion dripping from the nose in a 15-min period, found a marked reduction in secretion volume when IB pressurized aerosol, 40 µg/nostril, was given to normal volunteers before methacholine challenge. However, the reduction in secretion volume decreased from 80% to 40% when the challenge dose of methacholine increased, as can be expected with competitive receptor inhibition. In a study by Sjögren et al. (20), 40 µg and 100 µg/nostril of IB inhibited methacholine-induced secretions significantly compared with placebo, and 200 µg further inhibited the response and was significantly more effective than the two lower doses.

Baroody et al. (18), using a paper disc method for methacholine challenge and for measuring the secretory response, found similar results with IB aqueous spray. All doses tested were significantly better than placebo, but the highest dose (168 µg/nostril) was more effective than the lower doses (21, 42, and 84 µg/nostril) (Fig. 1). The inhibitory effect of the drug decreased with increasing dose of methacholine, as in the study of Borum (19).

The efficacy of IB pressurized aerosol, used by Borum (19) and by Sjögren et al. (20), and of the aqueous solution, used by Baroody et al. (18), cannot directly be compared, because the study designs were different. Recently, Borum et al. (21), however, made a direct comparison between the two drug formulations. The results showed that IB, 40 µg/nostril, delivered from a pressurized aerosol, has an inhibitory effect on the response to methacholine, which is both stronger and longer lasting than when the same dose is given as an aqueous solution (Fig. 2).

A similar trend, with regard to the duration of IB activity, appears when two different methacholine studies are compared. In the study of Borum (19), IB pressurized aerosol, 40 µg/nostril, still had a 50% inhibitory effect 8–12 hr after medication, whereas no effect was detectable 8 hr after the use of an aqueous solution, 168 µg/nostril, in the study of Wagenmann et al. (22). However, the two studies were performed with different design and methods.

The reason why there should be a difference between the two drug formulations is unknown, but it is possible that a higher dose of IB will be needed when patients are transferred from a pressurized aerosol to an aqueous spray.

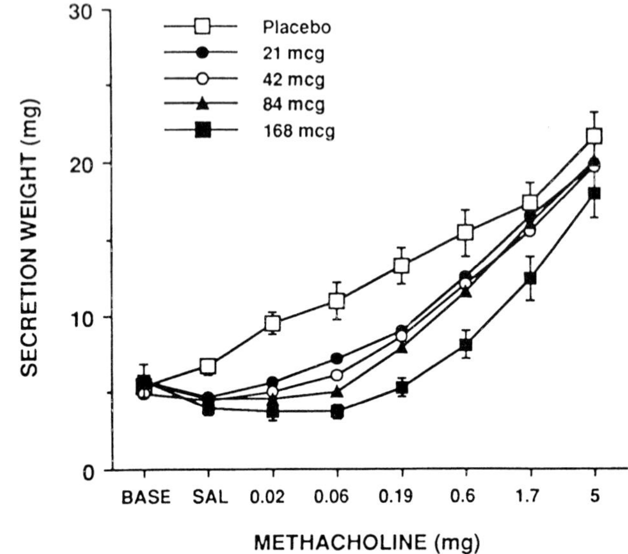

Figure 1 Dose-response curves of secretion weight after placebo and different doses of ipratropium bromide aqueous solution. (From Ref. 18.)

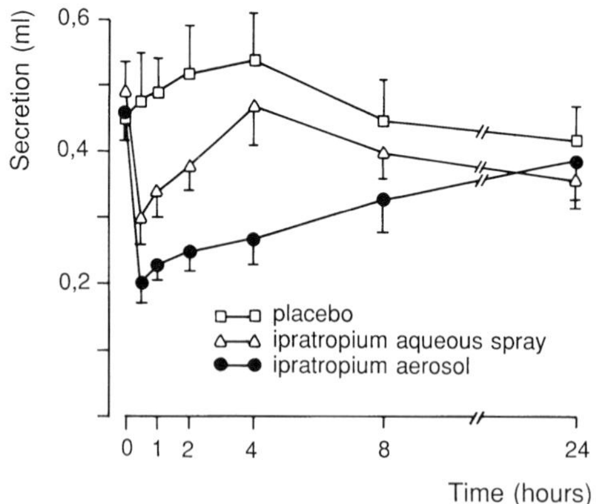

Figure 2 Volume of nasal secretions induced by methacholine challenge and effect of pretreatment with 80 µg ipratropium bromide given with two different formulations. (From Ref. 21.)

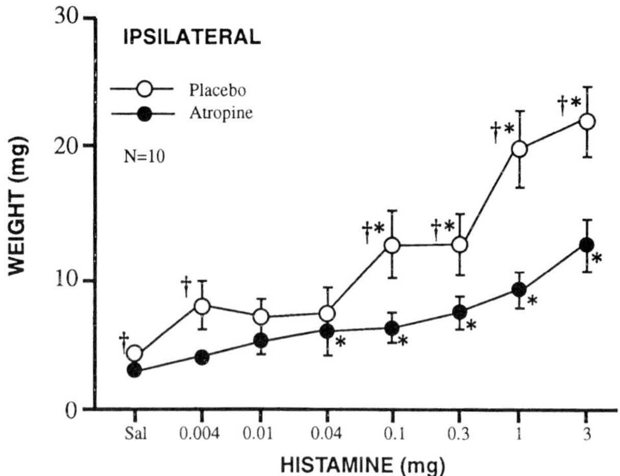

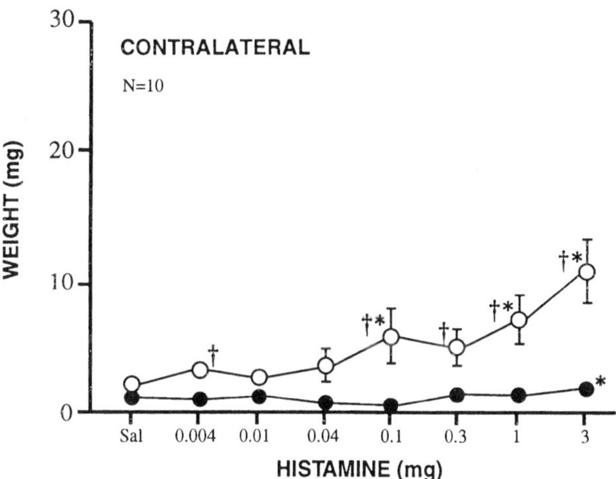

Figure 3 Effect of atropine premedication of both sides of the nose on ipsilateral and contralateral responses after stimulation of ipsilateral nasal cavity with histamine. (From Ref. 13.)

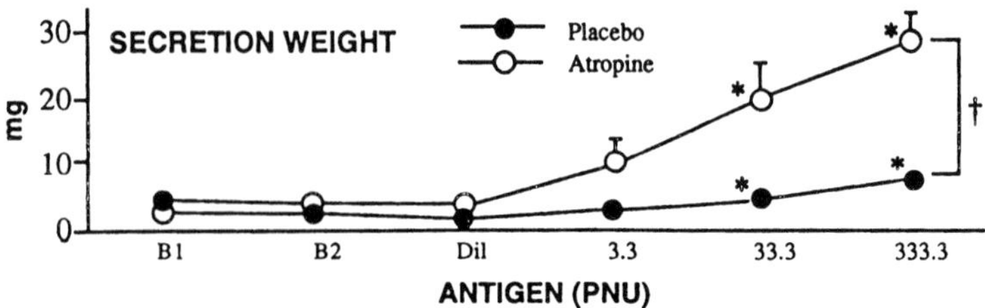

Figure 4 Effect of topical atropine premedication on ipsilateral changes after antigen challenge. (From Ref. 14.)

B. Histamine and Allergen

While unilateral challenge with methacholine induces unilateral secretion and no sneezing or blockage (18), challenge with histamine and with allergen induces sneezing, blockage, and bilateral secretion, with the contralateral volume being 40–65% of the ipsilateral (13,14,23) (Figs. 3–5). IB and atropine markedly reduce ipsilateral and almost abolish contralateral secretory response (13,14,23) (Figs. 3–5), which strongly supports the important role of parasympathetic reflexes in the nasal secretory response in allergic rhinitis. Anticholinergic medica-

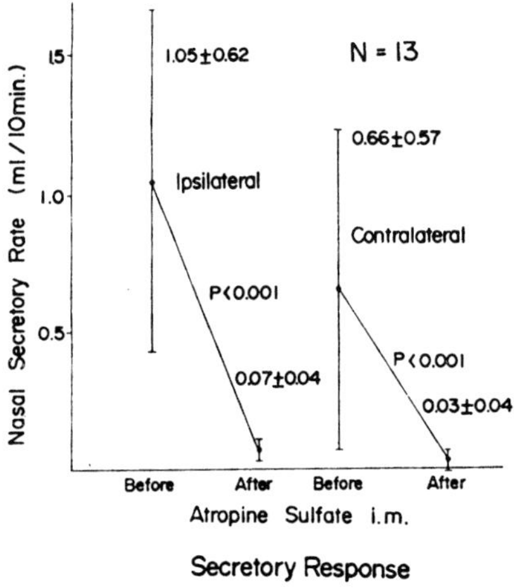

Figure 5 Effect of intramuscular atropine sulfate (1 mg/50 kg body weight) on nasal secretory response to unilateral antigen challenge. (From Ref. 23.)

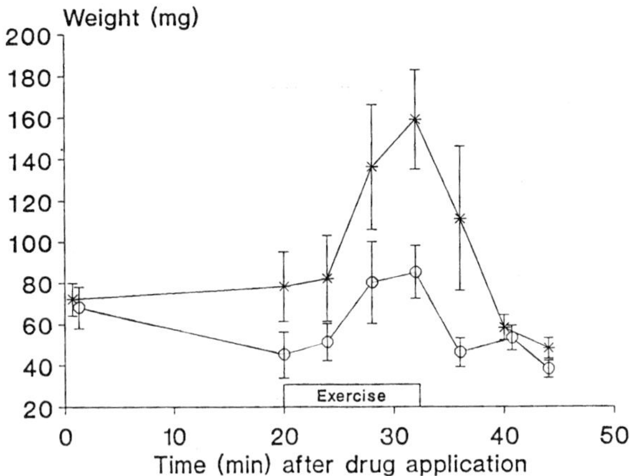

Figure 6 Exercise-induced nasal hypersecretion is blocked by pretreatment with ipratropium bromide (160 µg). Note, the effect of treatment on basic resting secretion. (From Ref. 25.)

tion has no effect on histamine- and allergen-induced itching, sneezing, or blockage.

C. Cold, Dry Air

Unilateral, experimental challenge with cold, dry air induces bilateral rhinorrhea, and the ipsilateral response is double the size of the contralateral response. Regardless of the side of application, atropine significantly reduces the secretory response by 60–70% (12), indicating that rhinorrhea induced by cold, dry air predominantly is mediated through parasympathetic pathways.

D. Exercise

Physical exercise, at ordinary room temperature, increases the amount of nasal secretions (24) and this increase can to a large extent be blocked by pretreatment with IB (25) (Fig. 6).

IV. Clinical Conditions

A. Perennial Nonallergic Rhinitis

An increasing number of placebo-controlled trials have all shown a significant effect of intranasal IB in patients with perennial nonallergic rhinitis. Both severity and duration of rhinorrhea is reduced, based on symptom scores and on the number of paper handkerchiefs used, but to a varying degree (Table 1). This variation between study results is probably due, at least in part, to differences in patient selection.

The majority of studies, in Europe and Canada, are carried out with the pressurized aerosol formulation of IB, whereas more recent studies from the United States are performed with the aqueous solution. There is a tendency toward a more marked effect of IB in the European/Canadian studies, as compared to the U.S. studies, but it is difficult to draw any definite conclusion because different daily doses, and dosing frequencies, have been used.

The results also indicate the existence of a dose-response relationship, and apparently higher doses of IB have been used in the common cold to get the same result as in perennial rhinitis.

In a study of Kirkegaard et al. (34) the double-blind protocol was followed by a period with a very high dose of IB pressurized aerosol in order to define the maximum potential of this type of treatment in perennial rhinitis. When the total daily dose of IB was increased from 320 µg to 1600 µg, the overall reduction of nose blowings was merely changed from 40% to 55%. In most patients the high dose only added to the local side effects, but a few patients with very severe rhinorrhea got added clinical benefit. While a few patients may need a dose higher than 320 µg/day, patients will usually reduce the dose when they are allowed to adjust it to fit their individual symptomatic requirement (33,43).

The high-dose study of Kirkegaard et al. (34) showed that, in perennial nonallergic rhinitis, at least half of all nose blowings are mediated by parasympathetic stimulation of nasal glands.

B. Perennial Allergic Rhinitis

Melzer et al. (37) gave IB aqueous spray (42 µg or 84 µg three times a day) to adults with perennial allergic rhinitis in a placebo-controlled study. Active treatment had a significant effect on severity and duration of rhinorrhea and on quality of life, with consistently greatest improvement in the group treated with the high dose. There was no effect on other rhinitis symptoms. The authors conclude that IB aqueous spray should be a useful addition to therapy in those patients in whom rhinorrhea is a major problem.

C. Cold Weather

Rhinitis patients, having hyperresponsive nasal airways, react with symptoms upon exposure to a series of nonspecific stimuli, including the inhalation of cold air. All individuals, however, will get some rhinorrhea upon exposure to cold air, and the effect of intranasal IB and atropine has been tested in two studies of normal persons. In a study of Østberg et al. (38), hospital staff members, walking around a frozen lake in winter, collected nasal discharge in preweighted paper handkerchiefs. Pretreatment with a very high dose of IB (400 µg from a pressurized aerosol) reduced the secretion weight by 73% (Fig. 7). Silvers (11) pretreated ski patrollers with intranasal atropine sulfate (0.005%), before cold exposure, and found a subjective improvement in 13/14, as compared to 0/14 in a placebo group. He concluded that anticholinergic medication can be helpful in "skier's nose."

D. Hot, Spicy Food

Hot, spicy food is also known to induce rhinorrhea in rhinitis patients and in normal persons. In the study of Østberg et al. (38) the normal volunteers, coming back to the laboratory from their promenade in the cold winter weather, consumed hot spicy soup, and the high dose of IB reduced the weight of the soup-induced secretion by 66% (Fig. 8). Raphael et al. (10) found that hot, spicy food increased the concentration of protein in nasal lavage fluid and took this as a measure of glandular hypersecretion. This "gustatory rhinitis" was reduced by 55–65% in seven volunteers pretreated with intranasal atropine sulfate.

Thus, it can be concluded that at least two-thirds of rhinorrhea, induced by cold air and by hot, spicy food, is mediated by parasympathetic reflexes and glandular cholinoceptors.

E. Common Cold

Borum et al. (39) treated patients with naturally occurring common cold with IB pressurized aerosol (320 µg/day) or placebo for 1 week. Watery rhinorrhea was significantly reduced but there was no effect on the amount of purulent discharge. The treatment was clinically beneficial only during the first days of the cold (Fig. 9) when rhinorrhea was profuse and predominantly watery.

Using a similar study design, Østberg et al. (40) gave a very high dose of IB pressurized aerosol (1600 µg/day) to define the maximum potential of this type of treatment in the common cold. Symptom scores and secretion weight were reduced by 56% and 58%, respectively, but this was at the expense of significant local side effects. An investigator score for the ability to pour the sampled nasal discharge, "pourability," was significantly lower in the IB group than in the placebo group (Fig. 10). When the watery rhinorrhea almost disappeared, the remaining discharge, dominated by mucopurulent secretions, seemed to change its physical characteristics and become highly viscoelastic. We can conclude that the IB-sensitive watery rhinorrhea is a product of parasympathetic stimulation of nasal glands, whereas this is not the case for the IB-resistant mucopurulent secretion. However, its obvious viscoelastic characteristics indicate that it also is a product of mucus-producing cells.

In two large U.S. studies of naturally acquired common cold (41,42) there

Table 1 The Antirhinorrhea Effect Obtained with Intranasal Ipratropium Bromide in Published Placebo-Controlled Trials

Disease/exposure (Ref.)	Number of patients	Drug, formulation	Dosage (µg)	Effect parameter	Symptom reduction (%)
Perennial nonallergic rhinitis					
Borum et al. (26)	20	PA	80 × 4	Symptom score	22
Bok et al. (27)	21	PA	80 × 4	Handkerchiefs	13
Jokinen and Sipila (28)	30	PA	80 × 4	Handkerchiefs	33
Malmberg et al. (29)	34	PA	80 × 4	Handkerchiefs	20
von Haacke et al. (30)	20	PA	80 × 4	Symptom score	28
Sjögren and Juhasz (31)	13	PA	80 × 4	Handkerchiefs	20
Knight et al. (32)	26	PA	80 × 4	Handkerchiefs	37
Dolovich et al. (33)	25	PA	80 × 4	Symptom score	42
Kirkegaard et al. (34)	36	PA	80 × 4	Nose blowings	40
		PA	400 × 4	Nose blowings	55
Druce et al. (35)	140	AS	42 × 2	Symptom score	17
		AS	84 × 2	Symptom score	21
Bronsky et al. (36)	233	AS	84 × 3	Symptom score	18
Perennial allergic rhinitis					
Melzer et al. (37)	123	AS	42 × 3	Symptom score	24
			84 × 3	Symptom score	35

Cold weather					
Østberg et al. (38)	14	PA	400 × 1	Weight	73
Hot, spicy food					
Østberg et al. (38)	14	PA	400 × 1	Weight	66
Common cold					
Borum et al. (39)	40	PA	80 × 4	Handkerchiefs	34
Østberg et al. (40)		PA	400 × 4	Weight	58
				Nose blowings	56
Dockhorn et al. (41)	321	AS	168 × 4	Weight	18
				Symptom score	22
Diamond et al. (42)	955	AS	84 × 3	Weight	13
				Symptom score	18
		AS	168 × 3	Weight	27
				Symptom score	24
		AS	336 × 3	Weight	27
				Symptom score	35

We have calculated the symptom reduction in percent based on mean values in tables and figures in the original publications.
PA, pressurized aerosol; AS, aqueous solution.

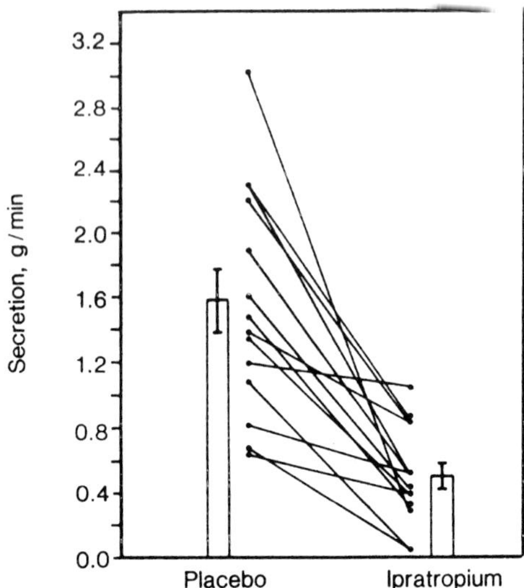

Figure 7   Amount of nasal secretions produced by exposure to cold air following pretreatment with ipratropium bromide (400 μg) pressurized aerosol or placebo. (From Ref. 38.)

has been a significant, but modest, effect of the IB aqueous solution, administered in various doses (Table 1; Fig. 11).

In experimental rhinovirus infection Gaffey et al. (44) showed that intranasally administered atropine methonitrate reduced nasal mucus production. However, in this study the dose of atropine methonitrate required to suppress rhinorrhea also produced systemic anticholinergic side effects. The same authors (45) failed to demonstrate any significant effect of IB pressurized aerosol, 80 μg three times daily, on mucus weight in experimental rhinovirus infection.

V.   Adverse Effects

A.   Systemic Side Effects

It is claimed that IB is poorly absorbed from the airway mucous membrane (7– 9) and that systemic side effects are less likely than when atropine sulfate is administered. It is in support of this statement that systemic anticholinergic effects only have been observed when a very high dose of IB (400 μg) has been given repeatedly (34,46).

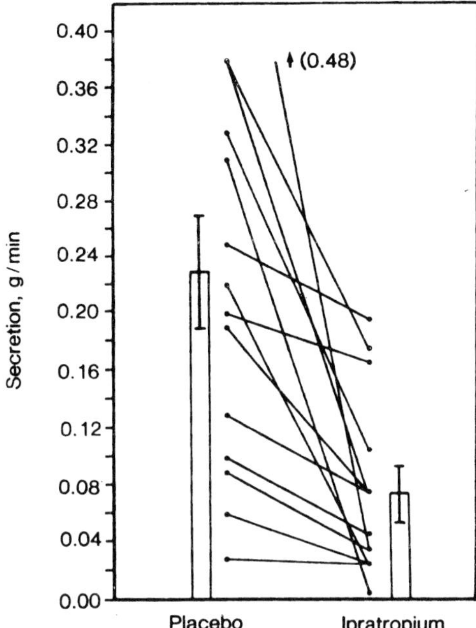

Figure 8 Amount of nasal secretions produced by ingestion of hot, spicy soup following pretreatment with ipratropium bromide (400 µg) pressurized aerosol or placebo. (From Ref. 38.)

After the use of 240–360 µg IB from a pressurized aerosol, Laurikainen et al. (47) and Kaila et al. (48) found measurable plasma levels with a peak within 30 min, but unfortunately these authors did not calculate bioavailability. Using the aqueous solution of IB (0.03%, 0.06%, and 0.12% strengths), Wood et al. (49) found a bioavailability of about 10%. While the clinical studies have shown that this absorbed dose is not associated with a significant risk of systemic adverse effects, when ordinary doses are used, it is uncertain whether intranasal anticholinergic medication can be effective without being absorbed, as the drug needs to reach the acini of the submucosal glands.

B. Local Side Effects

Long-term studies of intranasal IB have not disclosed any deleterious effect on the mucous membrane judged by symptom scores, rhinoscopy, methacholine challenge test, and olfactometry (32,33,43,50,51).

Although the nasal mucociliary transport rate is not reduced by ordinary

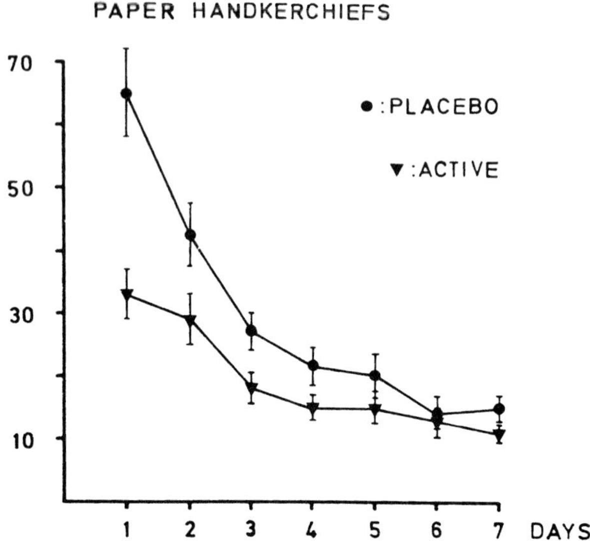

Figure 9 Number of paper handkerchiefs used in common cold patients treated with ipratropium bromide pressurized aerosol 80 μg qid and placebo. (From Ref. 39.)

(52) or by high-dose therapy with IB (34), a subjective sensation of nasal dryness can be a problem (Table 2), and this appears to be the dose-limiting factor for antirhinorrhea therapy with anticholinergic medication.

There is little doubt that a high dose of IB in a normal nose can give a sensation of dryness. This indicates that anticholinergic medication has an effect, not only on abnormal hypersecretion, but also on baseline secretory activity (25). However, an alternative explanation is that this effect on normal nasal physiology is mediated through an action on surface epithelial cells, which have a high number of muscarinic M3 receptors (53).

Also patients with perennial rhinitis and common cold can experience nasal dryness if they are treated in periods with no or few symptoms, which occurs, in particular, at night when secretory activity physiologically is low (54) (Fig. 12). The feeling of nasal dryness is unpleasant and can necessitate the insufflation of saline.

There are no controlled studies comparing the effects and side effects of IB as a pressurized aerosol and as an aqueous solution, but comparing the European/ Canadian studies with the more recent U.S. studies, one gets the impression that the sensation of dryness is less of a problem with the aqueous solution than with the pressurized aerosol. Bronsky et al. (36) hypothesize that such a difference is

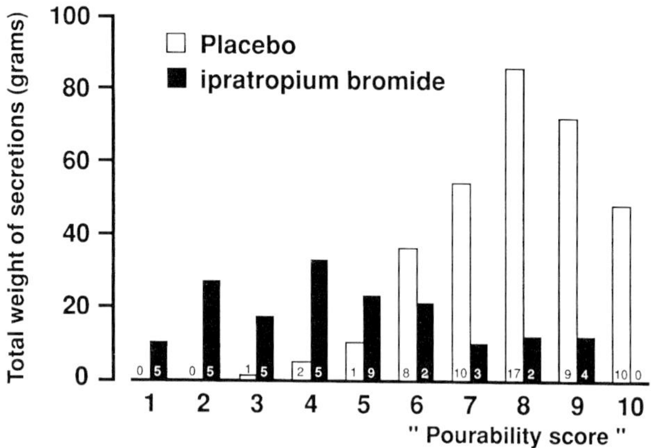

Figure 10 Score for "pourability" of nasal secretions in 50 common cold patients treated with either ipratropium bromide pressurized aerosol in a high dose (1600 µg/day) or placebo. A high score for the ability to pour the sampled nasal discharge indicates behavior like water and a low score behavior like a viscous gel. Columns represent total amount of secretions and the figures inside the columns indicate the number of samples. (From Ref. 40.)

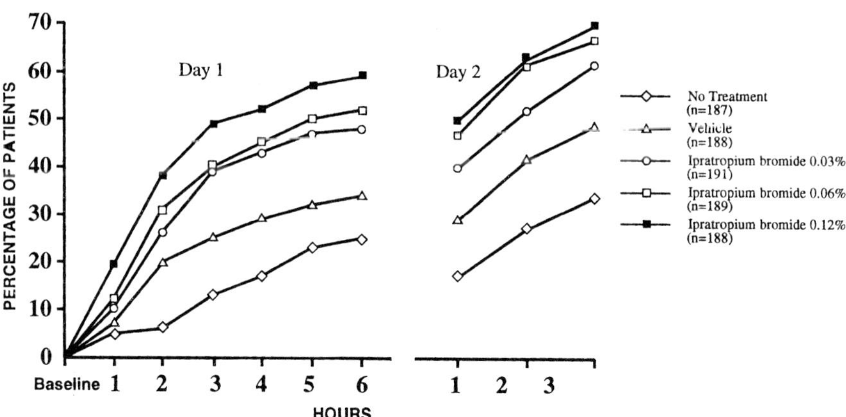

Figure 11 Percentage of common cold patients whose rhinorrhea symptoms improved to "very mild" or "none" on days 1 and 2. Ipratropium bromide aqueous solution was given as 84 µg, 168 µg, and 336 µg three times daily. (From Ref. 42.)

Table 2 Side Effects from Ipratropium Bromide Pressurized Aerosol in an Ordinary Dose and in a Very High Dose Only for Experimental Use

		Percentage of patients		
	Run-in	Placebo	Ipratropium bromide (80 µg qid)	Ipratropium bromide (400 µg qid)
Dryness of nose*,**	25 (8.1)	36 (15.8)	61 (31.2)	72 (49.6)
Dryness of mouth*	39 (21.6)	28 (17.6)	42 (23.2)	78 (50.0)
Dysuria*	3 (0.2)	6 (4.4)	11 (5.0)	28 (14.1)
Saccharine test (mean in min)	14.9	13.7	17.7	17.1

*$p < 0.01$ for column 1 versus column 4, and column 2 versus column 4.
**$p < 0.05$ for column 2 versus column 3.
The results of the questionnaire are presented as the percent of patients having the symptom and as percent of all days with the symptom (in parentheses).
Source: From Ref. 34.

due to "the drying properties of the propellant." An alternative explanation is differences in intranasal drug distribution and kinetics.

VI. Recommended Usage

Intranasal use of the anticholinergic agent IB can offer a useful treatment for watery rhinorrhea, but, as has been evidenced by many experimental and clinical studies, this treatment is monosymptomatic. It has no effect on itching, sneezing, or nasal blockage, nor will it be useful in patients with viscous mucus or purulent discharge from the nose or paranasal sinuses. In allergic rhinitis it cannot compete with nasal steroids, effective also on sneezing and blockage, or with antihistamines, effective also on sneezing and eye itching. However, IB has a documented effect on rhinorrhea also in allergic rhinitis (37) and in the United States it is approved for allergic and nonallergic perennial rhinitis in adults and children aged 12 years and older. Possibly, the added use of IB may be helpful in patients with severe rhinorrhea, if the effect of a steroid spray or an antihistamine has not been sufficient. However, the benefit of such combined treatment has not yet been documented.

The selection of patients is important for the response to anticholinergic therapy. Using the criteria in Table 3, Dolovich et al. (33) have identified a group of high responders, and they are the main target population for IB therapy.

In new patients, it is important to describe the quality and quantity of the

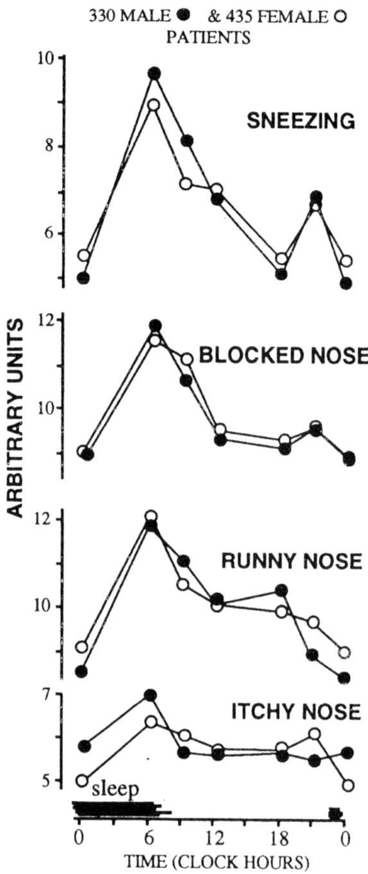

Figure 12 Day-night variation in occurrence and intensity of allergic rhinitis symptoms. (From Ref. 54.)

Table 3 Selection of High Responders to Ipratropium Therapy

1. Adults
2. Clear nasal discharge > 1 hr each day
3. No major problem with nasal blockage
4. No known allergic basis for the rhinitis
5. No satisfactory response to antihistamine or steroid spray

Source: Ref. 33.

nasal symptoms to determine the initial dose of IB and the dose frequency. The patients can later adjust the treatment to their individual, and changing, needs. Due to a marked diurnal variation of rhinorrhea, it is often preferable to give a high early-morning dose. Thereafter, many patients will require medication only on an as-needed basis, preferably before exposure to known trigger factors. A systematic four-times-a-day dosing will often result in unpleasant nasal dryness in the evening and at night, when the secretory activity is low. A sensation of dryness can also occur when a high dose of IB is necessary to combat an episode of severe rhinorrhea. The effect of the drug may outlast the length of the symptomatic episode, and in that case the use of a saline spray is beneficial.

Long-term treatment is not associated with the development of tachyphylaxis; on the contrary, there seems to be a tendency toward a reduced dose requirement of IB (43).

While the number of perennial rhinitis patients who need IB on a daily basis is low, the number of individuals who can benefit from occasional use is high. When watery rhinorrhea is a problem during a common cold, a sufficiently high dose of IB, at least as a pressurized aerosol, can "dry the nose," but a vasoconstrictor spray is needed to counteract blockage and a saline spray may be needed as well.

VII. Conclusions

It has been clearly shown that intranasal administration of IB can reduce the amount of watery rhinorrhea experimentally induced by methacholine, histamine, and allergen challenge, by exposure to cold air and spicy food, and in patients with perennial nonallergic rhinitis and common cold. It is a limitation that the treatment is monosymptomatic with no effect on sneezing and nasal blockage. Individual therapy, with the dosage being matched to the severity of the symptoms, is recommended to get the best therapeutic index between antirhinorrhea effect and a sensation of nasal dryness. It is probably preferable to give a high morning dose and only to supplement the treatment as required during the remainder of the day. The best effect is obtained when the spray is used before exposure to known provoking factors.

References

1. Wihl J-Å, Petersen BN, Petersen LN, Gundersen G, Breson K, Mygind N. Effect of the nonsedative H1-receptor antagonist astemizole in perennial allergic and nonallergic rhinitis. J Allergy Clin Immunol 1985; 75:720–727.
2. Cauna N, Cauna D, Hinderer KH. Innervation of the human nasal glands. J Neurocytol 1972; 1:49–60.

3. Uddman R, Änggård A, Widdicombe JG. Nerves and neurotransmitters in the nose. In: Mygind N, Pipkorn U, eds. Allergic and Vasomotor Rhinitis: Pathophysiological Aspects. Copenhagen: Munksgaard, 1987:50–62.

4. Bojsen-Møller F. Glandulae nasales anteriores in the human nose. Ann Otol 1965; 74:363–375.

5. Tos M. Distribution of mucus producing elements in the respiratory tract. Differences between upper and lower airway. Eur J Respir Dis 1983; 64(Suppl 128):269–279.

6. Persson CGA, Andersson M, Greiff L, et al. Airway permeability. Clin Exp Allergy 1995; 23:807–814.

7. Eugell DW. Clinical pharmacology and toxicology of ipratropium bromide. Am J Med 1986; 81(Suppl 5A):18–22.

8. Gross NJ. Ipratropium bromide. N Engl J Med 1988; 319:486–494.

9. Ensing K, de Zeeuw RA, Nossent GD, Koeter GH, Cornelissen PJG. Pharmacokinetics of ipratropium bromide after single dose inhalation and oral and intravenous administration. Eur J Clin Pharmacol 1989; 36:189–194.

10. Raphael G, Raphael MH, Kaliner M. Gustatory rhinitis: a syndrome of food-induced rhinorrhea. J Allergy Clin Immunol 1989; 83:110–115.

11. Silvers WS. The skier's nose: a model of cold-induced rhinorrhea. Ann Allergy 1991; 67:32–36.

12. Jankowski R, Philip G, Togias A, Naclerio RM. Demonstration of bilateral cholinergic secretory response after unilateral nasal cold, dry air challenge. Rhinology 1993; 31:97–100.

13. Baroody FM, Wagenmann MM, Naclerio RM. A comparison of the secretory response of the nasal mucosa to methacholine and histamine. J Appl Physiol 1993; 74:2661–2671.

14. Baroody FM, Ford S, Lichtenstein LM, Kagey-Sobotka A, Naclerio RM. Physiologic responses and histamine release after nasal antigen challenge: effect of atropine. Am J Respir Crit Care Med 1994; 149:1457–1465.

15. Okayama M, Mullol J, Baraniuk JN, et al. Muscarinic receptor subtypes in human nasal mucosa: characterization, autoradiographic localization, and function in vitro. Am J Respir Cell Mol Biol 1993; 8:176–187.

16. White MV. Muscarinic receptors in human airways. J Allergy Clin Immunol 1995; 95:1065–1068.

17. Borum P. Nasal methacholine challenge. A test for the measurement of nasal reactivity. J Allergy Clin Immunol 1979; 63:253–257.

18. Baroody FM, Majchel AM, Roecker MM, Roszko PJ, Zegarelli EC, Wood CC, Naclerio RM. Ipratropium bromide (Atrovent nasal spray) reduces the nasal response to methacholine. J Allergy Clin Immunol 1992; 89:1065–1075.

19. Borum P. Intranasal ipratropium: inhibition of methacholine induced hypersecretion. Rhinology 1978; 16:225–233.

20. Sjögren I, Jonsson L, Koling A, Jansson C, Österman K, Håkansson B. The effect of ipratropium bromide on nasal hypersecretion induced by methacholine in patients with vasomotor rhinitis. Acta Otolaryngol (Stockh) 1988; 106:453–459.

21. Borum S, Becker B, Mygind N, Borum P. Comparison between the effect of ipratropium bromide as a pressurized aerosol and an aqueous pump spray on methacholine-induced rhinorrhea. Rhinology 1997; 34:198–200.

22. Wagenmann M, Baroody FM, Jankowski R, Nadal JC, Roecker-Cooper M, Wood CC, Naclerio RM. Onset and duration of inhibition of ipratropium bromide nasal spray on methacholine-induced nasal secretions. Clin Exp Allergy 1992; 24:288–290.

23. Konno A, Togawa K, Fujiwara T. The mechanisms involved in onset of allergic manifestations in the nose. Eur J Respir Dis 1983; 64(Suppl 128):155–166.

24. Stanford CF, Stanford RL. Exercise induced rhinorrhea (athlete's nose). Br Med J 1988; 2:60.

25. Harris WE, Stanford CF, Giebaly K, Adair C, Alsuwaidan S, Nicholls DP, Stanford CF. The parasympathetic system in exercise-induced rhinorrhoea. Rhinology 1992; 30:21–23.

26. Borum P, Mygind N, Larsen FS. Intranasal ipratropium: a new treatment for perennial rhinitis. Clin Otolaryngol 1979; 4:407–411.

27. Bok HE, van Wijngaarden HA, Cornelissen PJG. Intranasal ipratropium bromide for paroxysmal rhinorrhoea. Eur J Respir Dis 1983; 64(Suppl 128):486–489.

28. Jokinen K, Sipila P. Intranasal ipratropium in the treatment of vasomotor rhinitis. Rhinology 1983; 21:341–345.

29. Malmberg H, Grahne B, Holopainen E, Binder E. Ipratropium (Atrovent) in the treatment of vasomotor rhinitis of elderly patients. Clin Otolaryngol 1986; 57:348–354.

30. von Haacke NP, Moore-Gillon V, Capel KH. Double-blind cross-over trial of ipratropium and placebo in chronic rhinorrhoea. Br Med J 1983; 287:1258–1259.

31. Sjögren I, Juhasz J. Ipratropium in the treatment of patients with perennial rhinitis. Allergy 1984; 39:457–461.

32. Knight A, Kazim F, Salvatori VA. A trial of intranasal Atrovent versus placebo in the treatment of vasomotor rhinitis. Ann Allergy 1986; 57:348–354.

33. Dolovich J, Kennedy L, Vickerson F, Kazim F. Control of the hypersecretion of vasomotor rhinitis by topical ipratropium bromide. J Allergy Clin Immunol 1987; 80:274–278.

34. Kirkegaard J, Mygind N, Mølgaard F, Grahne B, Holopainen E, Malmberg H, Brøndbo K, Røjne T. Ordinary and high-dose ipratropium in perennial non-allergic rhinitis. J Allergy Clin Immunol 1987; 79:585–590.

35. Druce HM, Spector SL, Fireman P, Kaiser H, Melzer EO, Boggs P, Wood CC, Paluch EP. Double-blind study of intranasal ipratropium bromide in nonallergic perennial rhinitis. Ann Allergy 1992; 69:53–60.

36. Bronsky EA, Druce H, Findley SR, Hampel FC, Kaiser H, Ratner P, Valentine MD, Wood C. A clinical trial of ipratropium bromide nasal spray in patients with perennial nonallergic rhinitis. J Allergy Clin Immunol 1995; 95:1117–1122.

37. Melzer EO, Orgel HA, Bronsky EA, Findlay SR, Georgitis JW, Grossman J, Ratner P, Wood CC. Ipratropium bromide aqueous nasal spray for patients with perennial allergic rhinitis: a study of its effect on their symptoms, quality of life, and nasal cytology. J Allergy Clin Immunol 1992; 90:242–249.

38. Østberg B, Winter B, Mygind N. Cold air-induced rhinorrhea and high-dose ipratropium. Arch Otolaryngol Head Neck Surg 1987; 113:160–162.

39. Borum P, Olsen L, Winter B, Mygind N. Ipratropium nasal spray: a new treatment for rhinorrhea in the common cold. Am Rev Respir Dis 1981; 123:418–420.

40. Østberg B, Borum P, Mygind N. Use of the cholinoceptor antagonist, ipratropium bromide as an indicator of reflex-mediated hypersecretion in the common cold. Rhinology 1997; 35:58–62.

41. Dockhorn R, Grossman J, Posner M, Zinny M, Tinkleman D. A. double-blind, placebo-controlled study of the safety and efficacy of ipratropium bromide nasal spray versus placebo in patients with the common cold. J Allergy Clin Immunol 1992; 90:1076–1082.

42. Diamond L, Dockhorn RJ, Grossman J, et al. A dose-response study of the efficacy and safety of ipratropium bromide nasal spray in the treatment of the common cold. J Allergy Clin Immunol 1995; 95:1139–1146.

43. Borum P, Mygind N, Larsen FS. Ipratropium treatment for rhinorrhoea in patients with perennial rhinitis. An open follow-up study of efficacy and safety. Clin Otolaryngol 1983; 8:267–272.

44. Gaffey MJ, Gwaltney JM Jr, Dressler WE, Sorrentino JV, Hayden FG. Intranasally administered atropine methonitrate treatment of experimental rhinovirus colds. Am Rev Respir Dis 1987; 135:241–244.

45. Gaffey MJ, Hayden FG, Boyd JC, Gwaltney JM Jr. Ipratropium bromide treatment of experimental rhinovirus infection. Antimicrob Agents Chemother 1988; 32:1644–1647.

46. Groth S, Dirksen H, Mygind N. The absence of systemic side-effects from high doses of ipratropium in the nose. Eur J Respir Dis 1983; 64(Suppl 128):490–493.

47. Laurikainen E, Koulu M, Kaila T, Scheinin L, Isalo E. Evaluation of the systemic anticholinergic activity of nasally administered ipratropium bromide. Rhinology 1988; 26:133–138.

48. Kaila T, Suonpää J, Grénman R, Isalo E. Vasomotor rhinitis and the systemic absorption of ipratropium bromide. Rhinology 1990; 28:83–89.

49. Wood C, Fireman P, Grossman J, Wecker M, MacGregor T. Product characteristics and pharmacokinetics of intranasal ipratropium bromide. J Allergy Clin Immunol 1995; 95:1111–1116.

50. Grossman J, Banov C, Boggs P, et al. Use of ipratropium bromide nasal spray in chronic treatment of nonallergic perennial rhinitis, alone and in combination with other perennial rhinitis medications. J Allergy Clin Immunol 1995; 95:1123–1127.

51. Kaiser HB, Findlay SR, Georgitis JW, et al. Long-term treatment of perennial allergic rhinitis with ipratropium bromide nasal spray 0.06%. J Allergy Clin Immunol 1995; 95:1128–1132.

52. Ohi M, Sakakura Y, Murai S, Miyoshi Y. Effect of ipratropium bromide on nasal mucociliary transport. Rhinology 1984; 22:241–246.

53. Baraniuk JN, Kaliner MA, Barnes PJ. Localization of m3 muscarinic receptor mRNA in human nasal mucosa. Am J Rhinol 1992; 6:145–148.

54. Smolensky MH, Reinberg A, Labrecque G. Twenty-four hour pattern in symptom intensity of viral and allergic rhinitis: treatment implications. J Allergy Clin Immunol 1995; 95:1084–1096.

18

Specific Immunotherapy for Allergic Rhinitis

**PASCAL DEMOLY, ANNE DES ROCHES,
and FRANÇOIS-BERNARD MICHEL**

Hôpital Arnaud de Villeneuve
Montpellier, France

JEAN BOUSQUET

Montpellier University
Montpellier, France

I. Introduction

Specific immunotherapy (SIT) for the treatment of allergic rhinitis was introduced in 1911 by Noon (1). Immunotherapy is still controversial since most protocols are devised empirically, some allergens are still poorly defined, the mechanisms of action of immunotherapy are not yet clear, the duration of treatment is poorly characterized, and the therapeutic index of SIT has been contested. In the 1980s, it was found that SIT was effective under optimal conditions including a demonstrated IgE-mediated disease, a high-quality extract, and an optimal allergen dose (2), but its safety was questioned as systemic reactions may become life-threatening (3–6). In the 1990s, pharmacoeconomic considerations also cause concerns since the costs for SIT may be greater than that of pharmacotherapy.

SIT is the only treatment, however, that may affect the natural course of the disease and prevent the onset of asthma. New routes of administration (nasal, sublingual, and oral) are currently being explored. In the future new formulations and the improvement of our knowledge on the basic mechanisms of allergic diseases may change our view of immunotherapy.

Table 1 Results of Double-Blind Placebo-Controlled Studies in Grass Pollen Allergy

Author	Species	Patient number A	P	Extract	Dose schedule	Protocol	Duration	Skin tests	Symptom-medication scores
Bousquet	Grass	15		Standardized	Rush	Pre + coseason	1 yr	$p < 0.01$	N: $p < 0.01$
	Grass	16	11	Formald. allergoid	Rush	Pre + coseason	1 yr	$p < 0.02$	N: $p < 0.05$
Bousquet	Grass	15	10	Formald. allergoid	Clustered	Pre + coseason	1 yr	$p < 0.001$	N: $p < 0.005$
Bousquet	Grass	18		Standardized	Rush	Pre + coseason	1 yr	$p < 0.01$	N,O,B: $p < 0.01$
	Grass	15	14	Formald. allergoid	Clustered	Pre + coseason	1 yr	$p < 0.04$	O,B: $0.05 < p < 0.01$
	Grass	13		HMW allergoid	Clustered	Pre + coseason	1 yr	$p < 0.005$	N,O,B: $p < 0.01$
Bousquet	Grass	39	18	HMW allergoid	Clustered	Pre + coseason	1 yr	$p < 0.05$	N,B: $0.005 < p < 0.01$
Bousquet	Grass	16	17	Standardized	Rush	Pre + coseason	1 yr	$p < 0.02$	N: $p < 0.02$
	Multiple species	16	17	Standardized	Rush	Pre + coseason	1 yr	NS	N: NS
Frankland	Grass	50	50	"Pollaccine"	Classic		1 yr		N: $p < 0.001$
		50	50	Purified antigen	Classic				N: $p < 0.001$
Grammer	Grass	18	18	Polymer. glutarald.	Classic	12 injections	12 wk		N: $p < 0.02$
Grammer	Grass	22	22	Polymer. glutarald.	Accelerated	13 injections	9 wk		N: $p < 0.05$
Mc Allen	Grass	47	23	Allpyral	Classic	?	1 yr		N,B: NS
		40		Depot preparation	Classic	?	1 yr		N,B: $p = 0.05$
Machiels	Grass	7	8	Ag-Ab complexes	Classic	Pre + coseason	3 mo		N: NS
Machiels	Grass	37	12	Ag-Ab complexes	Classic	Pre + coseason	3 mo		N,B: $p < 0.03$ and $p < 0.001$
Ortolani	Grass	8	8	Standardized	Classic	Preseason	1 yr		N: $p < 0.001$
Starr	Grass	42	10	Alum-pyridine	Classic	Preseason	1 yr		N: 79% improved
Varney	Grass	20	20	Standardized, alum	Classic	Pre + coseason	1 yr		N,B: $p < 0.01$
Weyer	Grass	17	16	Aqueous, then $Al(OH)_3$	Classic	Preseason	1 yr		N: Peak of season, $p < 0.03$

N: nasal; O: ocular; B: bronchial; HWM: high molecular weight; Ag-Ab: antigen-antibody.

Table 2 Results of Double-Blind, Placebo-Controlled Studies in Ragweed Pollen Rhinitis

Author	P	A	Extract	Schedule	Protocol	Dose	Duration	Symptom-medication scores
Arbesman	19	19	Repository	12 injections	Preseason	M: 4000 PNU	2 yr	NS vs. placebo
		22	Aqueous	12 injections	Preseason	M: 10,000 PNU	2 yr	Improved
Cockroft	21	22	Pollinex	4 injections	Preseason	M: 4000 Noon U	1 yr	Improved: A: 67%, P: 38%
Grammer	19	21	Polymer. glutarald	Classic	15 injections	M: 6250 PNU, C: 50,000 PNU	15 wk	$p < 0.02$
Hirsch	74	81	Aqueous	Rinkel	Pre + coseason	M: 27–41 PNU, 0.1–0.15 µg Antigen E	2 yr	NS for ragweed
Lichtenstein	24	24	Antigen E	Classic	Preseason	C: 17–800 µg	1 yr	$p < 0.01$
Lichtenstein	30	18	Antigen E	Classic	Preseason	1.0 mg	1 yr	$p < 0.01$
		21	Antigen E + K	Classic	Preseason	1.4 mg	1 yr	$p < 0.01$
		19	Crude Rw, aqueous	Classic	Preseason	C: 8800 PNU	1 yr	$p < 0.01$
Lowell	12	12	Aqueous	Classic	Preseason	Not stated	1 yr	$p < 0.01$
Meriney	10	10	Formald. allergoid	Classic	Preseason	C: 10,710 PNU	20 wk	$p < 0.01$
Van Metre	12	12	Aqueous	Rinkel	Pre + coseason	C = 94 ng Antigen E	3 mo	NS
Van Metre	17	15	Aqueous	Classic	Pre + coseason	C: 70 µg Antigen E	1 yr	$p < 0.01$
		18	Aqueous	Clustered	Pre + coseason	C: 17.5 µg Antigen E	1 yr	$p < 0.01$
Norman	21	21	Aqueous whole rw	Classic	Preseason	C: 9483 PNU per yr	4 yr	3rd, 4th yr; $p < 0.02$
		21	Antigen E	Classic	Preseason	C: 195,530 PNU per yr	4 yr	3rd, 4th yr: $p < 0.04$
Norman	21	20	Alum-precipitate	Classic	Preseason	C: 13,746 PNU (yr 1)	3 yr	$p < 0.006$
Norman		22	Formald. allergoid	Cluster	Preseason	C: 63,600 PNU (yr 1)	2 yr	$p < 0.01$
		22	Aqueous	Classic	Preseason	C: 2000 PNU (yr 1)	2 yr	$p < 0.01$

M: maximal dose, C: cumulative dose.

weight preparations are safer and as effective as the aqueous extracts or the low-molecular-weight formulations. Polyethylene glycol (PEG)-modified extracts represent another approach but the high expectations that followed animal studies were unfortunately not realized in humans (60).

Maintenance Dose

The maintenance dose is critical for the efficacy of SIT. Low-dose immunotherapy has been found ineffective during placebo-controlled studies (42,48,61) and should no longer be used. It has been suggested that patients should be given the "highest tolerated dose" with potent extracts (62,63) but severe systemic reactions were observed in many patients. Bousquet et al. (64,65) proposed use of an *optimal maintenance dose*, i.e., a dose inducing a change in cell reactivity and clinical efficacy but giving a low and acceptable rate of mild systemic reactions. Although a greater dose may increase the effectiveness of SIT, it is likely that side reactions would increase in number and be unacceptable in severity. Turkeltaub et al. suggested a similar approach for ragweed pollens (66).

Cross-Reactions Between Allergens

Many allergens share common epitopes leading to cross-reactivities that complicate the treatment of allergic diseases. Important cross-reactivities exist among pollens and it should be determined whether patients need to be treated by all the relevant species or only a few.

Concerning grass pollen SIT, it was proposed in Europe that a mixture of five to six common grasses, including timothy, would improve the efficacy of SIT. During the past decade, the use of a single allergen species has been favored in northern Europe. However this may not reflect a worldwide trend since pollens of some species such as Bermuda grass (*Cynodon dactylon*) or cereals do not completely cross-react with timothy.

Allergen mixtures also present problems. They may be less stable, more difficult to standardize, and the dilution of major epitopes in mixtures may lead to a low-dose SIT regimen. On the other hand, single allergen species may be less effective because relevant epitopes may be lacking.

Polysensitized Patients

The IgE immune response to environmental allergens is highly heterogeneous. Patients allergic only to grass pollens differ clinically and immunologically (67,68) from those allergic to many pollen species. A double-blind, placebo-controlled study compared the efficacy of SIT in patients allergic to grass or multiple pollen species (19). The results of the study indicated that grass-pollen-allergic patients, but not polysensitized patients, were protected. Using a higher allergen dose it might be possible to show efficacy in the polysensitized group but the rate of systemic reactions using standardized extracts might have been unacceptable.

Age of the Patients

For theoretical reasons, it is usually recommended to start SIT in children and adults and to avoid it in older subjects. SIT may be started in children under 5 years of age, but it is desirable to carefully evaluate the benefits since SIT leads to a greater number of systemic reactions in this age group. Systemic reactions, especially asthma, may be more severe. Additionally, most young children have not developed their allergenic sensitization.

During pregnancy, the severity of allergic diseases is often modified. SIT should not be started because of the risk of anaphylaxis on the unborn child. It may, however, be continued during pregnancy (69).

Safety

Life-threatening reactions occur with high-potency extracts and deaths have been reported. The rate of systemic reactions is greater with high-potency pollen extracts than with either nonstandardized extracts or high-molecular-weight preparations but does not differ from SIT performed with standardized extracts of other allergen species (6). Rush immunotherapy may expose to a higher risk of systemic reactions (65).

Duration

The duration of SIT is unknown. In inhalant allergy, data are lacking to support any definite conclusion, but it appears that a long-term treatment, at least 3 years, is required. For nasal symptoms, in a retrospective study, Mosbech and Osterballe (8) observed that the effect of grass pollen SIT lasted several years after its cessation. Grammer et al., using high-molecular-weight polymerized extracts, reached similar conclusions (7). However, prospective controlled studies are lacking and no definite conclusion can be drawn.

B. Other Routes for Allergen Administration

Efficacy

The usual route of administration of SIT is subcutaneous. Recent studies, however, have shown that alternative routes may be effective in reducing symptoms of rhinitis and medication needs. It must be stressed that only high allergen doses should be given (about 500 times greater than those achieving efficacy with the subcutaneous route) in those forms of immunotherapy.

Nasal immunotherapy was found to be effective in grass, ragweed, birch, and *Parietaria* pollen allergy in some but not all studies (70–87). Nasal inflammation was found to be reduced by SIT in *Parietaria* allergy (83).

Oral SIT was found to be ineffective in most trials in grass pollen allergy, possibly because these allergens are destroyed by digestive enzymes (88). In ragweed and birch pollen allergy, oral SIT was effective when very high allergen doses were administered (89–93).

Sublingual SIT was found to be effective in grass and *Parietaria* pollen allergy (94–96).

More studies are, however, needed to establish the efficacy of local SIT using high doses of standardized allergen extracts. The magnitude of efficacy of SIT using local routes also needs to be better studied and, in particular, it is necessary to compare subcutaneous and local SIT. We anticipate that local SIT will be less effective than subcutaneous SIT for a similar duration of treatment and a similar cumulative dose of allergen. On the other hand, the efficacy of a prolonged treatment may be similar. The addition of oral SIT to boost parenteral SIT may be effective, but more data are required since negative studies have been published (97–99).

Safety

Systemic or local reactions were uncommon with local administration of extracts. During nasal SIT, some patients complained about rhinitis symptoms during allergen insufflation, but when modified extracts were used, adverse reactions were rare. High-dose oral SIT was also associated with local reactions in the form of gastrointestinal symptoms. Sublingual SIT has been administered to thousands of patients and it is apparently well tolerated.

Compliance

The compliance to SIT is a prerequisite to achieve efficacy. It has long been known that compliance to subcutaneous SIT is poor. Compliance to local SIT is unknown but physicians who routinely use sublingual SIT estimate that it is better than compliance to subcutaneous SIT.

C. Indications for SIT in Pollen Allergy

SIT is indicated in severe rhinoconjunctivitis (10,11) in which pharmacotherapy insufficiently controls symptoms or produces undesirable side effects. On the other hand, SIT should not be started in mild to moderately severe pollinosis responding favorably to antihistamines and/or topical drugs, unless the season is long-lasting as is the case in southern Europe, South Africa, and California.

Since rhinoconjunctivitis is present in most, if not all, patients suffering from pollen allergy, and asthma occurs generally in the most severe patients, it is impossible to propose indications without considering all symptoms. It also appears that SIT is indicated when asthma during the pollen season complicates rhinoconjunctivitis (100) although this recommendation is not accepted by all investigators because of the increased risk of systemic reactions. British recommendations have proposed that patients with asthma should be specifically excluded (101), but this recommendation appears to be important only if asthma is moderately severe or severe.

IV. House Dust Mite Allergy

House dust mites of the genus *Dermatophagoides* are the cause of allergic rhinitis in patients with dust allergy, and a simple extract of house dust should no longer be used in the treatment of allergic patients. House dust mites are among the most prevalent perennial allergens throughout the world and have been shown to cause asthma, especially in childhood.

Few double-blind, placebo-controlled studies showing the efficacy of dust mite immunotherapy have been performed (102–110). With mite allergens, the indications for SIT are not firm but the treatment is indicated especially if the patient suffers from asthma. In rhinitis, a course of topical steroids is often required at the beginning of SIT since symptoms are due to both allergy and inflammation.

Nasal, oral, and sublingual SIT have been carried out using high allergen doses and efficacy was observed (111–114). Moreover, two studies using low-dose sublingual SIT have proven to be efficacious, but serious flaws in the design of the study and in the interpretation of the data do not make it possible to conclude that such a regimen is effective (115,116).

The indication for SIT in mite allergy is not easy to propose in rhinitis since many patients also suffer from asthma (12). Only patients with severe and long-lasting symptoms in whom nasal reactivity to house dust mites has been confirmed by a challenge may be treated. Moreover, it seems appropriate to exclude patients with chronic sinusitis (117).

V. Allergy to Animal Proteins

Although it has been recommended by the Position Papers of the European Academy of Allergy and Clinical Immunology (11) and WHO/IUIS (10) that allergen avoidance be preferred to SIT in animal dander allergy, SIT to cat or dog may occasionally be an alternative in occupational allergy and in children to whom the eviction of the animal may create an emotional problem.

Most studies have been carried out in asthma or using bronchial challenge as an effect parameter (118), and the clinical efficacy of cat or dog SIT remains to be ascertained in rhinitis since only one study has been conducted (119).

Oral and sublingual SIT have been carried out in cat-allergic patients (120,121). It was claimed that sublingual SIT was not effective since symptoms were improved in both the active and placebo groups, but the improvement was greater in the active group (121). Moreover, the only objective parameter of efficacy (nasal blockage index) was highly significantly improved in the treated group whereas it was unchanged in the placebo group (122).

The cloning and the characterization of the structure of major allergens make it possible to synthesize peptides having the structure of the native allergens. Among them, two *Felis domesticus* (cat) allergen (Fel d 1) peptides of 27 amino acids have been synthesized (Allervax Cat) (123). These peptides were shown to stimulate in vitro cat-specific T cells but were found to be unable to bind to cat-allergen-specific IgE. A few clinical trials have been performed and these two peptides have been found to protect patients against a cat room challenge in which nasal and bronchial symptoms were examined (125).

VI. Allergy to Molds

Molds often induce polysensitizations and the quality of extracts available is far from adequate for most species, so it is proposed to avoid mold SIT. However, efforts have been made to standardize extracts of some molds such as *Alternaria* and *Cladosporium*, and good-quality allergen extracts are now available (124). SIT with standardized *Cladosporium* (126–128) and *Alternaria* extracts (129) was therefore started and variable results obtained. In Nordic countries, patients treated with a standardized *Cladosporium* extract were polysensitized and SIT was found to be effective in challenges with the specific allergen but symptom-medication scores were only minimally improved. On the other hand, in the double-blind, placebo-controlled study of Horst et al. (129) performed over 1 year in 24 highly selected patients allergic only to *Alternaria*, both nasal challenges and symptom-medication scores were improved in the treated group and remained unchanged in the placebo group.

SIT with *Cladosporium* induced a high number of systemic reactions (126–128) whereas SIT with *Alternaria* was better tolerated, possibly because Horst et al. (129) attempted to define an optimal maintenance dose before starting SIT. Long-term safety of mold SIT has also been questioned and type III allergic reactions have been described (130).

These studies indicate that mold SIT may be effective in allergic diseases but they do not favor SIT with many mold species or with extracts of unknown quality. SIT should currently be restricted to a few patients allergic to *Alternaria* and/or *Cladosporium*.

VII. Immunotherapy with Other Extracts

SIT with extracts of undefined allergens (bacteria, *Candida albicans*, insect dusts, etc.) should no longer be used in clinical practice (10–13).

Acknowledgment

The authors thank Drs. W. Becker, H. Dhivert, F. Djoukhadar, A. Dotte, E. Frank, P. Godard, B. Guérin, A. Hejjaoui, B. Hewitt, J. Knani, L. Paradis, H. J. Maasch, L. Martinot, J. L. Ménardo, W. Skassa-Brociek, and R. Wahl and Mrs. M. Deltour for their help.

References

1. Noon L. Prophylactic inoculation against hay fever. Lancet 1911; 1:1572–1573.
2. Bousquet J, Michel F. Specific immunotherapy in allergic rhinitis and asthma. In: Busse W, Holgate S, eds. Asthma and Rhinitis. Oxford, UK: Blackwell Scientific Publications, 1995: 1309–1324.
3. Committee on Safety of Medicines. Desensitizing vaccines. Br Med J 1986; 293: 948.
4. Lockey RF, Benedict LM, Turkeltaub PC, Bukantz SC. Fatalities from immunotherapy (IT) and skin testing (ST). J Allergy Clin Immunol 1987; 79:660–677.
5. Norman PS. Safety of allergen immunotherapy. J Allergy Clin Immunol 1989; 84: 438–439.
6. Bousquet J, Michel FB. Safety considerations in assessing the role of immunotherapy in allergic disorders. Drug Safety 1994; 10:5–17.
7. Grammer LC, Shaughnessy MA, Suszko IM, Shaughnessy JJ, Patterson R. Persistence of efficacy after a brief course of polymerized ragweed allergen: a controlled study. J Allergy Clin Immunol 1984; 73:484–489.
8. Mosbech H, Osterballe O. Does the effect of immunotherapy last after termination of treatment? Follow-up study in patients with grass pollen rhinitis. Allergy 1988; 43:523–529.
9. Des-Roches A, Paradis L, Knani J, et al. Immunotherapy with a standardized *Dermatophagoides pteronyssinus* extract. V. Duration of efficacy of immunotherapy after its cessation. Allergy 1996; 51:430–433.
10. The current status of allergen immunotherapy (hyposensitisation). Report of a WHO/IUIS working group. Allergy 1989; 44:369–379.
11. Malling H, Weeke B. Immunotherapy. Position paper of the European Academy of Allergy and Clinical Immunology. Allergy 1993; 48(Suppl 14):9–35.
12. International consensus report on diagnosis and management of asthma. International Asthma Management Project. Allergy 1992; 47:1–61.
13. International consensus report on the diagnosis and management of rhinitis. Allergy 1994; 49(Suppl 19):1–33.

14. Frew AJ. Injection immunotherapy. British Society for Allergy and Clinical Immunology Working Party. Br Med J 1993; 307:919–923.

15. Des-Roches A, Paradis L, Menardo J-L, et al. Immunotherapy with a standardized Dermatophagoides pteronyssinus extract. VI. Specific immunotherapy prevents the onset of new senitizations in children. J Allergy Clin Immunol 1997; 99:450–453.

16. Rudd S. Immunotherapy compliance—a shot in the dark. Ann Allergy Asthma Immunol 1995; 74:195–198.

17. Bousquet J, Maasch H, Martinot B, Hejjaoui A, Wahl R, Michel FB. Double-blind, placebo-controlled immunotherapy with mixed grass-pollen allergoids. II. Comparison between parameters assessing the efficacy of immunotherapy. J Allergy Clin Immunol 1988; 82:439–446.

18. Bousquet J, Hejjaoui A, Soussana M, Michel FB. Double-blind, placebo-controlled immunotherapy with mixed grass-pollen allergoids. IV. Comparison of the safety and efficacy of two dosages of a high-molecular-weight allergoid. J Allergy Clin Immunol 1990; 85:490–497.

19. Bousquet J, Becker WM, Hejjaoui A, et al. Differences in clinical and immunologic reactivity of patients allergic to grass pollens and to multiple-pollen species. II. Efficacy of a double-blind, placebo-controlled, specific immunotherapy with standardized extracts. J Allergy Clin Immunol 1991; 88:43–53.

20. Creticos PS, Marsh DG, Proud D, et al. Responses to ragweed-pollen nasal challenge before and after immunotherapy. J Allergy Clin Immunol 1989; 84:197–205.

21. Iliopoulos O, Proud D, Adkinson N Jr, et al. Effects of immunotherapy on the early, late, and rechallenge nasal reaction to provocation with allergen: changes in inflammatory mediators and cells. J Allergy Clin Immunol 1991; 87:855–866.

22. Hedlin G, Silber G, Schieken L, et al. Attenuation of allergen sensitivity early in the course of ragweed immunotherapy. J Allergy Clin Immunol 1989; 84:390–399.

23. Frostad A, Bolle R, Grimmer Ø, Aas K. A new, well characterized, purified allergen preparation from timothy pollen. II. Allergenic in vivo and in vitro properties. Int Arch Allergy Appl Immunol 1978; 55:35–40.

24. Osterballe O. Immunotherapy in hay fever with two major allergens 19, 25 and partially purified extract of timothy grass pollen. A controlled double blind study. In vivo variables, season I. Allergy 1980; 35:473–489.

25. Viander M, Koivikko A. The seasonal symptoms of hyposensitized and untreated hay fever patients in relation to birch pollen counts: correlations with nasal sensitivity, prick tests and RAST. Clin Allergy 1978; 8:387–396.

26. Ortolani C, Pastorello EA, Incorvaia C, et al. A double-blind, placebo-controlled study of immunotherapy with an alginate-conjugated extract of *Parietaria judaica* in patients with Parietaria hay fever. Allergy 1994; 49:13–21.

27. Bousquet J, Hejjaoui A, Skassa-Brociek W, et al. Double-blind, placebo-controlled immunotherapy with mixed grass-pollen allergoids. I. Rush immunotherapy with allergoids and standardized orchard grass-pollen extract. J Allergy Clin Immunol 1987; 80:591–598.

28. Bousquet J, Maasch HJ, Hejjaoui A, et al. Double-blind, placebo-controlled immunotherapy with mixed grass-pollen allergoids. III. Efficacy and safety of unfraction-

ated and high-molecular-weight preparations in rhinoconjunctivitis and asthma. J Allergy Clin Immunol 1989; 84:546–556.

29. Frankland A, Augustin R. Prophylaxis of summer hay fever and asthma: a controlled trial comparing crude grass pollen extract with the isolated main protein components. Lancet 1954; 1:1055–1058.

30. Grammer LC, Shaughnessy MA, Suszko IM, Shaughnessy JJ, Patterson R. A double-blind histamine placebo-controlled trial of polymerized whole grass for immunotherapy of grass allergy. J Allergy Clin Immunol 1983; 72:448–453.

31. Grammer LC, Shaughnessy MA, Finkle SM, Shaughnessy JJ, Patterson R. A double-blind placebo-controlled trial of polymerized whole grass administered in an accelerated dosage schedule for immunotherapy of grass pollinosis. J Allergy Clin Immunol 1986; 78:1180–1184.

32. McAllen M. Hyposensitization in grass pollen hay fever. Acta Allergol 1969; 24: 421–431.

33. Machiels JJ, Buche M, Somville MA, Jacquemin MG, Saint-Remy JM. Complexes of grass pollen allergens and specific antibodies reduce allergic symptoms and inhibit the seasonal increase of IgE antibody. Clin Exp Allergy 1990; 20:653–660.

34. Machiels JJ, Somville MA, Jacquemin MG, Saint-Remy JM. Allergen-antibody complexes can efficiently prevent seasonal rhinitis and asthma in grass pollen hypersensitive patients. Allergen-antibody complex immunotherapy. Allergy 1991; 46:335–348.

35. Ortolani C, Pastorello E, Moss RB, et al. Grass pollen immunotherapy: a single year double-blind, placebo-controlled study in patients with grass pollen-induced asthma and rhinitis. J Allergy Clin Immunol 1984; 73:283–290.

36. Starr M, Weinstock M. Studies in pollen allergy. III. The relationship between blocking antibody levels, and symptomatic relief following hyposensitization with Allpyral in hay fever subjects. Int Arch Allergy 1970; 38:514–521.

37. Varney VA, Gaga M, Frew AJ, Aber VR, Kay AB, Durham SR. Usefulness of immunotherapy in patients with severe summer hay fever uncontrolled by antiallergic drugs. Br Med J 1991; 302:265–269.

38. Weyer A, Donat N, L'Heritier C, et al. Grass pollen hyposensitization versus placebo therapy. I. Clinical effectiveness and methodological aspects of a pre-seasonal course of desensitization with a four-grass pollen extract. Allergy 1981; 36:309–317.

39. Arbesman C, Reismann R. Hyposensitization therapy including repository: a double-blind study. J Allergy 1964; 35:12–17.

40. Cockroft D, Cuff M, Tarlo S, Dolovich J, Hargreave F. Allergen-injection therapy with glutaraldehyde-modified-ragweed pollen-tyrosine adsorbate. A double-blind trial. J Allergy Clin Immunol 1977; 60:56–62.

41. Grammer LC, Zeiss CR, Suszko IM, Shaughnessy MA, Patterson R. A double-blind, placebo-controlled trial of polymerized whole ragweed for immunotherapy of ragweed allergy. J Allergy Clin Immunol 1982; 69:494–499.

42. Hirsch SR, Kalbfleisch JH, Cohen SH. Comparison of Rinkel injection therapy with standard immunotherapy. J Allergy Clin Immunol 1982; 70:183–190.

43. Lichtenstein L, Norman P, Winkelwerder W. Clinical and in vitro studies on the role of immunotherapy in ragweed hay fever. Am J Med 1968; 44:514–524.

juvac) in patients with perennial rhinitis. II. Immunological aspects. Allergy 1990; 45:505–514.

109.   Corrado OJ, Pastorello E, Ollier S, et al. A double-blind study of hyposensitization with an alginate conjugated extract of *D. pteronyssinus* (Conjuvac) in patients with perennial rhinitis. 1. Clinical aspects. Allergy 1989; 44:108–115.

110.   Lofkvist T, Agrell B, Dreborg S, Svensson G. Effects of immunotherapy with a purified standardized allergen preparation of *Dermatophagoides farinae* in adults with perennial allergic rhinoconjunctivitis. Allergy 1994; 49:100–107.

111.   Tari MG, Mancino M, Monti G. Efficacy of sublingual immunotherapy in patients with rhinitis and asthma due to house dust mite. A double-blind study. Allergol Immunopathol Madr 1990; 18:277–284.

112.   Andri L, Senna G, Betteli C, Givanni S, Andri G, Falagiani P. Local nasal immunotherapy for *Dermatophagoides*-induced rhinitis: efficacy of a powder extract. J Allergy Clin Immunol 1993; 91:987–996.

113.   Fanales-Belasio E, Ciofalo A, Zambetti G, et al. Intranasal immunotherapy with *Dermatophagoides* extract: in vivo and in vitro results of a double-blind placebo-controlled trial. Rhinology 1995; 33:126–131.

114.   Giovane AL, Bardare M, Passalacqua G, et al. A three-year double-blind placebo-controlled study with specific oral immunotherapy to *Dermatophagoides:* evidence of safety and efficacy in paediatric patients. Clin Exp Allergy 1994; 24:53–59.

115.   Scadding G, Brostoff J. Low dose sublingual therapy in patients with allergic rhinitis due to house dust mite. Clin Allergy 1986; 16:493–499.

116.   Reilly D, Taylor M, Beattie N, et al. Is evidence for homeopathy reproducible? Lancet 1994; 344:1601–1606.

117.   Bousquet J, Hejjaoui A, Clauzel AM, et al. Specific immunotherapy with a standardized *Dermatophagoides pteronyssinus* extract. II. Prediction of efficacy of immunotherapy. J Allergy Clin Immunol 1988; 82:971–977.

118.   Bousquet J, Michel FB. Specific immunotherapy in asthma: is it effective? J Allergy Clin Immunol 1994; 94:1–11.

119.   Alvarez-Cuesta E, Cuesta-Herranz J, Puyana-Ruiz J, Cuesta-Herranz C, Blanco-Quiros A. Monoclonal antibody-standardized cat extract immunotherapy: risk-benefit effects from a double-blind placebo study. J Allergy Clin Immunol 1994; 93:556–566.

120.   Openheimer J, Areson JG, Nelson HS. Safety and efficacy of oral immunotherapy with standardized cat extract. J Allergy Clin Immunol 1994; 93:61–67.

121.   Nelson H, Oppenheimer J, Vatsia G, Buchmeier A. A double-blind, placebo-controlled evaluation of sublingual immunotherapy with standardized cat extract. J Allergy Clin Immunol 1993; 92:229–236.

122.   Bousquet J, Michel FB, Creticos PS. Sublingual immunotherapy for cat allergy. J Allergy Clin Immunol 1995; 95:920–921.

123.   Bond JF, Brauer AW, Segal DB, Nault AK, Rogers BL, Kuo MC. Native and recombinant Fel dI as probes into the relationship of allergen structure to human IgE immunoreactivity. Mol Immunol 1993; 30:1529–1541.

124.   Helm RM, Squillace DL, Yunginger JW. Production of a proposed international reference standard *Alternaria* extract. II. Results of a collaborative trial. J Allergy Clin Immunol 1988; 81:651–663.

125. Norman PS, Ohman JL, Long AA, et al. Treatment of cat allergy with T-cell reactive peptides. Am J Respir Crit Care Med 1996; 154:1623–1628.
126. Dreborg S, Agrell B, Foucard T, Kjellman NI, Koivikko A, Nilsson S. A double-blind, multicenter immunotherapy trial in children, using a purified and standardized *Cladosporium herbarum* preparation. I. Clinical results. Allergy 1986; 41:131–140.
127. Karlsson R, Agrell B, Dreborg S, et al. A double-blind, multicenter immunotherapy trial in children, using a purified and standardized *Cladosporium herbarum* preparation. II. In vitro results. Allergy 1986; 41:141–150.
128. Malling HJ, Dreborg S, Weeke B. Diagnosis and immunotherapy of mould allergy. V. Clinical efficacy and side effects of immunotherapy with *Cladosporium herbarum*. Allergy 1986; 41:507–519.
129. Horst M, Hejjaoui A, Horst V, Michel FB, Bousquet J. Double-blind, placebo-controlled rush immunotherapy with a standardized *Alternaria* extract. J Allergy Clin Immunol 1990; 85:460–472.
130. Kaad PH, Ostergaard PA. The hazard of mould hyposensitization in children with asthma. Clin Allergy 1982; 12:317–320.

19

Surgical Treatment

IAN S. MACKAY

Charing Cross Hospital
  and Royal Brompton Hospital
London, England

I. Introduction

Rhinitis may be allergic, infective, or associated with other miscellaneous factors and is characterised by nasal block, itching, sneezing, and nasal discharge. The ciliated mucous membranes lining the nose are continuous with the lining of the paranasal sinuses and it is rare for one to be involved without the other. Whatever the cause, inflammation will lead to obstruction of the nasal airway and interfere with the drainage and aeration of the sinuses, predisposing to further inflammation, and establishing a vicious cycle.

Nasal obstruction may also arise from structural abnormalities such as deviation of the nose and septum, nasal polyps, choanal atresia, enlarged turbinates, and adenoidal hypertrophy. Benign and malignant tumors of the nose and other sinister causes of rhinitis such as Wegener's granulomatosis and sarcoid need to be excluded, and watery rhinorrhea, particularly if unilateral or following an injury, suggests the possibility of a cerebrospinal fluid leak.

Surgery plays an important role in the management of primary structural abnormalities and may also be indicated when obstruction due to inflammation has failed to respond to medical treatment. Although medical treatment is often the first line of action, surgery is not necessarily indicated simply because medical treatment fails. A surgical opinion should be sought to exclude malignancy, particularly in patients with unilateral symptoms.

II. Adenoidal Hypertrophy

Adenoidal hypertrophy can be an important cause of catarrhal symptoms in children who present with a "snuffly nose," nasal obstruction, nasal speech, and snoring at night. Enlarged adenoids may be associated with large tonsils and there may be a history of otological symptoms with recurrent otitis media and otitis media with effusion (glue ear).

Adenoids can be difficult to assess; not all children will tolerate a postnasal mirror or endoscope and a lateral radiograph of the postnasal space can be misleading, but is the most reliable method of assessing the size of the adenoids (1). Adults rarely have any adenoidal tissue as this usually atrophies by late teens. Enlarged adenoid tissue in adults should raise suspicion of AIDS. If symptoms of adenoidal hypertrophy are severe, associated with otological symptoms, or there is any history to suggest associated sleep apnea, surgery should be considered.

III. Foreign Bodies

Unilateral nasal obstruction associated with a foul-smelling, purulent discharge, particularly in children, suggests the possibility of a foreign body. Occasionally bilateral foreign bodies are found and there may be a history of repeated insertion of these into both the nose and ears. Foreign bodies may at times be overlooked for many years and finally become calcified to form a rhinolith.

Many foreign bodies are not radiopaque, e.g., peas and other vegetable matter and plastic toys or beads, and are not demonstrated by X-ray. Careful endoscopic examination under local anesthesia or under a general anesthetic in an uncooperative child may be necessary to remove the object or to exclude the possibility.

IV. Choanal Atresia

Neonates are obligatory nose breathers and bilateral choanal atresia will present as a respiratory emergency at birth with the baby experiencing great difficulty with breathing and finding it impossible to feed. Crying relieves the breathing problem. A neonatal Waters airway is required to aid initial breathing and this should be taped securely into position. In addition, a nasogastric tube can be used to provide nourishment.

The time-honored method of radiographic investigation involves the use of contrast medium placed into both nasal fossae. This has now been replaced by axial computerized tomography (CT), which is particularly useful in demonstrating the extent of the atresia, which may be bony or membranous. Most cases will proceed to surgery within 24 hr, but the above measures will allow surgery to be delayed if the child's general health is unsatisfactory, which may occur if the child has other congenital defects as are found in as many as 60% of cases, notably the CHARGE association (2).

C   Colobomatous
H   Heart disease
A   Atresia of the choanae
R   Retarded growth and development (including central nervous system)
G   Genital hypoplasia (in males)
E   Ear deformities including deafness

Unlike bilateral choanal atresia, unilateral atresia is surprisingly easy to miss and the diagnosis is not infrequently made in adult life. The author has seen four patients who have undergone nasal surgery without the diagnosis being made. One patient underwent three separate surgical procedures: adenoidectomy, reduction of the inferior turbinates, and submucous resection of the septum by two different surgeons both of whom failed to make the diagnosis. This illustrates the importance of a careful endoscopic examination in all patients presenting with nasal obstruction, particularly when it is unilateral.

V. Hypertrophy of Turbinates

Before a surgical procedure is performed to reduce the bulk of the inferior turbinates, it is essential to make a diagnosis. This involves a careful history, examination (ideally endoscopic), and other investigations as indicated by the history, which may include skin prick tests, blood tests, and CT scanning of the sinuses. Many patients with chronic sinusitis may present with nasal "congestion," and medical or surgical treatment aimed at managing the sinusitis may be more helpful than reduction of the turbinates, which will often shrink once the chronic sinus condition has been treated.

Intraturbinal injection of repository corticosteroid has been widely used by otolaryngologists for more than 40 years, though the introduction of intranasal topical steroids has reduced the incidence of their usage. With these injections, there is a risk of visual loss following this procedure, which is thought to be due to retinal vasospasm or retrograde embolization of the injected material into the retinal circulation. Despite this, some authors continue to advocate its use with the following precautions: use a topical anesthetic, do not add anesthetic agents to the material to be injected, inject only the anterior tip of the inferior turbinate, and use freshly drawn material with steroid of small particle size and a fine needle (25 gauge or smaller) (3).

Extravagant claims are made for various methods of surgical reduction; whether this be by laser, surgical debrider, freezing, diathermy, trimming, or resecting, the aim of the procedure is to reduce the bulk of tissue of the inferior turbinate and thereby improve the airway. Why these procedures should affect the other symptoms of sneezing, itching, or watery rhinorrhea is puzzling despite the fact that some trials appear to demonstrate this (4–6).

Laser mucotomy of the inferior turbinates has been described by Englender (4), who reported 87 patients presenting with sneezing, rhinorrhea, or nasal block. All patients had failed either medical treatment or other surgical treatment. The anterior 2–3 cm of each inferior turbinate was vaporized with a CO_2 laser. The results were obtained using a questionnaire and followed up at 1 week, 2 months, and 12 months. Of these patients 93% found their nasal obstruction relieved, while 83% were "satisfied" with their sneezing and 87% no longer complained of rhinorrhea at 12 months.

Cook and associates (7) compared submucosal diathermy with CO_2 laser cautery to the inferior turbinates. They reviewed 23 patients and found that the improvement in the sensation of nasal airflow at 1 year compared with the preoperative state was significantly better in the laser group than in the submucosal diathermy group, but interestingly, there was no difference in the two groups as far as objective tests were concerned using peak nasal inspiratory flow rates and there is no mention of any change in other symptoms.

Trimming of the turbinates is certainly effective but may be associated with significant postoperative hemorrhage. Garth and associates (8), reviewing 214 patients undergoing surgical reduction of the inferior turbinates, found a 0.9% incidence of hemorrhage in a group undergoing anterior turbinectomy compared with a 5.8% incidence in those patients undergoing radical turbinectomy. Partial turbinectomy was associated with an incidence of 3.7% hemorrhage in another series reported by Mucci and Sismanis (6) but they were also able to demonstrate a 92% success rate for improving nasal obstruction with an average follow-up of 18 months.

Salam and Wengraf (5) compared total turbinectomy with conchoantropexy, an operation to relieve nasal obstruction by dislocating the inferior turbinate into the antrum after removal of the lateral nasal wall. While they found no significant difference in the efficacy of the two procedures, total turbinectomy was associated with more pain and long-term dryness and crusting. Lannigan and Gleeson (9) also reported good results using this technique. The outcome was evaluated in 12 patients all of whom reported success as demonstrated by a significant reduction in symptom scores for nasal obstruction.

Richtsmeier (10) has reported successful results using infrared coagulation of the inferior turbinates. Reduction of the turbinates using a power microcutting instrument to remove erectile soft tissue from the lateral and inferior borders of the inferior turbinates was reported by Davis and Nishioka (11), though no results were included!

No technique is likely to be useful for all patients and an attempt should be made to assess which one is likely to be most appropriate. If the enlarged turbinate does not respond to vasoconstriction, it is likely that the problem is related to a bulky turbinate bone, which may be reduced either by surgical trimming or by submucosal excision (turbinoplasty), which aims at removing bone but retaining the medial and some of the lateral surface mucosa.

Bulky posterior ends, which may be seen at endoscopy, may at times require excision. Where vasoconstrictors result in an improved airway, surgical scarring of the mucosa should be beneficial whether this be by infrared coagulation, laser, linear diathermy, submucosal diathermy, or submucosal multiple outfractures of the inferior turbinates.

The improvement following surgical reduction of the turbinates may be short-lived. Warwick-Brown and Marks (12) followed up a large series of patients undergoing submucosal diathermy, partial trimming, or radical trimming—all with or without outfracture of the turbinate bone—and found that although 82% felt their symptoms had improved at 1 month, only 41% remained symptom-free at 1 year, regardless of the technique used. These results were in accordance with those of Jones and Lancer (13) following submucosal diathermy. Mabry (3), however, was able to demonstrate a 75% success rate following ''turbinoplasty'' with a follow-up of 3 years or more. This technique involved submucosal reduction of the turbinate bone.

Wight et al. (14) compared the results of trimming the anterior portion of the inferior turbinate with a radical turbinectomy. The anterior end of the turbinate protrudes into the nasal valve area where it causes maximum obstruction. Rhinomanometry confirmed that although the nasal airway resistance was satisfactorily reduced in both groups, the symptom score was significantly better in those patients undergoing the more radical procedure.

Middle turbinates may contain a large air cell (concha bullosa), which may not only be associated with blockage of the ostiomeatal complex but at times cause marked limitation of nasal airflow. This deformity can be corrected simply under local or general anesthesia with endoscopic control, incising the lower edge of the turbinate with a sickle knife and removing the thin lateral lamella of bone (15).

VI. The Nasal Septum

Injury to the nose may result in a hematoma of the septum. This may be painful, but may occasionally be surprisingly painless, the patient presenting with bilateral nasal obstruction, a day or so after the incident. On examination there is smooth,

Many prosthetic devices have been used over the years, from quills and reeds to the silver wire alae nasi dilator used by Clement Francis. Davenport and associates (18) used a mold made with silicone putty, which is then cast in a clear acrylic resin through which a hole is drilled to provide an airway. More recently Breatherite plasters have gained popularity, particularly with sportsmen. A plaster is applied externally to the skin of the nose, which contains a strip of plastic the elasticity of which springs the lower lateral cartilages apart.

Surgical procedures include those that aim to modify existing cartilage and those requiring augmentation with cartilage grafts. Rettinger and Masing (19) noted that in many patients with alar collapse, the medial and lateral crura of the lower lateral cartilages lie in the same plane, and this is particularly true in the elderly patient with a drooping tip. They also observed the tension lines in a plastic model under polarized light. By rotating the two limbs of the model in opposite directions, they noticed that these tension lines were distributed over a larger surface increasing the stability of the system. By rotation of the lateral limb of the lower lateral cartilage in a cephalic direction, the distance between the medial and lower lateral crura is increased as is the tensile strength. Since the lateral crus of the lower lateral cartilage has to be dissected free to undertake this, there will also be a certain amount of scar tissue formation between the vestibular skin and the cartilage as well as the overlying skin of the nose and the cartilage, and this may also account for some of the increase in tensile strength.

In those cases where there is very weak cartilage, where it has been absorbed following trauma or removed during rhinoplasty, repositioning of cartilage is not possible and augmentation is required. Conchal cartilage harvested from the concha of the pinna (20) has proved a useful donor site; however, what is gained in tensile strength may be lost due to increased bulk in tissue in the early postoperative phase though this may improve with time.

IX. Paranasal Sinus Surgery

A century ago, Caldwell (21) demonstrated the possible importance of the middle meatus and anterior ethmoids as the key to sinus pathology. The work of Proetz (22), Hilding (23), Proctor (24), and Messerklinger (25) has supported this view and nowhere is this more true than with sinus problems arising secondarily to rhinitis, where inflammation of the mucosa may obstruct the middle meatus, predisposing to sinus infection, which in turn causes more inflammation— a vicious circle.

Obstruction of this ostiomeatal complex is particularly suited to functional endoscopic sinus surgery (FESS). The Messerklinger technique, popularized by Stammberger (26), aims at restoring the natural mucociliary clearance mechanism, drainage, and aeration of the sinuses by a minimally invasive technique, maintaining as much of the normal anatomy as possible. With the use of an endoscope, the surgery commences anteriorly and progresses posteriorly, superiorly, and laterally, but only as far as is necessary, concentrating particularly on the ostiomeatal complex, the anterior ethmoid, and its infundibulum. The endoscope affords the surgeon an exceptionally clear and well-illuminated field of vision with the added advantage of the ability to inspect recesses with angled distal lenses.

An endoscopic approach can be considered for the management of nasal polyposis, frontoethmoidal mucoceles, allergic fungal sinusitis, for the repair of cerebrospinal fluid leaks, orbital and optic nerve decompression, blow-out fractures, dacryocystorhinostomy, choanal atresia, hyposphysectomy, septal and turbinate surgery, management of epistaxis, drainage of periorbital abscess, and the management of certain circumscribed tumors. Only chronic or recurrent acute sinusitis is amenable to FESS, which attempts to reverse the pathophysiological processes by conservative surgery.

Many authors have reported excellent results following endoscopic sinus surgery (26–29). In a study undertaken by the author in collaboration with Lund, 650 patients were assessed with a follow-up in excess of 6 months following FESS; individuals were assessed as asymptomatic, improved, same, or worse and by individual symptom ranked into first, second, or third (30). Eighty-seven percent regarded themselves as asymptomic or improved, 11% were unchanged, and 2% worse. Evaluation of success, however, is beset with difficulties as patients may feel well despite a cavity that reveals obvious disease at endoscopic examination, and neither endoscopic nor CT findings correlate well with symptoms (31).

Some of the problems encountered in assessing results may be overcome by accurate staging of the extent of disease (32). The system suggested by the author and Lund scores the preoperative CT findings as 0 = no abnormality, 1 = partial opacification, 2 = total opacification for each of the sinus systems (maxillary, anterior and posterior ethmoidal, and sphenoid), and 0 or 2 for the ostiomeatal complex, giving a total score of 12 for each side. The greater the extent of disease, the worse one might expect the prognosis to be, and this has been confirmed by Kennedy (31). Those patients with a ''black halo'' on CT scanning (Fig. 2) would be expected to do better than patients with a ''white-out,'' or total opacity (Fig. 3).

X. Nasal Polyps

Nasal polyps result from inflammation of the mucosa of the nose and paranasal sinuses and are therefore likely to be related to rhinitis of any etiology: allergic, infective, structural (intense contact of mucosal surfaces), or other miscellaneous factors. The swollen, edematous mucosa prolapses down from the sinuses or clefts around the middle turbinate into the nasal airway, particularly from the ethmoids protruding through the middle meatus and presenting as smooth, round, pale, translucent swellings. The presenting symptoms will usually be nasal block

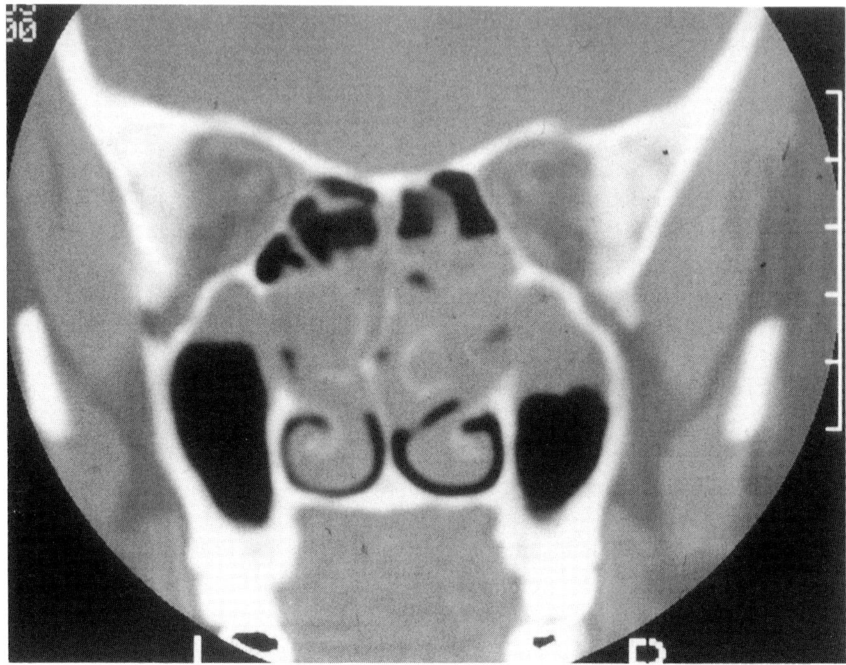

Figure 2 A "black halo" with polypoid mucosal hypertrophy in the region of the ostiomeatal complex, but healthy tissue beyond. An ideal case for functional endoscopic sinus surgery (FESS) and where one might expect an excellent outcome.

and poor sense of smell but there may be associated secondary symptoms due to sinusitis.

Polyps may be attached by a narrow pedicle or may appear as sessile, "cobblestoned" mucosal lining. The anterior end of the middle turbinate may swell to present a polypoidal appearance, but the inferior turbinates can be differentiated from polyps as the latter are insensitive and mobile on gentle probing. Benign polyps are usually bilateral. Children presenting with polyps should be regarded as having cystic fibrosis until proved otherwise.

Many patients with nasal polyposis will respond to medical treatment (33); surgery, however, plays an important role in the management when medical treatment fails to provide an adequate airway or when infections recur frequently. Malignancy should always be considered, particularly in unilateral cases, and all material removed at surgery must be sent for histological examination. Since surgical removal does not treat the underlying cause of nasal polyps, it is not surprising that polyps will often recur and postoperative treatment with topical corticosteroids would appear to be logical in attempting to reduce recurrence.

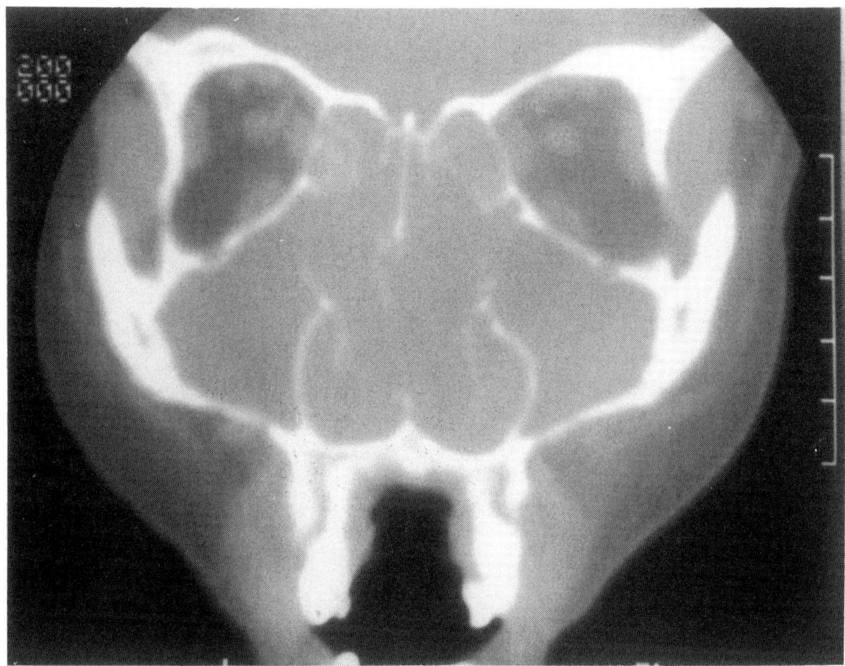

Figure 3 A "white-out" with total opacity of all sinuses. An endoscopic approach is still possible, but it will be more difficult to undertake a truly functional procedure and the outcome may be less favorable.

XI. Benign and Malignant Neoplasms

Both benign and malignant neoplasms may present with symptoms of rhinitis. One should be particularly suspicious of unilateral symptoms especially if these are associated with ominous symptoms of epistaxis, facial pain, numbness, or swelling of the face. Benign inflammatory nasal polyps may arise in the vicinity of more sinister pathology and one should be wary of taking a small anterior biopsy of tissue for histology as this may well be reported as a benign inflammatory polyp, when it is in fact obscuring a malignant lesion more posteriorly.

XII. Vidian Neurectomy

With the introduction of topical steroids, more effective and less sedating H_1 antagonists, and topical anticholinergics, the need for surgery to treat watery rhinorrhea has progressively decreased. Notwithstanding this, there is a small number of patients who, despite all attempts with medication, will continue to complain of this trying condition and for whom a surgical option may be considered.

Stimulation of the parasympathetic supply to the nasal mucosa results in watery rhinorrhea; dividing this supply should—and in many instances does—reduce nasal secretions. Malcomson (34) introduced resection of the vidian nerve via a transantral approach and this method was popularized by Golding-Wood (35).

Various other approaches have been described, including a septal approach (36) and a direct transnasal approach (37). Recently an endoscopic approach to the vidian nerve has been described (38). Whatever technique is used, any improvement may be short-lived, probably due to reinnervation. The transnasal technique has the advantage of being relatively quick and simple to undertake and can be repeated if necessary. In a series of 22 patients on whom this technique was used by the author and who were followed up for between 21 and 36 months, 13 (59%) remained better, 3 (14%) were the same while 6 (27%) regarded their symptoms as worse (39). A larger series of 258 patients were reported by Fernandes, who found that 88% of patients had a satisfactory result at 6 months or more (40).

XIII. Conclusions

Both medical and surgical treatment aim to control the symptoms of allergic and nonallergic rhinitis and can be complementary to one another. Surgical treatment plays an important role in the management of the primary symptoms of nasal blockage and may be useful for controlling obstinate watery rhinorrhea. Secondary symptoms that may result from obstruction of the paranasal sinuses in the middle meatus may be corrected by minimally invasive FESS.

While it is often reasonable to consider medication as the first line of action, surgical treatment will not necessarily be indicated simply because the former has failed. Some symptoms are no more likely to respond to surgery than to medical treatment. Conversely, many patients may best be managed by a combined medical and surgical approach and medical treatment may be particularly important in maintaining any improvement gained surgically, or in preventing recurrence. A combined medical and surgical clinic, staffed by physicians and surgeons who manage patients together, has proved to be an effective alliance that has benefited both the patients and the understanding of their practitioners (41).

References

1. Cohen D, Konak S. The evaluation of radiographs of the nasopharynx. Clin Otolaryngol 1985; 98:803–805.

2. Pagon RA, Graham JM, Zonna J, Yong S-L. Coloboma, congenital heart disease and choanal atresia with multiple anomalies: CHARGE association. J Paediatr 1981; 99:223–227.
3. Mabry R. Intranasal steroids in rhinology: the changing role of intraturbinal injection. Ear Nose Throat J 1994; 73:242–246.
4. Englender M. Nasal laser mucotomy (L-mucotomy) of the inferior turbinates. J Laryngol Otol 1995; 109:296–299.
5. Salam MA, Wengraf C. Concho-antropexy or total turbinectomy for hypertrophy of the inferior turbinates? A prospective randomised study. J Laryngol Otol 1993; 107: 1125–1128.
6. Mucci S, Sismanis A. Inferior partial turbinectomy: an effective procedure for chronic rhinitis. Ear Nose Throat J 1994; 73:405–407.
7. Cook JA, McCombe AW, Jones AS. Laser treatment of rhinitis—1 year follow-up. Clin Otolaryngol 1993; 18:209–211.
8. Garth RJN, Cox HJ, Thomas MR. Haemorrhage as a complication of inferior turbinectomy: a comparison of anterior and radical trimming. Clin Otolaryngol 1995; 20:236–238.
9. Lannigan FJ, Gleeson MJ. Antroconchopexy for surgical treatment of perennial rhinitis. Rhinology 1992; 30:183–186.
10. Richtsmeier WJ. Infrared coagulation of the inferior turbinate: a new treatment for refractory chronic rhinitis. Otolaryngol Head Neck Surg 1994; 111:674–679.
11. Davis WE, Nishioka GJ. Endoscopic partial inferior turbinectomy using a power microcutting instrument. Ear Nose Throat J 1996; 75:49–50.
12. Warwick-Brown NP, Marks NJ. Turbinate surgery; how effective is it? A long-term assessment. J ORL 1987; 49:314–320.
13. Jones AS, Lancer JM. Does submucosal diathermy to the inferior turbinates reduce nasal resistance to airflow in the long term? J Laryngol Otol 1987; 101:338–352.
14. Wight RG, Jones AS, Clegg RT. A comparison of anterior and radical trimming of the inferior nasal turbinates and the effects on nasal resistance to airflow. Clin Otolaryngol 1988; 13:223–226.
15. Cook PR, Begegni A, Bryant WC, Davis WE. Effect of partial middle turbinectomy on nasal airflow and resistance. Otolaryngol Head Neck Surg 1995; 113:413–419.
16. Fry JH. The pathology and treatment of haematoma of the nasal septum. Br J Plast Surg 1969; 22:331–336.
17. Cottle MH. Corrective Surgery on the Nasal Septum and External Pyramid. Chicago: American Rhinologic Society, 1960.
18. Davenport JC, Brain DJ, Hunt AT. Treatment of alar collapse with nasal prostheses. J Prosthet Dent 1981; 45:435–437.
19. Rettinger G, Masing H. Rotation of the alar cartilage in collapsed alae. Rhinology 1981; 19:81–86.
20. Walter C. Survey of the use of composite grafts in the head and neck region. Otolaryngol Clin North Am 1972; 10:571–602.
21. Caldwell GW. Disease of the accessory sinuses of the nose and an improved method of treatment for suppuration of the maxillary antrum. NY Med J 1893; 58:526–528.
22. Proetz AW. Essays on Applied Physiology of the Nose, 2nd ed. St. Louis: Annals Publishing Company, 1953.

II. Seasonal Allergic Rhinitis (Fig. 1)

A. Typical Symptoms in the Pollen Season

The diagnosis of seasonal allergic rhinitis or hay fever is usually easy to make based on its typical symptoms: itchy eyes and nose, sneezing, and watery rhinorrhea, which occur during the same months every year. In subtropical and tropical climates, pollen allergy may also cause perennial allergic rhinitis.

In most patients, no allergy testing is indicated, but when necessary, the

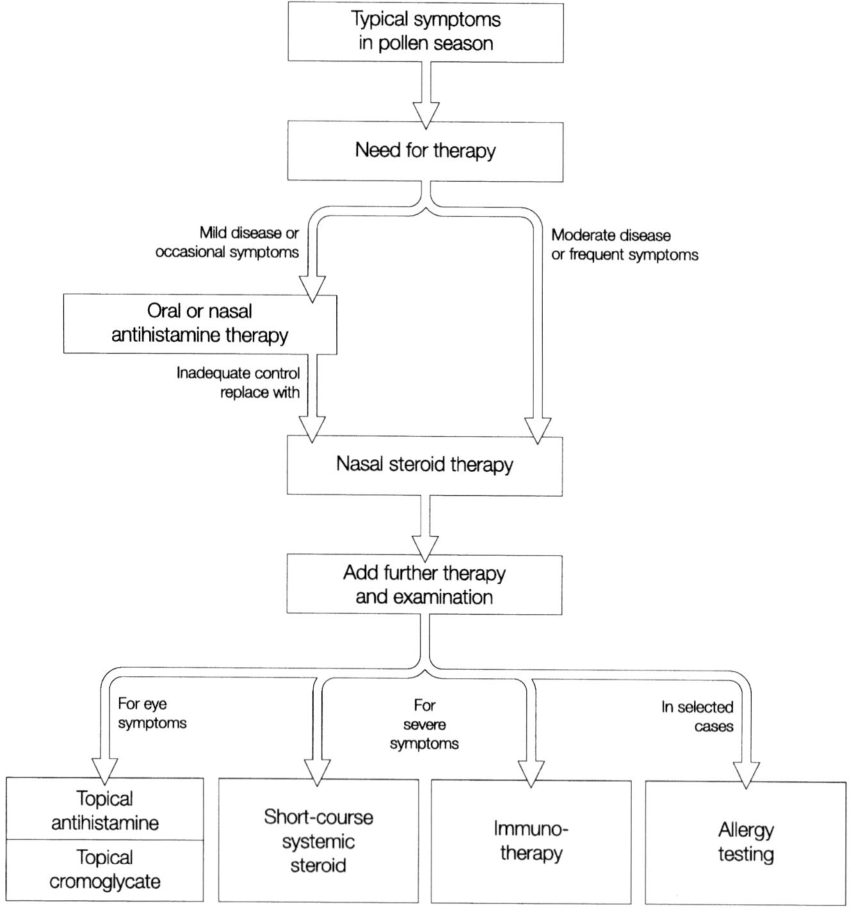

Figure 1   Management plan for seasonal allergic rhinitis.

diagnosis can be confirmed by skin testing or by RAST (Chapter 9). Allergy testing is indicated in patients with severe rhinitis symptoms or asthma in the season, in patients with perennial symptoms, and when immunotherapy is considered.

B. Need for Therapy

In patients with moderate to severe hay fever symptoms, the quality of life can be seriously impaired in the pollen season (see Chapter 8). In childhood and adolescence, the disease may lead to underperformance in school examinations, which are commonly held at the height of the grass pollen season.

Some exposure to pollen is inevitable, although excessive exposure can usually be avoided by common-sense measures, and by using air conditioning. As effective and safe therapies are available, the goal for treatment is no or minimal symptoms and a normal life without restrictions in the pollen season.

C. Antihistamine Therapy

When patients have a mild disease and pollen exposure is low, they will only have occasional symptoms and daily treatment is not indicated. Owing to their quicker onset of action, antihistamines are more suitable than corticosteroids (2–5).

Antihistamines can be applied topically to the eyes and nose or taken orally. Theoretically the advantage of topical treatment is that effect and side effects can be confined to the diseased organ. In addition, topical treatment has a faster onset of action (6). However, many patients prefer the convenience of oral therapy.

D. Nasal Steroid Therapy

In patients with moderate to severe disease and daily nasal symptoms, better effect is obtained with regular use of nasal steroid than with regular use of an antihistamine (7–9). The treatment is preferably begun early or before the start of the pollen season and continued during the entire season.

There exists no contraindication to a 2–3-month course of treatment (10). Thus, in hay fever, nasal steroids can be used as first-line therapy in patients with daily or frequent nasal symptoms, both in children and in adults (1).

E. Added Therapy for Eye Symptoms

Patients who use oral antihistamine as needed and those who are on nasal steroids often need eye drops to provide relief for eye itching. Those individuals who use oral antihistamines regularly usually have a good protection from eye symptoms.

The topically applied antihistamine levocabastine is more effective than cromoglycate and twice-daily use is sufficient (11). Contact lens wearers cannot use antihistamine eye drops, which contain benzalkonium chloride as a preservative.

F.   Added Therapy for Asthma Symptoms

Controlled studies have shown that nasal steroids have a moderate effect on asthma symptoms in the pollen season (12,13), and this may be sufficient in mild cases. Otherwise asthma symptoms need proper antiasthmatic therapy with inhaled steroid and an inhaled beta$_2$-agonist p.r.n.

G.   Added Therapy for Severe Rhinitis Symptoms

A steroid spray controls nasal symptoms in the large majority of patients but, as for any type of treatment, highly allergic patients can have breakthrough symptoms at the peak of the pollen season. In this situation, a short course of systemic steroid helps (1). This therapy is undoubtedly beneficial, but there are no controlled studies to prove an added efficacy of combined therapy and our knowledge of the dose of systemic steroid required is insufficient (see Chapter 14). An alternative approach is doubling the dose of the nasal steroid (14). The addition of an antihistamine, in the majority of cases, will not reduce nasal symptoms beyond what is obtain with nasal steroid therapy (7–9).

H.   Immunotherapy

A controlled study has shown immunotherapy to be highly efficient in hay fever patients, not controlled by drug therapy (15). Immunotherapy should be considered when systemic steroids are needed to control the disease.

III.   Perennial Rhinitis in Adults: Allergic and Nonallergic (Fig. 2)

A.   Symptoms Suggesting Rhinitis

In perennial allergic rhinitis the symptoms are largely the same as those of hay fever, but eye itching is less frequent and nasal blockage more prominent. In perennial nonallergic rhinitis, some patients sneeze frequently (''sneezers''), others predominantly suffer from nasal blockage (''blockers''), and others suffer only from watery rhinorrhea (''runners'').

B.   Examinations

Rhinoscopy, or preferably nasal endoscopy, is indicated in all patients with chronic nasal symptoms to exclude structural abnormalities and other diseases.

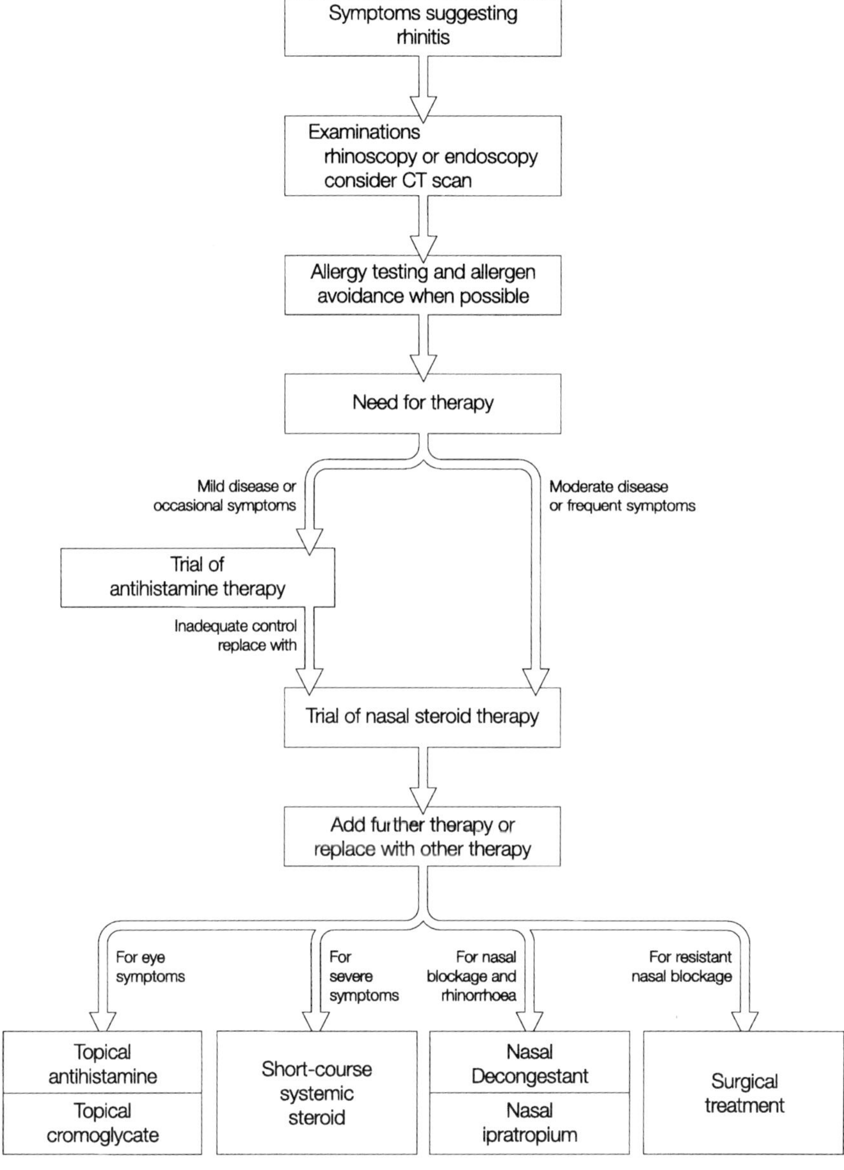

Figure 2 Management plan for perennial rhinitis in adults.

Computed-tomography (CT) imaging of the nose and paranasal sinuses is indicated in patients with chronic severe rhinitis not responding to treatment, when there is suspicion of malignancy or another serious disease, and before planning intranasal and sinus surgery (1).

C. Allergy Testing and Allergen Avoidance

Allergy testing is indicated in all patients with chronic rhinitis symptoms. Skin prick testing is the clinically most useful allergy test, but measurement of circulating IgE antibodies can be used in selected cases (see Chapter 9).

In principle, avoidance of allergens is the first measure to be recommended in allergic airway disease, but although it is desirable, it is not always practicable.

D. Drug Therapy

All patients with perennial allergic rhinitis and most patients with perennial non-allergic rhinitis benefit from drug therapy, which should be carefully selected based on the patient's diagnosis and symptomatology (Table 1).

E. Antihistamine Therapy

Antihistamines are used in patients with occasional and mild allergic symptoms. They have some effect in chronic allergic rhinitis but their role is less important in chronic rhinitis than in acute rhinitis and hay fever.

It may be worthwhile trying antihistamines for intermittent symptoms in patients with perennial nonallergic rhinitis, when sneezing is the dominant symptom (16,17).

Table 1 Drug Effect on Nasal Symptoms

	Symptom			
Drug	Sneezing	Rhinorrhea	Blockage	Reduced sense of smell
Antihistamines	++(+)	++	(+)	—
Oral vasoconstrictors	—	—	++	(+)
Nasal vasoconstrictors	−	−	+++	+
Cromoglycate	++	+	+	−
Intranasal steroids	+++	+++	++	+(+)
Systemic steroids	++(+)	++(+)	+++	+++
Ipratropium	−	++(+)	−	−

F. Nasal Steroid Therapy

Patients with daily symptoms will require anti-inflammatory therapy with a steroid spray, which is more effective in a chronic disease than antihistamines, in particular on nasal blockage (16). Patients with perennial allergic rhinitis will obtain considerable improvement from the steroid spray, and the same applies to most, but not all, patients with perennial nonallergic rhinitis. The latter group requires a 2-week therapeutic trial to determine whether the patient responds. When nasal blockage is pronounced, a short course of systemic steroid will increase the number of responders (18).

G. Further Therapy

When the rhinitis symptoms are severe, or in nonallergic patients who are not steroid responders, other therapies may be added. Such patients often have nasal obstruction due to structural abnormalities (''blockers'') or they have watery rhinorrhea as the only symptom (''runners'').

H. Systemic Steroids

In severe cases of rhinitis, systemic steroids are a valuable supplement to other therapies, and a short course can break vicious circles and give prolonged relief, especially with regard to nasal blockage (19). Systemic steroids should only be used as short-term therapy (2 weeks) in rhinitis, and not be given more frequently than every 3–4 months. Systemic steroids are not used for rhinitis in children, during pregnancy, or when there is a known contraindication.

I. Nasal Decongestants

Topical vasoconstrictors can be used with caution in selected patients with perennial rhinitis and serious nasal blockage: 1) when the patient starts a basic treatment with a topical steroid to ensure optimal drug distribution in the nose, and 2) when the patient has upper airway infection and sinusitis. Long-term treatment will result in the development of rhinitis medicamentosa, and regular use is therefore limited to 7–10 days (see Chapter 16).

Oral medication with alpha-adrenoceptor agonists has less effect on nasal patency than topical treatment but it can be used regularly without risk of rhinitis medicamentosa. It is, however, not elegant pharmacotherapy to constrict every blood vessel in the body to treat a stuffy nose, since the dosage needed is at the borderline of that which causes systemic side effects. In addition, there are many contraindications (see Chapter 16).

J. Ipratropium Bromide

Isolated watery rhinorrhea, not associated with sneezing, rarely responds to antihistamine or steroid therapy, but it can be reduced by topical application of the anticholinergic drug ipratropium bromide (see Chapter 17). The dosage must be adjusted to the severity of symptoms in order to optimize efficacy and minimize local adverse effects (a sensation of nasal dryness). Ipratropium can also serve as adjunctive treatment, in allergic rhinitis, to steroids and antihistamines if rhinorrhea remains.

IV. Perennial Allergic Rhinitis in Children (Fig. 3)

A. Symptoms and Signs Suggesting Rhinitis

In contrast to adults, children with perennial allergic rhinitis often have characteristic signs of chronic rhinitis.

B. Allergy Testing

All children with perennial symptoms should have allergy testing, and the importance of allergen avoidance must be emphasized to the parent to prevent the development of asthma.

C. Need for Therapy

Childrens' nasal symptoms are often ignored and allergic rhinitis may be under-diagnosed and undertreated. This is unfortunate, as simple and effective treatment is available.

D. Antihistamine Therapy

Antihistamines give effective relief for itch and sneezing (20,21). The drugs are usually given orally, but are also effective when given intranasally (20). There are very few controlled studies of efficacy, side effects, and dose-response relationships in children. Apparently, the oral dose required is relatively large, as children metabolize the drugs quicker than adults (22). Recently liquid forms of nonsedating antihistamines have become available.

E. Nasal Cromoglycate Therapy

Intranasal and intraocular sodium cromoglycate (cromolyn in the United States) has a weak anti-inflammatory activity, when used prophylactically (see Chapter 23). It gives a variable degree of symptom amelioration in allergic rhinoconjunc-

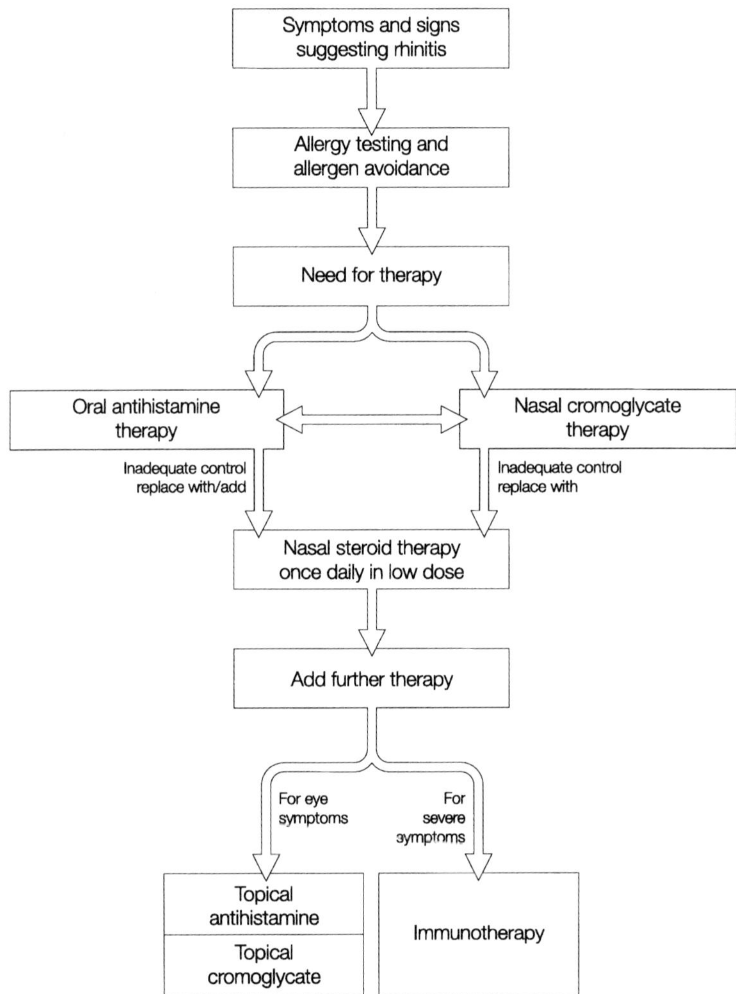

Figure 3 Management plan for perennial allergic rhinitis in children.

tivitis, but its relatively short duration of action (4–6-hr dosing) leads to poor patient compliance. As cromoglycate is free of recognized side effects, pediatricians often recommend it together with an antihistamine in children with perennial allergic rhinitis, but added effects of this combined therapy have not been demonstrated.

F. Nasal Steroid Therapy

While intranasal steroids can be used freely in hay fever with a short season, it is the opinion of some pediatricians that their regular use in children with perennial disease should be restricted to cases not controlled by other means. It is debatable, however, whether this restrictive attitude is in the best interest of the child. When a nasal steroid is used once daily in the lowest effective dose (half the adult dose), no clinically significant side effects on growth or other parameters have been shown to occur after use for more than 20 years (see Chapter 13).

V. Nasal Polyposis (Fig. 4)

A. Symptoms Suggesting Nasal Polyps

Nasal polyps, as a rule, develop in a patient who has suffered from perennial nonallergic (eosinophilic) rhinitis for some years. Nasal blockage gradually develops and can become complete. Impairment or loss of the sense of smell, and with that "taste," is characteristic.

B. Examination

In many patients, a simple rhinoscopy is sufficient for making the diagnosis, but nasal endoscopy gives a much better visualization of polyps, especially of small polyps in the middle meatus. A CT scan is always informative in patients with nasal polyposis and it is necessary before endonasal sinus surgery.

C. Need for Therapy

The disease can vary in severity from a single episode of nasal blockage to the most severe manifestation of eosinophil inflammation in the upper airways. With the exception of patients who have small polyps, diagnosed at a routine ear, nose, and throat examination, all patients with nasal polyps and symptoms need therapy.

D. Nasal Steroids

In most cases, it can be recommended to start treatment with a nasal steroid (23). If the symptoms have disappeared after treatment for 1 month, the nasal steroid can be continued as the only treatment.

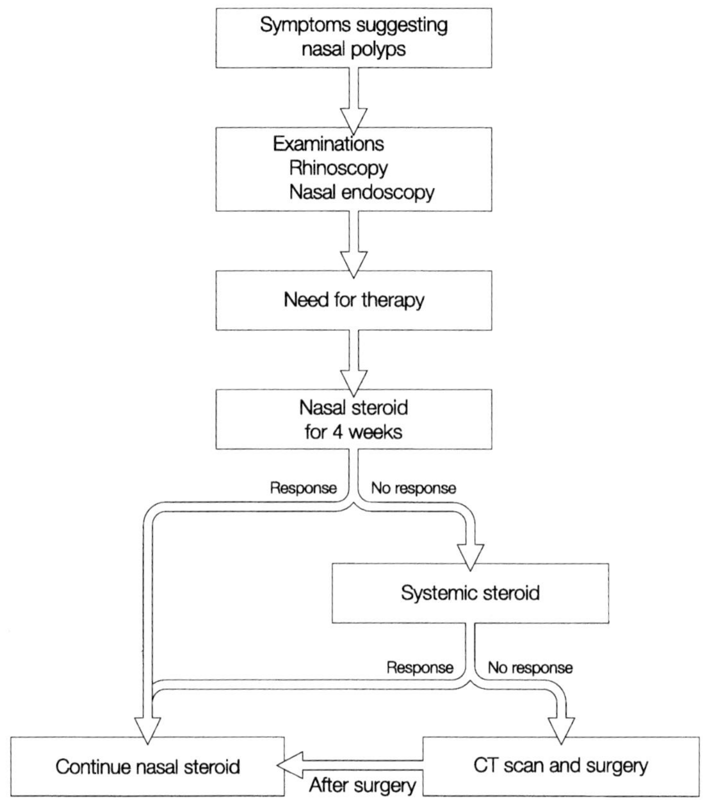

Figure 4 Management plan for nasal polyposis.

E. Systemic Steroids

Systemic steroids, in contrast to topical treatment, reach all parts of the nose and paranasal sinuses. Short courses of systemic steroids can be used in nasal polyposis to open up a blocked nose before therapy and when there is a temporary failure of spray treatment. In contrast to a steroid spray, systemic steroids have a marked effect on the sense of smell (24).

F. Surgery

Endonasal ethmoidectomy (functional endoscopic sinus surgery, FESS) is indicated in cases resistant to the above treatment schedule. Preoperative use of systemic steroids facilitates the surgery, and postoperative treatment with nasal steroids will retard the regrowth of polyps.

G. Combined Therapy

Thus, therapy is often a combination of: 1) long-term nasal steroid treatment, 2) short-term systemic steroid treatment, and 3) surgery.

References

1. Lund V. International Consensus Report on the Diagnosis and Management of Rhinitis. Allergy 1994; 49 (Suppl 19):1–34.
2. Horak F, Jäger S, Berger U. Onset and duration of the effects of three antihistamines in current use—astemizole, loratadine and terfenadine forte—studied during prolonged, controlled allergen challenges in volunteers. J Intern Med Res 1992; 20: 422–434.
3. Petersen LJ, Bindslev-Jensen C, Poulsen LK, Malling H-J. Time of onset of action of acrivastine in the skin of pollen-allergic subjects. Allergy 1994; 49:27–30.
4. Juniper E, Guyatt GH, Archer B, Ferrie PJ. Aqueous beclomethasone dipropionate in the treatment of ragweed-pollen induced rhinitis: further exploration of "as needed" use. J Allergy Clin Immunol 1993; 92:66–72.
5. Day JH, Buckeridge DL, Clark RH, Briscoe MP, Phillips R. A randomized, double-blind, placebo-controlled delivery study of the onset of action of aerosolized triamcinolone acetonide nasal spray in subjects with ragweed-induced allergic rhinitis. J Allergy Clin Immunol 1996; 97:1050–1057.
6. Stokes TC, Feinberg G. Rapid onset of action of levocabastine eye-drops in histamine-induced conjunctivitis. Clin Exp Allergy 1993; 23:791–794.
7. Juniper E, Kline PA, Hargreave FE, Dolovich J. Comparison of beclomethasone dipropionate aqueous nasal spray, astemizole, and the combination in the prophylactic treatment of ragweed pollen-induced rhinoconjunctivitis. J Allergy Clin Immunol 1989; 83:627–633.
8. Benincasa C, Lloyd RS. Evaluation of fluticasone propionate aqueous nasal spray taken alone and in combination with cetirizine in the prophylactic treatment of seasonal allergic rhinitis. Drug Invest 1994; 8:225–233.
9. Simpson RJ. Budesonide and terfenadine, separately and in combination, in the treatment of hay fever. Ann Allergy 1994; 73:497–502.
10. Mygind N, Lund V. Topical corticosteroid therapy of rhinitis. Clin Immunother 1996; 5:122–136.
11. Vermeulen J, Mercer M. Comparison of the efficacy and tolerability of topical levocabastine and sodium cromoglycate in the treatment of seasonal allergic rhinoconjunctivitis in children. Pediatr Allergy Immunol 1994; 5:209–213.
12. Reed CE, Marcoux JP, Welsh PW. Effects of topical nasal treatment for asthma. J Allergy Clin Immunol 1988; 81:1042–1047.
13. Corren J, Adinoff AD, Buchmeister AD, et al. Nasal beclomethasone prevents the

seasonal increase in bronchial responsiveness in patients with allergic rhinitis and asthma. J Allergy Clin Immunol 1992; 90:250–256.

14. Pedersen B, Dahl R, Richards DH, Jacques LA, Pichler W, Nykanen KN. Once daily fluticasone propionate aqueous nasal spray control symptoms of most patients with seasonal allergic rhinitis. Allergy 1995; 50:794–799.

15. Varney VA, Gaga M, Frew AJ, et al. Usefulness of immunotherapy in patients with severe summer hay fever uncontrolled by antiallergic drugs. Br Med J 1991; 302: 265–269.

16. Wihl J-Å, Petersen BN, Petersen LN, Gundersen G, Bresson K, Mygind N. Effect of the non-sedative H_1 receptor antagonist astemizole in perennial allergic and nonallergic rhinitis. J Allergy Clin Immunol 1985; 75:720–727.

17. van de Heyning PH, van Haesendonck J, Creten W, Rombaut N. Effect of topical levocabastine on allergic and non-allergic rhinitis. Allergy 1988; 43:386–391.

18. Cockcroft DW, MacCormack DW, Newhouse MT et al. Beclomethasone dipropionate in allergic rhinitis. Can Med Assoc J 1976; 15:523–526.

19. Borum P, Grønborg H, Mygind N. Seasonal allergic rhinitis and depot injection of a corticosteroid. Allergy 1987; 42:26–32.

20. Vermeulen J, Mercer C. Comparison of the efficacy and tolerability of topical levacabastine and sodium cromoglycate in the treatment of seasonal allergic rhinoconjunctivitis in children. Pediatr Allergy Immunol 1994; 5:209–213.

21. Lockhart JDF, Maneksha S. Children with allergies. Terfenadine suspension versus placebo. Practitioner 1983; 227:1313–1315.

22. Simons FE. New H_1-receptor antagonists: clinical pharmacology. Clin Exp Allergy 1990; 20 (Suppl 2):19–24.

23. Naclerio RM, Mackay I. Guidelines for the management of nasal polyposis. In: Mygind N, Lildholdt T, eds. Nasal Polyposis. An Inflammatory Disease and Its Treatment. Copenhagen: Munksgaard 1997:177–180.

24. Lildholdt T, Mygind N. Effect of corticosteroids on nasal polyps. Evidence from controlled trials. In Mygind N, Lildholdt T, eds. Nasal Polyposis. An Inflammatory Disease and Its Treatment. Copenhagen: Munksgaard 1997:160–169.

21

Nonallergic Rhinitis

ALKIS TOGIAS

The Johns Hopkins University
Baltimore, Maryland

I. Definition/Classification

''Nonallergic rhinitis'' is a term that can be applied to any disease of the nose presenting with obstructive and secretory symptoms, with or without hyperirritability, that does not have an allergic (IgE-mediated) etiology. This definition can be narrowed by allowing only chronic conditions to be included and, therefore, by excluding acute viral and acute bacterial infections (Figure 1).

A subcategory that includes treatable conditions with specific etiologies can be defined. Some, such as hypothyroidism, granulomatous and autoimmune diseases, and tumors, are rare. Other conditions, such as the rhinitis of pregnancy and anatomical abnormalities of the nasal passages, are much more frequent. Symptoms of rhinitis also appear as side effects of systemically administered pharmacological agents such as vasodilator antihypertensives, reserpine, oral contraceptives and other estrogens, and various antidepressants. As part of the classic hypersensitivity syndrome, aspirin and all the nonsteroidal anti-inflammatory drugs are frequently associated with nasal polyposis and chronic sinusitis and can cause severe asthma attacks; however, rhinitic attacks also occur (1). Finally, the term ''rhinitis medicamentosa'' applies to the rebound nasal obstruc-

"

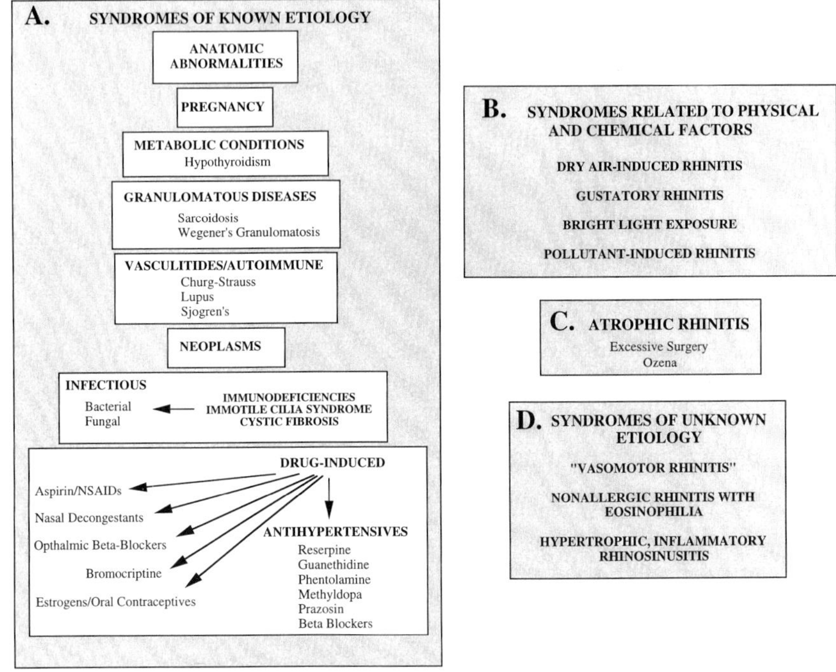

Figure 1 Nonallergic, chronic rhinitis: Classification.

tion and the pharmacological tolerance that the vasculature of the nose develops in a percentage of patients who, for some other reason, use topical decongestants (alpha-adrenergic agonists) chronically.

A number of illnesses that affect innate or acquired immunity predispose to chronic rhinitis of infectious origin, frequently associated with chronic or recurrent acute sinusitis. This category includes all forms of congenital and acquired immunodeficiencies, the immotile cilia syndrome (primary ciliary dyskinesia), and cystic fibrosis. In the latter two cases, the defective function of the nasal and sinus epithelium (thickened secretions and abnormal ciliary motility) is probably responsible for the development of chronic infections.

An interesting group of nonallergic rhinitis syndromes involves physical stimuli as triggers. These include inhalation of cold and dry air, ingestion of hot food, and exposure to bright light. Because the symptoms associated with these conditions can be experimentally reproduced, some knowledge of the pathophysiology of cold, dry air and hot-food-induced rhinitis has been generated (2,3).

Atrophic rhinitis represents a distinct nonallergic syndrome (4–6). The classic ozena characterized by severe crusting, epistaxis, and fetor is not frequently encountered in industrial countries anymore, but a less severe form that involves crusting and atrophic mucosal changes should be considered. Excessive nasal tissue removal by surgery aimed to relieve obstruction can result in this condition. In Egypt, South America, and some other nonindustrialized countries, *Klebsiella ozena* can be cultured from the nasal mucosa of patients with atrophic rhinitis. Atrophic changes in the nasal mucosa are seen more frequently in older individuals (7,8), but their clinical significance is unknown.

Little information is available on the effects of air pollutants and chemical sensitizers on the human nasal mucosa. Because of their well-known effects on the lower respiratory system, we should assume that some forms of nonallergic rhinitis may be causally related to or exacerbated by such factors. For example, it is interesting that chronic exposure to tobacco smoke and to outdoor air pollutants is associated with metaplastic changes in the nasal epithelium (9). The clinical significance of these effects has not been examined in detail, but the loss of functional nasal epithelium, under a mechanism similar to that of atrophic rhinitis, may have significant impact on the prevalence and severity of nonallergic nasal disease in industrialized countries.

What remains are a number of poorly defined nasal conditions of unknown etiology and pathophysiology that are generally difficult to treat. Most patients with nonallergic rhinitis are categorized under these conditions. Diagnostic workup is required to differentiate these syndromes from perennial allergic rhinitis because of similarities in the clinical presentation.

The term ''vasomotor rhinitis'' is frequently used to identify a large number of patients within this grouping. This term implies that the underlying cause is a vascular/neurological dysfunction of the mucosa. There are no scientifically sound data to support this notion and, therefore, the term is rather misleading (10). It is interesting that a significant percentage of patients with chronic fatigue syndrome also complain of rhinitic symptoms that are similar to those of patients with ''vasomotor rhinitis'' (11). It is not known, however, what percentage of patients who present with vasomotor rhinitis also have systemic symptoms compatible with chronic fatigue—in other words, whether this form of nonallergic rhinitis is, in essence, a localized manifestation of the intriguing chronic fatigue syndrome.

Within the subcategory of nonallergic rhinitis of unknown etiology, a syndrome that is characterized by nasal eosinophilia has been described (12,13). Even if this criterion separates a number of patients from the rest of the group, it is not clear that the clinical presentation of the nonallergic rhinitis with eosinophilia syndrome (NARES) has any consistent pattern.

Under the category of syndromes of unknown etiology falls another group of patients who suffer from chronic, inflammatory rhinosinusitis (14,15). Frequently, the term ''hyperplastic'' is added to the name of this syndrome to characterize the thickened mucosa that these patients develop as a result of their chronic inflammatory disease. The most characteristic aspect of these patients' history is the large number of sinus operations they have undergone, each time with limited success and with invariable recurrence. Frequently, these patients, in association with the rest of their nasal and sinus mucosal syndrome, suffer from recurrent nasal polyposis.

II. Epidemiology

Because of the lack of clear definitions it is difficult to obtain reliable epidemiological data. Nevertheless, it is interesting that the U.S. National Health Interview Survey data of 1983–1985 placed ''chronic sinusitis'' first in rank among the most common chronic conditions (16) with a prevalence of 13.5%. Since these surveys express the personal view of randomly selected individuals and since the symptomatology does not even allow physicians to separate between chronic sinusitis and the nonallergic rhinitis syndromes, a large number of cases reported as ''chronic sinusitis'' probably represent nonallergic rhinitis. Equally confusing is the report from the U.S. National Health and Nutrition Examination Survey II (1976–1980) according to which the prevalence of ''chronic rhinitis'' is 20.4% (17). Studies using allergy and otolaryngology clinic patient populations with chronic rhinitis report a 28–60% prevalence of nonallergic disease (12,18–21). These numbers are based on skin testing, and nonallergic rhinitis is an exclusion diagnosis. The high variability may be explained by the different techniques and reagents used in this procedure. No sound data on the distribution of the different syndromes within the nonallergic rhinitis patient population are available.

An interesting observation relates to the age of onset of nonallergic rhinitis, in comparison to its allergic counterpart. In a retrospective study involving 362, randomly selected, new patients with rhinitis who were evaluated at the Johns Hopkins Medical School allergy clinic (18), 70% of those diagnosed with nonallergic disease developed their condition in adult life. In contrast, this number was 31% for patients who were diagnosed with perennial and 26.5% with seasonal allergic rhinitis. From a different perspective, only 8.5% of patients who developed chronic rhinitis when younger than 20 years of age had nonallergic disease, this number increasing to 34.5% for all adults and to 62.5% for patients who developed the condition when older than 40. These data are in agreement with previously published work by Mygind et al. (19). The nature of the sample does not allow us to infer that the prevalence of nonallergic rhinitis is higher in older populations. However, it is tempting to speculate that a causal relationship between some forms of nonallergic rhinitis and aging may exist, with aging-related changes of the nasal mucosa predisposing for the development of these conditions.

III. Clinical Presentation/Diagnosis

A nasal ailment can present with a rather restricted variety of symptoms. As a result, the symptoms of nonallergic rhinitis are similar to those of its allergic, perennial counterpart. One should, therefore, expect that patients will complain of nasal congestion, rhinorrhea, posterior nasal drainage, pressure or pain over the sinuses, and occasional sneezing or pruritus. However, in the syndromes described below the problem is manifested with a single or a striking primary symptom.

Conditions that involve anatomical abnormalities, neoplasms, and granulomatous diseases mainly manifest with nasal obstruction; such presentation requires specific workup. Flexible and rigid endoscopy have become the mainstay of such workup. Notably, the suspicion of a neoplasm should increase if the obstructive symptoms are unilateral. In patients with anatomical obstruction, nasal/sinus symptoms can theoretically be potentiated as a result of either sinus ostial blockade due to the primary obstructive process or of changes in airflow pattern that increase local turbulence and may lead to hyperirritable ''hot spots'' in the mucosa. These areas may respond to nonspecific stimuli with diverse symptomatology. Various syndromes present with functional obstruction, that is with vascular congestion. This is classically seen in the topical-decongestant-induced rhinitis syndrome, in most of the other drug-induced rhinitides, in rhinitis of pregnancy, and in the nasal manifestation of hypothyroidism. Gustatory rhinitis involves rhinorrhea as its sole manifestation; the same symptom is the most prominent in cold, dry-air-induced rhinitis.

The best way to differentiate between nonallergic rhinitis of unknown etiology and allergic rhinitis is to perform specific tests to rule out the latter. These can be either skin testing or quantification of IgE antibodies against suspected allergens in the patient's serum. These diagnostic methods are discussed elsewhere in this volume. One should emphasize, however, that a good history will prove valuable in diagnosing nonallergic rhinitis (Fig. 2).

By definition, nonallergic rhinitis of unknown etiology is a chronic, perennial condition and the seasonal exacerbations classically seen in allergic disease are not generally encountered. However, virtually all individuals with chronic rhinitis, regardless of etiology, complain of symptoms related to abrupt changes in atmospheric conditions; the mechanism of this complaint is not understood. Also, patients suffering from cold, dry-air-induced rhinitis will have a seasonal, winter-related, presentation.

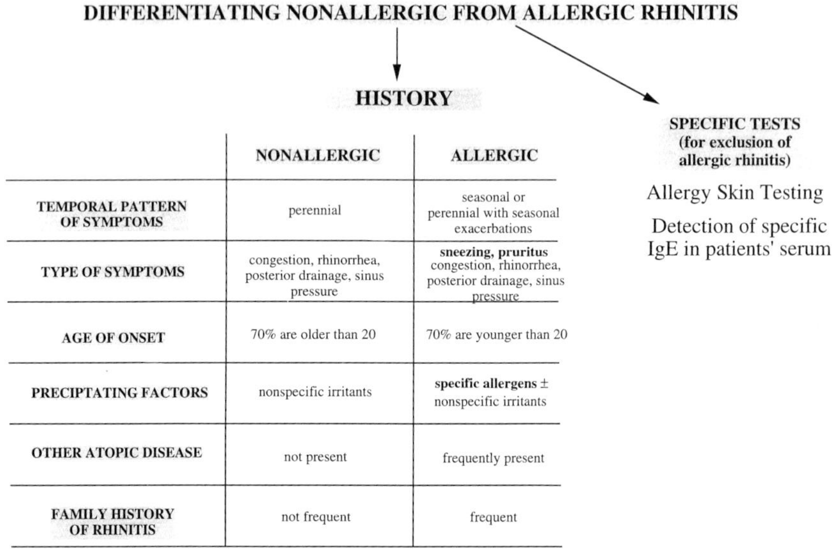

	NONALLERGIC	ALLERGIC
TEMPORAL PATTERN OF SYMPTOMS	perennial	seasonal or perennial with seasonal exacerbations
TYPE OF SYMPTOMS	congestion, rhinorrhea, posterior drainage, sinus pressure	**sneezing, pruritus** congestion, rhinorrhea, posterior drainage, sinus pressure
AGE OF ONSET	70% are older than 20	70% are younger than 20
PRECIPTATING FACTORS	nonspecific irritants	**specific allergens ±** nonspecific irritants
OTHER ATOPIC DISEASE	not present	frequently present
FAMILY HISTORY OF RHINITIS	not frequent	frequent

Figure 2   Differentiating nonallergic from allergic rhinitis.

In general, individuals who suffer from nonallergic rhinitis of unknown etiology, other than those in whom a distinct physical stimulus is the culprit, cannot indicate specific precipitating factors. Those who do, however, will blame nonspecific irritants such as smoke, strong odors, perfumes, and exposure to chemicals. This is in contrast to individuals with allergic rhinitis the majority of whom can relate acute episodes of rhinitis to a specific allergenic exposure (mowing the lawn, pets, dusting, etc.). The pitfall of such differentiation is that, secondary to chronic inflammation, patients with allergic rhinitis may also have a non-specifically hyperirritable mucosa.

As mentioned previously, information on the age of onset of chronic rhinitis can lean the balance toward the diagnosis of either nonallergic or allergic disease. The clinical presentation may also be somewhat different. Our retrospective study of the clinic patient population (18) has generated some additional information on this matter: Compared to perennial allergic rhinitis, a significantly lower percentage of patients with nonallergic disease complained of sneezing and conjunctival symptoms. On the other hand, symptoms related to sinus disease (headaches, facial pressure) were significantly more commonly encountered in the nonallergic group. No difference could be found between the two conditions with respect to the prevalence of rhinorrhea and nasal congestion.

We also found that patients with perennial allergic rhinitis had a significantly higher association of their disease with asthma, compared to the nonallergic group. Inversely, a significantly higher percentage of patients with nonallergic rhinitis gave a history of one or more prior episodes of sinusitis.

Another finding was that a history of asthma or chronic rhinitis in a first-degree relative was reported by a significantly higher percentage of patients with allergic disease. Surprisingly, approximately 40% of patients with nonallergic rhinitis gave the same report, a much higher percentage than would be expected by random probability, based on the prevalence of rhinitis or asthma. This finding suggests that some of the nonallergic rhinitis syndromes may have a familial predisposition and is worth further research as it may help us unveil the etiologies of these conditions.

IV. Pathophysiology

Our knowledge in this area is poor. Only in the syndromes in which the naturally occurring symptoms are inducible by a relevant stimulus in an experimental setting can specific pathophysiological information be obtained. In nonallergic rhinitis, these syndromes include cold, dry-air-induced and hot-food-related rhinitis, as well as the aspirin/nonsteroidal anti-inflammatory drug hypersensitivity syndrome.

When patients who complain of cold-air-induced rhinitis receive a nasal cold, dry-air inhalation challenge, they develop nasal symptoms whereas nonsensitive individuals do not (2). Our work in this field has demonstrated that mast cell-associated mediators are released in nasal secretions only in cold, dry-air responders after the challenge (2,22) and that unilateral cold, dry-air provocation leads to a secretory response bilaterally, indicating the generation of a neural reflex (23). It seems that the cold, dry-air-induced rhinorrhea is to a large degree the result of glandular parasympathetic stimulation as it is partially blocked by local application of atropine (24). The inflammatory mediators may have a contributing role in hypersecretion and may be even more important in the development of nasal congestion. In an attempt to explain the reason why only this group develops reactions to cold, dry air we demonstrated that only these patients show an increase in the osmolarity of nasal secretions after the provocation (25). At the same time, compared to controls, these individuals release more histamine in response to a hyperosmolar nasal challenge, whereas they do not differ with regard to nonspecific nasal reactivity assessed by provocation with histamine (26). Finally, we found that these patients shed a large number of epithelial cells in nasal lavage fluids following cold, dry-air challenge, compared to a nonsignificant effect in controls (27). Taken together, these observations suggest that, for a so-far-unknown reason, the nasal mucosa of cold, dry-air-sensitive patients has a defect in humidifying inhaled air at extreme conditions. As a result, the osmolarity of the epithelial lining fluid increases, epithelial desiccation and detachment occur, mast cells and irritant sensory nerves are activated, and a mucosal reaction ensues to restore the homeostasis of the tissue. Indeed, it has been well demonstrated that hyperosmolarity is a trigger for mast cell mediator release in vitro (28) and in vivo (29) and that it also activates nasal sensory nerve endings (30).

The picture is simpler in individuals who develop excessive rhinorrhea when eating spicy food. The reaction is purely neurogenic and parasympathetically mediated in that it is blocked by topical pretreatment with atropine (3) or ipratropium bromide (31). In pepper-spiced foods, the stimulatory substance is capsaicin, a potent stimulant of nociceptive sensory nerve endings (32).

A discussion on aspirin hypersensitivity is beyond the scope of this chapter but it is interesting that studies involving aspirin-sensitive patients show increased sulfidopeptide leukotriene generation in nasal lavage fluids following oral aspirin challenge (33). Also, the fact that respiratory reactions to aspirin challenge are attenuated by 5-lipoxygenase inhibitors and sulfidopeptide leukotriene receptor antagonists (34,35) is indicative of the central role of the leukotriene pathway of arachidonic acid metabolism in the aspirin hypersensitivity syndrome (36).

Several pathophysiological questions can be asked with respect to patients with nonallergic rhinitis of unknown etiology. First, it is important to know whether the nasal mucosa is in a hyperreactive state and, therefore, responds vigorously to all forms of nonspecific environmental stimulation resulting in rhinitic symptomatology. The above sentence contains a good clinical definition of nasal hyperresponsiveness; however, there is no standardized methodology for laboratory assessment. What complicates the matter is that, depending on the stimulus that is utilized to induce a nasal reaction, different elements of the nasal mucosa are activated. These include the glandular, vascular, and neuronal apparatus.

The second level of complexity lies in the fact that these mucosal elements may be activated directly or indirectly: for example, the submucosal glands can secrete mucus either upon direct stimulation of their muscarinic receptors with methacholine or through a neuronal reflex that is originated at a distant site (such as the contralateral nostril) using a sensory nerve stimulus (such as histamine or capsaicin). Furthermore, many stimuli used in these laboratory assessments have more than one action; when such stimuli are used, the type of outcome (for example, amount of nasal secretions vs. nasal airway resistance) will determine the type of reactivity that is being assessed.

On the basis of these considerations, the term ''hyperresponsiveness'' cannot be applied indiscriminately, but should be referred to particular mucosal elements. Also, to ensure the accuracy of statements regarding hyperresponsiveness, the above-mentioned methodological issues need to be adequately addressed. Unfortunately, it is rare to find any published work where this has been appropriately done.

Since methacholine is, in essence, a pure stimulus for glands, when the outcome involves nasal secretion, one can confidently state that glandular reactivity is being assessed. A study by Borum using nasal provocation with methacholine suggests that patients with nonallergic rhinitis of unknown etiology have glandular hyperreactivity (37). In his study, Borum included mainly patients with nonallergic rhinitis, without, however, providing any further subject characterization.

In studies involving nasal provocation with capsaicin, Stjärne et al. suggest that patients with nonallergic rhinitis (of the ''vasomotor'' type) have a higher secretory response than normal controls (38). This effect is more evident in those presenting with the main complaint of rhinorrhea (39). When capsaicin is used as a stimulus, it will not be evident whether the enhanced secretory outcome is due to an exaggerated neuronal response (which may involve the afferent, central, or efferent arm of a reflex arc), to an exaggerated glandular response, or even to an increased local release of neuropeptides that can directly stimulate the glandular epithelium (40).

In a study comparing the effect of nasal provocation with histamine on patients with nonallergic rhinitis of unknown etiology to that on patients with perennial allergic rhinitis and to normal controls, we found that the nonallergic group falls between the allergic and the normal individuals with respect to sneezing and to the vascular permeability response to the stimulus (Fig. 3) (41). Sneezing is a neurally mediated symptom, and the vascular permeability induced by histamine is most probably a direct effect of this autacoid on H_1 receptors on blood vessels (42).

Taken together, these published and unpublished data suggest that nasal hyperreactivity, possibly of glandular, vascular, and neuronal nature, is a factor in nonallergic rhinitis. If this is the case, one could explain the symptoms that patients with nonallergic rhinitis develop, when exposed to nonspecific atmospheric irritants. It is important to note, however, that the above data derive from relatively small numbers of patients and that, due to the classification/definition confusion, the clinical purity of the subjects who have participated in these studies is not established.

To complicate the picture, when we compared patients with perennial allergic rhinitis to those with nonallergic disease as well as to healthy controls with respect to their nasal responsiveness to capsaicin, we failed to find a difference between the nonallergic rhinitics and the controls in the capsaicin-induced symptoms or in the total protein, lysozyme, and albumin content of nasal secretions (43).

The observations regarding nasal mucosal hyperreactivity in nonallergic

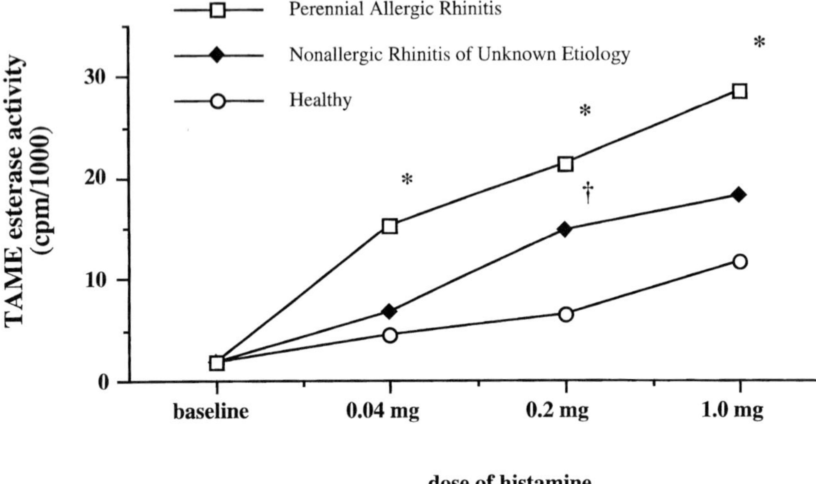

Figure 3 The effect of nasal provocation with histamine on three distinct groups of subjects. Median values are depicted. In this reaction, most of TAME-esterase activity represents the activity of plasma kallikrein and is, therefore, a marker of vascular permeability. cpm/1000: counts per minute $\times$ 10^{-3}; $*p < 0.001$, comparing the group with perennial allergic rhinitis to the normals; $\dagger p < 0.05$, comparing the group with nonallergic rhinitis to the normals.

rhinitis of unknown etiology lead to the question whether the underlying cause is chronic inflammation. In allergic airway disease, especially asthma, the relationship between mucosal inflammation and hyperresponsiveness is strong, albeit circumstantial. There is no question that active mucosal inflammation can exist in the nasal and sinus mucosal tissue of patients suffering from nonallergic, chronic hyperplastic rhinosinusitis. The characteristics of this inflammation have recently been described in a series of publications by Hamilos and colleagues (14,15,44). However, it is unknown whether this distinct group of patients exhibits elements of mucosal hyperresponsiveness. Characteristic mucosal eosinophilia exists in patients with NARES (12,45). Again, no data are available regarding mucosal hyperreactivity in this distinct group. A quite different picture is emerging in these patients whose nonallergic rhinitis of unknown etiology fits more the ''vasomotor rhinitis'' syndrome. Two groups of investigators have failed to identify, in nasal secretions or mucosal biopsies, any differences between these patients and healthy controls, with respect to cellular or biochemical markers of inflammation (11,46,47). It appears, therefore, that, in these individuals, the disorder is not of inflammatory nature, or, at least, not associated with chronic inflammation. If so, the above-described nasal mucosal hyperresponsiveness may have a totally different pathophysiological basis from that seen in chronic inflammatory disorders.

V. Management

In the subgroup of patients with well-documented etiologies such as anatomical abnormalities, tumors, systemic diseases, and drug-induced rhinitis, treatment should aim against the underlying problem. Therefore, discontinuation of the offending agent, surgical tumor removal, or anatomical correction may offer the solution to the problem.

Unfortunately, due to our general lack of knowledge regarding disease etiology and pathophysiology of most patients suffering from nonallergic rhinitis syndromes, the treatment of these conditions tends to be largely symptomatic and not very efficacious. Nevertheless, the relative efficacy of anti-inflammatory treatment with topical steroids has raised this modality to "first-line."

Mygind suggests that patients with perennial rhinitis should be generally categorized as "sneezers," "blockers," and "nose blowers" (48,49). In nonallergic rhinitis the first group is rather rare. It appears, however, that these patients may benefit by antihistamine treatment, as suggested by a study by Wihl et al. (49). It is unknown how histamine is released to cause sneezing in these patients. On the other hand, the "blockers" should benefit by systemic or local decongestant preparations. The details on this form of treatment are presented elsewhere in this book.

A. Ipratropium Bromide

Individuals who complain of excessive rhinorrhea and posterior nasal drainage have been treated in several studies with the local anticholinergic agent ipratropium bromide (50–52). This modality, which has demonstrated efficacy, is also discussed in another chapter. One should note that efficacy of this agent has been demonstrated in elderly patients with nonallergic rhinorrhea, a problem that probably affects large numbers in this age group (53). Posterior nasal drainage is much less responsive to treatment, compared to anterior rhinorrhea. Part of this problem may be secondary to the fact that we do not understand whether this uncomfortable symptom is the result of increased volume of secretions that follow the mucociliary clearance path in the nasopharynx, or whether it occurs as a result of thicker secretions that disturb mucociliary clearance and irritate sensory nerves. In the latter case, anticholinergic agents may increase, rather than improve, the problem.

Excessive rhinorrhea is, sometimes, dealt with by the surgical approach of vidian neurectomy, based on the series by Golding-Wood in 1961 (54). Although this approach is effective, the use of ipratropium bromide may eliminate its need. Furthermore, vidian nerve regeneration, leading to recurrence of rhinorrhea, appears to be a significant problem.

B. Topical Steroids

Topical steroids were tried in nonallergic rhinitis because of the enthusiasm generated by their efficacy in allergic disease. Although several studies have demonstrated clinical efficacy of these agents (55,56), a significant number of patients do not respond to this treatment. In trials involving both patients with perennial allergic rhinitis and those with nonallergic rhinitis, it is clear that the majority of responders belong to the allergic group whereas nonresponders tend to be nonallergic (57,58). This finding emphasizes the diversity of nonallergic rhinitis, which probably includes patients such as those with hyperplastic rhinosinusitis, whose problem is related to underlying mucosal inflammation (most of these should respond to steroids), and patients whose pathophysiology is noninflammatory.

An important finding from these studies is that the presence of eosinophilia in nasal secretions or scrapings, regardless of allergic status, is a positive prognostic factor for the efficacy of topical steroids (58,59). In this respect, it appears that nasal cytology may have a clinical application in nonallergic rhinitis, to provide information whether intranasal steroids are worth a therapeutic trial. One should be cautious, however, with cytological findings of neutrophilia. These cells may be abundant in all forms of inflammation, including infections, and corticosteroids will not be helpful in the latter situation.

C. Capsaicin

Several European investigators have published their experience regarding the effect of sensory defunctionalization with capsaicin, in patients with intractable, nonallergic rhinitis (38,60–65). The major problem with all these studies is that they are not placebo controlled, mainly because of the burning sensation that capsaicin generates when it is applied to the nose (66). The results of these nonrandomized, nonblinded studies are encouraging with improvement in symptomatology lasting from weeks to months. However, the symptoms invariably return and repeated capsaicin treatments will, theoretically, be required for long-term control of the problem. Studies regarding the efficacy and safety of repeated treatments have not been published.

As mentioned above, capsaicin activates mainly unmyelinated c-fibers and generates pain sensation and central nervous system reflexes (32). Repetitive local applications result in short-term neuronal defunctionalization, which can affect several forms of stimuli (other chemicals, warmth, mechanical stimulation). In the human nose, the duration of this effect appears to range from a few days to a few weeks (39,67). The mechanism of capsaicin-induced neuronal defunctionalization is not clear, although histological evaluation in animal tissues shows depletion of the sensory nerve content of neuropeptides, particularly tachykinins (32). In animal models, systemic administration of capsaicin leads to degeneration of some sensory nerves but, because of the reversibility of the desensitization phenomenon, there is no evidence that such neurotoxicity occurs with topical capsaicin administration in humans (39,67). However, this has to be more carefully investigated and confirmed.

VI. Conclusions

Nonallergic rhinitis is a common diagnosis that covers several nasal conditions. In the majority of patients, the etiology remains unknown. The physician's task is to detect those syndromes that are treatable with measures aiming at the underlying cause and to differentiate the other forms of nonallergic rhinitis from its allergic, perennial counterpart. The type of symptomatology may be helpful in selecting an appropriate treatment modality. Topical steroids, which are now used abundantly in nonallergic rhinitis, may be more effective if their selection is based on the presence of nasal eosinophilia. Researchers and practitioners should follow closely the ongoing clinical studies of long-term neuronal desensitization with capsaicin. Overall, nonallergic rhinitis is not understood and the available treatments are far from optimal. More research will be required to achieve significant impact on this condition.

Acknowledgment

This work was supported by NIH Grant R29 HL-48248.

References

1. Mathison DA, Stevenson DD. Hypersensitivity to nonsteroidal antiinflammatory drugs: indications and methods for oral challenges. J Allergy Clin Immunol 1979; 64:669–674.
2. Togias AG, Naclerio RM, Proud D, Fish JE, Adkinson NF, Kagey-Sobotka A, Norman PS, Lichtenstein LM. Nasal challenge with cold, dry air results in the production of inflammatory mediators: possible mast cell involvement. J Clin Invest 1985; 76: 1375–1381.
3. Raphael GD, Hauptschein-Raphael M, Kaliner MA. Gustatory rhinitis. Am J Rhinol 1989; 3:145–149.
4. Holopainen E. Nasal mucous membrane in atrophic rhinitis with reference to symptom free nasal mucosa. Acta Otolaryngol (Stockh) 1967; (Suppl 227): 26–47.

5. Mygind N, Thomsen J, Jorgensen MB. Ultrastructure of the epithelium in atrophic rhinitis. Acta Otolaryngol (Stockh) 1974; 78:106–112.

6. Fouad H, Afifi N, Fatt-hi A, El-sheemy N, Iskander I, Saif MNA. Altered cell mediated immunity in atrophic rhinitis. J Laryngol Otol 1980; 94:507–514.

7. Toppozada H. The human nasal mucosa in the menopause (a histochemical and electron microscopic study). J Laryngol Otol 1988; 102:314–318.

8. Koopman CF. Effects of aging on nasal structure and function. Am J Rhinol 1989; 3:59–62.

9. Calderon-Garciduenas L, Roy-Ocotla G. Nasal cytology in southwestern metropolitan Mexico City inhabitants: a pilot intervention study. Environ Health Perspect 1993; 101:138–144.

10. Mullarkey MF. The classification of nasal disease: an opinion. J Allergy Clin Immunol 1981; 67:251–252.

11. Ali M, Gaumond E, Yuta A, Clauw D, Baraniuk JN. Nonallergic rhinitis (NAR) of chronic fatigue syndrome (CFS). J Allergy Clin Immunol 1997; 99:S420 (abstract).

12. Mullarkey MF, Hill JS, Webb DR. Allergic and nonallergic rhinitis: their characterization with atttention to the meaning of nasal eosinophilia. J Allergy Clin Immunol 1980; 65:122–126.

13. Jacobs RL, Freedman PM, Boswell RN. Nonallergic rhinitis with eosinophilia (NARES syndrome). J Allergy Clin Immunol 1981; 67:253–262.

14. Hamilos DL, Plout M, Leung DY, Huston DP, Hamid QA. GM-CSF, IL-5 and RANTES mRNA expression and protein levels in chronic hyperplastic sinusitis with nasal polyposis. J Allergy Clin Immunol 1997; 99:S130 (abstract).

15. Hamilos DL, Leung DY, Wood R, Bean DK, Song YL, Schotman E, Hamid Q. Eosinophil infiltration in nonallergic chronic hyperplastic sinusitis with nasal polyposis (CHS/NP) is associated with endothelial VCAM-1 upregulation and expression of TNF-α. Am J Respir Cell Mol Biol 1996; 15:443–450.

16. Collins JG. Prevalence of selected chronic conditions, United States, 1983–85. NCHS advanced data 1988; 155:1–16.

17. Turkeltaub PC, Gergen PJ. The prevalence of allergic and nonallergic respiratory symptoms in the U.S. population: data from the second national health and nutrition examination survey, 1976–80 (NHANES II). J Allergy Clin Immunol 1988; 81:305.

18. Togias A. Age relationships and clinical features of nonallergic rhinitis. J Allergy Clin Immunol 1990; 85:182 (abstract).

19. Mygind N, Dirksen A, Johnsen NJ, Weeke B. Perennial rhinitis: an analysis of skin testing, serum IgE, and blood and smear eosinophilia in 201 patients. Clin Otolaryngol 1978; 3:189–196.

20. Viner AS, Jackman N. Retrospective survey of 1271 patients diagnosed as perennial rhinitis. Clin Allergy 1976; 6:251–259.

21. Wittig HJ, McLaughlin ET, Leifer KL, Bellott JD. Risk factors for the development of allergic disease: analysis of 2,190 patient records. Ann Allergy 1978; 41:84–88.

22. Proud D, Bailey GS, Naclerio RN, Reynolds CJ, Cruz AA, Eggleston PA, Lichtenstein LM, Togias AG. Tryptase and histamine as markers to evaluate mast cell activation during the responses to nasal challenge with allergen, cold, dry air, and hyperosmolar solutions. J Allergy Clin Immunol 1992; 89:1098–1110.

23. Philip G, Jankowski R, Baroody F, Naclerio RM, Togias A. Reflex activation of

nasal secretion by unilateral inhalation of cold dry air. Am Rev Respir Dis 1993; 148:1616–1622.

24. Cruz AA, Togias AG, Lichtenstein LM, Proud D, Kagey-Sobotka A, Naclerio RM. Local application of atropine attenuates the upper airway reaction to cold, dry air. Am Rev Respir Dis 1990; 141:A759 (abstract).

25. Togias AG, Proud D, Kagey-Sobotka A, Adams GK, Norman PS, Lichtenstein LM, Naclerio RM. The osmolality of nasal secretions increases when inflammatory mediators are released in response to inhalation of cold, dry air. Am Rev Respir Dis 1988; 137:625–629.

26. Togias AG, Lykens K, Kagey-Sobotka A, Eggleston PA, Proud D, Lichtenstein LM, Naclerio RM. Studies on the relationships between sensitivity to cold dry air, hyperosmolar solutions and histamine in the adult nose. Am Rev Respir Dis 1990; 141: 1428–1433.

27. Cruz AA, Naclerio RM, Proud D, Kagey-Sobotka A, Lichtenstein LM, Togias A. Epithelial cell detachment is observed during the nasal reaction to cold, dry air (CDA). J Allergy Immunol 1991; 87:147 (abstract).

28. Eggleston PA, Kagey-Sobotka A, Lichtenstein LM. A comparison of the osmotic activation of basophils and human lung mast cells. Am Rev Respir Dis 1987; 135: 1043–1048.

29. Silber G, Proud D, Warner J, Naclerio RM, Kagey-Sobotka A, Lichtenstein LM, Eggleston E. In vivo release of inflammatory mediators by hyperosmolar solutions. Am Rev Respir Dis 1988; 137:606–612.

30. Togias A, Lai G, Philip G. Hyperosmolar nasal challenge stimulates reflex nasal secretion. J Allergy Clin Immunol 1994; 93:217 (abstract).

31. Østberg B, Winther B, Mygind N. Cold air-induced rhinorrhea and high-dose ipratropium. Arch Otolaryngol Head Neck Surg 1987; 113:160–162.

32. Holzer P. Capsaicin: cellular targets, mechanisms of action, and selectivity for thin sensory neurons. Pharmacol Rev 1991; 43:143–201.

33. Ferrer NR, Howland WC, Stevenson DD, Spiegelberg HL. Release of leukotrienes, prostaglandins, and histamine into nasal secretions of aspirin-sensitive asthmatics during reaction to aspirin. Am Rev Respir Dis 1988; 137:847–854.

34. Christie PE, Smith CM, Lee TH. The potent and selective sulfidopeptide leukotriene antagonist, SK&F, inhibits aspirin-induced asthma. Am Rev Respir Dis 1991; 144: 957–958.

35. Dahlen B, Kumlin M, Margolskee DJ, Larsson C, Blomqvist H, Williams VC, Zetterstrom O, Dahlen SE. The leukotriene receptor antagonist MK-0679 blocks airway obstruction induced by inhaled lysine-aspirin in aspirin sensitive asthmatics. Eur Respir J 1993; 6:1018–1026.

36. Israel E, Fischer AR, Rosenberg MA, Lilly CM, Callery JC, Shapiro JO, Cohm J, Rubin P, Drazen JM. The pivotal role of 5-lipoxygenase products in the reaction of aspirin sensitive asthmatics to aspirin. Am Rev Respir Dis 1993; 148:1447–1451.

37. Borum P. Nasal methacholine challenge. A test for the measurement of nasal reactivity. J Allergy Clin Immunol 1979; 63:253–257.

38. Stjärne P, Lundblad L, Anggard A, Lundberg J. Local capsaicin treatment of the nasal mucosa reduces symptoms in patients with nonallergic nasal hyperreactivity. Am J Rhinol 1991; 5:145–151.

39. Stjarne P, Lundblad L, Lundberg J, Anggard A. Capsaicin and nicotine-sensitive afferent neurones and nasal secretion in healthy human volunteers and in patients with vasomotor rhinitis. Br J Pharmacol 1989; 96:693–701.

40. Baraniuk JN, Kaliner MA. Neuropeptides and nasal secretion. J Allergy Clin Immunol 1990; 86:620–627.

41. Togias A, Proud D, Kagey-Sobotka A, Lichtenstein LM, Naclerio RM. Cold dry air (CDA) and histamine (HIST) induce more potent responses in perennial rhinitics compared to normal individuals. J Allergy Clin Immunol 1991; 87:148 (abstract).

42. Togias AG, Proud D, Kagey-Sobotka A, Norman PS, Lichtenstein LM, Naclerio RM. The effect of a topical tricyclic antihistamine on the response of the nasal mucosa to challenge with cold, dry air and histamine. J Allergy Clin Immunol 1987; 79:599–604.

43. Sanico AM, Philip G, Proud D, Naclerio RM, Togias A. Comparison of nasal mucosal responsiveness to neuronal stimulation in nonallergic and allergic rhinitis: effects of capsaicin nasal challenge. Clin Exper Allergy 1998; 28:92–100.

44. Hamilos DL, Leung DY, Wood R, Cunningham L, Bean DK, Yasruel Z, Schotman E, Hamid O. Evidence for distinct cytokine expression in allergic versus nonallergic chronic sinusitis. J Allergy Clin Immunol 1995; 96:537–544.

45. Moneret-Vautrin DA, Hsieh V, Wayoff M, Guyot JL, Mouton C, Maria Y. Nonallergic rhinitis with eosinophilia syndrome a precursor of the triad: nasal polyposis, intrinsic asthma, and intolerance to aspirin. Ann Allergy 1990; 64:513–518.

46. Blom HM, Godthelp T, Fokkens WJ, Jan AK, Holm AF, Vroom TM, Rijntes E. Mast cells, eosinophils and IgE-positive cells in the nasal mucosa of patients with vasomotor rhinitis. Eur Arch Oto-Rhino-Laryngol 1995; 252:S33–S39.

47. Yuta A, Fujita K, Shimizu T, Ali M, Clauw D, Baraniuk JN. Elastase in nasal lavage of cystic fibrosis and chronic fatigue syndrome (CFS) subjects with nonallergic rhinitis (NAR). J Allergy Clin Immunol 1997; 99:S420 (abstract).

48. Mygind N. Perennial rhinitis. In: Nasal Allergy, 2nd ed. Oxford: Blackwell Scientific Publications, 1979:224–232.

49. Wihl JA, Petersen BN, Mygind N. The role of histamine in non-allergic perennial rhinitis. Acta Otolaryngol (Stockh) 1984; 214:99–102.

50. Sjøgren I, Juhasz J. Ipratropium in the treatment of patients with perennial rhinitis. Allergy 1984; 39:457–461.

51. Knight A, Kazim F, Salvatori VA. A trial of intranasal atrovent versus placebo in the treatment of vasomotor rhinitis. Ann Allergy 1986; 57:348–354.

52. Dolovich J, Mukherjee J, Salvatori VA. Intranasal ipratropium bromide to control the hypersecretion of vasomotor rhinitis: a dose response study. Am J Rhinol 1989; 3:221–224.

53. Malmberg H, Grahne B, Holopainen E, Binder E. Ipratropium (Atrovent) in the treatment of vasomotor rhinitis of elderly patients. Clin Otolaryngol 1983; 8:273–276.

54. Golding-Wood PH. Petrosal and vidian neurectory in chronic vasomotor rhinitis. J Laryngol 1961; 75:232–247.

55. McAllen MK, Langman MJ. A controlled trial of dexamethasone snuff in chronic perennial rhinitis. Lancet 1969; 1:968–971.

56. Malm L, Wihl JA. Intra-nasal beclomethasone dipropionate in vasomotor rhinitis. Acta Allergol 1976; 31:245–253.

57. Incaudo G, Schatz M, Yamamoto F, Mellon M, Crepea S, Johnson JD. Intranasal flunisolide in the treatment of perennial rhinitis: correlation with immunologic parameters. J Allergy Clin Immunol 1980; 65:41–49.

58. Small P. Beclomethasone dipropionate nasal aerosol in adult patients with ragweed seasonal rhinitis. Ann Allergy 1982; 49:20–22.

59. Balle VH, Pedersen U, Engby B. Allergic perennial and non-allergic, vasomotor rhinitis treated with budesonide nasal spray. Rhinology 1980; 18:135–142.

60. Lacroix JS, Buvelot JM, Polla BS, Lundberg JM. Improvement of symptoms of non-allergic chronic rhinitis by local treatment with capsaicin. Clin Exp Allergy 1991; 21:595–600.

61. Marabini S, Ciabatti G, Polli G, Fusco BM, Geppetti P, Maggi CA, Fanciullacci M, Sicuteri F. Effect of topical nasal treatment with capsaicin in vasomotor rhinitis. Regul Peptid 1988; 22:121 (abstract).

62. Marabini S, Ciabatti PG, Polli G, Fusco BM, Geppetti P. Beneficial effects of intranasal applications of capsaicin in patients with vasomotor rhinitis. Eur Arch Otorhinolaryngol 1991; 248:191–194.

63. Rajakulasingam K, Howarth PH. Topical capsaicin therapy in chronic rhinitis: a way forward? Clin Exp Allergy 1991; 21:531–532.

64. Saria A, Wolf G. Beneficial effect of topically applied capsaicin in the treatment of hyperreactive rhinopathy. Regul Peptid 1988; 22:167 (abstract).

65. Wolf G, Saria A. Capsaicin in the treatment of hyperreflectory rhinopathy (vasomotor rhinitis). VIII ISIAN meeting, Baltimore, MD. 1989 (abstract).

66. Philip G, Baroody FM, Proud D, Naclerio RM, Togias AG. The human nasal response to capsaicin. J Allergy Clin Immunol 1994; 94:1035–1045.

67. Geppetti P, Fusco BM, Marabini S, Maggi CA, Fanciullacci M, Sicuteri F. Secretion, pain and sneezing induced by the application of capsaicin to the nasal mucosa in man. Br J Pharmacol 1988; 93:509–514.

22

Nasal Polyps

BRENT A. SENIOR

Henry Ford Health System
Detroit, Michigan

DAVID W. KENNEDY

University of Pennsylvania Medical Center
Philadelphia, Pennsylvania

I. Introduction

The complaint of chronic sinusitis afflicted 14.7% of the U.S. population in 1993 (1). Nasal polyposis is said to affect nearly 5% of patients referred to otolaryngologists and 4% of patients referred to allergy clinics. Nasal polyposis is also said to affect 7% of patients with asthma (2). However, these figures probably underestimate the true prevalence. Identification of polyposis based upon anterior rhinoscopy will miss many of the subtle manifestations of the disease.

As a result of the high recurrence rate for nasal polyposis with traditional therapy and the significant morbidity that can occur, the overall societal and medical costs of the disease are significant. Glicklich, Bousquet, and others have evaluated the overall impact of chronic rhinosinusitis and rhinitis on the quality of life and demonstrated that the effects are greater than anticipated and, in fact, greater than those of a number of other chronic diseases that were previously thought to have greater impact (3,4).

Considering the frequency and morbidity of the disease, surprisingly little knowledge has been gained over the centuries since Hippocrates first used the word ''polyp'' to describe the ''many footed'' structure originating in the ethmoid sinuses (5). However, recently, with the introduction of nasal endoscopy and scientific advances in the fields of biochemistry, microbiology, and immunology, significant knowledge has been gained about nasal physiology and nasal polyposis. This has led to greater understanding of the etiology of nasal polyps, their physical origin, and ultimately their successful management.

Each of these issues will be discussed in this chapter, with an emphasis on successful management of the person suffering from nasal polyposis.

II. The Origin of Nasal Polyps

The topic of the origin of polyps has been, and remains, contentious. In the 1930s, the popular concept was that all nasal polyps were associated with allergy (6) as a result of the high concentration of eosinophils within polyps. This concept was accepted by most physicians until the 1970s and 1980s when investigators were unable to demonstrate an allergy linkage.

In 1989, Perkins likened some cases of nasal polyps to intrinsic asthma. He concluded that no cause-and-effect relationship existed between nasal polyps and allergic disease, agreeing with findings of other authors (7,8). Settipane and Chafee, using nonendoscopic techniques to examine over 6000 patients with asthma or allergic rhinitis, found nasal polyps in 13% of intrinsic nonallergic patients with asthma but only in 5% of allergic patients with asthma (9). Drake-Lee and Pitcher-Wilmott found no evidence of increased allergic disease in 200 patients admitted for polypectomy based on history, RAST findings, and skin testing (10). A later study found no higher incidence of allergic disease in those with nasal polyps than in controls (11). Studies such as these led Slavin to conclude that allergy is not a significant cause of nasal polyposis and, in the interest of health care cost containment, he recommends that allergy evaluation is not indicated (12). However, other authors believe that allergy is probably one predisposing cause of nasal polyposis (13,14).

While it now seems clear that strict systemic allergy as a cause of nasal polyposis is unlikely, Shatkin et al. have proposed a local mucosal allergic phenomenon in the absence of systemic allergy, as a potential cause of nasal polyposis and rhinitis (15). Specifically they performed a meta-analysis of nine studies comprised of 287 patients and identified 19% with specific IgE nasal mucosal allergy but no systemic allergy. The ultimate significance of this is unclear.

In the absence of allergy as a primary mechanism in the development of nasal polyps, other authors have identified additional factors. Indeed, recent literature has emphasized the importance of multiple environmental components that may contribute to increased mucosal reactivity throughout the upper airway, including the formation of polyps. For example, increasing air pollution has been implicated in the rise of nasal polyposis (16).

Ogawa proposed an aerodynamic component in polyp formation, noting that in patients with unilateral nasal polyps and septal deviation, polyps were more than twice as likely to be located on the concave side, the side of maximal airflow (17). According to this theory, the narrower diameter of the air space in the region of the middle turbinate results in Bernoulli's phenomenon and this negative pressure sucks the inflamed mucosa out into a polyp. However, it is unlikely that this is a primary mechanism.

Typically, nasal polyps arise on the lateral wall in the region of the ethmoid sinus. Less frequently they may occur from the middle turbinate medially, or from the region of the sphenoid sinus. Stammberger has used the term "contact site" to describe these common locations for the origin of polyps. In these narrow clefts even a tiny amount of mucosal edema, from whatever cause, results in mucosal contact, disordered mucociliary flow, and stagnation of mucus (18). He hypothesized a local neurogenic pathway for the occurrence of edema at these sites of contact. The chief contact sites are the frontal recess, the ethmoidal infundibulum, the lateral sinus, and the cleft between the ethmoidal bulla and the middle turbinate.

Antral choanal polyps typically have a cystic portion filled with cholesterol fluid within the maxillary sinus and extend out into the nose through an accessory ostium in the posterior fontanel. The portion within the nose is polypoid and the fluid filling it gelatinous. Is it possible that a portion of a cyst within a sinus cavity may become gelatinous as it extends into the nose and develop subsequent vascular ingrowth to form a polyp?

Larsen and Tos have demonstrated that, in autopsy specimens, polyps typically originate within the nose, adjacent to a sinus ostium (19,20). Is it possible that the intrasinus portion of the lesion may resolve in some cases and leave only a polyp? Certainly, on computerized tomography (CT) and at surgery, cells are often found to be enlarged and filled with polypoid mucosa.

Polyps have different histological and biochemical makeup from the adjacent lateral nasal wall mucosa, a fact that is not explained by aerodynamic theories. These changes do not represent simple edema of the nasal mucosa (21). Specifically polyps have no true seromucinous glands as seen in the middle and inferior turbinates, while the prominent cells of the polyp, eosinophils and mast cells, are found in greater concentration than in the inferior and middle turbinate (13). B lymphocytes, mast cells, and macrophages are all located in greater number in polyps than in adjacent nasal mucosa. The density of these cells is independent of the presence or absence of allergy in the patient (Fig. 1).

Recently, some authors have identified the presence of certain proinflammatory cytokines in the nasal mucosa of patients with allergic rhinitis, specifically interleukin 6 (IL-6), IL-8, and IL-1β (22). These same cytokines have been identified in individuals with common colds (23). IL-5 has now been identified in eosinophilic nasal polyps, suggesting a key role for this cytokine in the pathophysiology of polyps (24). Similarly the chemokine RANTES, a potent chemoattractant for eosinophils, lymphocytes, and monocytes, has been identified in the mucosa of human upper airways. Its presence has been postulated to play a relevant role in the pathogenesis of diseases such as asthma, rhinitis, as well as polyposis. Glucocorticoids have been found to inhibit its production (25).

We, along with other authors, feel that the pathogenesis of polyps is multivariate; they arise as an inflammatory growth controlled by the local microenvironment milieu. While atopy may be one predisposing component in this microenvironment, other factors, including physical, biochemical, immunological, and genetic, also appear to contribute. Dysfunction of the autonomic nervous system is thought by some to also play a role, although polyps have few nerve fibers themselves (26). In patients with aspirin intolerance, the arachidonic acid pathway appears to play a part with markedly elevated 5-lipoxygenase activity being found in polyps compared to adjacent inflamed mucosa (27). Infection also plays a role in this microenvironment as shown in the work of Norlander et al., illustrating the development of polyps in experimentally infected maxillary sinuses (28), though infection appears unlikely as the sole cause of polyp formation (29).

III. The Diagnosis of Nasal Polyps

Significant intranasal polyposis associated with subjective nasal congestion is not a difficult diagnosis (Fig. 2). Simple anterior rhinoscopy identifies such polyps without difficulty. More subtle polyps limited to the middle meatus including the bulla ethmoidalis, frontal recess, and/or uncinate process are more easily identified endoscopically. Indeed, comprehensive nasal endoscopy in all patients with polyps, even when easily seen on anterior rhinoscopy, may provide objective information with regard to extent of disease and preoperative planning, and with regard to the medical and surgical responses to therapy. Precise culture and biopsy can, when indicated, also be performed with ease in the clinic setting under endoscopic guidance. Subtleties of the appearance of the polyps noted with endoscopy may indicate a need to investigate for an etiology other than inflammatory.

When intranasal polyps are identified on examination, it is important to consider the possibility of associated disease (Table 1). Allergy evaluation is probably not necessary unless symptomatology is suggestive. ASA triad or Samter's triad, the syndrome of nasal polyposis/sinusitis, asthma, and aspirin intolerance, was first described by Widal in 1922 (30). Samter and Beers subsequently clarified the relationship (31). Patients tend to exhibit "panmucosal" reactivity with reactive mucosa throughout the airway including the tracheobronchial tree and sinuses. In this disorder sinus disease is frequently extensive, but can be successfully managed with aggressive medical and surgical therapy. Though controversial, a role for aspirin desensitization in successful management has been suggested by some authors (32).

In children, the presence of nasal polyps should raise other considerations, namely the possibility of cystic fibrosis or, if solitary, meningoencephalocele. The possibility of a meningoencephalocele can usually be evaluated by high-resolution CT and evaluation of the skull base for dehiscence. Magnetic resonance imaging (MRI) is confirmatory. Cystic fibrosis is one of the more frequent causes of nasal polyposis in children. The disorder has an autosomal recessive

Table 1 Diseases Associated with Nasal Polyps

Cystic fibrosis
ASA triad
Kartagener's syndrome
Young's syndrome
Immunodeficiency
Allergic disease
Fungal sinusitis
Tumor
  Inverted papilloma
  Juvenile nasopharyngeal angiofibroma
  Esthesioneuroblastoma
  Carcinoma
  Sarcoma
  Meningioma
Antral choanal polyps
Meningoencephalocele

inheritance and occurs in 1/2000 live births with an estimated 12 million carriers in the United States. The defect has now been localized to the 7q31–32 gene locus with a diversity of phenotypes possible. With genetic screening, more cases are being identified. Adults with a history of significant sinus disease and polyposis since childhood, should be investigated for the presence of cystic fibrosis, particularly if the secretions are the typical creamy purulent material seen in this disease (33) (Fig. 3). Genetic screening in this situation is more sensitive than sweat testing (34).

The identification of unilateral nasal polyposis should raise the possibility of either allergic fungal sinusitis or inverting papilloma (Fig. 4). The latter, or even an occult malignancy, may also lurk within diffuse polyposis. Rigid intranasal endoscopy may thus, by pinpointing polyp origin and improving identification of polyp appearance, improve diagnostic accuracy. On CT, particular attention should be paid to the presence of bone erosion, although bone expansion or erosion may also occur with benign nasal polyposis. As in other forms of sinusitis, CT is best performed after medical management, to delineate the underlying chronic disease component, rather than the secondary or acute changes.

MRI is advisable when there is a skull base erosion adjacent to an area of sinus opacity. In this situation MRI enables the differentiation of sinus disease eroding the skull base from a meningocele or encephalocele. In the presence of tumors, MRI may also be of assistance in delineating the tumor from retained secretions and secondary inflammatory disease.

IV. Medical Management

A. Intranasal Corticosteroids

Inflammatory nasal polyposis, like chronic sinusitis, is primarily a medical disease. Surgery alone, without aggressive medical therapy, will typically fail.

Corticosteroids are central to medical therapy for patients with intranasal polyposis. Nearly all patients will require intranasal steroids and these should be initiated as first-line therapy in an attempt to gain medical control and avoid surgical intervention. If surgery is subsequently required, long-term postoperative treatment with corticosteroid nose sprays has been shown to reduce the tendency for recurrence (35–38). Current preparations in the United States include beclomethasone dipropionate, triamcinolone acetonide, budesonide, and fluticasone propionate, and mometasone furoate monohydrate. All preparations appear effective at reducing polyps, though clinical observation has found that fluticasone and budesonide have the greatest efficacy. Various propellants and additives in the preparations occasionally limit the acceptability of the medicines to some patients; however, after about 8 years following surgery, we have observed that nearly 75% of our patients remain on intranasal steroid without complication.

Following surgery, the most common site of persistent disease is the frontal recess. In this situation the application of steroid drops (e.g., Decadron 0.1% solution) in the head-inverted position (Moffit's position) may be beneficial in obtaining maximum local activity. Local intralesional injection of deposteroids is also effective, but rare instances of visual loss have occurred, significantly lessening enthusiasm for this type of intervention.

B. Oral Corticosteroids

Oral steroids are an important weapon in our armamentarium for the treatment of nasal polyposis. While many patients and practitioners agree with Davison's observation in 1945 that ''steroid dependence is a pair of dirty words'' (39) leading to hesitancy in prescribing, their beneficial effects can at times be remarkable. Frequently a rapid taper of steroid is all that is required to achieve a significant shrinkage of the polyps. However, others will benefit from prolonged low-dose therapy for, in many patients, polyps are very sensitive to the lower doses of steroid.

When combined with surgery, steroids are typically given at moderate dosages dependent on the extent of disease (30–40 mg prednisone once a day) for about 3 or 4 days prior to surgery to reduce the mucosal reactivity and vascular congestion, as well as to shrink the polyps for improved surgical exposure. This is particularly important in the asthmatic where the steroids also serve to stabilize the bronchial hyperreactivity prior to surgery. Dosages are then gradually tapered over the course of some weeks following the surgery while the sinus cavity heals. Most commonly, the patient is weaned off entirely but in occasional cases may require a very low chronic dose.

Potential side effects of short courses of steroids include insomnia, increased appetite, and mood swings: higher levels of energy at higher doses with low energy levels and depressed mood at lower levels. Although rare, rapid hip osteonecrosis has also been reported with short courses of steroids. The side effects of prolonged steroid usage are well known and include osteopenia, cataracts, and Cushing's disease. Great care must be taken in administering oral steroids to those with diabetes mellitus, psychiatric disorders, glaucoma, and hypertension.

C. Antibiotics

The relationship between polyps and sinusitis is critical and the presence of inflammation may be a strong trigger for polyp disease. Nearly all patients with nasal polyposis have some concurrent sinusitis. This becomes exacerbated when polyps cause osteomeatal obstruction and the secondary infection may trigger further polyp growth, resulting in a vicious cycle. Antibiotics may therefore be included in the initial medical treatment regimen of patients with nasal polyposis. While antibiotics covering *Streptococcus pneumoniae*, *Hemophilus influenzae*, and *Moraxella cattarhalis* are essential, in the setting of chronic sinusitis, coverage for anaerobic organisms may also be important. Recent evidence also supports additional coverage for gram-negative enteric organisms, at least in the tertiary care setting (40). In patients who have been on several prior courses of antibiotics, direct endoscopic culture is recommended to exclude the presence of resistant organisms.

V. Surgical Management

A. Indications

Surgical therapy for nasal polyps is effective as an adjunct to medical therapy in selected situations. Although the presence of nasal polyps alone is not an indication for surgery, surgery is indicated in patients whose quality of life is hampered by their polyp disease despite appropriate medical therapy. This may include chronic nasal congestion, continued or recurrent infections as well as patients who are developing increasing sinus disease, bone erosion, mucoceles, or other complications. Patients with worsening asthma and who have increasing medication requirements also often benefit from surgery, particularly if there is significant intercurrent infection. However, in general we only recommend surgery for asthma if there are also significant sinus complaints. Performing surgery for hyposmia, in patients with polyposis resistant to medical therapy, is more questionable. Although short-term recovery of olfaction typically occurs, the long-term results are less certain.

B. Surgical Approach

Traditional surgical approaches for the management of polyposis have included simple intranasal polypectomy where polyps themselves are removed without intent to remove surrounding sinus structures. The procedure can be performed in the operating room under general anesthesia or local anesthesia or in the outpatient clinic setting. In patients with localized involvement in the nose and little sinus disease, a combination of limited polypectomy with prolonged medical therapy may provide extended relief. However, in patients with significant sinus involvement a more complete operation is usually preferred, to avoid a rapid recurrence of the symptomatology and to avoid continued progression of the sinusitis.

In patients with significant sinus involvement, surgical therapy is directed at the sinuses involved with either ethmoidectomy alone or, more typically, complete procedures addressing disease in the sphenoid, maxillary, and frontal sinus areas.

The traditional approach for polyps of the maxillary sinus was the Caldwell-Luc procedure. Originally described 1893, the procedure entails anterior maxillotomy via a gingival-buccal incision (41). Traditional headlight approaches to the ethmoid, sphenoid, and frontal sinuses, both intranasal and external, have also been used with success. However with the advent of the improved visualization made possible by the endoscope, endoscopic sinus procedures have now generally become the treatment of choice.

Powered instrumentation using microdebriders originally developed for temporomandibular joint surgery have also offered a significant advance to the endoscopic sinus surgeon in the setting of massive polyposis (42). The instruments consist of an electrically powered disposable blade, which is ensheathed and open only through a small window on the side and tip, while the remainder of the tip is blunt. Oscillation of the blade is accompanied by continuous suction through a hollow shaft removing debris and blood from the operative field. The sharp, oscillating blade allows for cutting of the polypoid mucosa while leaving adjacent tissue intact, thus reinforcing the concept of mucosal preservation. Probably the most significant advantage of the soft tissue shaver in the setting of nasal polyps is its continuous suction and ability to maintain a bloodless field. This improves visualization and potentially, therefore, safety during the procedure (Fig. 5).

The endoscopic surgical approach as described by Kennedy et al. (43) is briefly outlined below. General anesthesia as well as local anesthesia with sedation have both been used successfully in the management of this disease. However, we generally still favor local anesthesia with sedation because it is well tolerated, bleeding is minimized, and the ability to monitor the patient and to monitor any pain provides an additional margin of safety. As noted previously, when indicated, patients are treated with antibiotics and oral steroids in the immediate preoperative period, to minimize infection, shrink the polyps, and reduce mucosal hyperreactivity. The pretreatment with steroids assumes greater importance in patients with asthma.

At the beginning of surgery, irrespective of the type of anesthesia utilized, routine intranasal injections are performed with a solution of 1% lidocaine with 1/100,000 epinephrine into the lateral nasal wall and into the region of the sphenopalatine ganglion. The latter injection can be performed transnasally, but, in the presence of severe polyposis, is typically best performed transorally through the greater palatine foramen. Gross polypoid disease is most conveniently and rapidly removed with the microdebrider, taking care not to traumatize the mucosa of the lateral nasal wall, turbinates, and septum. In an individual who has not had previous surgery, we then proceed with infundibulotomy and uncinectomy. The bulla is resected identifying the lamina papyracea, a constant landmark in all cases, whether revision or not. The basal lamella is entered inferiorly and posterior cells opened. The skull base, a second critical landmark, is typically identified within the posterior ethmoid.

If the sphenoid sinus is to be opened, the natural ostium is identified by the Lanza technique. The ostium is identified from within the ethmoid sinus, by first identifying the superior meatus medially and then resecting the inferior third of the superior turbinate. This allows direct visualization of the sphenoid ostium without the necessity to work through the nasal cavity. The natural opening is then enlarged. Dissection is now carried in a posterior-to-anterior direction along the skull base using cutting instrumentation such as the Black Star through-cutting instruments (Xomed Surgical Products, Jacksonville, FL) to minimize mucosal loss. Mucosal preservation is a major goal in all cases, even those with massive polypoid disease and revision cases. Dissection is continued into the frontal recess and the frontal sinus is opened using through-cutting giraffe instruments such as those produced by SSI Surgical Instruments (Nashville, TN). Finally the natural ostium of the maxillary sinus is identified and enlarged.

Previous surgery (including polypectomy) that may have altered surgical anatomy requires variations on these standard techniques; however, in all procedures two anatomical landmarks need to be identified clearly: the lamina papyracea and the skull base. Both landmarks are constant regardless of previous surgery or extensive disease. Mucosal preservation is strongly emphasized in all cases in order to leave a mucosa-lined cavity at the completion of the procedure. Preservation of the mucosa results in more rapid healing with less scarring and less crusting during the postoperative period. Mucosal preservation becomes critical in the frontal recess, if postoperative frontal recess stenosis is to be avoided.

In all cases of diffuse disease, a complete ethmoidectomy needs to be performed with the removal of all bony partitions. Any remaining septae may act as foci of chronic infection postoperatively, precipitating localized persistence of polyp disease and eventually more diffuse recurrence. In addition, the middle turbinate must be evaluated for the presence of osteitic bone and overlying polyp formation. If significantly involved in the disease process, it is best resected.

Following surgery, patients are treated with aggressive medical and surgical care. Topical steroids are usually resumed quickly in the postoperative period. Appropriate culture-directed or broad-spectrum antibiotics are administered until the cavity is completely mucosalized on endoscopic evaluation. The time table for tapering the oral steroids is dependent on both the extent of disease seen preoperatively and the postoperative appearance on endoscopic examination. Typically in diffuse polyposis they are tapered over a course of several weeks.

Regular postoperative visits are essential to control the tendency toward recurrence of polyps. Small recurrent polyps may be debrided endoscopically under topical anesthesia in the clinic. Adhesions are also removed to create a widely patent sinus cavity. Any loose fragments of bone, or areas of poorly viable bone, are identified and removed. Such bone frequently appears to result in persistent inflammation and overlying polyp formation. The aim is to treat any persistent disease before it again becomes symptomatic because, by the time symptoms recur, the disease could again be extensive. Evidence of infection is also readily identified endoscopically, and antibiotics are rapidly initiated to prevent further polyp growth.

If more significant polyp regrowth is seen on follow-up evaluation, aggressive medical therapy with increased dosage of topical steroids, antibiotics, and possibly also a tapering course of oral steroids can be initiated. If such therapy proves unsuccessful, CT scanning may identify any hidden cells that have not been exenterated. If the CT confirms that all cellular partitions have indeed been removed, subsequent management is usually only medical. On the other hand, if bony fragments and residual partitions are identified, revision surgery may be indicated.

While topical and sometimes oral steroids, along with antibiotics, are mainstays in controlling polypoid disease and preventing recurrence, a variety of other agents have been analyzed targeting certain biochemical features of polyps in an attempt to prevent postsurgical recurrence. For example, the presence of leukotrienes C4 and D4 in polyp fluid (35) has suggested a possible role for leukotriene-blocking agents, while lysine acetylsalicylate (44) and furosemide (45) have also both been experimentally assessed. In preliminary reports, both medications appear to show some efficacy at preventing polyp recurrence.

VI. Results of Medical and Surgical Therapy for Nasal Polyps

While some authors have concluded that "surgery for polyposis is doomed to failure" (46), our experience has shown that with intensive medical and surgical management of nasal polyposis as outlined above, it is possible to bring lasting relief to a significant percentage of patients, even those significantly afflicted with their disease (Fig. 6). Data from the senior author indicate that over 85% of patients operated on with the techniques of functional endoscopic sinus surgery for chronic sinusitis and/or nasal polyps report marked subjective improvement in their symptoms at an average follow-up of 18 months (47). Indeed it is our impression that, if the ethmoid cavity can be kept free of significant disease following surgery, the degree of mucosal reactivity slowly decreases over time. Thus, although the patient may require intensive medical management and debridement for months, or even years, following surgery, the tendency to form recurrent disease decreases over time with maximal therapy, and the degree of medical intervention can slowly be reduced.

In our earlier study, the primary prognostic factor for complete resolution of disease was the extent of sinus involvement at the time of surgery. A history of prior surgery, the presence of asthma, or aspirin sensitivity (ASA triad) did not, per se, appear to adversely affect outcome once the patients were stratified for the extent of disease. However, while subjective outcome appears good in polyp disease, relatively few patients have completely normal-appearing cavities on endoscopic exam at 18 months post surgery. Of those patients with polyps confined to the middle meatus alone, 42% exhibited some areas of mucosal abnormality (scarring, erythema, discharge, mucosal hypertrophy, or polypoid change) on endoscopy. With diffuse polypoid disease, the incidence of postoperative mucosal abnormalities rose to 76% (47). However, with early identification of such endoscopic abnormalities, surgical intervention consisting of minor debridements in the office setting, combined with medical therapy, can be initiated and long-term excellent subjective results can be maintained. With careful follow-up and postoperative care, we find that revision surgery is rarely necessary (4%).

VII. Conclusions

Nasal polyposis is a multifactorial disease. In its more diffuse manifestations, it appears to represent a diffuse, nonspecific mucosal inflammation and is closely related to asthma. Although there may be a prior atopic history, allergy evaluation at the time of presentation is frequently unremarkable. Familial predisposition appears to be significant, but the disease is frequently initiated with an upper respiratory tract infection.

The treatment of nasal polyps remains primarily medical and has been revolutionized by the use of topical nasal steroids, although antibiotics and oral steroids are also an important part of the treatment armamentarium. Other medical therapies such as furosemide, lysine acetylsalicylate, and leukotriene antagonists may be helpful in medical management, but further studies are required.

Surgery is currently reserved for patients who are medical failures or who would otherwise require prolonged oral steroid therapy. In general, we recommend that all diseased sinuses be exenterated at the time of surgery and we feel that with this approach and with detailed postoperative care, this disease, and the tendency to reform polyps, can be slowly reversed.

Finally, nasal polyposis can be a frustrating disease for the patient who is afflicted, as well as for the treating physician. However, we strongly disagree that a patient with nasal polyposis is doomed to multiple surgical procedures. If both the patient and the physician are willing to commit to detailed postoperative care and medical therapy, the disease can often be reversed in even the most recalcitrant cases. The postoperative care may need to be intensive, is sometimes prolonged, and may involve local debridement in addition to an intensive medical regimen. However, we believe that with such therapy, a slow resolution of the underlying mucosal inflammation can frequently be achieved.

References

1. National Center for Health Statistics, Benson V, Marano M. Current estimates for the National Health Interview Survey—1993. In: Vital and Health Statistics, Vol 10. Washington, DC: Government Printing Office, 1995:190.
2. Maran A, Lund V. Clinical Rhinology. New York: Thieme Medical Publishers, 1990: 95.
3. Gliklich R, Metson R. The health impact of chronic sinusitis in patients seeking otolaryngologic care. Otolaryngol Head Neck Surg 1995; 113:104–109.
4. Bousquet J, Bullinger M, Fayol C, Marquis P, Valentin B, Burtin B. Assessment of quality of life in patients with perennial allergic rhinitis with the French version of the SF-36 Health Status Questionnaire. J Allergy Clin Immunol 1994; 94:182–188.
5. Josephson JS. The role of endoscopic sinus surgery for the treatment of nasal polyposis. Otolaryngol Clin North Am 1989; 22:831–840.
6. Kern R, Schenck H. Allergy: a constant factor in the etiology of so-called mucous nasal polyps. J Allergy 1933; 4:485–497.
7. Perkins JA, Blakeslee DB, Andrade P. Nasal polyps: a manifestation of allergy? Otolaryngol Head Neck Surg 1989; 101:641–645.
8. Pulido V, Garcia-Calderon PA. Some immunological parameters in serum and nasal secretion in subjects with vasomotor and allergic rhinitis and nasal polyps—a comparative study. Rhinology 1983; 21:29–37.
9. Settipane G, Chafee F. Nasal polyps in asthma and rhinitis: a review of 6,037 patients. J Allergy Clin Immunol 1977; 59:17–21.

10. Drake-Lee A, Pitcher-Wilmott R. The clinical and laboratory correlates of nasal polyps in cystic fibrosis. Int J Pediatr Otorhinolaryngol 1982; 4:209–220.

11. Drake-Lee A, Lowe D, Swanston A, Grace A. Clinical profile and recurrence of nasal polyps. J Laryngol Otol 1984; 98:783–793.

12. Slavin R. Allergy is not a significant cause of nasal polyps. Arch Otolaryngol Head Neck Surg 1992; 118:771 (letter).

13. Bernstein JM, Gorfien J, Noble B. Role of allergy in nasal polyposis: a review. Otolaryngol Head Neck Surg 1995; 113:724–732.

14. Keith P, Dolovich J. Allergy and nasal polyposis. In: Mygind N, Lildholdt T, eds. Nasal Polyposis: An Inflammatory Disease and Its Treatment. Copenhagen: Munksgaard, 1997:68–77.

15. Shatkin JS, Delsupehe KG, Thisted RA, Corey JP. Mucosal allergy in the absence of systemic allergy in nasal polyposis and rhinitis: a meta-analysis. Otolaryngol Head Neck Surg 1994; 111:553–556.

16. Suonpaa J, Antila J. Increase of acute frontal sinusitis in southwestern Finland. Scand J Infect Dis 1990; 22:563–568.

17. Ogawa H. A possible role of aerodynamic factors in nasal polyp formation. Acta Otolaryngol (Stockh) 1986; (Suppl 430):18–20.

18. Stammberger H. Functional Endoscopic Sinus Surgery: The Messerklinger Technique. Philadelphia: BC Decker, 1991.

19. Larsen PL, Tos M. Origin of nasal polyps. Laryngoscope 1991; 101:305–312.

20. Larsen P, Tos M. Site of origin of nasal polyps. Transcranially removed nasoethmoidal blocks as a screening method for nasal polyps in autopsy material. Rhinology 1995; 33:185–188.

21. Tos M, Mogensen C, Thompson J. Nasal polyps in cystic fibrosis. J Laryngol Otol 1977; 91:827–835.

22. Bachert C, Wagenmann M, Hauser U. Proinflammatory cytokines: measurement in nasal secretion and induction of adhesion receptor expression. Int Arch Allergy Appl Immunol 1995; 107:106–108.

23. Roseler S, Holtappels G, Wagenmann M, Bachert C. Elevated levels of interleukins IL-1 beta, IL-6 and IL-8 in naturally acquired viral rhinitis. Eur Arch Oto-Rhino-Laryngol 1995; (Suppl 1):S61–S63.

24. Bachert C, Wagenmann M, Hauser U, Rudack C. IL-5 synthesis is upregulated in human nasal polyp tissue. J Allergy Clin Immunol (submitted).

25. Stellato C, Beck L, Gorgone G, Proud D, Schall T, Ono S, Lichtenstein L, Schleimer R. Expression of the chemokine RANTES by a human bronchial epithelial cell line. Modulation by cytokines and glucocorticoids. J Immunol 1995; 155:410–418.

26. Sasaki Y, Nakahara H. Innervation of human nasal polyps. Rhinology 1985; 23:195–199.

27. Smith DM, Gerrard JM, White JG. Comparison of arachidonic acid metabolism in nasal polyps and eosinophils. Int Arch Allergy Appl Immunol 1987; 82:83–88.

28. Norlander T, Fukami M, Westrin KM, Stierna P, Carlsoo B. Formation of mucosal polyps in the nasal and maxillary sinus cavities by infection. Otolaryngolo Head Neck Surg 1993; 109:522–529.

29. Jacobs RL, Freda AJ, Culver WG. Primary nasal polyposis. Ann Allergy 1983; 51:500–505.

30. Falliers C. First complete description of the aspirin idiosyncrasy-asthma-nasal polyposis syndrome. J Asthma 1987; 24:297–300.

31. Samter M, Beers R. Concerning the nature of intolerance to aspirin. J Allergy 1967; 40:281–293.

32. Sweet J, Stevenson D, Simon R, Mathison D. Long-term effects of aspirin-desensitization-treatment for aspirin-sensitive rhinosinusitis-asthma. J Allergy Clin Immunol 1990; 85:59–65.

33. Thaler E, Smullen S, Kennedy D. Adult cystic fibrosis presenting with nasal polyposis and chronic sinusitis. Am J Rhinol 1994; 8:237–239.

34. Kingdom T, Lee K, Cropp G. Chronic sinusitis and a negative sweat test in a patient with cystic fibrosis. Am J Rhinol 1995; 9:225–228.

35. Drake-Lee AB. Medical treatment of nasal polyps. Rhinology 1994; 32:1–4.

36. Drettner B, Ebbesen A, Nilsson M. Prophylactive treatment with flunisolide after polypectomy. Rhinology 1982; 20:149–158.

37. Ruhno J, Andersson B, Denburg J, Anderson M, Hitch D, Lapp P, Vanzieleghem M, Dolovich J. A double-blind comparison of intranasal budesonide with placebo for nasal polyposis. J Allergy Clin Immunol 1990; 86:946–953.

38. Lildholdt T, Rundcrantz H, Lindqvist N. Efficacy of topical corticosteroid powder for nasal polyps: a double-blind, placebo-controlled study of budesonide. Clin Otolaryngol 1995; 20:26–30.

39. Davison F. Chronic sinusitis and infectious asthma. Arch Otolaryngol 1969; 90:110–115.

40. Bolger W. Gram negative sinusitis: an emerging clinical entity? Am J Rhinol 1994; 8:279–284.

41. Caldwell G. The accessory sinus of the nose, and an improved method of treatment for suppuration of the maxillary antrum. NY Med J 1893; 58:526–528.

42. Setliff R, Parsons D. The ''hummer'': new instrumentation for functional endoscopic sinus surgery. Am J Rhinol 1994; 8:275–278.

43. Kennedy DW, Zinreich SJ, Rosenbaum AE, Johns ME. Functional endoscopic sinus surgery. Arch Otolaryngol 1985; 111:576–582.

44. Giampiero P, Paolo B, Eleonora N, Domenico S, Giuseppe P, Giuseppina S, Giovanna F, Rita PL. Intranasal treatment with lysine acetylsalicylate in patients with nasal polyposis. Ann Allergy 1991; 67:588–592.

45. Passali D, Lauriello M, Ferrara A, Bernstein J. Medical therapy for the prevention of relapsing nasal polyposis: a pilot study on the use of furosemide by inhalation. Am J Rhinol 1996; 10:187–192.

46. Biedlingmaier JF. Endoscopic sinus surgery with middle turbinate resection: results and complications. Ear Nose Throat J 1993; 72:351–355.

47. Kennedy D. Prognostic factors, outcomes and staging in ethoid sinus surgery. Laryngoscope 1992; 102:1–18.

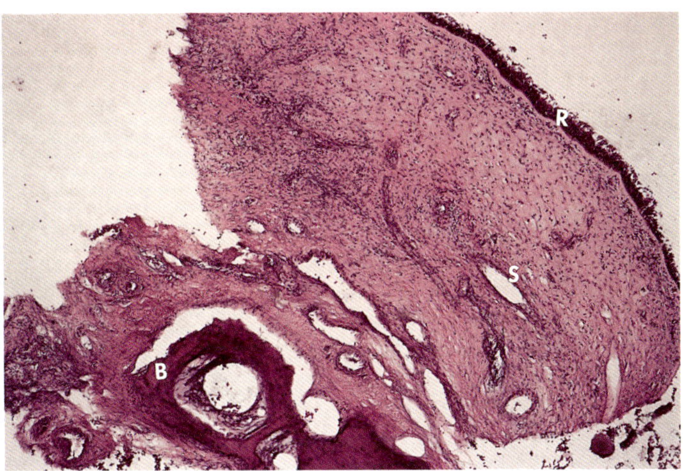

Figure 1 Photomicrograph of polypoid ethmoid mucosa illustrating histological features including overlying respiratory mucosa (R), loose stroma, and inflammatory infiltrate. Venous sinusoids (S) are seen adjacent to a fragment of bone (B). Overall bland architecture is in contrast to mucosa overlying the turbinates where tissue is filled with blood vessels.

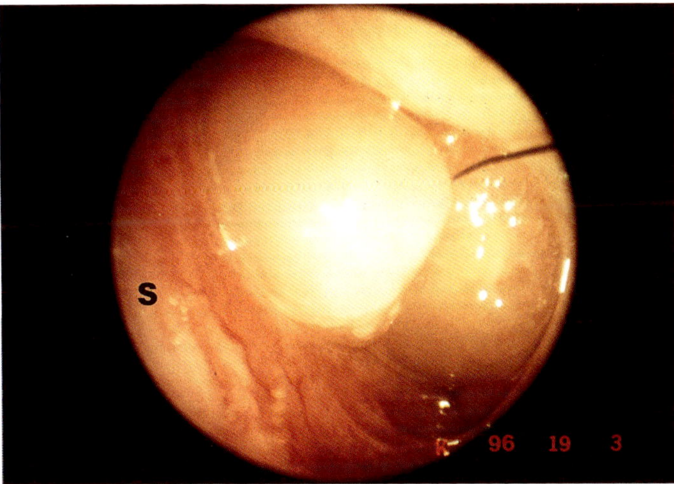

Figure 2 Endoscopic view of the left nasal cavity showing massive nasal polyps. Note the typical avascular, glistening, boggy appearance of inflammatory polyps. S = nasal septum.

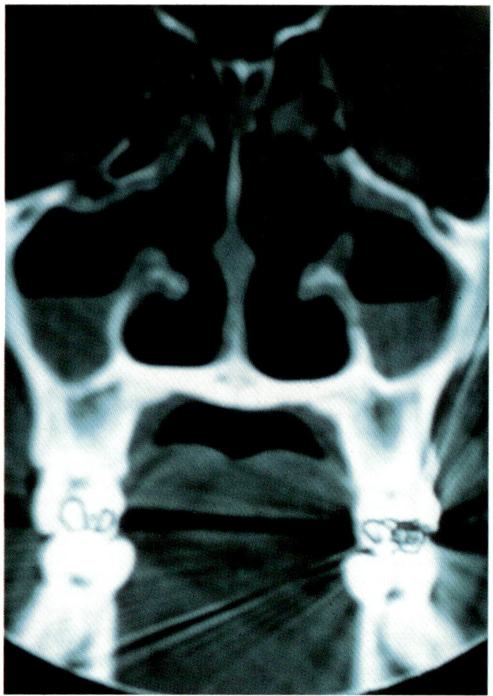

Figure 3 CT scan in the coronal axis through the sinuses in a 33-year-old with "chronic bronchitis" and refractory nasal polyposis and sinusitis despite aggressive medical and surgical therapy. Pulmonary disease was discovered to have been present since childhood. Genetic screening for cystic fibrosis was found to be positive.

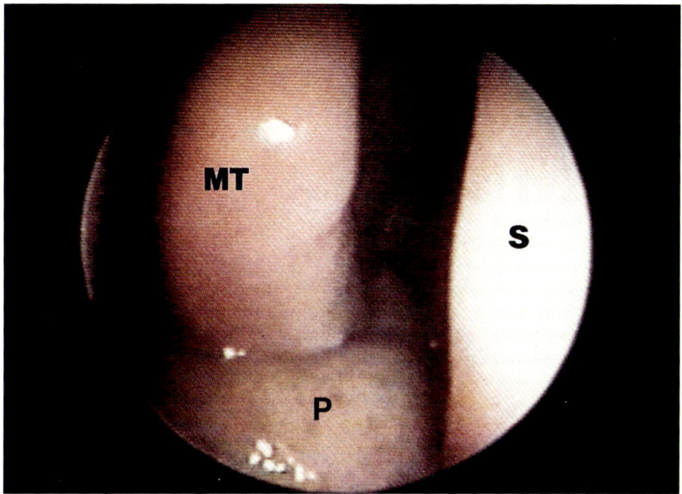

Figure 4   Endoscopic view of the right nasal cavity in a 16-year-old male with unilateral nasal polyposis. Polyp (P) was noted to be firm, friable and extending into the region of the sphenopalatine foramen laterally and into the nasopharynx posteriorly. Pathology in the operating room confirmed juvenile nasopharyngeal angiofibroma. S = septum; MT = middle turbine.

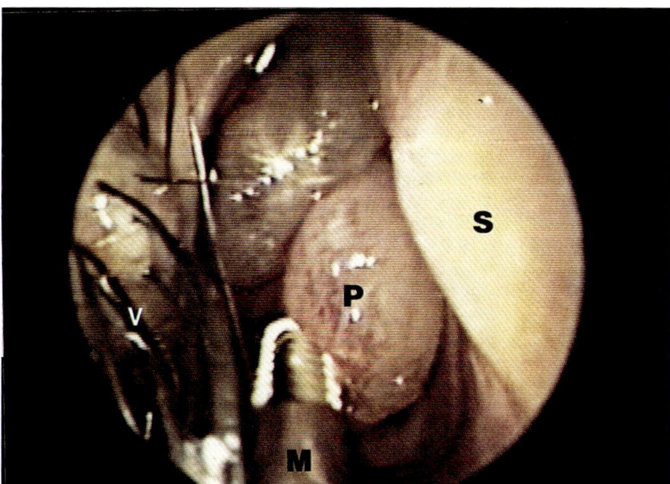

Figure 5   Endoscopic view in the right nasal cavity illustrating the use of the microdebrider for the resection of nasal polyps. Continuous suction allows the polyps to be resected with minimal bleeding while sharp cutting action preserves normal adjacent mucosa. V = vibrissae; M = microdebrider; S = septum; P = polyps.

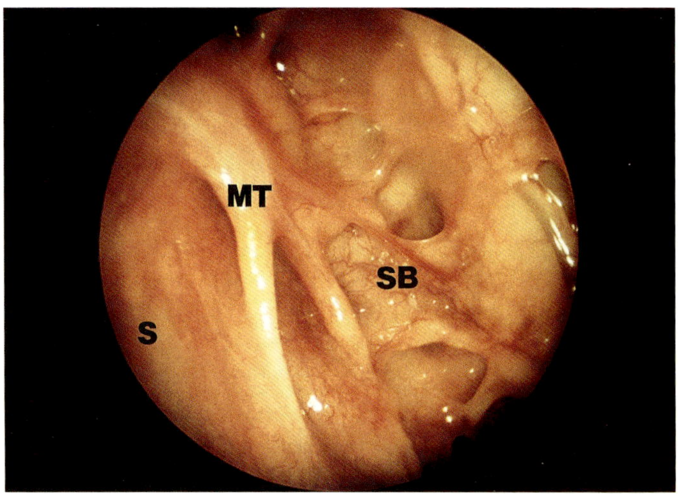

Figure 6 Endoscopic view looking up into the left ethmoidectomy cavity in a 57-year-old woman with ASA triad who presented with massive nasal polyps extruding through both nares. Photo illustrates appearance of the cavity nearly four years post-operatively. She required perioperative oral steroids in a slowly tapering course several weeks post-operatively to a baseline of prednisone 5 mg every other day for control of her asthma and remains on that dose. In addition, she continues to use an intranasal corticosteroid spray. S = septum; MT = middle turbinate remnant; SB = skull base.

23

Rhinitis in Children

PHILIP FIREMAN

Children's Hospital of Pittsburgh and
  University of Pittsburgh School of Medicine
Pittsburgh, Pennsylvania

I. Introduction

Rhinitis, allergic and nonallergic, is the most common chronic illness affecting children with peak prevalence in the adolescent and young adult (1). As a chronic condition, rhinitis, especially allergic rhinitis in childhood, is unique since most other chronic illnesses such as hypertension, diabetes, arthritis, and cardiovascular diseases increase their prevalence in the older adult population. The most recent surveys in the United States and Europe indicate that rhinitis in childhood is becoming even more frequent (2–4). This changing pattern of rhinitis in children will probably manifest itself with increased nasal disease in adults in the next 10–20 years. If true, this projected increase in chronic rhinitis will also manifest itself with increased health care costs.

Because rhinitis in the absence of one of its complications is not associated with mortality or hospitalizations, many clinicians tend to trivialize the child with chronic rhinitis. However, 2 million or more schoolday absences have been attributed to allergic rhinitis alone. Therefore, for the children or their parents, chronic rhinitis is not a trivial disease. This chapter will emphasize those aspects of rhinitis that are important for the pediatric patient and those clinicians who care for these children.

II. Classification and Epidemiology

A classification of rhinitis is shown in Table 1. Infectious rhinitis, which is typically viral, is often referred to as a ''common cold'' or upper respiratory infection (URI). Acute infectious rhinitis is much more common in children than adults. Whereas, children average six or more URI episodes per year, the adult averages two or three. In a recent telephone survey the duration and frequency of the complications of URI were studied in children aged 1–3 years (5). URIs were found to last longer in children aged 1–2 years in day care settings (8.9 days) than in children in home care or small care groups (6.6 days). The percentage of URI that lasted more than 15 days ranged from 6.5% for children 1–3 years of age in home care to 13.1% for these same-aged children in day care, perhaps suggesting the complication of sinusitis. Otitis media as a complication of the URI was also more frequent in children less than 1 year in the day care settings (43.1%) as compared to home care (27.4%).

Allergic rhinitis can be episodic or perennial; when symptoms recur annually during certain months, the syndrome is called seasonal allergic rhinitis (see Table 1). Typically, seasonal allergic rhinitis does not develop until after the child has been sensitized by two or more pollen seasons. Seasonal allergic rhinitis is frequently referred to as ''hay fever'' or a summer cold. These descriptive terms are misleading and should be discarded because fever is not a symptom associated with allergic rhinitis and neither hay nor the common cold virus is incriminated in the etiology of this syndrome.

Until recently, the prevalence of allergic rhinitis in the general population had been considered to be about 10%, with the peak incidence in the postadolescent teenage child. In 1974, Broder and colleagues, in their often-quoted retrospective study of a well-defined population in Tecumseh, Michigan, found the

Table 1 Classification of Rhinitis

1. Infectious rhinitis
    a. Acute
    b. Chronic
2. Allergic rhinitis
    a. Seasonal
    b. Perennial
3. Nonallergic, noninfectious rhinitis
    a. Structural
    b. Cholinergic (vasomotor)
    c. Nonallergic rhinitis with eosinophilia (NARES)
    d. Hormonal

incidence of hay fever (seasonal allergic rhinitis) to increase during childhood from less than 1% during infancy to an incidence of 4–5% from ages 5 to 9 years to 9% during adolescence to 15–16% after adolescence (6). The incidence of allergic rhinitis remained constant in the young adult but gradually declined during the middle years and in the elderly. Even though seasonal allergic rhinitis is infrequent in the very young child, perennial allergic rhinitis has been recognized in infancy and even in the neonate. The Tecumseh study also indicated that seasonal allergic rhinitis is almost twice as common as perennial allergic rhinitis. For reasons that are not clear, more male than female children are affected with allergic rhinitis prior to adolescence, whereas females are more often affected with nasal allergy after adolescence. Race and socioeconomic factors are not thought to be important factors in the expression of allergic rhinitis.

The perception that rhinitis, especially allergic rhinitis, is more common than previously thought is supported by studies that showed increased prevalence in Switzerland from 0.28% in 1928 to 10% in 1985 (2). Also prevalence of allergic rhinitis increased from 4.4% in 18-year-old Swedish army recruits in 1971 to 8.4% in 1981 (3). An even larger prevalence was identified in Tucson, Arizona during a recent prospective longitudinal study of the natural history of allergic rhinitis in children (4). A cohort of 747 healthy children in a health maintenance organization were followed from birth. By the age of 6, 42% of children had physician-diagnosed allergic rhinitis. Children whose rhinitis began in the first year of life had more respiratory symptoms at age 6 and were more likely to have a diagnosis of asthma. Early introduction of foods or formula, heavy maternal cigarette smoking in the first year of life, and higher IgE, as well as prenatal allergic disorders, were associated with early development of rhinitis. Risk factors for allergic rhinitis that remained significant in a multivariate model included maternal history of allergy and IgE greater than 100 IU/ml at age 6. The ratio odds for allergic rhinitis as compared to nonallergic rhinitis were significantly higher only among those with high IgE and in those families who had dogs. This study needs to be confirmed in another U.S. community to make certain that this was not a unique local phenomenon in Arizona, which has attracted many allergic patients and experienced a large population increase in past 50 years. This may have increased the genetic expression of allergy.

The prevalence of the types of nonallergic, noninfectious rhinitis listed in Table 1 is not well studied. The incidence of deviated nasal septum is not described in children. Nasal polyps are uncommon in children except in cystic fibrosis and are not thought to be increased in children with allergic rhinitis. The nonallergic rhinitis with nasal eosinophil syndrome (NARES) is much more common in adults but has been described in children. A hormonal basis for rhinitis has been described in childhood both in children with thyroid dysfunction and in pregnant adolescents.

III. Etiology

The development of allergic rhinitis requires two conditions: (1) the atopic familial predisposition to develop allergy and (2) exposure of the sensitized child to the allergen. Children are not born with allergies, but if genetically predisposed (atopic), they do have the capacity to develop symptoms spontaneously through repeated exposure to allergens in their environment.

Inhalants, which are the principal allergens responsible for allergic rhinitis in children, may be present outdoors and indoors. These microscopic airborne particles include the pollens from weeds, grasses, and trees, mold spores, animal products, and environmental dusts, with exposure either at home, school, recreational, or occupational.

Seasonal allergic rhinitis is primarily induced by pollens from the germination of ''nonflowering'' vegetation. In the temperate climates, the most important are tree pollens in the spring, grass pollens in the late spring and early summer, and ragweed in the late summer and early fall. Recreational activities during childhood are associated with greater pollen exposure than in adults. Since there is variation from one geographic area to another, it is necessary for each clinician to become familiar with the pollination patterns in his region. ''Flowering'' vegetation, such as roses and fruit blossoms, rarely causes allergic rhinitis because these pollens are too heavy to be airborne and germination is facilitated by the action of bees and other insects.

In warm climates, mold spores may be airborne year round, but in climates in which snow and freezing occur in the winter months, airborne mold spores are present intermittently during the spring, summer, and fall until there is significant frost. In some children with perennial allergic rhinitis and asthma, mold spores may be a significant inhalant allergen indoors.

The principal allergen in house dust can vary, but the major portion is due to the various species of house dust mite, *Dermatophagoides*. The specific house dust mite allergens have been identified in its cuticle and feces.

Animal epidermal danders, as well as salivary proteins, urinary proteins, feces, and feathers, especially from pets such as cats, dogs, and birds, but also the cockroach, are potential inhalant allergens.

Most allergens, including the pollens, have not been completely chemically characterized, and each consists of multiple antigenic determinants. Food allergens are of lesser importance in the etiology of allergic rhinitis but cannot be ignored, especially in young children (7). Patients can be sensitive to one or multiple allergens. Although it is a well-established fact that exposure to an allergen is necessary to develop sensitivity and symptoms, it is not known why allergic individuals with the same exposure become sensitive to certain allergens but not to others. The threshold of reactivity to each allergen varies greatly from one patient to another; certain individuals react to small allergenic challenges, and others tolerate a large allergen dose before developing symptoms.

In addition to allergens, other nonallergenic factors can contribute to the development of nasal symptoms. These include aerosolized cosmetics, cigarette smoke, industrial fumes, and changes in temperature, humidity, and barometric pressure (8). Psychological and social stresses and anxiety may also aggravate nasal symptoms (9). The importance of these additional contributory factors varies greatly from child to child and should not be neglected in patient management.

Even though it is not possible to predict with certainty the potentially atopic patient, the familial nature of allergic rhinitis has been recognized for years, and a positive family history of atopy has been noted in 50–75% of allergic children (10). Despite several extensive retrospective family and twin studies, there is no agreement as to the hereditary pattern in atopic diseases. Most investigators feel that several genetic loci are involved in the expression of allergic disease, and inheritance is multifactorial. Immunological studies have isolated some of these genetic influences. Elevated serum levels of IgE are sometimes associated with certain allergic diseases, and a recessive genetic influence has been suggested (10).

Animal studies have shown that synthesis of specific antibodies to well-characterized antigens is controlled in part by immune response (Ir) genes, which are linked to the major tissue histocompatibility locus (HLA). The seasonal family studies by Levine and co-workers more than 20 years ago suggested that ragweed allergic rhinitis and immune responses to purified ragweed antigen E were linked to a particular HLA haplotype in successive generations of allergic families (11). Recent studies have suggested in several family cohorts in England that the gene for the specific IgE responses resides on chromosome 11, but this has not been confirmed (12). Another genetic locus has been suggested on chromosome 5.

IV. Symptoms and Signs

Initial symptoms in seasonal allergic rhinitis progress from frequent sneezing and nasal pruritus to rhinorrhea and finally to nasal obstruction. Children with perennial allergic rhinitis have more nasal stuffiness and obstruction than sneezing and pruritus. These symptoms not only vary considerably from season to season but also differ markedly at various times of night and day. Many children complain of early-morning and late-evening symptoms, and their sleep can frequently be interrupted because of nasal obstruction. Children complain of not only nasal pruritus but also itching of the eyes, throat, and ears. Many children constantly rub the nose with the hand or arm in an effort to relieve the nasal itch and perhaps to improve the nasal obstruction. Other children may press the palm of the hand upward against the nose in an "allergic salute." Constant rubbing of the nose often leads to the development of a transverse nasal crease, a horizontal groove across the lower third of the nose.

With nasal obstruction the child will be a constant mouth breather and snoring will be a prominent nighttime symptom. It has been suggested that constant mouth breathing may contribute to the development of orofacial dental abnormalities requiring orthodontic procedures, but this has not been established definitively (13).

Seasonal allergic rhinitis is frequently accompanied by allergic conjunctivitis with lacrimation, bilateral ocular pruritus, bilateral watery ocular secretions, and photophobia. Symptoms involving the adjacent sinuses may also be evident, especially maxillary discomfort or headaches when the symptoms of nasal obstruction are severe.

In children with eustachian tube dysfunction, allergic rhinitis may contribute to the development of otitis media with effusion. Some children may complain of a feeling of fullness or a popping sound in their ears. A hearing loss in a child with chronic or perennial allergic rhinitis should raise the suspicion of a conductive hearing deficit associated with otitis media with effusion.

Loss of sense of smell and taste may also be described. Children may also manifest symptoms of generalized malaise, irritability, and fatigue; these symptoms are often difficult to differentiate from the side effects of the frequently used sedating antihistamine therapy. This is especially so in the nonverbal child. There can also be the paradoxical side effect of hyperactivity in the child. In the school-age child therapy with sedating antihistamines can contribute to decreased performance in learning skills (14).

Patients with seasonal pollinosis describe a gradual increase in the severity of symptoms as the season progresses, especially on dry, windy days. At times, children can experience a continuation of the symptoms beyond the pollen season, and many clinicians feel that repeated exposure to allergens increases the reactivity of the nasal mucosa so that ordinarily innocuous allergen and other environmental exposures can produce symptoms in the "primed" nasal mucosa.

The pattern of the patient's symptoms frequently distinguishes those with seasonal from those with perennial allergic rhinitis, especially in temperate climates with obvious seasonal climatic changes. In the warmer subtropical climates, the seasonal pollen pattern may not be obvious, since the grass pollen season extends over many months and mold spores can remain in the air throughout the year. The arid southwestern United States was traditionally pollen free, but the advent of irrigation and increased vegetation has changed that clinical impression. Ragweed tends to grow at the edges of cultivated farm fields as well as playing fields and playground. It also grows along highways and tends to cause increased symptoms during automobile trips. Even though airborne pollens spread for miles, increased concentrations of pollens are noted in areas of high plant density, and patients frequently complain of more symptoms in areas of high pollen density. If there is direct contact with a substantial quantity of pollen, such as playing and rolling in grass, children may have significant symptoms including angioedema, especially of the eyes and throat, and, on occasion, urticaria.

Although frequently incriminated, ingested foods are an uncommon documented cause of allergic rhinitis in the child. However, in studies of children with severe atopic dermatitis, Sampson and co-workers, using double-blind, placebo-controlled challenges, have documented upper and lower respiratory signs and symptoms in 20–30% of these highly allergic study subjects (15).

The clinician should take a very careful environmental history and survey in all patients who complain of intermittent or year-round symptoms that do not fit the usual seasonal pattern previously described. In general, these patients with year-round symptoms are much more of a diagnostic challenge than those with only intermittent complaints. The almost continuous exposure to house or school-room inhalants may induce perennial symptoms because congestion of the mucosal tissues may not have the opportunity to subside or return to normal during the few hours free of allergen exposure. It is also in these patients that the nonallergenic environmental factors tend to contribute to the symptoms: these additional nonallergenic factors include changes in barometric pressure, temperature, and humidity and aerosolized irritants such as cigarette smoke, chalk dust, combustion fumes, and aerosolized cosmetics.

With development of the allergic reaction, clear nasal secretions will be evident, and the nasal mucous membranes will become edematous without much erythema. The mucosa appears boggy and blue-gray. With continued exposure to the allergen, the turbinates will appear to be not only congested but also swollen, and they will obstruct the nasal airway. If nasal obstruction is present, it may be necessary to shrink the mucosa with a vasoconstrictor to document the absence of nasal polyps, which may complicate allergic rhinitis but are relatively uncommon in allergic rhinitis, occurring in less than 0.5% of patients (16).

Conjunctival edema and hyperemia are frequent findings in patients with associated conjunctivitis. Allergic rhinitis patients with significant nasal obstruction and venous congestion, particularly children, may also demonstrate edema and darkening of the tissues beneath the eyes. These so-called ''allergic shiners'' are not pathognomonic for allergic rhinitis; they also can be seen in patients with recurrent or persistent nasal venous stasis of any other cause such as adenoidal hypertrophy. The conjunctiva may also demonstrate a lymphoid follicular pattern with a cobblestone appearance.

Nasal obstruction will cause mouth breathing, which can give the appearance of the adenoidal facies attributed to adenoidal hypertrophy. Pallor of the palatine and pharyngeal tissues is also evident, and on occasion small follicular lymphoid hyperplasia is evident on the posterior pharyngeal surface without regional cervical lymphadenopathy or tonsillar hypertrophy. Purulent secretions can be evident in the allergic child in the presence of secondary infections of the nose or sinuses.

V. Laboratory Studies

The nasal secretions of children with allergic rhinitis usually contain increased numbers of eosinophils. Eosinophilia may not be present in patients not recently exposed to specific allergens or in the presence of a superimposed infection. Steroids can significantly reduce eosinophilia, but antihistamine therapy has no significant effect on nasal eosinophils. The usefulness of nasal eosinophilia is, in large part, dependent on the technique used to obtain the specimens and preparation of the slides for examination. It is difficult to quantify nasal eosinophilia accurately, and more than 3% eosinophils seen on stained smear of expelled nasal secretions is considered an increase. Analysis of the nasal cytology obtained by gently pressing down on the mucosal surface of the inferior turbinate with a flexible plastic nasal probe can be helpful in the differential diagnosis of selected patients with recurrent rhinitis (17). Increased mucosal basophils, mast cells, or both are found in varying proportions in allergic rhinitis and nonallergic eosinophilic rhinitis. Infection is usually evidenced by a predominance of neutrophil leukocytes on the nasal smear.

Although several methods of measuring nasal airway resistance by rhinomanometry have been developed in the past few years, the diagnostic usefulness of quantifying this parameter in children is yet to be established and documented.

Laboratory confirmation of specific IgE antibody synthesis to specific allergens is helpful but not mandatory in every patient with seasonal allergic rhinitis. These laboratory tests should be considered in those patients in whom the presence of a seasonal pattern is not clear-cut. In other patients, it can be helpful to confirm the clinical impression with documentation of specific IgE antibodies by in vivo skin testing or in vitro serum immunoassay testing to reinforce the importance of environmental control. Skin testing with the suspected allergens is mandatory in all patients prior to initiation of immunotherapy with allergy extracts because the intensity of the local wheal-and-flare skin reaction will be utilized as a guide in determining the initial dose of allergen. Clinicians should be selective in the use of allergens for skin testing and should employ only *common* allergens of potential clinical importance in their patients. The most useful allergens in the study of allergic rhinitis in children are the pollens, molds, house dust mite, and cat and dog danders. Allergens used for skin testing should be selected on the basis of prevalence in the patient's area of the country and the environment in which he or she lives.

There is no need to test for allergy to foods in children with clear-cut seasonal allergic rhinitis; food allergy skin testing should be reserved for those children whose conditions are diagnostic problems, with intermittent or perennial symptoms. The major problem with skin testing, especially for food allergens, has been the lack of potency, stability, and purity of the allergen solutions. The crude, undefined composition of allergens often produces false-positive reactions secondary to an irritating effect on the skin. It is well known that great care must be used in interpreting the results of food skin testing because there is often a discrepancy between the production of clinical symptoms and positive skin reactions to foods. If allergy testing is indicated, there is no need to test with a multitude of allergens. The clinician should selectively use those allergens which best correlate with the history.

To avoid false-negative skin tests, antihistamine drugs should be withheld for 36 hr before skin tests are performed. Prick skin testing usually precedes intradermal skin testing; the specifics of skin testing are outlined in standard allergy textbooks (18). Skin testing in children can be performed as early as 1 month of age but positive skin tests for allergens with seasonal exposure such as pollens should not be performed before 2 or 3 years of age.

As mentioned earlier, the in vitro serum immunoassay (RAST, FAST, ELISA) tests for assessing the presence of serum IgE antibodies to various allergens has been employed as a diagnostic aid in allergic rhinitis. For certain allergens, these tests have been shown to be as reliable as skin tests; however, their cost has been a major disadvantage. In addition, skin testing is 10–20% more sensitive than the serum immunoassays. Table 2 compares the usefulness of allergy skin testing as compared to serum IgE antibody testing.

Nasal provocation tests are rarely utilized in assessing rhinitis in children. The sublingual challenge with allergen is not a useful diagnostic tool for allergic

Table 2 Comparison of Skin Testing and In Vitro Serum Assays for Specific IgE Antibodies

Skin test	Serum immunoassay
Less expensive	No patient risk
Greater sensitivity	Patient convenience
Wide allergen selection	Not influenced by drugs
Results available immediately	Results are quantitative
Will detect non-IgE-mediated allergic reactions	Preferable to skin testing in: Patients with dermographism Patients with widespread dermatitis Uncooperative children

rhinitis, in the opinion of this author. The in vitro cytotoxic leukocyte test with foods and other allergens was shown not helpful as a laboratory test in controlled studies and is not recommended (19).

VI. Differential Diagnosis

Children who present to the clinician with complaints of rhinorrhea and nasal obstruction may have symptoms not only of allergy but also of infections, foreign bodies, structural changes, drug reactions, or neoplasms. Nasal infections are usually characterized by burning and redness of the nasal mucosa and a purulent discharge. Without doubt, the common cold virus is the most frequent cause of URI, and at its outset a viral URI with its clear watery rhinorrhea and sneezing resembles allergic rhinitis. Redness of the nasal mucosa is characteristic of URI and distinguishes it from allergic rhinitis. After several days, the purulent nature of the nasal discharge clearly identifies the presence of infection, or in a confusing clinical situation, demonstration of the predominance of neutrophils on a smear of nasal secretions will confirm that impression. One must realize that nasal infections can be superimposed on allergic rhinitis.

Nasal obstruction and rhinorrhea, usually purulent, can also occur with foreign objects in the nares. However, usually the symptoms are unilateral, and this differentiates the presence of foreign objects from allergic or infectious rhinitis.

Another cause of unilateral nasal obstruction may be deviation of the nasal septum or a neoplasm; both conditions are detectable on visual examination of the nasal airway.

Nasal obstruction can also occur because of nasal polyps, which may not be associated with allergic disease but can be associated with cystic fibrosis or, rarely, with aspirin sensitivity. Polyps can usually be demonstrated by inspection and the use of a vasoconstrictor to reduce the local edema that may obscure the nasal polyps.

The most common drug rhinopathy is rhinitis medicamentosa following intranasal topical administration of vasoconstrictors for more than 1 week. The mucosa becomes erythematous and edematous, unlike the situation seen in allergic rhinitis. It is important to question patients carefully to diagnose this condition, because some patients will consider the use of nose drops insignificant in their medical history. Frequently, the seasonal allergic rhinitis or the URI for which the topical vasoconstrictor was initially applied has subsided by the time it is recognized that the problem is being perpetuated by the topical therapy. Another cause for nasal congestion is pregnancy, which may be considered in appropriate adolescent patients.

The aforementioned conditions can usually be differentiated from allergic rhinitis, but the separation of allergic from nonallergic perennial rhinitis is often complicated. Nonallergic rhinitis may occur during childhood but more often is seen in adults. It temporally simulates the perennial type of allergic rhinitis, but no immunological etiology can be implicated.

When nasal eosinophilia is present, but the allergist is unable to document specific IgE antibodies by serum or skin testing, the syndrome is diagnosed as nonallergic rhinitis with eosinophilia (NARES). NARES is much less common in children than in adults.

Vasomotor rhinitis is a nonallergic form of persistent nasal disease also manifested by watery rhinorrhea and nasal obstruction. Eosinophils are not seen in nasal secretions, and increased mast cells and basophils are not detected in the nasal epithelium. Vasomotor rhinitis is a vague category of chronic or intermittent nasal disease usually seen in older children and adults and more common in females than males. Because its pathogenesis is ill defined, it does not lend itself to a specific definition. The patient complains of overresponsiveness of the nose to minimal changes of air temperature, obnoxious odors, and often change in position of the head. Some patients seem to have unusual awareness of their symptoms and complain disproportionately to their magnitude.

VII. Therapy

Successful therapy of allergic rhinitis involves three primary considerations: (1) identification and avoidance of the specific allergens and other contributory factors, (2) pharmacological management, and (3) immunotherapy to alter the patient's immune response to the allergen.

A. Identification and Avoidance

Complete avoidance of the allergens is the best therapy for allergic disease because without exposure to allergens the allergic reaction will not take place. Once the specific allergens that are responsible for the symptoms are identified, each patient should make some effort to reduce the exposure to these allergens. Elimination of exposure to an animal dander by removal of a pet from the house may provide complete or partial relief of symptoms. Avoidance of more ubiquitous allergens such as pollens, dust, and molds may be more difficult.

Children who are sensitive to grass pollens should avoid increased exposure through gardening and grass cutting during the grass pollen season. Camping trips and picnics in the countryside should be postponed by ragweed-sensitive patients during the ragweed pollen seasons until another time of the year. Pollen rubbed into the nose and eyes can produce severe local edema, a point particularly important to remember in dealing with children, who often play outdoors in close contact with pollinating plants. Therefore, allergic patients should avoid direct contact with pollinating plants.

House dust control measures, especially in the bedroom, can often be an effective treatment for patients allergic to house dust mite. These measures include providing rubberized or plastic airtight enclosures for mattresses and box springs; the use of synthetic bedding fabrics; and the removal of carpets, stuffed toys or stuffed furniture, heavy drapery, and dust catchers, such as bookshelves and record cabinets, from the bedroom. Washing bedclothes in hot water ($>130°F$) will kill the mite and is recommended for all dust mite laden items. Thorough weekly cleaning and vacuuming of the bedding and rugs in the bedroom effectively reduces the house dust mite allergen concentration.

Electrostatic precipitrons or HEPA filters can be installed in central forced-air heating and cooling systems, and these can substantially reduce not only house dust but also pollens and other airborne particles. Single-room air conditioners, which recirculate the air, can also effectively reduce pollen in the bedroom. Because single-room electrostatic precipitron units are less effective and may generate irritating ozone, they are not recommended. Mold-sensitive patients should be advised against raking leaves, since the outdoor molds, especially *Alternaria* and *Hormodendrum*, thrive on dead leaves and cut vegetation. Damp basements and moist wallpaper, as well as glass-enclosed shower stalls, are often sources of molds in the home, and removal of the source of moisture will eliminate mold proliferation. If the moisture cannot be eliminated, mold retardants can be incorporated into the house paints or used in washing the walls. Molds in damp basements can be reduced by aerosolized paraformaldehyde or other antifungal agents. It is unfortunate that many parents do not have sufficient motivation to carry out adequate avoidance procedures to control their children's symptoms.

B. Pharmacological Management

Antihistamines

If the child cannot completely avoid the allergen, the symptoms can be controlled with medications in most cases. Antihistamines are preferred for treating mild to moderate allergic rhinitis. The antihistamines function by competing with histamine, the principal mediator of allergic rhinitis, for the H_1 receptor on sensory nerves, endothelial cells, and smooth muscle cells (in asthma) (20). There are several groups of antihistamines, which differ in chemical structure and in action. Antihistamines are classified into two major groups; the first-generation (classic) antihistamines, which are lipophilic, enter the central nervous system and cause sedation. The newer (second-generation), nonsedating antihistamines are lipophobic and tend not to enter the central nervous system (Table 3). Therefore, the clinician should become familiar with the use of one or more antihistamines in each of the listed groupings.

The effectiveness of the classic antihistamines is frequently hampered by their side effects, which include drowsiness, lethargy, interference with perfor-

Table 3 Representative Antihistamines for Oral Therapy of Allergic Rhinitis

Generic name	Brand name	Sedative effect
First generation		
Alkylamines		
Chlorpheniramine	Chlor-Trimeton	Mild
Dexchlorpheniramine	Polaramine	Mild
Brompheniramine	Dimetane	Moderate
Triprolidine	Actidil	Moderate
Ethylenediamines		
Tripelennamine	Pyribenzamine	Moderate
Methapyrilene	Histadyl	Moderate
Ethanolamines		
Diphenhydramine	Benadryl	Marked
Carbinoxamine	Clistin	Moderate
Doxylamine	Decapryn	Moderate
Second generation		
Fexofenadine	Allegra	None
Astemizole	Hismanal	None
Loratadine	Claritin	None
Cetirizine	Zyrtec	Minimal

mance tasks in school, cholinergic effects or dryness, and less often hyperactivity. Adolescents should be warned to be wary of bicycle, motorcycle, or automobile traffic after taking classic antihistamines.

The pharmacokinetics of the antihistamines are listed in Table 4. Whereas the active metabolite of terfenadine, fexofenadine, has a half-life similar to the parent terfenadine, the active metabolite of astemizole has a much more prolonged half-life of more than 1 week and clinically has a prolonged effect in patients for many weeks after being discontinued. Since terfenadine and astemizole are metabolized in the liver, their metabolism may be prolonged in patients with liver disease or if taken with an inhibitor of the P450 cytochrome oxidase such as ketoconazole or erythromycin (Table 5). Terfenadine and astemizole should not be given together with ketoconazole or erythromycin because of the possibility of prolonged metabolism increasing blood levels of the antihistamines and inducing a rare cardiac arrhythmia, torsades de pointes.

Vasoconstrictors

Antihistamines provide good symptomatic control of pruritus, sneezing, and rhinorrhea but do not relieve congestion or stuffiness. When nasal obstruction is a prominent symptom, an alpha-adrenergic decongestant, such as phenylephrine,

Table 4 Pharmacokinetics of H_1 Antihistamines and Their Pharmacological Active Metabolites

H_1 receptor antagonist	Peak level (hr)	Half-life (hr)	Clearance rate (ml/min/kg)
Terfenadine	1.0	18	NA
Fexofenadine[a]	3.0	17	600
Astemizole	0.6	26	1500
N-Desmethylastemizole[a]	NA	228	NA
Loratadine	1.0	11	200
Descarboethoxyloratadine[a]	1.5	17	NA
Cetirizine	1.0	7.4	1.0
Acrivastine	0.9	1.4	4.6
Chlorpheniramine	2.8	28	1.8

[a]Indicates the active metabolite and values are those for healthy young adults; values are means. NA, not available.

phenylpropanolamine, or pseudoephedrine, can be used individually or in combination with an antihistamine to alleviate nasal mucosal engorgment, to decrease the nasal obstruction, and to improve the upper airway ventilation. Sometimes, it is necessary to employ one or more trials of an antihistamine or antihistamine-decongestant combination to ascertain the most effective preparation for each patient.

Topical nasal alpha-adrenergic vasoconstrictors usually provide prompt symptomatic relief but should not be used for more than 1 week. Many patients, after some weeks of using a topical decongestant, will develop so-called rebound vasodilatation and at times habituation. It is necessary to discontinue nose drops to relieve this "rhinitis medicamentosa."

Table 5 Factors Affecting Metabolism of Antihistamines

Half-lives prolonged
  Hepatic dysfunction
  Microsomal oxygenase inhibitors
    Ketoconazole
    Erythromycin
    Others
  Elderly patients
  Renal disease (cetirizine, acrivastine)
Half-lives shortened
  Children (?)

Topical Corticosteroids

If symptoms cannot be controlled with antihistamines, decongestants, and avoidance, clinicians utilize intranasal topical corticosteroid therapy. In pediatric patients, the risk-to-benefit ratio of treating even severe allergic rhinitis with oral or parenteral corticosteroids is so high that we feel that those routes of administration are usually contraindicated. However, aerosol topical corticosteroids, especially for short-term seasonal use, have proved useful in children and adolescents. According to the product description, they are not recommended in infants or children less than 6 years, but according to anecdotal experience, clinicians have used them in children as young as 2 years of age. There was no suppression of longitudinal growth in children or suppression of the children's response to ACTH in the efficacy and safety trials of these intranasal steroids prior to Food and Drug Administration approval in the United States. However, intranasal budesonide, given in a dosage of 200 µg twice daily but not once daily, may suppress short-term bone growth as measured by knemometry (21). Therefore, these safety issues may require better definition in children who chronically use intranasal corticosteroids. An intranasal corticosteroid should be given once daily in the morning in the lowest dosage that can control the symptoms.

Currently available in the United States are five topical intranasal steroids: beclomethasone dipropionate, flunisolide, triamcinolone, budesonde, and fluticasone propionate. Each of these five agents were efficacious as compared to placebo but there are no head-to-head trials that recommend one versus another.

Beclomethasone dipropionate and triamcinalone are available as a metered-dose inhaler or an aqueous pump spray, which is better tolerated by some adults and especially young children. The other topical steroids that effectively control symptoms of allergic rhinitis include budesonide, available as a metered-dose inhaler (and an aqueous spray outside the United States), and funisolide and fluticasone propionate, available as a pump spray. These topical agents appear to achieve better compliance in adults than in children, perhaps because adults tolerate the inconvenience or discomfort associated with the intranasal delivery systems better than children.

Cromolyn

Another topical aerosol anti-inflammation pharmacological agent that has gained acceptance for the treatment of allergic rhinitis is cromolyn sodium (sodium cromoglycate), which is believed to inhibit the release of mediators from mast cells. Although European investigators have found the drug to be effective in 75% of patients treated, such high efficacy has not been reported in a study of allergic rhinitis patients in the United States (22). Since there are minimal potential or deleterious side effects associated with the use of intranasal topical cromolyn as compared with intranasal corticosteroids, cromolyn should be considered in children who require continuous long-term therapy. However, the need for spraying 4 times daily considerably reduces patient compliance, especially in children who need to carry the spray with them at school.

C. Immunotherapy

If symptomatic drug therapy and avoidance cannot adequately control symptoms or inadvertently provoke significant side effects, immunotherapy (hyposensitization) with allergen solutions should be considered. Before proceeding with immunotherapy, the physician should institute a comprehensive investigation of the causative factors, and the patient's history of symptoms should be closely correlated with the presence of specific IgE antibodies, determined either by skin test results or by an in vitro immunoassay. Positive results of skin or blood tests that do not confirm the clinical presentation are considered false-positive reactions and are not used as criteria for immunotherapy. the abuse and the use of these false-positive test results contribute to unnecessary and unsuccessful immunotherapy.

In several double-blind studies, immunotherapy or hyposensitization injections with solutions of pollen have been shown to be effective in reducing the symptoms of allergic rhinitis (23). More recently, immunotherapy has been shown to decrease the mediators of inflammation in nasal secretions following intranasal allergen provocation challenge in patients with allergic rhinitis. Studies of the clinical efficacy of nonpollen immunotherapy with house dust, molds, and animal dander allergens in perennial allergic rhinitis are not as conclusive as those reported for seasonal allergy (24).

There is no place for immunotherapy with allergens that can be easily removed or avoided. This is especially true for food allergens. The use of animal danders for immunotherapy should be limited to those individuals who cannot avoid exposure to animal allergens. Even though it is not known precisely how immunotherapy promotes clinical improvement in allergic rhinitis, studies have shown a reasonable relationship between the higher doses of allergens administered, a decrease in specific IgE antibodies as measured by RAST over a period of months, an increase in IgG-blocking antibodies, an increase in the number of allergen-specific suppression T lymphocytes, and a reduction in the release of histamine in vitro (25–27).

After the decision is made to initiate immunotherapy, the clinician should carefully select the allergens to be employed. The clinical history should be correlated with skin test results, and the magnitude of the local skin reaction should be a guide to the dose of allergen to initiate injection therapy. This author does not agree with the suggestion that immunotherapy be initiated based on the results of in vitro serum immunoassay. Not only does this hypothesis lack adequate documentation and clinical confirmation, but also it contributes to remote provision of clinical care by nonphysician health providers who do not see or examine the patient. End-point titration skin testing has also been recommended as a guide for initiation of immunotherapy, but this suggestion adds significantly to the cost of skin testing and also requires better documentation as well as confirmation prior to widespread acceptance.

Immunotherapy may be expected to provide significant clinical improvement in 80–90% of children with pollen-induced allergic rhinitis. If improvement is not obtained after a 2-year trial with immunotherapy, the patient should be reevaluated, and discontinuation of immunotherapy should be considered. Duration of immunotherapy injections in children who achieve clinical benefits is dependent on the patient's overall clinical response. In the presence of clinical improvement, the child should be given the opportunity to see whether the clinical benefits are sustained after the allergy immunotherapy is discontinued. These patients should be given the opportunity to stop their immunotherapy after approximately 3–5 years of injections.

Many children with allergic rhinitis tend to improve with time, but they are not "growing out" of the allergy because improvement is not related to physical growth but to an as yet undefined immunological tolerance. It has been claimed that immunotherapy in children for seasonal allergic rhinitis may reduce their chances of developing pollen-induced asthma, but this report is open to some questions and has never been confirmed (28).

In general, patients with seasonal allergic rhinitis are more responsive to immunotherapy than those with perennial allergic rhinitis. The factors responsible for clinical improvement are multiple. Certain patients have exacerbations of symptoms after a spontaneous or induced remission for several seasons, and immunotherapy can be reinstituted without complication. Overall, the prognosis of allergic rhinitis, with or without therapy, is better than that for nonallergic and vasomotor rhinitis.

VIII. Conclusions

Rhinitis, allergic and nonallergic, is the most common chronic condition that affects children with peak prevalence in adolescents. The prevalence of allergic rhinitis in children has been reported to have increased the past 10 years in both the United States and Europe. Whether this is due to enhanced recognition or an increase in absolute number of patients has not yet been defined. Upper respiratory viral infections (common cold) are the most common cause of nonallergic rhinitis. The genetic and familial basis of allergic rhinitis is multifactorial and newly developed molecular biological technology will help in better defining its heredity. The definition of IgE-mediated immunological mechanisms in the pathogenesis of allergic rhinitis has enhanced diagnosis by specifically identifying the specific inhalant allergens responsible for provoking the allergic reaction. However, the patient's history and physical examination are most important in establishing the diagnosis of allergic rhinitis. The therapy of allergic rhinitis consists of (1) avoidance of specific causative allergens, (2) appropriate pharmacotherapy, and (3) immunotherapy. Much progress has been made in improving the pharmacotherapy of allergic rhinitis. The introduction of the second-generation (less sedating) antihistamine and intranasal corticosteroids has benefited many patients. For those patients not improved with environmental control and pharmacotherapy, allergen immunotherapy may be indicated. Although not a fatal condition, rhinitis has significant impact on quality of life and deserves appropriate diagnostic and therapeutic management.

Acknowledgment

This work was supported in part by NIH Grants RO1AI19262 and MO1RR00084.

References

1. Newacheck PN, Stoddard JJ. Prevalence and impact of multiple childhood chronic illnesses. J Pediatr 1994; 124:26–28.
2. Wütrich B. Epidemiology of the allergic diseases: are they really on the increase? Int Arch Allergy Appl Immunol 1989; 90:3–10.
3. Aberg N. Asthma and allergic rhinitis in Swedish conscripts. Clin Exp Allergy 1989; 19:59–63.
4. Wright AL, Holberg CJ, Murtney FD, et al. Epidemiology of physician diagnosed allergic rhinitis in children. Pediatrics 1994; 94:895–901.
5. Wald ER, Guerra N, Byers C. Upper respiratory tract infections in young children: duration and frequency of complications. Pediatrics 1991; 98:129–37.
6. Broder I, Higgins MW, Mathews KP, et al. Epidemiology of asthma and allergic rhinitis in a total community, Tecumseh, Michigan. III. Second survey of community. J Allergy Clin Immunol 1974; 53:127.
7. Johnstone DE. Food allergy in children under two years of age. Pediatr Clin North Am 1969; 6:211.
8. Brown EB, Ipsen J. Changes in severity of symptoms of asthma and allergic rhinitis due to air pollutants. J Allergy 1968; 41:254.
9. Wolf S, Holmes TH, Treuting T, et al. An experimental approach to psychosomatic phenomenon in rhinitis and asthma. J Allergy 1950; 21:1.
10. Huang SH, Marsh DG. Immunogenetics of allergic disease In: Middleton E Jr, Reed CF, Ellis EF, eds. Allergy. Principles and Practice. St. Louis: CV Mosby, 1993:60–72.
11. Levine BB, Strembas RH, Fotino M. Ragweed hayfever, genetic control and linkage to HL-A haplotypes. Science 1972; 178:1201.
12. Cookson W, Sharp PA, Fauci JA, et al. Linkage between immnoglobulin E responses underlying asthma, rhinitis and chromosome 11q. Lancet 1989; 1:1292.

13. Bresolin D, et al. Mouth breathing in children: its relationship to dentofacial development. Am J Orthodont 1993; 83:334–340.

14. Simons FE, et al. Adverse central nervous system effects of older antihistamine in children. Pediatr Allergy Immunol 1996; 7:22–27.

15. Bock SA, Atkins FM. Patterns of food hypersensitivity during 16 years of double blind placebo controlled food challenges. J Pediatr 1990; 117:561–567.

16. Caplin I, Haynes FT, Spohn J. Are nasal polyps an allergic phenomenon? Ann Allergy 1971; 29:631.

17. Meltzer EO, Zeiger RS, Schatz M, et al. Chronic rhinitis in infants and children. Pediatr Clin North Am 1983; 39:847.

18. Norman PS. In vivo methods of study of allergy: skin and mucosal tests, techniques and interpretation. In: Middleton E, Reed CD, Ellis EF, eds. Allergy: Principles and Practice. St. Louis: CV Mosby, 1978:256.

19. Liberman P, Crawford L, Bjelland J, et al. Controlled study of the cytotoxic food tests. J Allergy Clin Immunol 1974; 53:89.

20. Paton WDM. Receptors for histamine. In: Schacter M, ed. Histamine and Antihistamines. International Encyclopedia of Pharmacology and Therapeutics. Oxford: Pergamon Press, 1973:Vol 1.

21. Wolthers OD, Pedersen S. Short term growth in children with allergic rhinitis treated with oral antihistamines and intranasal glucocorticoids. Acta Pediatr 1993; 82:635–640.

22. Handelman NI, Friday GA, Schwartz HJ, et al. Cromolyn sodium, nasal solution in the prophylactic treatment of pollen-induced seasonal allergic rhinitis. J Allergy Clin Immunol 1977; 59:237.

23. Sadan N, Rhyne MB, Mellitis ED, et al. Immunotherapy of pollinosis in children. N Engl J Med 1969; 280:623.

24. Van Metre TE Jr, Adkinson NF Jr. Immunotherapy for aeroallergen disease. In: Middleton E Jr, ed. Allergy: Principles and Practice. St. Louis: CV Mosby, 1993: 1489–1509.

25. Creticos PS, Van Metre TE Jr, Mordinez MR, et al. Dose response of IgE and IgG antibodies during ragweed immunotherapy. J Allergy Clin Immunol 1983; 73:94.

26. Tamir R, Costracone JM, Rocklin RE. Generation of suppressor cells in atopic patients during immunotherapy that modulate IgE synthesis. J Allergy Clin Immunol 1987; 79:591.

27. Creticos PS, Marsh DG, Proud D, et al. Responses to ragweed-pollen nasal challenge before and after immunotherapy. J Allergy Cli Immunol 1989; 84:197.

28. Johnstone DE, Dutton A. The value of hyposensitization therapy for bronchial asthma in children: a 14 year study. Pediatrics 1968; 42:793.

24

Rhinitis and Asthma

WILLIAM W. BUSSE

University of Wisconsin Medical School
Madison, Wisconsin

I. Introduction

Asthma and rhinitis are common respiratory diseases that often coexist. Furthermore, and of considerable interest, is the possibility that the severity of asthma is influenced by the activity of rhinitis, and other upper airway diseases. The influence and interaction between asthma and rhinitis exist with allergic rhinitis, sinusitis, and viral upper respiratory infection. These observations raise the possibility that events in the upper airway can influence lower airway disease severity and/or parallel similar events that occur throughout the respiratory tract. The following discussion will focus on the hypothesis that upper respiratory diseases, i.e., allergic rhinitis, sinusitis, or upper respiratory viral infections, influence or promote asthma. Evidence will be reviewed to suggest that events in the upper airway can enhance the severity of asthma and treatment of upper airway disease can reduce the severity of asthma.

II. Interaction Between Allergic Rhinitis and Asthma

Allergic rhinitis and asthma occur together more often than would be expected by chance alone. The prevalence of allergic rhinitis in subjects with asthma ranges from 28 to 50% (1,2). This compares to a prevalence of allergic rhinitis of 10–20% in the general population. Moreover, the prevalence of asthma in hay-fever subjects is 13–38% (1,2); this compares to an estimated prevalence of 5–10% in the general population. These statistics, in particular the high incidence of allergic rhinitis in asthma, are not totally surprising. The allergic mechanisms in both disease states are similar, the allergens that provide symptoms in asthma and allergic rhinitis parallel one another, and the mediator and cellular responses to allergen exposure have similar patterns. However, what is intriguing, and largely unanswered, is the possibility that allergic events in the upper airway, i.e., active rhinitis, can influence lower airway physiology.

Ramsdale et al. (3) used methacholine and isocapnic hyperventilation to measure bronchial hyperresponsiveness in 25 subjects with rhinitis who did not have a diagnosis of asthma. In six subjects,the provocative concentration (PC_{20}) of methacholine that decreased the FEV_1 by 20% was less than 8 mg/ml, in a range of responsiveness found in asthma. There were four additional subjects whose PC_{20} was in the 8–16 mg/ml range. These observations indicate that bronchial responsiveness is increased in subjects with rhinitis. Many interpretations of these data exist including the possibility that the 10 subjects with increased bronchial responsiveness have subclinical asthma. It is also possible that these findings suggest that rhinitis may be a risk factor for asthma and activation of lower airway disease may be an eventual consequence of inflammatory processes in the upper airway. Furthermore, the observations of Ramsdale et al. (3) also raise the possibility that airway hyperresponsiveness is a feature of allergic upper airway disease that may be influenced by factors that intensify rhinitis.

Studies by Corren and associates (4) expand upon the relationship between allergic rhinitis and lower airway dysfunction. In a randomized, crossover design study, these investigators performed nasal challenges with either placebo or antigen. They were careful to prevent introduction of antigen into the lower airway during the nasal challenges. In the 10 subjects studied, nasal allergen challenge provoked an increase in nasal blockade within 30 min of the allergen challenge, when compared to placebo. Baseline levels of airway responsiveness to methacholine were similar on the 2 days of challenge. Normally, there is a diurnal reduction in airway responsiveness in early and late afternoon. This expected decrease in airway responsiveness was seen on the days the subjects were given the placebo nasal challenge. When antigen was used in the nasal challenge, the diurnal variation in bronchial responsiveness was lost and the results suggest an increase in airway responsiveness (Fig. 1).

A number of explanations were put forth by these investigators to explain the link between upper airway allergic responses and the provoked lower airway dysfunction. The possibilities by which active allergic nasal disease can elicit changes in lung function include (1) elicitation of a nasal-bronchial reflex, (2) absorption of mediators or chemotactic factors into the general circulation and

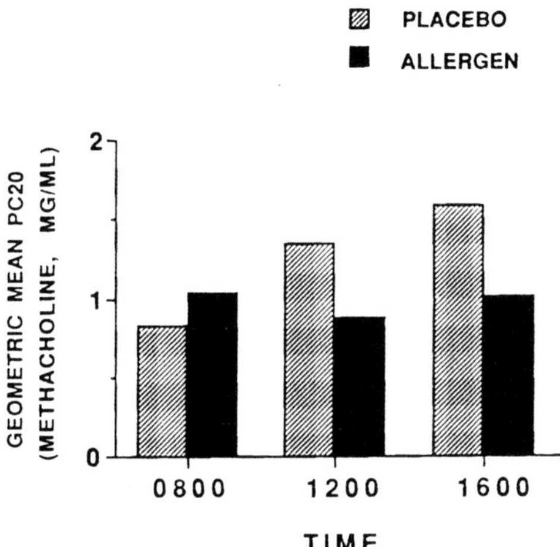

Figure 1 Effect of nasal challenge on bronchial reactivity, expressed as the mean of PC_{20} to inhaled methacholine, comparing change from baseline (0800) for placebo versus allergen ($p = 0.01$). (From Ref. 4.)

transport to the lungs, (3) postnasal drainage of inflammatory mediators to the lower airways, and (4) diminished β-adrenergic responsiveness (4,5). The observations by Corren et al. did not establish the causes for lower airway changes.

To extend these observations, Madonini et al. (6) evaluated the seasonal exposure to antigen on bronchial responsiveness to inhaled carbachol in subjects with allergic rhinitis. Twenty-seven subjects with allergic rhinitis were identified for study. Bronchial provocation with carbachol was performed on two occasions: after the grass pollination season (baseline level of airway responsiveness) and during the time of grass pollination. Preseasonally, three subjects had a PD_{20} carbachol value of <1 mg, which is the usual range found for asthma. Six subjects had a PC_{20} value of 1–2 mg carbachol and the remaining subjects failed to reach a 2-mg cumulative dose of carbachol. However, when measures of bronchial responsiveness were determined during the pollination season, a distinctly different pattern of response was found. Although 10 subjects still failed to respond to a cumulative carbachol dose of 2 mg, that is, remained ''nonasthmatic,'' 13 individuals (48%) now responded in the asthma range.

Although these studies do not identify a mechanism by which lower airway function changes, the observations suggest that alterations in bronchial responsiveness may identify those individuals with ''future asthma'' or patients who may be at risk to become symptomatic with asthma with appropriate allergen exposure.

Insight into mechanisms by which upper airway reactions influence lower airway disease can be obtained from animal studies. Bellofiore et al. (7) used sensitized Brown Norway rats to assess the contribution of upper and lower airways to the changes in pulmonary resistance after inhalation of antigen. In these studies, upper and lower airway resistance to inhaled antigen was determined when the allergen was inhaled through the nose and through a tracheostomy. After inhalation of antigen through the nose, both upper and lower airway resistance increased. Furthermore, the changes in resistance in the upper and lower airway were highly correlative when antigen was given via the nasal route; in contrast, when the antigen, ovalbumin, was introduced through the tracheostomy, lower, but not upper, airway resistance increased. To explore possible mechanisms by which the upper airway allergic response enhanced lower airway function, the animals were pretreated with inhaled atropine. Atropine blocked the increase in lower airway resistance following application of ovalbumin to the upper airway. The investigators interpreted these results to suggest that when rats inhale antigen through the nose, the predominant reaction occurs in the upper airways and the lower airways responses are mediated, in part, by cholinergic mechanisms. Whether similar changes occur in humans with allergic rhinitis is not established. However, those observations suggest that modification of upper airway allergic disease may affect bronchial function.

To extend these observations to treatment effects of the upper airway on lower airway function, Aubier et al. (8) conducted the following study. Eleven allergic rhinitis patients were identified with the aim of the study to compare the effect of an identical dose of nasal or bronchial corticosteroid treatment on bronchial hyperresponsiveness. In this study, the patients received an aerosol dose of 400 µg/day beclomethasone dipropionate into the nose or a similar dose into the lower airway for 2 weeks. After 2 weeks of intranasal beclomethasone, bronchial responsiveness significantly decreased; in contrast, no change in lower airway responsiveness followed 2 weeks of treatment to the lower airway (Fig. 2).

There were a number of surprising results in this study. First, bronchial responsiveness has been shown to improve with bronchial treatment in other studies (9); perhaps the limited treatment time explains these differences. Second, a short course of nasal steroids significantly modified lower airway function but did not affect baseline pulmonary function. These end-points indicate an effect that is not directly on the airways. Although they did not specifically address the subject, the authors did not feel that a ''nasobronchial'' reflex was responsible for the observed changes. However, they did not provide an explanation for their findings.

Additional evidence that upper airway treatment can affect lower bronchial function comes from a study by Watson et al. (10). Twenty-one subjects (aged 7–17 years) with perennial allergic rhinitis and asthma, and airway hyperrespon-

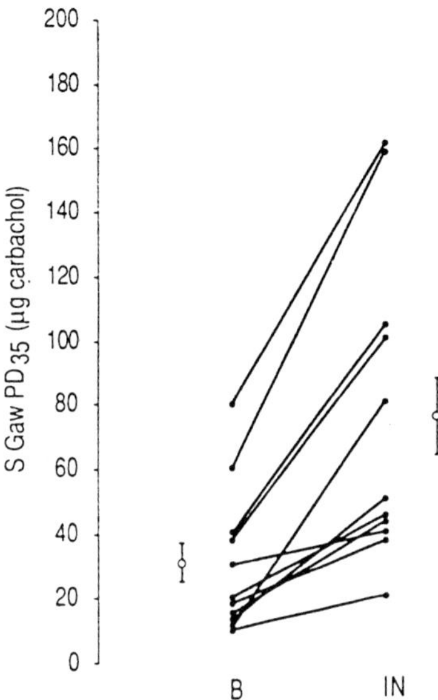

Figure 2 Individual (closed circles) values of SGaw PD_{35} in pollen-allergic patients measured as baseline (B) and after 2 weeks of nasal administration of intranasal beclomethasone dipropionate (IN). Open circle represent the group mean values ($\pm$SEM). (From Ref. 8.)

siveness (PC_{20}) of less than 8 mg/ml methacholine, were recruited and treated with beclomethasone dipropionate (400 µg/day) or placebo (Fig. 3). The results parallel those of Aubier et al. (8). As expected, rhinitis symptom scores decreased significantly on treatment with nasal steroids. There was also a trend for asthma scores to decrease even though asthma was very mild in these individuals. Most relevant to our discussion was the significant improvement in bronchial responsiveness that followed 4 weeks of nasal corticosteroid treatment. The authors indicate that the steroid benefit is not related to deposition of medication into the lungs as less than 2% was found to enter the chest. Second, it is unlikely that systemic absorption of corticosteroids gave the generalized effect on the airway. Other possibilities include a suppression of upper airway inflammation and with this change a diminished airway signal for inflammation.

Not all nasal anti-inflammatory therapy will affect lower airway dysfunction. Reed et al. (11) studied 120 adult patients with seasonal allergic rhinitis. Of these, 58 had a history of asthma during the ragweed pollen season. The enrolled subjects were treated with intranasal placebo, cromolyn sodium, flunisolide, or beclomethasone dipropionate. All active forms of treatment were more

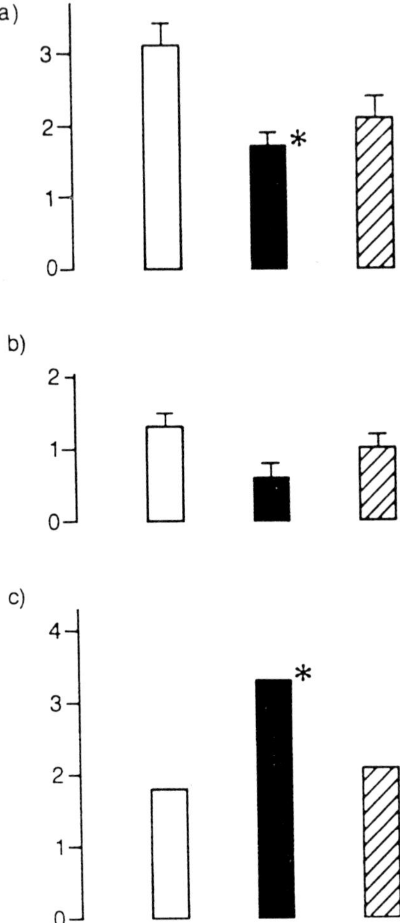

Figure 3 Effect of treatment of global assessments: baseline (open bars), intranasal aqueous beclomethasone dipropionate (closed bars), and placebo (hatched bars). (a) Rhinitis scores decreased significantly after corticosteroid treatment. (b) Asthma symptom scores showed no significant difference. (c) Mean PC_{20} methacholine increased significantly after intranasal corticosteroid treatment ($*p = 0.04$). (From Ref. 10.)

effective than placebo in reducing nasal symptoms of allergic rhinitis. However, only the topical corticosteroids were effective in diminishing asthma symptoms. The authors speculate that one explanation for the benefit of the nasal steroids on asthma is a restoration of normal nasal physiology. As a consequence of these changes, nasal functions, including warming, humidification, and filtration of airborne allergens, particularly ragweed pollen, occur and with this, lesser amounts of antigen enter the lower airway.

The studies quoted all have a common theme: upper airway allergic disease can significantly influence lower airway function. What remains to be fully established is the mechanism associated with worsening of bronchial responsiveness with activation of allergic rhinitis, and the converse, improvement of asthma features with corticosteroid treatment of active allergic upper airway disease.

III. Sinusitis and Asthma

Sinusitis is a complication of severe rhinitis and viral upper respiratory infections (12). A frequent sequela in patients with existing asthma is a worsening of lower airway disease with sinusitis (13). Rachelefsky et al. (14) were early observers of this relationship in children. Forty-eight children with asthma were identified to have chronic daytime and nighttime symptoms of cough and wheeze. All of these individuals were under active treatment for asthma. Sinus Water's radiographs revealed abnormalities in all 48 children: mucosal thickening, maxillary sinus opacification, or air-fluid levels. All children were empirically treated with antibiotics. At the completion of antibiotic treatment, nearly 80% had normal sinus radiographs. Of those tested, 67% now had normal pulmonary functions. Finally, at the completion of treatment, only 21% required bronchodilator treatment. Although limited in its scope, this study provides some evidence that sinusitis, like allergic rhinitis, can affect lower airway disease.

Brugman and co-workers (15) developed a rabbit model to identify mechanisms associated with lower airway changes in sinusitis. Rabbits have well-developed maxillary sinuses, which are accessible for treatment. In this study, 6-month-old New Zealand white rabbits had lower airway physiology measured including bronchial responsiveness. Maxillary sinuses were then injected with the active complement component C5a to cause an inflammatory process. Following the C5a injection, the rabbits had an increase in bronchial responsiveness.

To extend these studies and attempt to characterize mechanisms for these changes, the following experiments were conducted. Animals received C5a in the knee bursa to determine whether an ''off-site'' inflammatory response could elicit lower airway changes. In addition, rabbits were intubated prior to the C5a injection, injected but kept in the head-down position, or injected in the head-down position and then maintained in the upright position. Only in the animals who were upright and not intubated were changes in bronchial responsiveness to the C5a injection noted.

These observations, with obvious limitations, suggest that ''drainage'' of material to the lower airway may contribute to changes in airway function. Whether it is mediators, cytokines, or other factors has not been established, nor has it been identified that inflammatory factors are generated in the sinuses and directly enter the lower airway. Nonetheless, sinusitis exacerbates asthma and the search for a mechanism continues.

IV. The Effect of Viral Respiratory Infections on Asthma

In older children and young adults, upper respiratory tract infections are a major cause of wheezing. Duff and colleagues at the University of Virginia (16) evaluated children who presented to an emergency room with acute episodes of wheezing. In children less than 2 years of age, nearly 70% of those presenting with wheezing had virus grown on culture of their airway secretions; respiratory syncytial virus was the major infection associated with wheezing in these young children. In contrast, children greater than 2 years of age with wheezing had virus cultured in only 30% of such episodes, and the respiratory virus detected in these children was rhinovirus. Since rhinovirus is an infection of the upper airways, it underscores the focus of this discussion—upper airway events influence lower airway function.

To further evaluate this situation, the investigators calculated the odds ratio for wheezing in these two groups of children. In children greater than 2 years of age, allergy and the presence of virus were the risk factors associated with wheezing. These studies indicate an age-dependent relationship between the infecting virus and the possibility that the coexistence of allergic disease is a major risk factor for children over 2 years of age to wheeze with respiratory infections.

Johnston and colleagues (17) at Southampton evaluated 108 children, aged 9–11 years, over a 13-month period. In this study population, episodes of increased asthma or symptoms of an upper respiratory infection were noted by the subjects and evaluated by measurements of lung function and collection of airway secretions for virus culture and virus RNA. Over 80% of the wheezing episodes in these children were associated with viral respiratory infections. Furthermore, using the technique of RT-PCR, rhinovirus was noted in 60% of the wheezing episodes. The observations by Johnston and his co-workers indicate the importance of upper respiratory tract infections to asthma exacerbations. This study underscores the importance of viral upper respiratory infections to exacerbations of wheezing in children.

V. Mechanisms of Rhinovirus-Induced Wheezing

A number of mechanisms have been proposed to explain how respiratory viruses induce asthma including a direct cytopathic effect of the virus upon the lower airway. If respiratory viruses replicate in the lower airway, they could damage airway epithelium and alter lung function, including an increase in airway responsiveness. Other possible causative factors include the generation of upper airway mediators and their aspiration into the lower airway, release of proinflammatory cytokines by viruses into the airway, and reflex bronchospasm secondary to infection of the upper airway.

To address the effect that rhinoviruses may have on airway inflammation, Lemanske et al. (18) evaluated the effect of a rhinovirus upper respiratory tract infection on bronchial responsiveness and the airway response to inhaled allergen in 10 individuals with allergic rhinitis. The investigators found the experimental rhinovirus infection to increase airway responsiveness to inhaled histamine as well as the immediate airway response to inhaled antigen.

More importantly, Lemanske and co-workers (18) observed that the frequency of late allergic reactions to inhaled allergen increased during the acute rhinovirus infection. Prior to the infection, one of 10 subjects had a late allergic reaction. At the time of the acute infection, eight of the 10 subjects had late reaction to an allergen challenge. Furthermore, when evaluated 4 weeks after recovery from the viral respiratory infection, five of seven individuals continued to have a late reaction to allergen challenge. These observations suggest that one mechanism by which respiratory viruses promote airway hyperresponsiveness and the possibility of wheezing is through an enhancement of those factors that cause the development of the late allergic reaction, a model for allergen-driven inflammation.

In a subsequent study, Calhoun and co-workers (19) used bronchoscopy and segmental challenge of the airway with antigen to evaluate the effects of a rhinovirus infection on allergic inflammatory response in the airway. In this study, subjects were seen on three separate occasions: (1) precold, (2) during acute respiratory infection, and (3) 3–4 weeks post infection. During each study period, the subjects had two bronchoscopies. At the first bronchoscopy, antigen was introduced into the airway and lavage was performed immediately afterward. This approach evaluated the effect of antigen on the acute allergic response, which is characterized by mast cell activation and mediator release. Forty-eight hours later bronchoscopy was repeated, and the same airway segments were identified and relavaged. The timing of this procedure allowed for the measurement of those features associated with late allergic reactions, i.e., the inflammatory response. When bronchoscopy and antigen challenge were conducted during the acute rhinovirus upper respiratory tract infection, mast cell histamine release to antigen was increased. More importantly, eosinophil recruitment measured 48 hr after antigen challenge was also greater during the acute virus infection. The increase in eosinophil recruitment was still detected 4 weeks after the acute respiratory infection. These studies suggest that an experimental rhinovirus infection of the upper airway promotes allergen-driven inflammatory responses in the lower airway and this enhancement in the response to antigen is seen predominantly in those features associated with the late allergic inflammatory response, i.e., eosinophils.

VI. Conclusions

Rhinitis can have a significant influence on lower respiratory problems, including asthma. There is clear evidence that activation of allergic rhinitis, the development of sinusitis, or acquisition of a viral upper respiratory infection can enhance asthma symptoms. Conversely, treatment of allergic rhinitis can be beneficial to asthma. A major goal needs to be an identification of the mechanism by which rhinitis can worsen asthma.

References

1. Sibbald B, Strachen DP. Epidemiology of rhinitis. In: Busse WW, Holgate ST, eds, Asthma and Rhinitis. Boston: Blackwell Scientific Publications, 1995: 32–43.
2. Wesbie ER. Epidemiology of hayfever and perennial allergic rhinitis. Monogr Allergy 1987; 21:1–20.
3. Ramsdale EH, Morris MM, Robert RS, Hargreave FE. Asymptomatic bronchial hyperresponsiveness in rhinitis. J Allergy Clin Immunol 1985; 75:573–577.
4. Corren J, Adinoff AD, Irvin CG. Changes in bronchial responsiveness following nasal provocation with allergen. J Allergy Clin Immunol 1992; 89:611–618.
5. Adinoff AD, Irvin CG. Upper respiratory tract disease and asthma. Semin Respir Med 1987; 8:308–314.
6. Madonini E, Briatico-Vangosa G, Pappacoda A, Maccagui G, Cardani A, Saporiti F. Seasonal increase of bronchial reactivity in allergic rhinitis. J Allergy Clin Immunol 1987; 79:358–363.
7. Bellofiore S, DiMara GU, Martin JG. Changes in upper and lower airway resistance after inhalation of antigen in sensitized rats. Am Rev Respir Dis 1987; 136:363–368.
8. Aubier M, Levy J, Clerici C, Neukirch F, Herman D. Different effects of nasal and bronchial glucocorticosteroid administration on bronchial hyperresponsiveness in patients with allergic rhinitis. Am Rev Respir Dis 1992; 146:122–126.
9. Ryan G, Latimer KOM, Juniper EF, Roberts RS, Hargreave FE. Effect of beclomethasone dipropionate on bronchial responsiveness to histamine in controlled nonsteroid-dependent asthma. J Allergy Clin Immunol 1985; 75:25–30.
10. Watson WTA, Becker AB, Simons FER. Treatment of allergic rhinitis with intranasal corticosteroids in patients with mild asthma, effect on lower airway responsiveness. J Allergy Clin Immunol 1993; 91:97–101.
11. Reed CE, Marcoux JP, Welsh PW. Effects of topical nasal treatment on asthma symptoms. J Allergy Clin Immunol 1988; 81:1042–1047.
12. Kern EB. Sinusitis. J Allergy Clin Immunol 1984; 73:25–31.

13. Druce HM, Slavin RG. Sinusitis: a critical need for further study. J Allergy Clin Immunol 1991; 88:675–677.
14. Rachelefsky GS, Katz RM, Siegel SC. Chronic sinus disease with associated reactive airway disease in children. Pediatrics 1984; 73:526–529.
15. Brugman SM, Larsen GC, Henson PM, Honor S, Irvin CG. Increased lower airways responsiveness associated with sinusitis in a rabbit model. Am Rev Respir Dis 1993; 147:314–320.
16. Duff AL, Pomeranz ES, Gelber LE, Rice GW, Farris H, Hayden FG, Platts-Mills TAE, Heymann PW. Risk factors or acute wheezing in infants and children: viruses, passive smoke, and IgE antibodies to inhalant allergens. Pediatrics 1993; 92:535–540.
17. Johnston SL, Pattemore PK, Sanderson G, Smith S, Lawn F, Josephs L, Symington P, O'Toole S, Myint SH, Tyrell DAJ, Holgate ST. Community study of role of viral infections in exacerbations of asthma in 9–11 year old children. Br Med J 1995; 310:1225–1228.
18. Lemanske RF Jr, Dick EC, Swenson CA, Vrtis RF, Busse WW. Rhinovirus upper respiratory infection increases airway hyperreactivity and late asthmatic reactions. J Clin Invest 1989; 83:1–10.
19. Calhoun WJ, Dick EC, Schwartz LB, Busse WW. A common cold virus, rhinovirus 16, potentiates airway inflammation after segmental antigen bronchoprovocation in allergic subjects. J Clin Invest 1994; 94:2200–2208.

25

Rhinitis and Otitis

PAUL VAN CAUWENBERGE and DE-YUN WANG

University Hospital Ghent
Ghent, Belgium

I. Introduction

Rhinitis and otitis media are both inflammatory diseases, one of the nasal cavity and the other of middle ear mucosa. The etiology and pathogenesis of these two diseases are multifactorial and the exact mechanisms of both disease processes are not fully understood, though there is continuity of the mucous membrane from the nose to the tympanic cavity via the eustachian tube. Nasal and middle ear diseases are both frequent health problems and they may often occur at the same time in the patients.

During the last decades, the etiological relationship between rhinitis and otitis media, especially the role of allergy in otitis media with effusion (OME), has been the subject of much controversy. Uncontrolled studies report the incidence of respiratory allergy in children with OME to range from 4% to over 90% (1).

Many important questions still need to be firmly answered; for example, does a child with allergic rhinitis have a high incidence of middle ear disease? If true, which kind of therapeutic strategy should be implicated in these children? Can OME be cured by treating the underlying nasal or sinus infection?

To better understand these entities, it is important to know the pathophysiological mechanism by which allergy or other nasal pathologies influence middle ear disease. On the other hand, there is a need to perform longitudinal epidemiological studies on these diseases with a comparable or standardized methodology. In this way, a more accurate assessment of the etiological relationship between these two common diseases can be achieved.

In this chapter, we discuss the definition and the etiology of these two diseases, as well as their potential relationship in different pathophysiological conditions.

II. Definition and Classification of Rhinitis and Otitis Media

Rhinitis is defined as an inflammation of the lining of the nose, characterized by one or more of the following symptoms: nasal congestion, rhinorrhea, sneezing, and itching (2). Rhinitis has been classified into three categories: (1) allergic rhinitis, i.e., seasonal and perennial; (2) infectious rhinitis, i.e., acute and chronic, or specific and nonspecific; (3) others such as idiopathic, nonallergic rhinitis with eosinophilia syndrome (NARES), occupational, hormonal, and drug-induced rhinitis, and rhinitis caused by irritants, food, emotional, and atrophic factors.

Otitis media is an inflammation of the middle ear without reference to etiology or pathogenesis (3). The types of otitis media have been classified as: (1) otitis media without effusion, i.e., present in the early stages of acute otitis media but may also be found in the stage of resolution of acute otitis media or may even be chronic; (2) acute otitis media (AOM), i.e., acute suppurative or purulent otitis media; (3) otitis media with effusion (OME), which can be serous, mucoid, or purulent; (4) atelectasis of the tympanic membrane.

III. Infectious Rhinitis and Otitis Media

Infectious rhinitis (common cold) is probably the most common disease in humans. Children below the age of 7 years have six to seven episodes of common cold per year (4); adults have fewer episodes, although there is a wide range of individual data. Infectious rhinitis is usually of viral origin, rhinoviruses and coronaviruses being the most common species in adults, while in children parainfluenza, respiratory syncytial virus (RSV), and adenoviruses also play a major role (5).

Complications of infectious rhinitis are more commonly seen in children. AOM is the most common complication; 90% of the AOM cases in children under 3 years are preceded or accompanied by a viral rhinitis (6). In adults, acute sinusitis is a more frequent complication of a common cold than AOM.

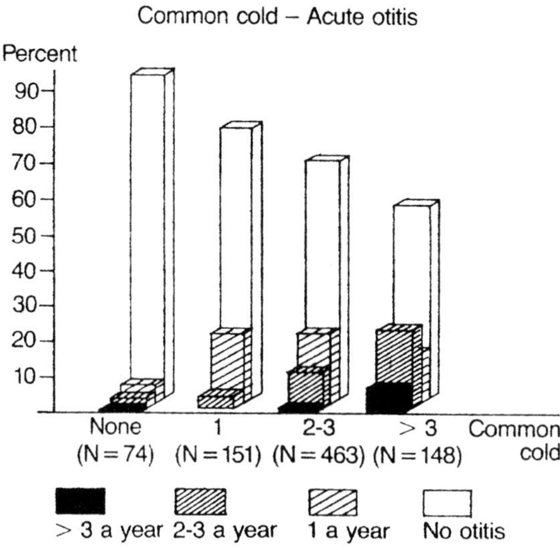

Figure 1 Relationship between the annual incidence of common cold and that of acute otitis media.

A. The Ghent Epidemiological Study

We investigated more than 2000 preschool children in order to study the relationship between rhinitis and otitis media. A highly significant correlation was found between the annual frequency of common cold and that of AOM ($p < 0.001$, both with the multiple linear regression analysis and with the chi-square test) (Fig. 1). In children who did not have a common cold during the previous year, the chance of being free from AOM was about 90%. This, however, dropped to 55% in children who had four or more episodes of common cold during the previous year.

In the same study, the relationship between nasal infection and middle ear disorders was also demonstrated by evaluating the tympanometric results against several nasal parameters, i.e., annual frequency of common cold, the time between the last episode of common cold and ear disease, and the rhinoscopic findings. The number of flat tympanograms increased with the number of annual common colds ($p < 0.01$). The highest prevalence of OME is seen 5–8 weeks after the last episode of common cold. After this period, there is a progressive improvement of the middle ear status. The correlation between tympanometric findings and the annual frequency of common cold is not as strong as that between the annual episodes of AOM and of common cold, indicating that OME probably

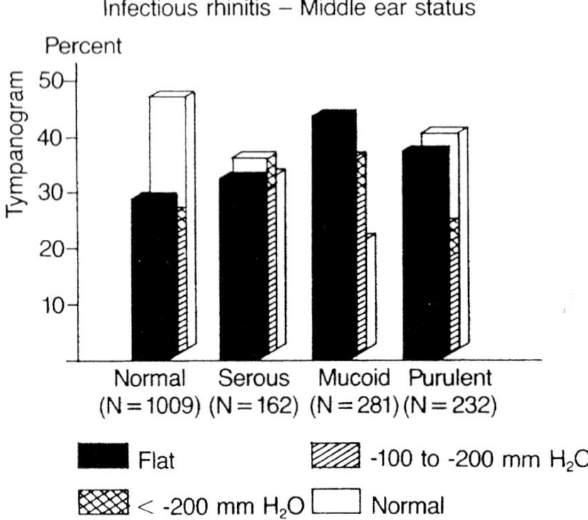

Figure 2 Relationship between rhinoscopic and tympanometric findings in a selected group of children, with special regard to the character of nasal secretions.

involves more factors in its pathophysiology than AOM and that the influence of the annual frequency of common cold on OME is indirect.

When plotting the tympanometric results against the overall rhinoscopic findings (with special regard to the signs of nasal infection), we found that in all types of infectious rhinitis the number of normal tympanograms was reduced (Fig. 2). Rhinitis with viscid mucoid secretions was more frequently associated with flat curves and negative middle ear pressure than rhinitis with purulent or watery hypersecretion. The investigation of infectious rhinitis was performed on a selected group of children ($n = 842$), which explains the higher number of pathological typanograms compared to the whole group of children screened.

From these data we concluded that there is a well-defined, strong correlation between nasal infection and the middle ear status.

B. Possible Mechanisms

The nose is situated at the ''front line'' of the respiratory tract and it is continuously exposed to different environmental agents. Therefore, rhinitis is one of the most common diseases that may occur at any age.

A properly functioning eustachian tube (ventilation, protection, drainage, and clearance) is important in maintaining a normal middle ear. It is not surprising that a nasal infection involving the continuous mucosa at the eustachian tube is involved in the pathogenesis of AOM.

It has been shown that pathogenic bacteria (*Streptococcus pneumoniae, Hemophilus influenzae, M. catarrhalis*) are found in the nasopharynx in 97% of patients with AOM, with organisms corresponding to those isolated from middle ear effusion in 69% (7). The nasopharyngeal microorganism may enter the middle ear through the eustachian tube. This may be facilitated by nose blowing or closed-nose swallowing (Toynbee maneuver), or by aspiration into the middle ear as a result of negative middle ear pressure.

In many cases, especially in older children, chronic effusion may appear without any evidence of preceding acute otitis media. It has been shown, however, that middle ear effusions are not sterile, and that they contain the same spectrum of microorganisms as is found in acute effusions (8). In these cases, the fluid is produced by the middle ear mucosa in response to subclinical antigenic stimulation rather than by an overt acute infectious process (8).

Viruses are frequently the cause of acute episodes of upper respiratory tract infection in childhood and often precede the development of eustachian tube obstruction and otitis media. The potential mechanisms of virus-induced bacterial otitis media has been explained by Bernstein (9) (Fig. 3). RSV is the most common virus found in the middle ear fluid and in the nasopharynx in the winter months in younger children. RSV has a propensity to produce IgE-associated antibody, which can attach either to nasopharyngeal cells or to mast cells in the nasopharynx. Persistence of virus or recurrence of viral infection with RSV may produce IgE-antibody immune complexes on the surface of mast cells with release of histamine and other mediators, which may result in eustachian tube edema and consequent eustachian tube dysfunction. RSV may also impair ciliary function and neutrophil function and then lead to bacterial invasion of the middle ear cavity with bacterial organisms.

IV. Allergy and Otitis

The role of allergy as an etiological factor in the pathophysiology of OME is still controversial. In 1973 Miglets found 19 published papers, the earliest one from 1952, in which the authors expressed strong opinions that allergy plays an important, if not major, role in the pathogenesis of OME (10). On the other hand, not everybody supported this concept. Senturia stated that there was a lack of evidence to substantiate the claim of an allergic etiology for the great majority of cases of OME (11). The reason for this controversy is probably the bias in the study design, especially in the selection of the study population. To perform a critical epidemiological study, a strict clarification of the different pathological conditions in these organs, appropriate selection criteria of the study population, and a well-defined control group are indispensable.

Until 1975, there were no clinical studies available in which an unselected

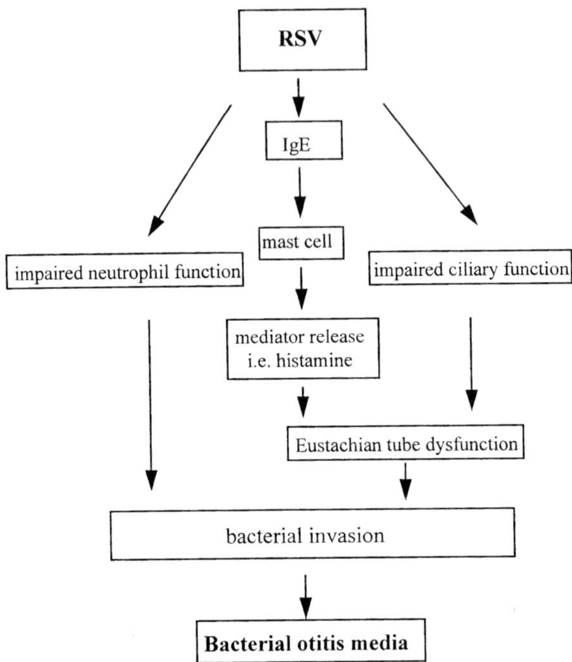

Figure 3 Potential mechanism of viral-induced bacterial otitis media, according to Bernstein (9).

group of children from an otology practice was screened both for allergy and for OME. Before that period it was assumed by many otologists and allergists that allergy should be ranked high on the list of factors predisposing to OME.

In 1975, Reisman and Bernstein (12) published the first report on the relationship between allergy and OME arising in an unselected group of children from an otology practice: 23% of the children who were tested for OME had an atopic disease; this figure was only slightly higher than could be expected from a random examination of unselected children. These findings were confirmed by De (13) and Ruokonen et al. (14) whereas Kjellman et al. (15) found the incidence of atopic disease in their material to be significantly higher ($p < 0.001$) than in an unselected control group. We can state, however, that from all the clinical studies it is obvious that the incidence of allergy in children with OME is, at most, slightly greater than might be expected in the general population.

A. The Relationship Between Allergy and OME

The actual percentage of patients with serous otitis media who exhibit atopic symptoms varies widely. The highest percentage (94%) was reported by Lecks

Table 1   Relationship Between Allergy and Middle Ear
Condition in 353 Children Who Underwent Nasal Fiberscopy,
Tympanography, and Skin or Serum RAST Test for the
Common Aeroallergens

	Allergy ($n = 98$)	Nonallergy ($n = 255$)
Normal	77 (79%)	133 (52%)
OME	21 (21%)	122 (48%)

A negative relationship exists (chi-square test, $p < 0.001$) between the two
parameters studied.

(1961). However, he was dealing with a selected group of serous otitis patients,
since a large percentage (84%) were adenoidectomy failures (10). On the basis
of the world literature and laboratory investigations at the Children's Hospital
of Buffalo, Bernstein found that otitis media is associated with allergy in 35–
40% of cases (9). In an 18-month follow-up study, Irander et al. (16) found that
the number of episodes of AOM was higher and the duration of episodes of OME
was longer in 13 infants with respiratory tract allergy, as compared with 14 allergic children with only skin manifestations and with 25 nonatopic children. The
authors concluded that middle ear morbidity during the first 18 months of life
is more common in atopic children with asthma than in nonatopic infants and
early appearance of nasal metachromatic cells is associated with middle ear infection (16).

In a study of 817 children (mean age 6 years) who underwent fiberscopic
examination of the nasal and nasopharyngeal cavities and tympanometry, 353
children had been tested by skin or serum RAST testing for the common aeroallergens (D-Y. Wang et al., unpublished data). The chi-square test was performed
to investigate the relationship between allergy and the occurrence of OME. Table
1 shows that the incidence of OME (21%) in children with allergy was even
lower than in the nonallergic group (48%). These children were referred for fiberscopy from a pediatric ear, nose, and throat outpatient clinic because of complaints of nasal obstruction, OME, or other complaints (sleep apnea and recurrent
bronchitis) which in the opinion of pediatrician could be related to adenoid hypertrophy. On the other hand, allergy was observed in only 14% of children (21 of
143) with OME.

In a previously reported epidemiological study in children ($n = 2360$ ears)
with allergic diseases and otitis media in Ghent, there was no statistically significant difference in middle ear findings between allergic children and those who
were reported to be free of allergy (17). When the allergic children were divided
into three subgroups: allergic rhinitis, allergic asthma, and atopic dermatitis, it
was noted that OME was more prevalent in children with atopic dermatitis than

in nonallergic children or children with a respiratory allergy. The higher number of OME cases in children with atopic dermatitis, which is usually not a type I allergic reaction, suggests that other disease processes may be involved. The data obtained from this large population study suggest that allergic rhinitis and asthma are not a major predisposing factor to OME.

B. The Relationship Between Food Allergy and OME

The relationship between food allergy and OME is not yet fully understood. It has been suggested that the food immune complexes, particularly with dairy products, may be an important factor, especially in the otitis-prone child less than age 2 years (9).

C. Possible Mechanisms

The relationship between allergy and otitis media, if any, is not fully understood. Histologically, the nasal cavity and middle ear cavity are covered by a similar respiratory mucosa. Hence, there probably is a similarity of mucosal response to the same etiological and pathogenic factors between these two sites. In some studies, it was found that many lymphocytes, plasma cells, macrophages, leukocytes, and other inflammatory cells accumulated in inflamed middle ear mucosa, but only a few mast cells were found in the normal middle ear mucosa (18,19). Mogi et al. reported that mast cells in the tubotympanum of guinea pigs are mainly located in areas covered by ciliated and secretory epithelium. Even though the number was small, mast cells were even found in fetal tubotympani that had received no antigenic stimuli (20).

It is known that the mast cell is a key cell in the allergen-induced immediate response. A question that has been discussed for several decades is whether the middle ear can be considered an allergic ''shock organ.'' This has been studied in only a few definite experimental animal studies. Miglets (10) passively sensitized 15 squirrel monkeys with human serum containing IgE antibodies to ragweed pollen. Then powered ragweed antigen was insufflated into the left eustachian tube and middle ear, three time per day for 4 days, via a blunt, 27-gauge needle, to evaluate the initial response of the middle ear and eustachian tube to the antigen. An unsensitized group was used as control. The results showed that a relatively acellular effusion similar to serous otitis media was produced by this direct challenging method. This study demonstrated that the middle ear has the capability of acting as an allergic ''shock organ.'' On the contrary, Doyle et al. (21) failed to confirm this finding by use of a noninvasive challenging method. In their experiment pollen allergen was insufflated into the middle ear of sensitized rhesus monkeys using a small Politzer's bag via the nose and eustachian tube. In this way, the pollen reached the tympanic cavity. They suggested that the inflammation of middle ear mucosa and production of middle ear effusion demonstrated in the study by Miglets was due to infection secondary to the traumatized catheterization of the eustachian tube.

There is, however, a lack of information with regard to humans. The concept that the middle ear mucosa can act as an allergic "shock organ" in normal life is not generally accepted, because in natural circumstances the middle ear mucosa is not directly exposed to aeroallergens. When an intranasal antigen challenge is performed in guinea pigs, an important infiltration of eosinophils and mast cells as well as edema formation could be found in the mucous membrane lining the nose, nasopharynx, and eustachian tube near the pharyngeal orifice, but not in the rest of the eustachian tube (20). Some studies demonstrated a tubal dysfunction occurring after intranasal challenge with allergen (22,23) and histamine (24) in atopic patients.

It has been demonstrated that increased concentrations of mediators such as histamine, leukotriene C_4, and eosinophil cationic protein (ECP) have been found in the nasal secretions not only in atopic patients after nasal allergen challenge outside the season, but also in patients with ongoing allergic rhinitis (25). These mediators are potent inflammatory agents.

The role of IgE-mediated hypersensitivity in the development of OME has been reviewed by Bernstein (9). He felt that IgE-mediated hypersensitivity, or allergy, represents only one variable in a complex disease entity. Bacterial infection, viral infection, and mucociliary clearance are important variables that may be effected by the allergic response. Some studies have demonstrated a localized inflammatory process within the middle ear itself (26,27). Hurst and Venge (26) found abnormally elevated levels of ECP in the middle ear fluid in 87% of patients with OME. There was no correlation between an individual's ear and serum levels of ECP, or between effusion ECP and serum IgE.

Although there exists a relationship between nasal allergic inflammation and otitis media caused by a dysfunction of the eustachian tube (Fig. 4), we should take into consideration that there exists a difference in peak prevalence with respect to the age distribution between these two diseases. Otitis media is most common during early childhood (28), whereas the clinical expression of allergic rhinitis is not common before the age of 5 years (2).

V. Conclusions

Rhinitis and otitis media are both common health problems and they may appear together in a patient. The pathogenic mechanisms of these diseases involve a spectrum of multifactorial elements such as bacteria, viruses, and allergens. Acute bacterial or viral rhinitis is often associated with middle ear disease, particularly in young children. Eustachian tube dysfunction, however, is the most common etiology of otitis media. IgE-mediated allergic reaction is a common cause of

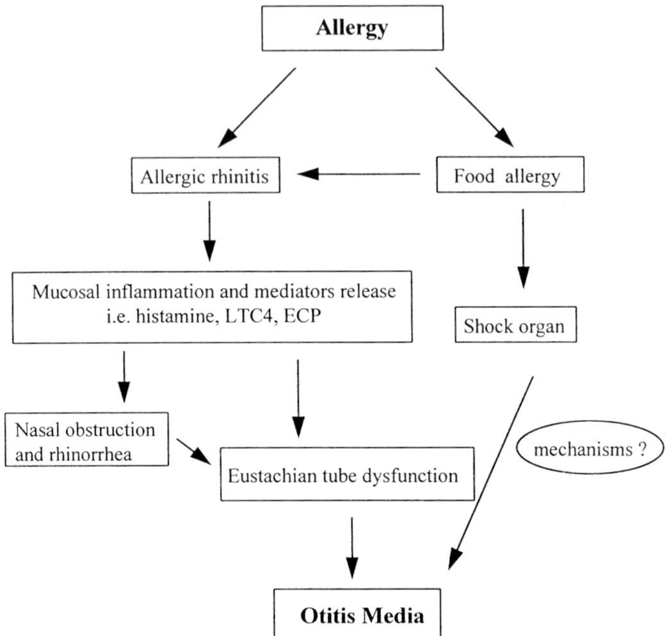

Figure 4 Mechanisms by which allergy may exert its influence on otitis media (hypothetical).

rhinitis, but it represents only one etiological factor of otitis media. The middle ear mucosa itself is rarely a target tissue for allergic processes, although the biochemical mediators released during nasal allergic reactions most likely produce eustachian tube edema and inflammation. Over a long period this chronic inflammatory response, along with viral or bacterial infection, may produce middle ear effusion. On the other hand, in patients with OME, atopy may be responsible for recurrences and maintenance of the middle ear disease in some patients.

References

1. Corey JP, Adham RE, Abbass AH, Seligman I. The role of IgE-mediated hypersensitivity in otitis media with effusion. Am J Otolaryngol 1994; 15:138–144.
2. Lund V. International consensus report on the diagnosis and management of rhinitis. Allergy 1994; (Suppl 19):5–34.
3. Bluestone CD, Klein JO. Otitis media, atelectasis, and eustachian tube dysfunction.

In: Bluestone CD, Stool SE, Kenna MA, eds. Pediatric Otolaryngology, 3rd ed. Philadelphia: WB Saunders, 1996:388–582.

4. Van Cauwenberge P. Epidemiology of common cold. Rhinology 1985; 23:273–282.
5. Gwaltney JM, Hayden FG. The nose and infection. In: Proctor DF, Andersen I, eds. The Nose. Amsterdam: Elsevier, 1982:339–342.
6. Van Cauwenberge P, Ingels K. Rhinitis: the spectrum of the disease. In: Busse WW, Holgate ST, eds. Asthma and Rhinitis. Boston: Blackwell Scientific Publications, 1995:6–12.
7. Howie VM, Ploussard JH. Simultaneous nasopharyngeal and middle ear exudate cultures in otitis media. Pediatr Dig 1971; 13:31–35.
8. Gates GA, Muntz HR, Gaylis B. Adenoidectomy and otitis media. Ann Otol Rhinol Laryngol 1992; 101:24–32.
9. Bernstein J. The role of IgE-mediated hypersensitivity in the development of otitis media with effusion: a review. Otolaryngol Head Neck Surg 1993; 109:611–620.
10. Miglets A. The experimental production of allergic middle ear effusions. Laryngoscope 1973; 83:1355–1384.
11. Senturia BH. Allergic manifestations in otologic disease. Laryngoscope 1960; 70:287–297.
12. Reisman RE, Bernstein JM. Allergy and secretory otitis media. Pediatr Clin North Am 1975; 22:251–257.
13. De PR. Secretory otitis media and allergic rhinitis. J Laryngol 1980; 94:185–189.
14. Ruokonen J. Holopainen E, Palva T, Backman A. Secretory otitis media and allergy. Allergy 1981; 36:59–68.
15. Kjellman NIM, Synnerstad B, Hansson LO. Atopic allergy and immunoglobulins in children with adenoids and recurrent otitis media. Acta Paediatr Scand 1976; 65:593–600.
16. Irander K, Borres MP, Björkstén B. Middle ear disease in relation to atopic disease and nasal metachromatic cells in infancy. Int J Pediatr Otorhinolaryngol 1993; 26:1–9.
17. Van Cauwenberge P, Ingels K. Rhinitis and otitis. In: Mygind N, Naclerio RM, eds. Allergic and Non-allergic Rhinitis. Copenhagen: Munksgaard, 1993:189–193.
18. Albiin N, Hellström S, Stenfors L-E, Cerne A. Middle ear mucosa in rats and humans. Ann Otol Rhinol Laryngol 1986; 95(Suppl 126):1–15.
19. Lim DJ, Mogi G. Mucosal immunology of the middle ear and Eustachian tube. In: Ogra PL, Strober W, Mestecky J, McGhee JR, Lamm ME, Bienenstock J, eds. Handbook of Mucosal Immunology. San Diego, CA: Academic Press, 1994:599–606.
20. Mogi G, Tomonaga K, Watanabe T, Chaen T. The role of type I allergy in secretory otitis media and mast cells in the middle ear mucosa. Acta Otolaryngol (Stockh) 1992; (Suppl 493):155–163.
21. Doyle WJ, Takahara T, Fireman P. The role of allergy in the pathogenesis of otitis media with effusion. Arch Otolaryngol Head Neck Surg 1985; 111:502–506.
22. Ackerman MN, Friedman RA, Doyle WJ, Bluestone CD, Fireman P. Antigen-induced eustachian tube obstruction: an intranasal provocative challenge test. J Allergy Clin Immunol 1984; 73:604–609.
23. Skoner DP, Doyle WJ, Chamovitz AH, Fireman P. Eustachian tube obstruction after

intranasal challenge with house dust mite. Arch Otolarygol Head Neck Surg 1986; 112:840–842.

24. Tomonaga K, Kurono Y, Mogi G. The role of nasal allergy in otitis media with effusion. A clinical study. Acta Otolaryngol (Stockh) 1988; (Suppl 458):41–47.

25. Wang D, Clement P, Smitz J, De Waele M, Derde M-P. Correlations between concentrations, inflammatory cells and mediators concentrations after nasal allergen challenge and during natural allergen exposure. Int Arch Allergy Appl Immunol 1995; 106:278–285.

26. Hurst DS, Venge P. The presence of eosinophil cationic protein in middle ear effusion. Otolarygol Head Neck Surg 1993; 108:711–722.

27. Yellon RF, Leonard G, Marucha P, et al. Characterization of cytokines present in middle ear effusion. Laryngoscope 1992; 101:165–169.

28. Faden H, Bernstein JM, Brodsky L, et al. Otitis media in children. I. The systemic response to nontypable *Haemophilus influenzae*. J Infect Dis 1989; 160:999–1004.

26

Future Therapies for Allergic Diseases
of the Airways

ROBERT P. SCHLEIMER

The Johns Hopkins University
  School of Medicine
Baltimore, Maryland

I. Introduction

Five main systems serve as potential targets for antiallergic therapies in the airways: the vasculature, the nervous system, mucus-secreting tissues, smooth muscle, and immune and inflammatory processes. This review is not intended to consider all of the possible new approaches to modifying these five systems, but rather to focus primarily on the immune and inflammatory processes that participate in a central fashion in antigen-induced rhinitis. An attempt is made to consider new therapies that are at present at a variety of stages of development, from early preclinical to late clinical trials. Some of the discussion will consider strategies being developed for the treatment of allergic asthma. These studies are applicable to upper airways allergic inflammation insofar as the underlying process that produces the response is similar.

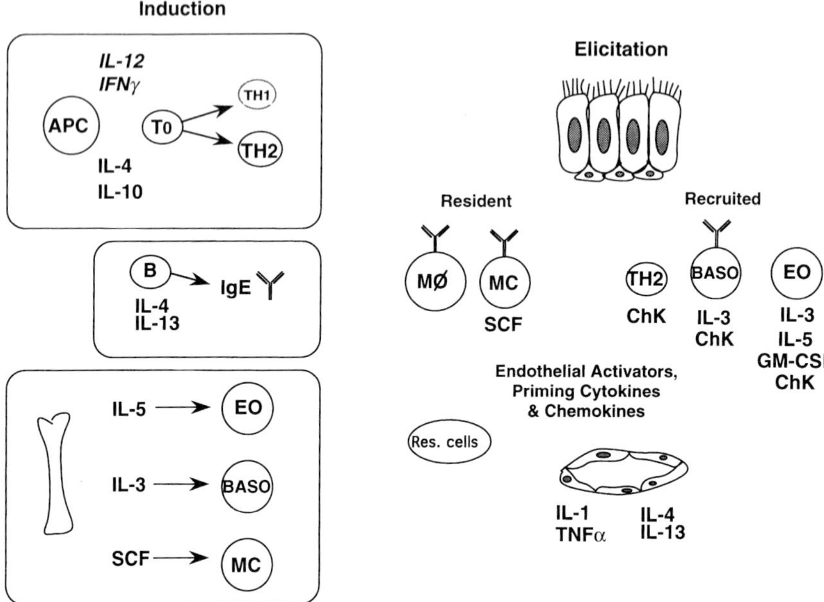

Figure 1 The role of cytokines in allergic airway inflammation. Primary cytokine targets for antiallergic therapy are indicated for the induction phase (left) and the elicitation phase (right) of allergic airway inflammation. Cytokines shown in upper panel of induction are stimulatory (Roman type) and suppressive (italics) for the development of TH2 cells. For further explanation see text.

II. Strategies to Suppress the Allergic Inflammatory Response

A. Cytokine-Directed Approaches

Induction Versus Elicitation

Immune and inflammatory responses are overlapping, but distinct entities. Allergic inflammation involves the *induction* of sensitivity to allergens via generation of antigen-specific T cells and antigen-specific IgE (Fig. 1). Other components of induction include generation by the bone marrow of precursors or mature forms of eosinophils, basophils, mast cells, and lymphocytes. *Elicitation* involves reexposure to antigen in a previously sensitized individual, an event that is followed by the traditional allergic response including mast cell degranulation, and the recruitment and activation of immune and inflammatory cells at the site of secondary exposure to antigen. Several cytokine targets are now known to be involved in both induction and elicitation, which makes them particularly attractive as therapeutic targets.

One such cytokine, IL-4, is involved in the generation of specific IgE antibodies, expression of IgE receptors, and activation of endothelium for recruitment of lymphocytes, eosinophils, and basophils from the circulation at sites of allergic inflammation (1).

Another centrally involved cytokine is IL-5, which not only appears to be important for development and generation of eosinophils in the bone marrow, but also is involved in recruitment of mature eosinophils to local tissue sites as well as maintenance of eosinophil survival in the airways (2).

Shown in Figure 1 on the left are cytokines involved in regulation of various inductive processes. In the top panel, preferential induction of TH2-type cells is thought to be promoted by the presence of IL-4 (and IL-13), as well as IL-10 (3). The two cytokines shown in italics, IFNγ and IL-12, favor the development of TH1 and thus are suppressive to TH2 development (4). IL-18 shares this property.

In the middle panel, B-cell synthesis of IgE is shown to be promoted by IL-4 and IL-13, while the lower panel indicates the cytokines that are important growth factors for eosinophils, basophils, and mast cells, including IL-5, IL-3, and stem-cell factor, respectively (3,5).

On the right hand of Figure 1 are shown cytokines that participate in cell recruitment and influence the behavior of resident and recruited cells in an already sensitized individual. These include endothelial-activating cytokines (IL-1, TNFα, IL-4, IL-13), eosinophil-priming cytokines (IL-3, IL-5, GM-CSF), and chemokines (RANTES, MCP-3, MCP-4, MCP-5, eotaxin) (6).

Central Cytokine Targets

Inhibition of the action of cytokines presents unique problems to the development of new therapeutics since cytokines are relatively large protein molecules that function at low concentrations and have a high affinity for their specific receptors.

It has been generally difficult to disrupt cytokine pathways with low-molecular-weight receptor-blocking drugs. For that reason a number of alternative approaches have been pursued (Fig. 2). One approach is to attempt to inhibit the synthesis of the target cytokine. This is difficult to do in a cytokine-specific way. Recently Lee et al. have developed cytokine synthesis anti-inflammatory drugs (CSAIDs), which target p38, an important protein kinase in the induction of IL-1 and TNF gene expression (7). Antisense oligonucleotides have been explored as another way to achieve this result.

More companies or investigators have pursued approaches that diminish the concentration of active cytokine either in the circulation or at local tissue sites. One method by which this has been achieved utilizes soluble receptors (often dimerized and linked with immunoglobulin heavy chains) (8). A similar

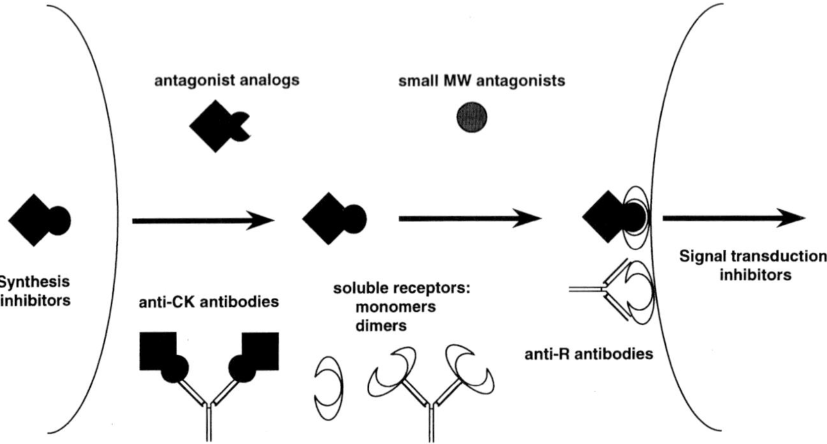

Figure 2 Approaches to the disruption of a cytokine-receptor system.

approach involves using antibodies directed against the cytokines. For use in humans, these antibodies are usually ''humanized,'' a process by which the complementarity determining regions (CDR) from high-affinity mouse monoclonal antibodies are grafted onto the framework structure of human immunoglobulins to diminish the immunogenicity of the reagent.

Blocking of the actions of a cytokine at its specific receptor can be achieved with the use of antireceptor antibodies, avoiding those that activate the receptor. Antireceptor antibodies can theoretically cause destruction of the target cell, however, and rapid recycling of receptors may defeat the efficacy of antireceptor antibodies.

Development of receptor antagonists of a cytokine is often sought. One way by which this is achieved is to develop mutated cytokine molecules or identify naturally occurring cytokine analogs that bind to the receptor but have no intrinsic activity and therefore act as competitive antagonists (9). The preferred method to disrupt cytokine pathways is to develop a low-molecular-weight drug that is orally active and binds specifically to the receptor in question with high affinity and with no intrinsic activity. While this has been difficult to date, recent successes in the chemokine area are encouraging. Development of drugs that disrupt the postreceptor signal transduction events is an active area (see below).

Discussion in this section will focus on three main classes of cytokines that are involved in allergic reactions. Discussion of these three classes of cytokines can be found in other reviews, so their relevance to allergic inflammation will only be briefly considered here (6). In many cases, some or all of the above-listed approaches are being pursued. Only selected examples will be presented.

Eosinophil-Priming Cytokines

The cytokines IL-5, IL-3, and GM-CSF cause eosinophils to respond much more vigorously to their usual stimuli, resulting in exaggerated adhesion, migration, and activation (10,11).

Studies on expression in human disease have led to the belief that IL-5 is the most central eosinophil-priming cytokine. Although it was believed that IL-5 is the primary eosinophilopoietic factor, recent experience with IL-5 knockout mice revealed that an IL-5-independent subset of eosinophils exists (12,13).

Evidence has been presented that eosinophils in the circulation and/or airways of patients with allergic airways disease are in a steady state of priming, presumably under the influence of these cytokines (14,15). Thus, priming cytokines are involved in both the generation and activation of eosinophils.

The development of antagonists has been an important goal of the biomedical and pharmaceutical communities. To this point, GM-CSF and IL-5 have been the major targets for developmental work. Work from the laboratory of Lopez, Vadas, and colleagues has led to the development of GM-CSF analogs with a single amino acid substitution that bind to the receptor with high affinity but do not stimulate target cells (personal communication). These molecules have proven effective as antagonists in vitro and are now undergoing trials in vivo. Likewise, Huston et al. and Chaiken et al. have focused on developing IL-5 antagonists based on modification of the native IL-5 molecule (9,16). These studies have shown that a monomeric IL-5 can be produced that binds to and functionally activates the receptor. It is hoped that in the near future mutagenesis studies will yield effective antagonists of the IL-5 system.

Several studies in the literature have shown that antibodies to IL-5 can cause a drastic decrease in eosinophils in parasitic and experimental allergic disorders in animals (17,18). One such antibody, TRFK5, has been used extensively in models of allergic airways disease in guinea pigs and primates (18–20). A related antibody, which has recently been humanized, is now entering clinical trials in humans for asthma.

The anti-IL-5 antibody has been found not only to dramatically suppress eosinophil infiltration at the site of antigen challenge, but also to virtually completely block changes in airways reactivity induced by antigen challenge for up to 6 months after a single administration (20). While in the long term antibodies to IL-5 may not prove to be the best methodology to disrupt the IL-5 pathway, these studies represent an exciting "proof of concept" test that will determine the therapeutic promise of disrupting the IL-5 system in allergic airways disease.

Based upon current dogma, it is reasonable to expect that immunoregulatory cytokines that favor the development of TH1 may have therapeutic value in allergic reactions of the airways. Thus, IFNγ has been indirectly shown to shift the response of rodents to TH1 in vivo (39,40). In humans, inhalation of IFN has been found to have modest effects on eosinophil numbers in the airways (41,42).

Recent studies with IL-12 have shown that administration along with antigen can dramatically shift T cells to the TH1 subset and block the occurrence of antigen-induced bronchial hyperreactivity (39,43,44). In parasite models IL-12 has been shown to promote TH1-mediated immunity to *Schistosoma mansoni*. Subsequent studies with IFNγ knockout mice indicate that the protective effect of IL-12 is indirect through induction of IFNγ (39). While this might indicate that IL-12 would not be superior to IFNγ as a therapeutic agent in allergic inflammation, the fact that IL-12 has a greater half-life than IFNγ favors IL-12 in this regard.

Recently, IL-12 administration has been used in an animal model of antigen-challenged allergic inflammation in the airways and found to dramatically inhibit the production of TH2-type cytokines and the associated inflammatory infiltration with leukocytes and changes in airways reactivity (43). The possibility of neonatal immunization to produce an early shift in T-cell compartments, away from the TH2 subtypes, is now being explored. In light of the recognized ability of immunotherapy to produce modest shifts in T-cell subtypes away from TH2 and toward TH1 (45), it is not unreasonable to suggest that promoting that activity by combining immunotherapy with cytokines that favor development of TH1 (e.g., IFNγ or IL-12) would succeed (see below).

B. Cell Adhesion Molecule Targets

Over the last 15 years awareness of the existence and functional relevance of adhesion molecules in inflammatory diseases has grown exponentially. Huge strides have been made in identifying, cloning, sequencing, and characterizing a large array of adhesion molecules belonging primarily to several families, including the selectins, the integrins, the immunoglobulin supergene family, and the cadherins (24).

Adhesion molecules are now known to be involved in most biological processes involving both sessile and motile cells. Adhesion molecules therefore represent an important target area for development of new therapeutic entities with its own unique set of challenges. For example, adhesion molecule binding is almost exclusively multivalent. When two cells bind via adhesion molecules, the number of interactions can be dozens, hundreds, or even possibly thousands of ligand pairs between the two cells.

Blocking the resulting high-avidity binding is a daunting task, especially with low-molecular-weight compounds. This problem notwithstanding, a number of antagonists have been developed, including antibodies, soluble ligands, peptides, and even organic compounds that mimic the binding sites (24). This section will consider the adhesion molecules relevant to allergic airways inflammation by family.

Selectins

The primary selectins are P- and E-selectin, which are expressed on endothelium, and L-selectin, which is expressed on leukocytes. Selectins are thought to be involved in rolling of leukocytes on the blood vessel wall prior to firm adhesion and transendothelial migration. Selectins recognize oligosaccharides, especially sLe^x and related sugars, which can be found on a variety of counterligands, some of which are glycolipids or glycoproteins.

Selectin interactions have been disrupted with soluble oliogosaccharides, antibodies, and small compounds that mimic the lectin ligand (24). An antibody directed against E-selectin has been found to be useful in blocking neutrophil recruitment in lower airways allergic inflammation in the monkey (46). Other forms of lung injury models have been found by Mulligan et al. to be inhibited by antibodies against P-selectin or E-selectin, as well as soluble sLe^x oligosaccharides (47–52). Several models of inflammation have been found to be disrupted by selectin antagonists or knockouts of selectin genes, especially the double knockout of P-selectin and E-selectin (53–55).

Intravital microscopic and in vitro studies have suggested that histamine-induced expression of P-selectin may be important for early rolling of leukocytes in inflammatory processes that involve mast cell activation (56). Thus, P-selectin may be a particularly attractive target for development of antiallergic drugs.

Integrins and Immunoglobulin Supergene Family Members

Integrins thought to be involved in cell recruitment include the β2 integrin family, whose members are β2 (CD18) combined with either αL (LFA-1), αM (Mac-1), αX (P150/95), or αD.

Many integrins bind to members of the immunoglobulin supergene family, as well as numerous arginine-glycine-aspartic acid (RGD)-containing counterligands. Integrins are thought to be important in the firm adhesion that follows rolling of leukocytes, as well as in transendothelial migration and anchorage within the extravascular tissues (57,58).

Notable in the context of allergic disease among the β1 integrins is the heterodimer of α4 and β1 (CD49, CD29). This integrin is responsible for the binding of eosinophils and lymphocytes to VCAM-1 and fibronectin. Considerable evidence implicates VLA-4 in cell recruitment during allergic reactions (59). Another relevant integrin is α4β7, which is felt to be important in binding of eosinophils and lymphocytes to MAdCAM, the mucosal addressin found in gut lymph nodes.

Several studies have attempted to disrupt integrins and their counterligands in models of allergic inflammation. Wegner et al. showed that an antibody against ICAM-1 blocked recruitment of eosinophils to the lung of monkeys (60). In related studies, antibodies against β2 integrins were found not to inhibit recruitment, but appeared to block activation of eosinophils within the lung parenchyma.

Several laboratories have attempted to disrupt the VLA-4/VCAM-1 interaction by using either antibodies against VCAM-1, antibodies against VLA-4, or the fibronectin CS-1 peptide, which also blocks the interaction of VLA-4 with VCAM-1. In most cases, disruption of the VLA-4/VCAM-1 system has been found to inhibit recruitment of eosinophils and/or lymphocytes to sites of allergic inflammation in mice, guinea pig, monkeys, rabbits, and sheep (36,61–64).

A series of low-molecular-weight cyclic peptide inhibitors of VLA-4 has been developed, but not yet tested in allergic reactions (65). There is some indication that low-molecular-weight organic compounds that inhibit this binding interaction may soon be available from the pharmaceutical industry. Recent studies have shown that basophils and eosinophils express a considerable amount of the newly recognized β2 integrin αD, which is a counterligand for ICAM-3, another member of the immunoglobulin supergene family. The function of αD is as yet unknown.

C. Immunotherapy

The use of injection of allergens to prevent allergic reactions dates back to the 19th century and originally springs out of the huge success with vaccination to prevent infectious diseases. Anaphylaxis was discovered by Portier and Richet in experiments attempting to prevent allergic reactions to jellyfish venom. To this day, anaphylaxis is the greatest impediment to this form of therapy. In many cases, immunotherapy can successfully quench allergic disease. It is generally held to be effective in seasonal allergic rhinitis, but its efficacy in asthma and other allergic diseases is more controversial (66).

Studies of immunotherapy against experimental challenge indicate preferential inhibition of the late-phase response and the associated cellular infiltration and activation of cytokine-producing cells. Several approaches have been taken to avoid anaphylaxis. One is to use modified antigens that are not recognized by antibodies against the native antigen, but that provide the primary peptides that induce either immunization and subtype shifting of T cells or T-cell tolerance (67).

This same basic idea has been pursued recently using peptides found in the major allergen from cat. In these experiments, T-cell epitopes (relatively small peptides) are used for immunization since IgE antibodies do not recognize the peptides (68). While peptide immunotherapy has had some success, there have been interesting, but paradoxical systemic reactions to the vaccine. Since IgE is not responsible, one interpretation of this is that peptide-activated T cells by themselves may be adequate to promote allergic inflammation of sufficient magnitude to cause physiological responses.

Recently another immunological approach to immunotherapy of allergic diseases has been the utilization of anti-IgE. In this case, an antibody has been produced that is directed against an epitope of IgE that is masked when bound by the high-affinity IgE receptor (69,70). These antibodies therefore do not cross-link the IgE which is receptor associated, and do not cause mast cell activation. This approach has had significant early success, preventing both cutaneous and airways reactions to experimental antigen challenge. As mentioned above in reference to treatment with anti-IL-5, it may be best to view this as a test for "proof of concept" rather than a therapy with potential for long-term utility. If anti-IgE is found to be effective against asthma or rhinitis, this will hopefully spur the industry to develop traditional drugs that can reduce the level of IgE by other mechanisms.

Recently, a novel approach of immunotherapy has been developed by Raz et al. that utilizes plasmids containing cDNA for the antigen in question (71). Immunization of mice with a plasmid containing a cDNA sequence for β-galactosidase preferentially induced $IgG_{2\alpha}$ antibodies and did not induce formation of IgE antibodies, in contrast to antigen injected in either saline or alum, which induced IgE. When T-cell subsets were analyzed in these mice, it was found that IL-4 and IL-5 production was virtually nonexistent after immunization with the plasmid antigen preparation, while antigen in alum induced substantial production.

In animals that had been previously sensitized with antigen in alum, a boost with antigen cDNA in plasmid initiated a de novo IFNγ response and suppressed the production of IL-5, and to some extent IL-4. This treatment was found to lead to a steady decline in IgE levels in the presensitized animals (71).

The mechanism of this novel form of immunotherapy is not known, but one reasonable explanation is that when antigen is synthesized by antigen-presenting cells following engulfment of cDNA, the antigen-presenting cells treat that antigen as if it were a viral antigen. That is to say that major histocompatibility class I molecules are used rather than class II for antigen presentation. Preferential induction of TH1 cells and cytotoxic T cells may result. Alternatively, the antigen preparation may regulate IgE levels indirectly, via simulation of production of IFNγ either directly or secondarily via IL-12 induction. Either of these events can lead to a shift of T cells from TH2 to TH1. A potential pitfall of this type of approach is that the cDNA may remain in tissues and transfected cells and may produce antigen for an extended period. The profound effect of this type of immunotherapy is compelling, and the results of clinical trials will be of great interest.

D. Immune/Inflammatory Targeted Treatments

To this point, new therapies primarily utilizing macromolecules have been considered. The challenges are great in attempts to overcome the physical interactions and/or functional actions of adhesion molecules or the cytokine network. A number of attractive targets besides cytokines, chemokines, and adhesion molecules may have potential value in development of new therapies to treat allergic diseases of the upper or lower airway. In general, these targets have the added advantage that they are amenable to development of low-molecular-weight drugs.

Antihistamines

Antihistamines have been exceedingly valuable in the treatment of a variety of allergic conditions, especially those associated with nasal, conjunctival, and cutaneous itch. Topical antihistamines have been utilized with success for treatment of ophthalmic symptoms associated with hay fever and topically in the treatment of rhinitis (72,73).

Cyclooxygenase Inhibitors

Traditional nonsteroidal anti-inflammatory drugs (NSAIDs) have been known to have anti-inflammatory and analgesic properties for years. Cyclooxygenase type 1 (Cox-1) has been known to be the target of NSAIDs. Recently, another form of this enzyme, Cox-2, which is inducible during inflammatory responses, has been discovered (74,75). Several companies are developing drugs that specifically inhibit Cox-2 but not Cox-1. These drugs avoid the gastrointestinal and antiplatelet effects and, it is hoped, will be useful in diseases such as rheumatoid arthritis, which respond to nonspecific cyclooxygenase inhibitors such as aspirin. It is suspected that the beneficial effects of aspirin are largely the result of inhibition of Cox-2. Although NSAIDs are not effective in allergic airway disease, trials would probably be worthwhile since prostanoids arising from Cox-1 and Cox-2 may have counterregulatory actions.

11β-Hydroxysteroid Dehydrogenase

Compounds derived from licorice have been known to have anti-inflammatory actions in gut mucosa for many decades and recently have been shown to inhibit an enzyme that degrades cortisol to cortisone (76). Nasal lavage and bronchoalveolar lavage studies utilizing a highly sensitive gas chromatographic (GC) mass spectrometric assay have shown that endogenous cortisol is degraded in the airway lumen (R. Schleimer, W. Hubbard, et al., unpublished observations). Since endogenous cortisol is likely to play an important regulatory role in allergic reactions in the airways and skin, local inhibition of 11β-hydroxysteroid dehydrogenase (11β-HSD) may have some utility. Inhibitors of 11β-HSD such as carbenoxolone and glycyrrhetinic have been proposed to have potential value as anti-inflammatory compounds in the airways (76,77).

Nitric Oxide Synthase

Nitric oxide (NO) is an atypical autacoid that is a gas that can diffuse rapidly and exert regulatory effects on nerve, muscle, and vasculature. NO was originally recognized as an endothelial-dependent relaxing factor that can relax vascular smooth muscle but is also now recognized to be a mediator of inflammation and toxicity to pathogenic organisms (78–80).

NO synthase, like cyclooxygenase, is now known to have at least two forms, one of which is induced during inflammation (78–80). Since recent studies in asthma have shown a large increase of the inducible form of NO synthase (iNOS), presumably in the epithelium of the airways of asthmatics, NO synthase is now considered to be a potential target of anti-inflammatory drug development (81,82). Studies with glucocorticoids have shown a reduction of NO synthase and exhaled NO in asthmatics following treatment (81).

Inhibitors of Receptors for Tachykinins

Tachykinins are peptides involved in communication between nerves and vasculature as well as other parenchymal cells. At present, five tachykinins and three receptors have been recognized and development of specific inhibitors of some tachykinin receptors has been achieved at several companies with the hope that they will block neuronally mediated inflammation. Calcitonin gene-related peptide (CGRP), a related peptide, and its receptor have also been implicated in neurogenic inflammation and are targets for drug development. While the tachykinins substance P and neurokinin A induce vascular leak in human skin and nose, the importance of tachykinins in allergic airways disease is still unknown.

Leukotriene Antagonists

Leukotrienes are felt to play an important role in modulation of muscle, vasculature, and possibly nerve function in the upper and lower airways. For this reason, a number of companies have developed leukotriene antagonists, which are now available in the clinic or in advanced clinical trials for treatment of asthma (83).

Traditionally, leukotrienes have been considered central mediators of bronchospasm in asthma, but recent studies suggest that sulfidopeptide leukotrienes are possibly also involved in leukocyte recruitment in antigen challenge models in both humans and animals (84). Leukotriene administered by aerosol has been shown to potently stimulate persistent eosinophil accumulation (87). This accumulation, as expected, is blocked by leukotriene antagonists.

Leukotrienes are also known to regulate microvascular permeability and are potent stimuli for mucus secretion and mucociliary transport as well as airways smooth muscle proliferation. Finally, leukotrienes may have some effects on the function of lower airways by modulating the activity of afferent nerves (85,86).

Leukotriene antagonists in turn have been found to attenuate antigen-induced increases in bronchoalveolar lavage eosinophils (88). The mechanism by which leukotrienes achieve this is unknown but could involve activation of P-selectin expression on the endothelium. Clearly, these studies, which have focused on the lower airways, justify a study of intranasal leukotriene antagonists in models of allergic rhinitis.

Neutral Endopeptidase

Neutral endopeptidase is an enzyme that degrades a variety of inflammatory peptides including bradykinin and tachykinins, and may be important in the regulation of the action of a number of proinflammatory peptides. Direct administration of neutral endopeptidase is presently being tested for potential therapeutic benefit in upper airways inflammation.

Phosphodiesterase Type 3 and 4 Inhibitors

Cyclic adenosine monophosphate (cAMP) was first identified as an activator of intermediary metabolism in liver or muscle. In the 1960s it was observed that cAMP suppresses immune and inflammatory cells, and it was demonstrated that drugs like theophylline have some anti-inflammatory properties (albeit at high concentrations), probably by virtue of elevating cAMP as a result of inhibiting the phosphodiesterases responsible for its elevation (89).

Dozens of phosphodiesterases (PDE) and isotypes are now known to exist and pursuit of specific inhibitors of PDE type 3 and 4 has been motivated by a desire to separate the anti-inflammatory properties of PDE inhibitors from many of the side effects on the heart and central nervous system (90).

Although emesis has been a nagging side effect for many of the presently chosen lead compounds, promising compounds have been developed that are effective in inhibiting antigen-induced airways inflammation. With present awareness of at least five isotypes of PDE3 it is hoped that even better selective inhibitors can be developed. Since theophylline has been shown to have anti-inflammatory effects in the upper airways, study of these compounds in rhinitis is worthwhile.

Signal Transduction Pathways

The understanding of signal transduction pathways is key to a complete awareness of the interaction between a cell and its microenvironment. Both tyrosine and serine-threonine kinases are now known to be important in several signal transduction pathways.

The MAP kinase pathway is known to be important in cytokine-induced responses, including proliferation and activation, in a number of cells. Targets of signaling kinases and phosphatases are numerous. In some cases, specific domains on the intracellular portion of cell surface molecules involved in signaling, known as sarc homology (SH) domains, have been recognized.

In addition, the ultimate targets of many signal transduction pathways are transcription factor molecules whose function is to regulate gene expression. Several biotechnology companies are vigorously targeting pathways of signal transduction and transcriptional regulation with the hope of identifying pathways that are specifically involved in key biological events in inflammation.

Some of the major transcription factors that are being targeted include AP-1 and NFκB, both of which are thought to be involved in inflammation. In addition, specific components in the pathways that activate these particular transcription factors, including the jun kinase and IκB kinase, are being pursued as potential anti-inflammatory drug targets. Other molecular targets include SH2 and SH3 domain recognition sites, various components of the MAP kinase pathway, and isotypes of protein kinase C and G proteins, thought to be involved in early signal transduction.

The main challenge for drug development utilizing these strategies will be finding targets or compounds whose action is limited to the desired biological response and not related responses whose disruption could lead to undesired effects.

Type 2 Muscarinic Receptors

The type 2 muscarinic receptor has been shown to regulate acetylcholine release and control airway smooth muscle responses. Eosinophil major basic protein has been suggested to block this receptor and exacerbate cholinergic responses; this has been proposed to be an important mechanism of eosinophil-mediated airways reactivity (91). While selective type 2 muscarinic agonists may have some utility in lower airways allergic diseases, their value in allergic rhinitis is uncertain. Studies with a variety of stimuli have determined that reflex vascular leak does occur in the upper airways, however.

Glucocorticoids

Glucocorticoids have become a mainstay of treatment for upper airways allergic inflammation with the development of intranasal preparations that have a high degree of efficacy and minimal toxicity.

Although inhaled glucocorticoids are extremely valuable in the management of asthma, the pharmaceutical industry continues to attempt to develop better and safer inhaled glucocorticoids (92). Some of the approaches include glucocorticoids that have a longer residence time in the lung, either by virtue of delivery in liposomes or other vehicles, or by virtue of improved lipid solubility (92).

Attempts have been made to develop glucocorticoids that are metabolized even more rapidly than the present generation of drugs following absorption into the blood stream. Many of these steroids were not effective in the lower airways, however, in part perhaps due to an overly short tissue half-life.

As our understanding of the molecular mechanism of glucocorticoid action inside the cell improves, it is hoped that it will be possible to develop drugs that achieve the anti-inflammatory effects without the side effects. This is now more than just a dream, since it is now believed that many or most of the side effects are due to binding of glucocorticoid receptor complex to the glucocorticoid response element (GRE) in the promoter of induced genes, while most of the anti-inflammatory effects appear to be due to interactions between the glucocorticoid-receptor complex and transcription factors, including AP-1 and NFκB (93). In the nose, toxicity of absorbed steroid is generally not problematic. The goal for this type of research is therefore a more effective topical glucocorticoid.

E. Other Approaches

Apoptosis

Research over the last two decades has elucidated natural pathways by which cell death occurs. Cells undergoing programmed cell death usually display typical pathological features, referred to as apoptosis, which can be distinguished from necrotic cell death.

Apoptosis is characterized by a shrinking of cytoplasm and nucleus, blebbing of nuclear membrane, fragmentation of DNA, and other characteristic changes (94,95). Ultimately this leads to expression of adhesion molecules on the surface of the apoptotic cell, which rapidly induce engulfment and destruction by neighboring phagocytic cells. This last feature of apoptosis is key, in that it leads to removal of the dying cell without release of damaging or toxic cellular biomolecules.

A number of pathways have been described that induce apoptosis. These include a family of cellular proteins that either protect or subject the cell to apoptosis, including bc12, bcl-xl, bcl-xs, bax, p53, c-myc, certain IL-1b-converting-enzyme-like (ICE) proteases (caspases), and others. On the cell surface are several molecules that can induce a cell to enter apoptosis following engagement. These include fas and CD69.

The therapeutic potential of apoptosis is obvious but has not been extensively exploited in allergic disease. In the case of allergic inflammation, eosinophils and allergen-specific T cells are two cell types in which intentional induction of apoptosis could have potential therapeutic benefit. In the case of the eosinophil, antibodies to fas have been shown to induce apoptosis in vitro (96). In allergen-induced inflammation of the lower airways in animals, anti-fas has been found to induce disappearance of eosinophils rather rapidly (97). Likewise, anti-CD69 causes eosinophil apoptosis in vitro (98).

Glucocorticoids are known to induce apoptosis of eosinophils and this may be one of their important therapeutic mechanisms (99,100). Some companies are now searching for molecules that can induce apoptosis in eosinophils or other relevant cells. Recently, lidocaine has been shown to induce eosinophil apoptosis and ameliorate even severe steroid-dependent asthma (101).

In the upper airways, nasal polyposis is one disease in which exploitation of apoptotic pathways could be particularly beneficial. It has been suggested that the central role of IL-5 in this disease is to block eosinophil apoptosis. If this is true, topical IL-5 antagonists could have particular value in treatment of rhinitis or polyposis.

Gene Therapy

The concept of gene therapy was originally developed to treat genetic diseases in which a deficiency in a single enzyme or protein was responsible for disease. Early targets of this type of approach include adenosine deaminase deficiency and cystic fibrosis. In the latter, targeting of the CFTR gene using various types of viral vectors such as adenovirus has been employed.

While gene therapy remains in its infancy, and many technical hurdles have yet to be overcome, including the development of ideal viral vectors and the requirement of proliferation for targeted cells, the approach has interesting potential application to allergic diseases of the airways. It is possible to envision inhaled gene therapy in which the delivered gene could either downregulate the cellular inflammation or shift the paradigm of TH2 to TH1 in the upper or lower airways.

III. Therapies Targeting Other Systems

The upper airways are among the most highly vascularized tissues in the body and new compounds that can effectively and directly regulate vessel tone and/or permeability would have potential value as antirhinitic medications. Likewise, secretory cells are inviting targets for the development of new therapies for upper airways inflammation.

IV. Conclusions

A number of exciting new therapeutic strategies are now under development and testing at all stages including early basic studies, and all phases of clinical testing of safety and efficacy. The wheels of progress are thus steadily turning and it is anticipated that in 10 years the therapeutic management of diseases of the upper airways will be quite different and, it is hoped, significantly improved from the approaches used today.

References

1. Finkelman FD, Katona IM, Urban JF, Holmes J, Ohara J, Tung AS, Sample JG, Paul WE. IL-4 is required to generate and sustain in vivo IgE responses. J Immunol 1988; 141:2335–2341.
2. Sanderson CJ. Interleukin-5, eosinophils, and disease. Blood 1992; 79:3101–3109.
3. Mosmann TR, Coffman RL. TH1 and TH2 cells: different patterns of lymphokine secretion lead to different functional properties. Annu Rev Immunol 1989; 7:145–173.
4. Murphy E, Shibuya K, Hosken N, Openshaw P, Maino V, Davis K, Murphy K, O'Garra A. Reversibility of T helper 1 and 2 populations is lost after long-term stimulation. J Exp Med 1996; 183:901–913.
5. Witte ON. Steel locus defines new multipotent growth factor. Cell 1990; 63:5–6.
6. Schleimer RP, Beck L, Schwiebert L, Stellato C, Bochner BS. Inhibition of inflammatory cell recruitment by glucocorticoids: cytokines as primary targets. In: Schleimer RP, Busse WW, O'Byrne P. Topical Glucocorticoids in Asthma: Mechanisms and Clinical Actions. New York: Marcel Dekker, 1997:203–238.
7. Lee JC, Laydon JT, McDonnell PC, et al. A protein kinase involved in the regulation of inflammatory cytokine biosynthesis. Nature 1994; 372:739–746.
8. Ensle K, Schulz G. Regulation of interleukin-4 activity by soluble interleukin-4 receptors. J Clin Lab Anal 1995; 9:450–455.
9. Carter DB, Deibel MR, Dunn CJ, et al. Purification, cloning, expression and biological characterization of an interleukin-1 receptor antagonist protein. Nature 1990; 244:633–670.
10. Lopez AF, Williamson DJ, Gamble JR, et al. Recombinant human1 granulocyte-macrophage colony-stimulating factor stimulates in vitro mature human neutrophil and eosinophil function, surface receptor expression, and survival. J Clin Invest 1986; 78: 1220–1228.
11. Silberstein DS, Austen KF, Owen WF Jr. Hemopoietins for eosinophils. Hematol/Oncol Clin North Am 1989; 3:511–533.
12. Foster PS, Hogan SP, Ramsay AJ, Matthaei KI, Young IG. Interleukin-5 deficiency abolishes eosinophilia, airways hyperreactivity, and lung damage in a mouse asthma model. J Exp Med 1996; 183:195–201.
13. Kopf MF, Brombacher F, Hodgkin PD, et al. IL-5-deficient mice have a develop-

mental defect in CD5+ B-1 cells and lack eosinophilia but have a normal antibody and cytotoxic T cell responses. Immunity 1996; 4:15–24.

14. Calhoun WJ, Bates ME, Schrader L, Sedgwick JB, Busse WW. Characteristics of peripheral blood eosinophils in patients with nocturnal asthma. Am Rev Respir Dis 1992; 145:577–581.

15. Virchow JC, Oehling A, Boer L, Hansel TT, Werner P, Matthys H, Blaser K, Walker C. Pulmonary function, activated T cells, peripheral blood eosinophilia, and serum activity for eosinophil survival in vitro: a longitudinal study in bronchial asthma. J Allergy Clin Immunol 1994; 94:240–249.

16. Li J, Cook R, Dede K, Chaiken I. Single chain human interleukin-5 and its asymmetric mutagenesis for mapping receptor binding sites. J Biol Chem 1996; 271: 1817–1820.

17. Coffman RL, Seymour BWP, Hudak S, Jackson J, Rennick D. Antibody to interleukin-5 inhibits helminth-induced eosinophilia in mice. Science 1989; 245:308–310.

18. Mauser PJ, Pitman A, Witt A, et al. Inhibitory effect of the TRFK-5 anti-IL-5 antibody in a guinea pig model of asthma. Am Rev Respir Dis 1993; 148:1623–1627.

19. Kung TT, Stelts DM, Zurcher JA, et al. Involvement of IL-5 in a murine model of allergic pulmonary inflammation: prophylactic and therapeutic effect of an anti-IL-5 antibody. Am J Respir Cell Mol Biol 1995; 13:360–365.

20. Mauser PJ, Pitman AM, Fernandez X, Foran SK, Kreutner W, Egan RW, Chapman RW. Effects of an antibody to interleukin-5 in a monkey model of asthma. Am J Respir Crit Care Med 1995; 152:467–472.

21. Devos RG, Plaetinck R, Cornelis S, Guisez Y, Van der Heyden J, Tavernier J. Interleukin-5 and its receptor: a drug target for eosinophilia associated with chronic allergic disease. J Leuk Biol 1995; 57:813–819.

22. Bochner BS, Schleimer RP. The role of adhesion molecules in human eosinophil and basophil recruitment. J Allergy Clin Immunol 1994; 94:427–438.

23. Bochner BS, Schleimer RP. Endothelial cells and cell adhesion. In: Kaplan AP, ed. Allergy, 2nd ed. Orlando, FL: WB Saunders, 1997:251–276.

24. Peebles RS, Bochner BS, Schleimer RP. Pharmacologic regulation of adhesion molecule function and expression. In: Ruffolo RR, Hollinger MA, eds. Inflammation: Mediators and Pathways. Boca Raton, FL: CRC Press, 1995:29–97.

25. Mullarkey MF, Leiferman KM, Peters MS, et al. Human cutaneous allergic late-phase response is inhibited by soluble IL-1 receptor. J Immunol 1994; 152:2033–2041.

26. Watson ML, Smith D, Bourne AD, Thompson RC, Westwick J Cytokines contribute to airway dysfunction in antigen-challenged guinea pigs—inhibition of airway hyperreactivity, pulmonary eosinophil accumulation, and tumor necrosis factor generation by pretreatment with an interleukin-1 receptor antagonist. Am J Respir Cell Mol Biol 1993; 8:365–369.

27. Lukacs NW, Strieter RM, Chensue SW, Widmer M, Kunkel SL. TNF-alpha mediates recruitment of neutrophils and eosinophils during airway inflammation. J Immunol 1995; 154:5411–5417.

28. Schall TJ. Biology of the RANTES/SIS cytokine family. Cytokine 1991; 3:165–183.

29. Baggiolini M, Dahinden CA. CC chemokines in allergic inflammation. Immunol Today 1994; 15:127–133.
30. Stellato C, Beck LA, Gorgone GA, Proud D, Schall TJ, Ono SJ, Lichtenstein LM, Schleimer RP. Expression of the chemokine RANTES by a human bronchial epithelial cell line: modulation by cytokines and glucocorticoids. J Immunol 1995; 155:410–418.
31. Kwon OJ, Jose PJ, Robbins RA, Schall TJ, Williams TJ, Barnes PJ. Glucocorticoid inhibition of RANTES expression in human lung epithelial cells. Am J Respir Cell Mol Biol 1996; 12:488–496.
32. Beck LA, Stellato C, Beall LD, Schall TJ, Leopold D, Bickel CA, Baroody F, Bochner BS, Schleimer RP. Detection of the chemokine RANTES and endothelial adhesion molecules in nasal polyps. J Allergy Clin Immunol 1996; 98:766–780.
33. Davies RJ, Wang JH, Trigg CJ, Devalia JL. Expression of GM-CSF, IL-8 and RANTES in bronchial epithelium of mild asthmatics is down-regulated by inhaled beclomethasone dipropionate. Int Arch Appl Allergy 1994; 107:428–429.
34. Schwiebert LM, Stellato C, Schleimer RP. The epithelium as a target of glucocorticoid action in the treatment of asthma. Am J Respir Crit Care Med 1996; 154:S16–S20.
35. Gimbrone MA, Obin MS, Brock AF, et al. Endothelial interleukin-8: a novel inhibitor of leukocyte-endothelial interactions. Science 1989; 246:1601–1605.
36. Gonzalo J-A, Lloyd CM, Kremer L, Finger E, Martinez-A C, Siegelman MH, Cybulsky M, Gutierrez-Ramos J-C. Eosinophil recruitment to the lung in a murine model of allergic inflammation. The role of T cells, chemokines, and adhesion receptors. J Clin Invest 1996; 98:2332–2345.
37. Mosmann TR, Cherwinski H, Bond MW, Giedlin MA, Coffman RL. Two types of murine helper T cell clone. I. Definition according to profiles of lymphokine activities and secreted proteins. J Immunol 1986; 136:2348–2357.
38. Romagnani S. Human T_{H1} and T_{H2} subsets: doubt no more. Immunol Today 1991; 12:256–259.
39. Wynn TA, Jankovic D, Hieny S, Zioncheck K, Jardieuy P, Cheever AW, Sher A. IL-12 exacerbates rather than suppresses T helper 2-dependent pathology in the absence of endogenous IFN-γ. J Immunol 1995; 154:3999–4009.
40. Li X-M, Chopra RK, Chou T-Y, Schofield BH, Wills-Karp M, Huang SK. Mucosal IFN-γ gene transfer inhibits pulmonary allergic responses in mice. J Immunol 1996; 157:3216–3219.
41. Boguniewicz M, Martin RJ, Martin D, Gibson U, Celniker A, Williams M, Leung DYM. The effects of nebulized recombinant interferon-γ in asthmatic airways. J Allergy Clin Immunol 1995; 95:133–135.
42. Nakajima H, Iwamoto I, Yoshida S. Aerosolized recombinant Interferon-gamma prevents antigen-induced eosinophil recruitment in mouse trachea. Am Rev Respir Dis 1993; 148:1102–1104.
43. Gavett SH, O'Hearn DJ, Li X, Huang S-K, Finkelman FD, Wills-Karp M. Interleukin 12 inhibits antigen-induced airway hyperresponsiveness, inflammation, and Th2 cytokine expression in mice. J Exp Med 1995; 182:1527–1536.
44. Wynn TA, Cheever AW, Jankovic D, Poindexter RW, Caspar P, Lewis FA, Sher A.

An IL-12-based vaccination method for preventing fibrosis induced by schistosome infection. Nature 1995; 376:594–596.

45. Durham SR, Ying S, Varney VA, Jacobson MR, Sudderick RW, Mackay IS, Kay AB, Hamid QA. Grass pollen immunotherapy inhibits allergen-induced infiltration of CD4+ T lymphocytes and eosinophils in the nasal mucosa and increases the number of cells expressing messenger RNA for interferon-gamma. J Allergy Clin Immunol 1996; 97:1356–1365.

46. Gundel RH, Wegner CD, Torcellini CA, Clarke CC, Haynes N, Rothlein R, Smith CW, Letts LG. Endothelial leukocyte adhesion molecule-1 mediates antigen-induced acute airway inflammation and late-phase airway obstruction in monkeys. J Clin Invest 1991; 88:1407–1411.

47. Mulligan MS, Varani J, Dame MK, Lane CL, Smith CW, Anderson DC, Ward PA. Role of endothelial-leukocyte adhesion molecule 1 (ELAM-1) in neutrophil-mediated lung injury in rats. J Clin Invest 1991; 88:1396–1406.

48. Mulligan MS, Polley MJ, Bayer RJ, Nunn MF, Paulson JC, Ward PA. Neutrophil-dependent acute lung injury—requirement for P-selectin (GMP-140). J Clin Invest 1992; 90:1600–1607.

49. Mulligan MS, Smith CW, Anderson DC, Todd RF, Miyasaka M, Tamatani T, Issekutz TB, Ward PA. Role of leukocyte adhesion molecules in complement-induced lung injury. J Immunol 1993; 150:2401–2406.

50. Mulligan MS, Paulson JC, Defrees S, Zheng ZL, Lowe JB, Ward PA. Protective effects of oligosaccharides in P-selectin-dependent lung injury. Nature 1993; 364:149–151.

51. Mulligan MS, Lowe JB, Larsen RD, Paulson J, Zheng ZL, Defrees S, Maemura K, Fukuda M, Ward PA. Protective effects of sialylated oligosaccharides in immune complex-induced acute lung injury. J Exp Med 1993; 178:623–631.

52. Mulligan MS, Watson SR, Fennie C, Ward PA. Protective effects of selectin chimeras in neutrophil-mediated lung injury. J Immunol 1993; 151:6410–6417.

53. Bullard DC, Kunkel EJ, Kubo H, et al. Infectious susceptibility and severe deficiency of leukocyte rolling and recruitment in E-selectin and P-selectin double mutant mice. J Exp Med 1996; 183:2329–2336.

54. Tang T, Frenette PS, Hynes PO, et al. Cytokine-induced meningitis is dramatically attenuated in mice deficient in endothelial selectins. J Clin Invest 1996; 97:2485–2490.

55. Frenette PS, Mayadas TN, Rayburn H, et al. Susceptibility to infection and altered hematopoiesis in mice deficient in both P- and E-selectins. Cell 1996; 84:563–574.

56. Kubes P, Kanwar S. Histamine induces leukocyte rolling in post-capillary venules. J Immunol 1994; 152:3570–3577.

57. Butcher EC. Leukocyte-endothelial cell recognition: three (or more) steps to specificity and diversity. Cell 1991; 67:1033–1036.

58. Springer TA. Traffic signals on endothelium for lymphocyte recirculation and leukocyte emigration. Annu Rev Physiol 1995; 57:827–872.

59. Bochner BS, Ebisawa M, Knol EF, Yamada T, Georas SN, Liu MC, Schleimer RP. Mechanisms of eosinophil accumulation during allergic inflammation. In: Nadel J, Pozzi E, Venge P. Eosinophils and Bronchial Smooth Muscle Cells. Milan: Masson Italia, 1995:81–95.

60. Wegner CD, Gundel RH, Reilly P, Haynes N, Letts LG, Rothlein R. Intercellular adhesion molecule-1 (ICAM-1) in the pathogenesis of asthma. Science 1990; 247: 456–459.

61. Weg VB, Williams TJ, Lobb RR, Nourshargh S. A monoclonal antibody recognizing very late activation antigen-4 inhibits eosinophil accumulation in vivo. J Exp Med 1993; 177:561–566.

62. Abraham WM, Sielczak MW, Ahmed A, et al. a_4-integrins mediate antigen-induced late bronchial responses and prolonged airway hyperresponsiveness in sheep. J Clin Invest 1994; 93:776–787.

63. Metzger WJ, Ridger V, Tollefson V, Arrhenius T, Gaeta FCA, Elices M. Anti-VLA-4 antibody and CS-1 peptide inhibitor modifies airway inflammation and bronchial airway hyperresponsiveness in the allergic rabbit. J Allergy Clin Immunol 1994; 93:A183.

64. Nakajima H, Sano H, Nishimura T, Yoshida S, Iwamoto I. Role of vascular cell adhesion molecule-1/very late activation antigen-4 and intercellular adhesion molecule-1/lymphocyte function-associated antigen-1 interactions in antigen-induced eosinophil and T-cell recruitment into the tissue. J Exp Med 1994; 179:1145–1154.

65. Nowlin DM, Gorcsan F, Moscinski M, Chiang SL, Lobl TJ, Cardarelli PM. A novel cyclic pentapeptide inhibits a4b1 and a5b1 integrin-mediated cell adhesion. J Biol Chem 1993; 268:20352–20359.

66. Norman PS. Current status of immunotherapy for allergies and anaphylactic reactions. Adv Intern Med 1996; 41:681–713.

67. Marsh DG, Lichtenstein LM, Campbell DH. Studies on ''allergoids'' prepared from naturally occurring allergens. I. Assay of allergenicity and antigenicity of formalinized rye group I component. Immunol 1970; 18:705–722.

68. Norman PS, Ohman JL, Long AA, et al. Treatment of cat allergy with T-cell reactive peptides. Am J Respir Crit Care Med 1996; 154:1623–1628.

69. Shields RL, Whether WR, Zioncheck K, O'Connell L, Fendly B, Presta LG, Thomas D, Saban R, Jardieu P. Inhibition of allergic reactions with antibodies to IgE. Int Arch Allergy Appl Immunol 1995; 107:308–312.

70. Haak-Frendscho M, Robbins K, Lyon R, Shields R, Hooley J, Schoenhoff M, Jardieu P. Administration of an anti-IgE antibody inhibits CD23 expression and IgE production in vivo. Immunology 1994; 82:306–313.

71. Raz E, Tighe H, Sato Y, Corr M, Dudler JA, Ropman M, Swain SL, Spiegelberg JL, Carson DA. Preferential induction of a Th1 immune response and inhibition of specific IgE antibody formation by plasmid DNA immunization. Proc Natl Acad Sci USA 1996; 93:5141–5145.

72. Pipkorn U, Bende M, Hedner J, Hedner T. A double-blind evaluation of topical levocabastine, a new specific H1 antagonist in patients with allergic conjunctivitis. Allergy 1985; 40:491–496.

73. Schata M, Jorde W, Richarz-Barthauer U. Levocabastine nasal spray is better than sodium cromoglycate and placebo in the topical treatment of seasonal allergic rhinitis. J Allergy Clin Immunol 1991; 87:873–878.

74. Kujubu DA, Fletcher BS, Varnum BC, Lim RW, Herschman HR. TIS10, a phorbol ester tumor promoter-inducible mRNA from Swiss 3T3 cells, encodes a novel pros-

taglandin synthase/cyclooxygenase homologue. J Biol Chem 1991; 266:12866–12872.

75. Xie W, Chipman JG, Robertson DL, Erikson RL, Simmons DL. Expression of a mitogen-responsive gene encoding prostaglandin synthase is regulated by mRNA splicing. Proc Natl Acad Sci USA 1991; 88:2692–2696.

76. Schleimer RP. Potential regulation of inflammation in the lung by local metabolism of hydrocortisone. Am J Respir Cell Mol Biol 1991; 4:166–173.

77. Schleimer RP, Kato M. Regulation of lung inflammation by local glucocorticoid metabolism—a hypothesis. J Asthma 1992; 29:303–317.

78. Lyons CR, Orloff GJ, Cunningham JM. Molecular cloning and functional expression of an inducible nitric oxide synthase from a murine macrophage cell line. J Biol Chem 1992; 267:6370–6374.

79. Xie Q-W, Cho JJ, Calaycay J, Mumford RA, Swiderek KM, Lee TD, Ding A, Troso T, Nathan C. Cloning and characterization of inducible nitric oxide synthase from mouse macrophages. Science 1992; 256:225–228.

80. Lowenstein CJ, Glatt CS, Bredt DS, Snyder SH. Cloned and expressed macrophage nitric oxide synthase contrasts with the brain enzyme. Proc Natl Acad Sci USA 1992; 89:6711–6715.

81. Barnes PJ, Liew FY. Nitric oxide and asthmatic inflammation. Immunol Today 1995; 16:128–130.

82. Shaul PW, North AJ, Wu LC, Wells LB, Brannon TS, Lau KS, Michel T, Margraf LR, Star RA. Endothelial nitric oxide synthase is expressed in cultured human bronchiolar epithelium. J Clin Invest 1994; 94:2231–2236.

83. Holgate ST, Bradding P, Sampson AP. Leukotriene antagonists and synthesis inhibitors: new directions in asthma therapy. J Allergy Clin Immunol 1996; 98:1–13.

84. Hay DWP, Torphy TJ, Undem BJ. Cysteinyl leukotrienes in asthma: old mediators up to new tricks. TIPS 1995; 16:304–309.

85. Underwood DC, Osborn RR, Newsholme SJ, Torphy TJ, Hay DWP. Persistent airway eosinophila after leukotriene (LT) D4 administration in the guinea pig: modulation by the LTD4 receptor antagonist, pranlukast, or an IL-5 monoclonal antibody. Am J Respir Crit Care Med 1996; 154:850–857.

86. Undem BJ, Weinreich D. Electrophysiological properties and chemosensitivity of guinea pig nodose ganglion neurons in vitro. J Auton Nerv Syst 1993; 44:17–34.

87. Ellis JL, Undem BJ. Role of peptidoleukotrienes in capsaicin-sensitive sensory fibre-mediated responses in guinea-pig airways. J Physiol 1991; 436:469–484.

88. Foster A, Chan CC. Peptide leukotriene involvement in pulmonary eosinophil migration upon antigen challenge in the actively sensitized guinea pig. Int Arch Allergy Appl Immunol 1991; 96:279–284.

89. Lichtenstein LM, Margolis S. Histamine release in vitro: inhibition by catecholamines and methylxanthines. Science 1968; 161:902–903.

90. Torphy TJ, Murray KJ, Arch JRS. Selective phosphodiesterase isozyme inhibitors. In: Page CP, Metzger WJ, eds. Drugs and the Lung. New York: Raven Press, 1994: 397–447.

91. Jacoby DB, Gleich GJ, Fryer AD. Human eosinophil major basic protein is an endogenous allosteric antagonist at the inhibitory muscarinic M2-receptor. J Clin Invest 1993; 91:1314–1318.

92. Brattsand R, Axelsson BI. Basis of airway selectivity of inhaled glucocorticoids. In: Schleimer RP, Busse WW, O'Byrne P, eds. Inhaled Glucocorticoids in Asthma: Mechanisms and Clinical Actions. New York: Marcel Dekker, 1997:351–379.

93. Karin M, Saatciouglu F. Negative transcriptional regulation by the glucocorticoid receptor is responsible for the antiinflammatory activity of glucocorticoids. In: Schleimer RP, Busse WW, O'Byrne PM. Inhaled Glucocorticoids in Asthma: Mechanisms and Clinical Actions. New York: Marcel Dekker, 1997:29–52.

94. Wyllie AH. Apoptosis: death gets a brake. Nature 1994; 369:272–273.

95. Cohen JJ, Duke RC. Apoptosis and programmed cell death in immunity. Annu Rev Immunol 1992; 10:267–293.

96. Matsumoto K, Schleimer RP, Saito H, Iikura Y, Bochner BS. Induction of apoptosis in human eosinophils by anti-fas antibody treatment in vitro. Blood 1995; 86:1437–1443.

97. Tsuyuki S, Bertrand C, Erard F, Trifilieff A, Tsuyuki J, Wesp M, Anderson GP, Coyle AJ. Activation of the fas receptor on lung eosinophils leads to apoptosis and the resolution of eosinophilic inflammation of the airways. J Clin Invest 1995; 96:2924–2931.

98. Walsh GM, Williamson ML, Symon FA, Willars GB, Wardlaw AJ. Ligation of CD69 induces apoptosis and cell death in human eosinophils cultured with granulocyte-macrophage colony-stimulating factor. Blood 1996; 87:2815–2821.

99. Lamas AM, Marcotte GV, Schleimer RP. Human endothelial cells prolong eosinophil survival. Regulation by cytokines and glucocorticoids. J Immunol 1989; 142:3978–3984.

100. Schleimer RP, Bochner BS. The effects of glucocorticoids on human eosinophils. J Allergy Clin Immunol 1994; 94:1202–1213.

101. Gleich GJ, Hunt LW, Bochner BS, Schleimer RP. Glucocorticoid effects on human eosinophils. In: Schleimer RP, Busse WW, O'Byrne PM. Topical Glucocorticoids in Asthma: Mechanisms and Clinical Actions. New York: Marcel Dekker, 1997:279–308.

AUTHOR INDEX

Gaya, A, 226, 247
Gayler, B, 202, 206, 208, 212, 213, 216
Gaylis, B, 449, 455
Gebbers, JO, 186, 197
Gefter, MA, 53, 61
Geha, RS, 110, 111, 122
Gelber, LE, 55, 62, 440, 443
Georas, SN, 465, 477
Georgitis, JW, 318, 320, 323, 326,
    330, 331, 340, 347, 348
Geppetti, P, 72, 91, 392, 393, 397
Gergen, PJ, 383, 394
German, DF, 37, 44
Gerrard, JM, 402, 411
Gerth van Wijk, R, 134, 142
Ghezzo, H, 151, 160
Gibson, U, 464, 476
Giebaly, K, 317, 330
Giedlin, MA, 463, 476
Giklich, RE, 213, 218
Gilbert, AN, 291, 306
Gill, FF, 187, 197
Gillen, MS, 230, 249
Gillespei, CA, 242, 254
Gillis, S, 117, 127
Gilson, BS, 136, 143
Gimbrone, M, 115, 125
Gimbrone, MA, 114, 125, 463, 476
Giotakis, I, 230, 248
Gislason, D, 55, 62
Giuseppe, P, 408, 412
Giuseppina, S, 408, 412
Givanni, S, 341, 350
Glaser, J, 149, 160
Glass, M, 113, 124
Glatt, CS, 468, 479
Gleeson, MJ, 356, 364
Gleich, G, 192, 199
Gleich, GJ, 116, 126, 340, 348, 471,
    473, 479, 480
Gliklich, R, 399, 410
Glinert, R, 55, 62
Gluck, U, 186, 197
Gluckman, JL, 87, 93
Goa, KL, 270–272, 275, 280, 287

Godthelp, T, 111, 119, 123, 129, 190,
    198, 223, 224, 246, 390, 396
Goff, J, 120, 132
Golbert, TM, 338, 347
Golding-Wood, PH, 364, 365, 391, 396
Goldmsith, CH, 136, 143
Goldstein, S, 340, 348
Golembesky, HE, 179, 194
Golovich, MS, 120, 132
Gomez, E, 112, 118, 123, 130, 185,
    191, 196, 198, 222, 245
Gomez, EG, 230, 248
Gomez, G, 235, 250
Gonzalo, JA, 463, 476
Gorcsan, F, 466, 478
Gordon, J, 119, 130
Gorevic, PG, 117, 128
Gorfien, J, 400, 411
Gorgone, G, 401, 411
Gorgone, GA, 463, 476
Gott, JP, 117, 127
Gottbert, L, 236, 251
Grace, A, 32, 42, 400, 411
Graf, P, 233, 249, 302, 303, 309
Graf, W, 256, 257, 263
Graham, D, 80, 82, 89, 93, 94
Graham, DE, 89, 94
Graham, JM, 355, 364
Grahne, B, 238, 253, 318, 320, 322,
    324, 326, 330, 391, 396
Grammer, LC, 69, 90, 334, 335, 339,
    343, 345
Grant, J, 88, 93
Grant, JA, 117, 128
Graveson, S, 54, 62
Gray, L, 3, 4, 20
Graziani, D, 226, 247
Green, J, 55, 62
Green, W, 38, 42
Green, WF, 53, 61
Greenly, R, 335, 346
Greenstone, M, 364, 365
Gregen, PJ, 67, 89
Greico, MH, 335, 346
Greiff, L, 230, 249, 312, 329

SUBJECT INDEX